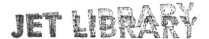

Joint Education and Training Library

This book is to be returned on or before the last date stamped below. Overdue charges will be incurred by the late return of books.

Renew in person, by phone (01270 612538, or internal x2538/2705) or online at: http://libcat.chester.ac.uk (NHS staff ask for password)

Fabry Disease

Deborah Elstein · Gheona Altarescu · Michael Beck
Editors

Fabry Disease

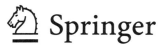 Springer

Editors
Deborah Elstein
Gaucher Clinic
Shaare Zedek Medical Center
Bayit Street 12
91034 Jerusalem
Israel
elstein@szmc.org.il

Gheona Altarescu
Genetics Unit
Shaare Zedek Medical Center
Bayit Street 12
91031 Jerusalem
Israel
gheona@szmc.org.il

Michael Beck
Children's Hospital
University of Mainz
Langenbeckstrasse 1
55131 Mainz
Germany
Dr.M.Beck@t-online.de

ISBN 978-90-481-9032-4   e-ISBN 978-90-481-9033-1
DOI 10.1007/978-90-481-9033-1
Springer Dordrecht Heidelberg London New York

Library of Congress Control Number: 2010930427

Springer is part of Springer Science+Business Media (www.springer.com)

There is no medicine like hope, no incentive so great, and no tonic so powerful as expectation of something better tomorrow.

(Orison Swett Marden)

This is the first textbook dedicated solely to Fabry disease. Fabry disease unfortunately is a multi-system disease that is incompletely treated by the currently available enzyme replacement therapies. The often significant lag in achieving the correct diagnosis, the myriad of symptoms and signs, the suffering that the patient experiences on so very many levels, and the social ramifications for family and friends, all underscore the complexity of this disease and the inherent need for a better understanding of the pathological mechanisms underlying its expression.

The section on pre-clinical studies highlights the various directions that have been undertaken to improve diagnosis and identification of disease-specific features. The clinical chapters represent the most current evaluations by experts that should allow the uninitiated as well as the treating physician to appreciate the spectrum of disease-specific manifestations. And finally, the chapters assessing the various aspects of treatment are of importance for physician and patient alike.

We have had the good fortune to include chapters by many of the most prominent clinicians and researchers in the field, men and women who have been involved with Fabry disease for many decades and whose dedication has been unstinting. It is to the patients and those concerned with their welfare that this book is dedicated in the hope that the near future will provide insight into the disease and thereby improved treatment of its symptoms.

Contents

Contributors

Johannes M.F.G. Aerts Department of Medical Biochemistry, Academic Medical Center, University of Amsterdam, Amsterdam, The Netherlands, j.m.aerts@amc.uva.nl

Francisco Allegue Department of Dermatology, University Hospital of Vigo, Vigo, Spain, francisco.allegue.rodriguez@sergas.es

Gheona Altarescu Medical Genetics Institute, Shaare Zedek Medical Center, Jerusalem, Israel, gheona@szmc.org.il

Maryam Banikazemi Columbia University School of Medicine, New York, NY, USA, mb3186@columbia.edu

Soraya Barrera Department of Pathology and Neuropathology, University Hospital of Vigo, Vigo, Spain, sbarcab@yahoo.es

Michael Beck Children's Hospital, University of Mainz, Mainz, Germany, Dr.M.Beck@t-online.de

Robin L. Bennett Division of Medical Genetics, Department of Medicine, UWMC Medical Genetics Clinic, University of Washington Medical Center, Seattle, WA, USA, robinb@u.washington.edu

Roscoe O. Brady National Institute of Neurological Disorders and Stroke, National Institutes of Health, Bethesda, MD, USA, bradyr@ninds.nih.gov

Tobias Böttcher Medical Faculty, Albrecht-Kossel-Institute for Neuroregeneration, University of Rostock, Rostock, Germany, tobias.boettcher@med.uni-rostock.de

T. Andrew Burrow Division of Human Genetics, Cincinnati Children's Hospital Medical Center, Cincinnati, OH, USA; Department of Pediatrics, University of Cincinnati College of Medicine, Cincinnati, OH, USA, Thomas.Burrow@cchmc.org

Joe T.R. Clarke Department of Pediatrics, Division of Clinical and Metabolic Genetics, Hospital for Sick Children and University of Toronto, Toronto, ON,

Canada; Service de génétique, Département de pédiatrie, Centre hospitalier universitaire de Sherbrooke, Sherbrooke, QC, Canada, jtrc@sickkids.ca

Ales Dudesek Department of Neurology, University of Rostock, Rostock, Germany, alesdudesek@gmx.de

Milan Elleder First Faculty of Medicine, Institute of Inherited Metabolic Disorders, Charles University, Prague, Czech Republic, melleder@cesnet.cz

Carmen Fachal Department of Pathology and Neuropathology, University Hospital of Vigo, Vigo, Spain, Carmen.Fachal.Bermudez@sergas.es

Jian-Qiang Fan Pfantastic Medical Research Institute, Cresskill, NJ, USA, jfan@pfantastic.com

Jose M. Fernandez Department of Clinical Neurophysiology, University Hospital of Vigo, Vigo, Spain, Jose.Maria.Fernandez.Rodriguez@sergas.es

Manuela Födinger Institute of Laboratory Medicine, Sozialmedizinisches Zentrum Süd, Vienna, Austria, manuela.foedinger@wienkav.at

Andreas Gal Institut für Humangenetik, Universitätsklinikum Hamburg-Eppendorf, Hamburg, Germany, gal@uke.de

Scott C. Garman Department of Chemistry, University of Massachusetts, Amherst, MA, USA; Department of Biochemistry & Molecular Biology, University of Massachusetts, Amherst, MA, USA, garman@biochem.umass.edu

Dominique P. Germain Medical Genetics, Centre de référence de la maladie de Fabry et des maladies héréditaires du tissu conjonctif, U.F. de Génétique Médicale, Hôpital Raymond Poincaré (AP-HP), Garches, France; University of Versailles – St Quentin en Yvelines (UVSQ), Versailles, France, dominique.germain@rpc.aphp.fr

Ehud Goldin Medical Genetics Branch, National Human Genome Research Institute, National Institutes of Health, Bethesda, MD, USA, goldine@mail.nih.gov

Gregory A. Grabowski Division of Human Genetics, Cincinnati Children's Hospital Medical Center, Cincinnati, OH, USA; Department of Pediatrics, University of Cincinnati College of Medicine, Cincinnati, OH, USA, greg.grabowski@cchmc.org

Abigail I. Guce Department of Chemistry, University of Massachusetts Amherst, Amherst, MA, USA, aguce@chem.umass.edu

C.E.M. Hollak Department of Internal Medicine/Endocrinology and Metabolism, Academic Medical Center, AZ Amsterdam, The Netherlands, c.e.hollak@amc.uva.nl

Robert J. Hopkin Division of Human Genetics, Cincinnati Children's Hospital Medical Center, University of Cincinnati College of Medicine, Cincinnati, OH, USA, rob.hopkin@cchmc.org

Martin Hřebíček First Faculty of Medicine, Institute of Inherited Metabolic Disorders, Charles University, Prague and General University Hospital, Prague, Czech Republic, martin.hrebicek@lf1.cuni.cz

D.A. Hughes Lysosomal Storage Disorders Unit, Department of Academic Haematology, Royal Free Hospital and University College Medical School, London, UK, d.hughes@medsch.ucl.ac.uk

Satoshi Ishii Faculty of Medicine, Oita University, Oita, Japan, ishiists@hotmail.com

Christoph Kampmann University Medicine, Johannes Gutenberg University Mainz, Mainz, Germany, kampmann@uni-mainz.de

Jana Ledvinová First Faculty of Medicine, Institute of Inherited Metabolic Disorders, Charles University, Prague and General University Hospital, Prague, Czech Republic, jana.ledvinova@lf1.cuni.cz

Aleš Linhart Department of Internal Medicine, Carl's University, Prague, Czech Republic, ales.linhart@lf1.cuni.cz

G.E. Linthorst Department of Internal Medicine/Endocrinology and Metabolism, Academic Medical Center, Amsterdam, The Netherlands, g.e.linthorst@amc.nl

Jan Lukas Medical Faculty, Albrecht-Kossel-Institute for Neuroregeneration, University of Rostock, Rostock, Germany, jan.lukas@med.uni-rostock.de

Atul Mehta Department of Haematology, Royal Free Hospital, University College London, School of Medicine, London, UK, atul.mehta@royalfree.nhs.uk

Beatriz San Millan Department of Pathology and Neuropathology, University Hospital of Vigo, Vigo, Spain, Beatriz.San.Millan.Tejado@sergas.es

Omid Motabar Medical Genetics Branch, National Human Genome Research Institute, National Institutes of Health, Bethesda, MD, USA, motabaro@mail.nih.gov

Carmen Navarro Department of Pathology and Neuropathology, University Hospital of Vigo, Vigo, Spain, c.navarro.fb@gmail.com; cnavfer@sergas.es

João Paulo Oliveira Departments of Pathology, Medicine and Human Genetics, Faculty of Medicine, Hospital São João, Porto, Portugal, oliveira@med.up.pt

Catherine H. Orteu Department of Dermatology, Royal Free Hospital, London, UK, Cate.orteu@royalfree.nhs.uk; kateorteu@hotmail.com

Saida Ortolano Department of Pathology and Neuropathology, University Hospital of Vigo, Vigo, Spain, saida.ortolano@sergas.es

Gregory M. Pastores Departments of Neurology and Pediatrics, New York University School of Medicine, New York, NY, USA, gregory.pastores@nyumc.org

Carlos E. Prada Division of Human Genetics, Cincinnati Children's Hospital Medical Center, University of Cincinnati College of Medicine, Cincinnati, OH, USA, carlos.prada@cchmc.org

Annick Raas-Rothschild Department of Human Genetics and Metabolic Diseases, Hadassah Hebrew University Medical Center, Ein Kerem, Jerusalem, Israel, annik@hadassah.org.il

Julian A.J. Raiman Division of Clinical and Metabolic Genetics, Hospital for Sick Children, Toronto, ON, Canada, julian.raiman@sickkids.ca

Uma Ramaswami Department of Paediatrics, Addenbrooke's Hospital, Cambridge, UK, uma.ramaswami@addenbrookes.nhs.uk

Arndt Rolfs Medical Faculty, Albrecht-Kossel-Institute for Neuroregeneration, University of Rostock, Rostock, Germany, arndt.rolfs@med.uni-rostock.de

Perri Segal Department of Human Genetics and Metabolic Diseases, Hadassah Hebrew University Medical Center, Ein Kerem, Jerusalem, Israel, perri.segal@mail.huji.ac.il

James A. Shayman Department of Internal Medicine, University of Michigan, Ann Arbor, MI, USA, jshayman@umich.edu

Ellen Sidransky Medical Genetics Branch, National Human Genome Research Institute, National Institutes of Health, Bethesda, MD, USA, sidranse@mail.nih.gov

Andrea Sodi Eye Clinic, University of Florence, Florence, Italy, andrea.sodi@unifi.it

Gere Sunder-Plassmann Division of Nephrology and Dialysis, Department of Medicine III, Medical University Vienna, Vienna, Austria, gere.sunder-plassmann@meduniwien.ac.at

Susana Teijeira Department of Pathology and Neuropathology, University Hospital of Vigo, Vigo, Spain, susana.teijeira.bautista@sergas.es

Carmen Valbuena Departments of Pathology, Medicine and Human Genetics, Faculty of Medicine, Hospital São João, Porto, Portugal, valbuena@med.up.pt

David G. Warnock Division of Nephrology, Department of Medicine, University of Alabama, Birmingham, AL, USA, dwarnock@uab.edu

Michael West Department of Medicine, Dalhousie University, Halifax, Canada, michael.west@cdha.nshealth.ca

Catharina Whybra-Trümpler Universitätskinderklinik der Johannes Gutenberg Universität Mainz, Langenbeckstr. 1, Mainz, Germany, c.whybra@web.de

Bryan Winchester Biochemistry Research Group, UCL Institute of Child Health at Great Ormond Street Hospital, University College London, London, UK, b.winchester@ich.ucl.ac.uk

Elisabeth Young Biochemistry Research Group, UCL Institute of Child Health at Great Ormond Street Hospital, University College London, London, UK, lissy@younglis.freeserve.co.uk

Wei Zheng NIH Chemical Genomics Center, NHGRI, NIH, Bethesda, MD, USA, wzheng@mail.nih.gov

Fabry Disease – An Overview

Roscoe O. Brady

Major Signs and Symptoms

Fabry disease is an X-linked hereditary metabolic storage disorder. It is a multi-system condition characterized by reddish-purple maculopapular lesions on the skin (angiokeratoma corporis diffusum), corneal opacities (cornea verticillata), hypohidrosis, gastroenteritis, chronic airflow obstruction, reduced kidney function leading to end-stage renal disease, left ventricular hypertrophy, premature myocardial infarctions and early-onset of strokes. The occurrence of these abnormalities varies in their extent and frequency in males with this condition. They are generally less prevalent in females with the disorder, but there are notable exceptions.

Pathological Biochemistry

Fabry disease is caused by the accumulation of excessive quantities of members of the class of lipids called sphingolipids that have the long chain aminoalcohol sphingosine as their common structural moiety (Fig. 1a). A long chain fatty acid is bound to the nitrogen atom on carbon atom two of sphingosine forming the structure called ceramide. Linked to carbon atom one of the sphingosine portion of ceramide are varying numbers of sugars forming glycosphingolipids. The most prevalent accumulating material in patients with Fabry disease is globotriaosylceramide (Gb3) that was previously called ceramidetrihexoside (Fig. 1b) [1]. Additional accumulating substances are digalactosylceramide that is especially present in kidneys (Fig. 1c) and globotriaosylsphingosine (lyso-Gb3) (Fig. 1d) [2]. Based on the discoveries of the enzymatic defects in Gaucher disease [3] and in Niemann-Pick disease [4], it was predicted that the metabolic defect in Fabry disease was due to insufficient activity of an enzyme that catalyzes the hydrolytic cleavage of the terminal galactose from

R.O. Brady (✉)
National Institute of Neurological Disorders and Stroke, National Institutes of Health, Bethesda, MD, USA
e-mail: bradyr@ninds.nih.gov

Fig. 1 Accumulating glycosphingolipids in patients with Fabry disease. The core component is the long chain amino alcohol sphingosine

A. $CH_3\text{-}(CH_2)_{12}\text{-}CH=CH\text{-}CH\text{-}CH\text{-}CH_2OH$
$\quad\quad\quad\quad\quad\quad\quad\quad\quad\quad | \quad |$
$\quad\quad\quad\quad\quad\quad\quad\quad\quad\quad OH \ NH_2$

Sphingosine

B. **Sphingosine-Glucose-Galactose-Galactose**
$\quad\quad\quad |$
Fatty Acid

Globotriaosylceramide (Gb_3)

[also known as Ceramidetrihexoside]

C. **Sphingosine-Galactose-Galactose**
$\quad\quad\quad |$
Fatty Acid

Digalactosylceramide

D. **Sphingosine-Glucose-Galactose-Galactose**

Globotriaosylsphingosine

[also known as Lyso-Gb3]

Gb3 [5]. Because the chemical synthesis of Gb3 had not been accomplished at that time, the entire Gb3 molecule was labeled with ^3H using a technique what was known as the Wilzbach procedure [6]. The compound to be labeled is exposed to a high level of ^3H in a sealed ampoule under increased pressure for 7 days. The uniformly labeled radioactive product was purified extensively until background radioactivity was sufficiently low that it could be used as a substrate to detect an enzyme that might be involved in its catabolism. A survey of rat tissues revealed that the small intestine contained the highest level of specific catabolic activity [7]. That source was therefore used for the purification of the enzyme ceramidetrihexosidase that catalyzes the cleavage of the terminal molecule of galactose from Gb3. The cause of the accumulation of pathological quantities of Gb3 was quickly shown to be due to insufficient activity of ceramidetrihexosidase [8] (Fig. 2). Because the bond between the two molecules of galactose in Gb3 is in the α-anomeric configuration, ceramidetrihexosidase was subsequently termed α-galactosidase A. Since patients with both Gaucher disease and Niemann-Pick disease showed some detectable residual glucocerebrosidase and sphingomyelianse activity, it was somewhat surprising to find that the activity of ceramidetrihexosidase in the intestinal biopsies from the two Fabry patients that were examined was undetectable. This situation was later seen in approximately 45% of the hemizygous Fabry males examined in my Branch at the National Institutes of Health. Although the catabolism of digalactosylceramide and lyso-Gb3 catalyzed by α-galactosidase A appears not to have been specifically examined, the elevated levels of these substances in patients with reduced or absent α-galactosidase A activity implies that they are catabolized

The catabolism of Gb3 is initiated by the enzyme α-galactosidase A.

Sphingosine-Glucose-Galactose-Galactose + H$_2$O →
I
Fatty Acid

Sphingosine-Glucose-Galactose + Galactose
I
Fatty Acid

The enzymatic defect in Fabry disease.

Sphingosine-Glucose-Galactose-I-Galactose + H$_2$O →II
I
Fatty Acid

Fig. 2 The catabolism of Gb3 is initiated by the enzyme α-galactosidase A

by this enzyme. Based on very slow rate of hydrolysis of glucosylsphingosine catalyzed by gluocerebrosidase compared with glucocerebroside [9], one might deduce that the enzymatic cleavage of the terminal molecule of galactose from lyso-Gb3 might be much slower than that of Gb3. Because galactosylsphingosine (lyso-galactocerebroside) [10] and glucosylsphingosine (lyso-glucocerebroside) [11] have been shown to by highly cytotoxic, the toxicity of lyso-Gb3 may be anticipated to be considerably greater than Gb3.

Pathophysiology

Glycosphingolipids are found in the plasma cell membranes of most of the cells in the body. However, the turnover of red blood cells has emerged as a major contributor to the pathophysiology of Fabry disease. Except for persons with the pk and p red blood cell groups, the principal glycosphingolipid in erythrocyte stroma is globotetraosylcermide (Gb4), frequently referred to as globoside (Fig. 3). When red blood cells become senescent, they are removed from the circulation by tissue macrophages such as the Kupffer cells in the liver. All of the membranous components of the phagocytized cells are degraded enzymatically in subcellular organelles called lysosomes. Lysosomes contain a series of consecutively acting

Sphingosine-Glucose-Galactose-Galactose-N-Acetylgalactosamine
I
Fatty Acid

Globotetraosylceramide

[also called Globoside]

Fig. 3 Structure of the most prevalent glycosphingolipid in human red blood cell stroma

enzymes that biodegrade ingested membrane components as well as an acidic mileu at which these catalysts are maximally active. The catabolism of the major red blood cell membrane globotetroasylceramide (globoside) is initiated by the enzyme hexosaminidase B forming globotriaosylceramide (Gb3). Because of insufficient α-galactosidase A activity, pathological quantities of Gb3 accumulate throughout the body of patients with Fabry disease. The importance of a constant source of sphingoglycolipids originating from the stroma of senescent red blood cells was substantiated in experiments with a mouse model of Fabry disease. A significant accumulation of Gb3 occurs in the organs and tissues of mice when α-galactosidase A activity is eliminated [12]. However, the mice had a normal life span and showed no major manifestations of Fabry disease such as strokes, myocardial infarctions or renal disease. The reason for the absence of the typical Fabry phenotype was soon discovered [13]. Red blood cells in the C57BL/6 × 129/Svj hybrid strain of mice used for knocking out α-galactosidase A do not contain a detectable quantity of either Gb4 (globoside) or Gb3. They therefore have some resemblance to human blood group p that do not contain Gb3 or Gb4 in their red blood cells due to absence of Gb3 synthase that catalyzes the addition of galactose from UDP-galactose to ceramidelactoside [14]. If the findings in the α-galactosidase A –/– mouse models of Fabry disease can be extrapolated to humans, it would seem unlikely that a reduction or lack of α-galactosidase A activity in blood group p humans would cause the array of pathological manifestations conventionally associated with Fabry disease.

Therapy

Enzyme Replacement

Since many of the salient aspects of Fabry disease are discussed in detail in various chapters in this book, I should like to restrict my further remarks to a consideration of strategies for the treatment for patients with this disorder. Because of the extraordinarily beneficial effects of enzyme replacement therapy (ERT) in patients with Gaucher disease [15–17], this stratagem was high on the list of approaches to try to improve the lives of patients with Fabry disease. Even before ERT was undertaken in patients with Gaucher disease, an investigation along this line was carried out in patients with Fabry disease. In an effort to maximally reduce the possibility of sensitizing patients to the exogenous protein, a human source of ceramidetrihexosidase (α-galactosidase A) was considered desirable. An examination of fresh human placental tissue revealed that it contained this enzyme and was therefore used as the source [18]. When this enzyme was infused into two patients with Fabry disease, a rapid reduction of Gb3 in the circulation occurred [19]. The level of Gb3 returned to the pre-infusion value by 48 h following the administration of the enzyme. Additional preliminary ERT trials were carried out with α-galactosidase A preparations obtained from human spleen and plasma [20]. Variations in enzyme kinetics and the extent of reduction of plasma Gb3 levels that were observed with the two isoforms were attributed to differences in sialylation and phosphorylation of these enzymes that are glycoproteins.

It was apparent that only limited quantities of α-galactosidase A could be obtained from sources such as these. Two biotechnology corporations began to prepare α-galactosidase A recombinantly. One of these was Transkaryotic Therapies, Inc., Cambridge MA, which subsequently became Shire Human Genetic Therapies, Inc. α-Galactosidase A was initially produced in a cultured human skin fibroblast cell line using a proprietary gene-activation technique. Intravenous administration of this preparation of α-galactosidase A to patients with Fabry disease caused a mean decrease of 31% of hepatic Gb3 and 38% decrease of urinary Gb3 [21]. Encouraged by these findings, larger quantities of α-galactosidase A were produced in a genetically engineered continuous human cell line. A randomized controlled trial with this preparation was conducted with 26 male patients with Fabry disease [22]. Recipients of the enzyme experienced a decrease in the severity of neuropathic pain and an increase of the quality of life. The recipients also had an approximately 50% reduction of plasma Gb3; a decrease of inulin clearance; an increase of creatinine clearance; improvement of cardiac conduction and gain of body weight. There was also a particularly striking increase in the number of normal kidney glomeruli and a reduction of the number of glomeruli with mesangial widening in the recipients. This preparation of α-galactosidase A is called Replagal. It is also known as agalsidase alfa (see Chapter 25 by Pastores). The dose used in patients is 0.2 mg/kg of body weight intravenously every 2 weeks.

The Genzyme Corporation, Cambridge, MA, used transduced Chinese hamster ovary cells to produce recombinant α-galactosidase A. This preparation is called agalsidase beta (Fabrazyme) (see Chapter 26 by Hopkin). It is administered at a dose of 1 mg/kg of body weight every other week. The initial trial with agalsidase beta revealed clearance of Gb3 from microvascular endothelial deposits in the kidney, skin and heart and reduction of plasma and urinary Gb3. Although seroconversion was observed in 88% of the recipients, it was concluded that it did not affect efficacy end points [23].

Based on these observations, agalsidase alfa and agalsidase beta were approved for the treatment of patients with Fabry disease in Europe and a number of other countries. However, only agalsidase beta was approved in the United States. Despite more than 8 years of availability of this therapy, complete restoration of health in patients with Fabry disease remains to be achieved. An encouraging possibility concerning the ultimate benefit of enzyme therapy for patients with Fabry disease might be derived from the finding that increasing the frequency of administration of α-galactosidase A from bi-weekly to weekly may slow the decline of renal function [24]. This observation, coupled with delay of onset of renal insufficiency in patients with mild mutations in the α-galactosidase A gene, prompted the deduction that there may be a need for a continuous presence of α-galactosidase A in cells [25]. Perhaps the most obvious approach to achieving this condition is gene therapy that is commented on later.

Molecular Chaperone Therapy

The discovery that certain small molecule inhibitors of α-galactosidase A can increase the catalytic activity of some of the mutated forms of this enzyme [26–30] has prompted a major investment into the identification and assessment of such agents that may be therapeutically useful (see Chapter 29 by Fan). Although this approach appears to be reasonable, the large proportion (~45%) of nonsense mutations in the α-galactosidase A gene in patients with Fabry disease results in no detectable residual enzyme (vs. and 31). This situation precludes a large number of patients with Fabry disease from benefiting from this treatment. In order to identify patients who might be helped by molecular chaperone therapy, a rapid procedure was developed to assess the degree of enhancement of α-galactosidase A catalytic activity by a molecular chaperone [32]. Application of this technique should assist in deciding who might benefit from chaperone therapy.

Substrate Reduction Therapy

Substrate reduction therapy (SRT) is accomplished by blocking a specific enzymatic step in the biosynthesis of an accumulating substance. Partially blocking the addition of glucose to ceramide to form glucocerebroside has been shown to provide benefit to some patients with Gaucher disease [33]. It is an approved therapy for certain patients with this disorder. More recently an improved inhibitor of glucocerebroside biosynthesis has been produced and is in clinical trial [34]. It was considered to be of interest in Fabry disease to examine the effect of blocking the addition of glucose to ceramide that would result in reducing the formation of Gb3. Therefore, the effect of a strong inhibitor of glucocerebroside biosynthesis was examined in Fabry mice [35]. A reduction of Gb3 of approximately 50% was observed in the kidneys, liver and heart following 8 weeks of intra-peritoneal administration of the inhibitor. The precise mechanism of clearance of Gb3 from the organs of mice lacking α-galactosidase A has not been established. Nevertheless, further examination of SRT appears warranted in patients with Fabry disease.

Gene Therapy

The availability of α-galactosidase A–/– knock-out mice [12] made it possible to undertake a number of critical experiments in regard to eventual gene therapy in patients with Fabry disease [36]. Pertinent findings in these investigations include significant reductions of accumulated Gb3 following a single injection of a recombinant adeno-associated viral vector containing a modified chicken α-actin promoter. At 6-months after administration of the vector, the elevated Gb3 in the liver and spleen were found to be normal levels. There was an 85% reduction in the heart and a 66% reduction in the lung [37]. Kidneys showed an 82% reduction at 2 months.

However, at 6 months, the amount of Gb3 in this organ had returned to 60% of the pre-treatment level. Gene therapy for Fabry disease and many other metabolic storage disorders has been significantly delayed by the occurrence of insertional mutagenesis following the use of a retroviral vector that caused leukemia in several human recipients [38–40]. Hopefully, the use of self-inactivating lentival vectors in stem cell-derived erythroid cells [41–43] may reduce oncogenic hazards associated with gene therapy and successful treatment for patients with Fabry disease will be realized.

The Future

I should like to touch on two additional potential approaches to treat patients with Fabry disease and other hereditary metabolic disorders. The first is the use of reagents to induce exon skipping in the considerable number of patients with Fabry disease who have nonsense mutations that disrupt the open-reading frame for α-galactosidase A causing a lack of enzyme. Aminoglycosides have been tried to induce exon skipping in a number of instances, particularly with regard to the treatment of Duchenne muscular dystrophy. However, the near-toxic levels required of these agents has limited their use. Recently, an examination of antisense oligonucleotides and several derivatives has been undertaken [44] as well as studies with viral vectors containing small nuclear RNAs [45] to induce exon skipping. Whether this approach is feasible for patients with Fabry disease remains to be determined.

An additional possibility that has yet to be shown to be clinically effective is homologous recombination. There are a number of potential advantages if this technique becomes useful [46]. This approach is under extensive consideration for the treatment of hemoglobinopathies [47]. Successful application of this strategy to treat a hereditary metabolic storage disorder remains to be demonstrated.

References

1. Sweeley CC, Klionsky B (1963) Fabry's disease: classification as a sphingolipidosis and partial characterization of a novel glycolipid. J Biol Chem 238:3148–3150
2. Aerts JM, Groener JE, Kuiper S et al (2008) Elevated globotriaosylsphingosine is a hallmark of Fabry disease. Proc Natl Acad Sci USA 105:2812–2817
3. Brady RO, Kanfer JN, Shapiro D (1965) Metabolism of glucocerebrosides. II. Evidence of an enzymatic deficiency in Gaucher's disease. Biochem Biophys Res Commun 18:221–225
4. Brady RO, Kanfer JN, Mock MB, Fredrickson DS (1966) The metabolism of sphingomyelin. II. Evidence of an enzymatic deficiency in Niemann-Pick disease. Proc Natl Acad Sci USA 55:366–369
5. Brady RO (1966) Sphingolipidoses. N Engl J Med 275:312–318
6. Wilzbach KE (1956) Tritium-labeling by exposure of organic compounds to tritium gas. J Am Chem Soc 79:1013
7. Brady RO, Gal AE, Bradley RM, Martensson E (1967) The metabolism of ceramidetrihexosides. I. Purification and properties of an enzyme which cleaves the terminal galactose molecule of galactosylgalactosylglucosylceramide. J Biol Chem 242:1021–1026

8. Brady RO, Gal AE, Bradley RM, Martensson E, Warshaw AL, Laster L (1967) Enzymatic defect in Fabry's disease. Ceramidetrihexosidase deficency. N Engl J Med 276:1163–1167

9. Pentchev PG, Brady RO, Hibbert SR, Gal AE, Shapiro D (1973) Isolation and characterization of glucocerebrosidase from human placental tissue. J Biol Chem 248:5256–5261

10. Suzuki K (1998) Twenty-five years of the "psychosine hypothesis". A personal perspective of its history and present status. Neurochem Res 23:251–259

11. Schueler U, Kolter T, Kaneski CR, Blusztajn JK, Herkenham M, Sandhoff K, Brady RO (2003) Toxicity of glucosylsphingosine (glucopsychosine) to cultured neuronal cells: a model system for assessing neuronal damage in Gaucher disease Type 2 and 3. Neurobiol Disease 14:595–601

12. Ohshima T, Murray GJ, Swain WD et al (1997) α-Galactosidase A deficient mice: a model of Fabry disease. Proc Natl Acad Sci USA 94:2540–2544

13. Ohshima T, Schiffmann R, Murray GJ et al (1999) Aging accentuates and bone marrow transplantation ameliorates metabolic defects in Fabry disease mice. Proc Natl Acad Sci USA 96:6423–6427

14. Furukawa K, Iwamura K, Uchikawa M et al (2000) Molecular basis for the p phenotype. J Biol Chem 275:37752–37756

15. Barton NW, Brady RO, Dambrosia JM et al (1991) Replacement therapy for inherited enzyme deficiency – macrophage-targeted glucocerebrosidase for Gaucher's disease. N Engl J Med 324:1464–1470

16. Grabowski GA, Barton NW, Pastores G et al (1995) Enzyme therapy in Gaucher disease Type 1: comparative efficacy of mannose-terminated glucocerebrosidase from natural and recombinant sources. Ann Int Med 122:33–39

17. Brady RO (2006) Enzyme replacement therapy for lysosomal diseases. Ann Rev Medicine 57:283–296

18. Johnson WG, Brady RO (1972) Ceramidetrihexosidase from human placenta. Methods Enzymol XXVIII:849–856

19. Brady RO, Tallman JF, Johnson WG et al (1973) Replacement therapy for inherited enzyme deficiency: use of purified ceramidetrihexosidase in Fabry's disease. N Engl J Med 289:9–14

20. Desnick RJ, Dean KJ, Grabowski G, Bishop DF, Sweeley CC (1979) Enzyme therapy in Fabry disease. Differential in vivo plasma clearance and metabolic effectiveness of plasma and splenic a-galactosidase A isozymes. Proc Natl Acad Sci USA 76:5326–5330

21. Schiffmann R, Murray GJ, Treco D et al (2000) Infusion of α-galactosidase A reduces tissue globotriaosylceramide storage in patients with Fabry disease. Proc Natl Acad Sci USA 97:365–370

22. Schiffmann R, Kopp JB, Austin HA et al (2001) Enzyme replacement therapy in Fabry disease. A randomized controlled trial. JAMA 285:2743–2749

23. Eng CM, Guffon N, Wilcox WR et al (2001) Safety and efficacy of recombinant human a-galactosidase A replacement theapy in Fabry's disease. N Engl J Med 345:9–16

24. Schiffmann R, Askari H, Timmons M et al (2007) Weekly enzyme replacement therapy may slow decline of renal function in patients with Fabry disease who are on long-term biweekly dosing. J Am Soc Nephrol 18:1576–1583

25. Schiffmann R (2009) Fabry disease. Pharmacol Ther 122:65–77

26. Fan J-Q, Ishii S, Asano N, Suzuki Y (1999) Accelerated transport and maturation of lysosomal a-galactosidase A in Fabry lymphoblasts by an enzyme inhibitor. Nat Med 5:112–115

27. Yam GH-F, Bosshard N, Zuber C, Steinmnn B, Roth J (2006) Pharmacological chaperone corrects lysosomal storage in Fabry disease caused by trafficking-incompetent variants. Am J Physiol Cell Physiol 290:C1076–C1082

28. Shin S-H, Murray GJ, Kluepfel-Stahl S et al (2007) Screening for pharmacological chaperones in Fabry disease. Biochem Biophys Res Commun 359:168–173

29. Sugawara K, Tajima Y, Kawashima I et al (2009) Molecular interaction of imino sugars with human a-galactosidase: insight into the mechanism of complex formation and pharmacological chaperone action in Fabry disease. Mol Genet Metab 96:233–238

30. Benjamin ER, Flanagan JJ, Schillinig A et al (2009) The pharmacological chaperone 1-deoxygalactonojirimycin increases alpha-galactosidase A levels in Fabry patient cell lines. J Inherit Metab Dis 32:424–440
31. Desnick RJ, Ioannou YA, Eng CM (2001) α-Galactosidase A deficiency: Fabry disease. In: Scriver CR, Beaudet AL, Sly WS Valle D (eds) The metabolic and molecular bases of inherited disease, 8th edn. McGraw-Hill, New York, pp 3733–3774
32. Shin SH, Kluepfel-Stahl S, Cooney AM et al (2008) Prediction of response of mutated α-galactosidase A to a pharmacological chaperone. Pharmacogenet Genomics 18:773–780
33. Cox T, Lachmann R, Hollak C et al (2000) Novel oral treatment of Gaucher's disease with N-butyldeoxynojirimycin (OGT 918) to decrease substrate diosynthesis. Lancet 355:1481–1485
34. McEachern KA, Fung J, Komarnitsky S et al (2007) A specific and potent inhibitor of glucosylceramide synthase for substrate inhibition therapy of Gaucher disease. Mol Genet Metabol 91:259–267
35. Abe A, Gregory S, Lee L et al (2000) Reduction of globotriaosylceramide in Fabry disease mice by substrate deprivation. J Clin Invest 105:1563–1571
36. Jung S-C, Han IP, Limaye A et al (2001) Adeno-associated viral vector-mediated gene transfer results in long-term enzymatic and functional correction in multiple organs of Fabry mice. Proc Nat Acad Sci USA 98:2676–2681
37. Park J, Murray GJ, Limaye A et al (2003) Long-term correction of globotriaosylceramide storage in Fabry mice by recombinant adeno-associated virus-mediated gene transfer. Proc Nat Acad Sci USA 100:3450–3454
38. Hacein-Bey-Abina S, Garrigue A, Wang GP et al (2008) Insertional oncogenesis in 4 patients after retrovirus-mediated gene therapy of SCID-X1. J Clin Invest 118:3132–3142
39. Howe SJ, Mansour MR, Schwarzwaelder K et al (2008) Insertional mutagenesis combined with acquired somatic mutations causes leukemogenesis following gene therapy of SCID-XI patients. J Clin Invest 118:3143–3150
40. Kohn DB, Sadelain M, Glorioso JC (2003) Occurrence of leukaemia following gene therapy of X-linked SCID. Nat Rev 3:477–488
41. Moreau-Gaudry F, Xia P, Jiang G et al (2001) High-level erythroid-specific gene expression in primary human and murine hematopoietic cells with self-inactivating lentiviral vectors. Blood 98:2664–2672
42. Chang AH, Stephan MT, Sadelain M (2006) Stem cell-derived erythroid cells mediate long-term systemic protein delivery. Nature Biotechnology 24:1017–1021
43. Enquist IB, Nilsson E, Mansson J–E et al (2009) Successful low-risk hematopoietic cell therapy in a mouse model of Type 1 Gaucher disease. Stem Cells 27:736–744
44. Heemskerk HA, de Winter CL, de Kimpe SJ et al (2009) In vivo comparison of 2'-O-methyl phosphorothioate and morpholino antisense oligonucleotides for Duchenne muscular dystrophy exon skipping. J Gene Med 11:257–266
45. Goyenvalle A, Babbs A, van Ommen GJ, Garcia L, Davies KE (2009) Enhanced exon-skipping induced by U7 snRNA carrying a splicer silencer sequence: promising tool for DMD therapy. Mol Ther 17:1234–1240
46. Porteus M (2007) Using homologous recombination to manipulate the genome of human somatic cells. Biotechnol Genet Eng Rev 24:195–212
47. Sadelain M, Boulad F, Lisowki L, Moi P, Riviere I (2008) Stem cell engineering for the treatment of severe hemoglobinopathies. Curr Mol Med 8:690–697

Fabry Disease – A Patient Perspective

Jack Johnson

The weekend has arrived that I had designated for myself to begin writing about Fabry disease. I apologize, but do not feel well enough to do this right now.

Several days have passed and I can now continue. Things not going as planned is just one aspect of living with Fabry disease. It can be very difficult to make plans of any kind at times. Even feeling well enough to keep scheduled doctor appointments can be difficult for some, but enough about that for now.

I would like to disclose that unlike other distinguished authors in this book I have no formal medical training. What degree of expertise I may kindly be attributed with comes from personal experience as patient with a Fabry disease and many years of contact with numerous individuals in the Fabry community, including patients, care givers and members of the medical community.

Fabry disease is known as a rare disease and meeting others that suffer from the condition certainly can be a very unusual occurrence. This not withstanding that Fabry disease is not so rare when it affects you or your family. Some individuals may be the only person affected in a family, while others may have parents, children, aunts, uncles and additional extended family members with the disease. One thread that runs throughout this varied community is a feeling of loneliness.

So many patients suffer for years or even decades not knowing what is wrong. They may feel isolated because no one understands what they are going through. Patients go from doctor to doctor. They receive some diagnosis or another thinking an answer has been found. The treatment regimen that is begun does not provide the improved health as expected. Instead frustration replaces the hope that was previously conveyed. This cycle of disappointments for some patients is too much and they retreat from the medical community denying that their problems still persist.

Many patients who suffer don't recognize that the medical establishment is not geared to train each physician to recognize every condition. Nor has the medical establishment done a very good job at having its members reveal this lack of pertinent information to patients.

Some patients are ultimately rewarded by being persistent enough to keep seeking answers until the puzzle pieces are in place. Other patients eventually develop

---

This title is edited by Michael J. Russo

significant organ involvement which points a specialist in the right direction, too frequently via a biopsy. A very few patients actually manage to be directed to a physician knowledgeable about Fabry disease at a point early enough in the progression of the disease to impact symptoms and possibly alter the disease course. Whatever the specific route, receiving that correct diagnosis is the pivotal point that leads to another universal thread: diagnosed patients finally have a name for what has been plaguing them and that small bit of data provides some level of relief.

Once the initial diagnosis has been made, it can lead to a domino affect as additional family members are diagnosed. While some sense of relief may be felt learning the name of what is causing their myriad symptoms, initially it can also be quite frightening. With this information newly-diagnosed patients may look at older relatives and worry that they too will follow the same path. Patients may be afraid of the future after learning about the impact Fabry disease can have on one's health.

Denial is another regrettable possibility that may develop after being diagnosed or even after a relative's diagnosis. Too many patients have stories about a relative who says his/her health problems have nothing to do with Fabry disease although s/he may have already been diagnosed or are at genetic risk for the condition. These individuals may say that they don't need to worry about Fabry disease because they have been getting along well enough so far (Nothing went wrong yesterday so there is no reason to think it will be worse tomorrow). Other individuals may not be able to accept the probability that s/he may have passed a serious disease like Fabry disease on to their children.

For most patients, the first symptoms of Fabry disease occur during childhood or adolescence. Children continue to play and run like they have on so many other days, but then comes the time when intense pain surges through their feet. They crumple to the ground crying just wanting the pain to go away. This pain is unlike anything they have ever experienced and may disappear within a few minutes. Perhaps, their first symptom is complaint of a fever. The youngster's mother is not able to stop the fiery burning pain in her child's hands and feet.

The emergency room physician, pediatrician, or family doctor finds nothing unusual during an examination and chalks the complaints up to growing pains, some other common aliment, or suggests that perhaps the child just doesn't want to be in physical education class anymore and is making all this up.

After a number of episodes at school, classmates often stop believing that these spells of distress are genuine. A child may even be called a 'crybaby' by his teacher. Lack of understanding from parents or siblings also takes its toll. Some patients may conclude that the best way to cope with this is to stop talking about their symptoms all together. Even if it is acknowledged that a child has Fabry disease, these issues may be impossible to control or avoid.

The intensity of pain that Fabry disease can inflict on the body may be incredibly difficult to convey to others. This pain can vary from person to person and the types of pain experienced by a single individual may vary greatly during any given day. Oftentimes, one particular day or perhaps several consecutive days, remain clearly fixed in the patient's mind.... not because of the pain, but rather because for that brief period, absolutely no Fabry pain was present. These occasions are few and far between.

At first it may not be obvious what precipitating event is responsible for the onset of pain, but in time it frequently becomes clearer, especially with the onset of the more severe episodes. Common factors include: over-exertion, getting too hot, or stress to the body from temperature changes, hot or cold. Fevers are frequent triggers and some patients have recurring fevers with no apparent cause. Changes in the weather can cause increased pain. This may be associated with seasonal changes such as the onset of spring, or pain may be brought on by a strong weather front passing through. The stresses of daily living may also cause an episode of pain.

Another common complaint is a degree of 'background pain'; this is so prevalent and chronic that when asked about the presence of discomfort or pain, the patient may take a moment to realize that there is a level of pain that is always there. This pain may be uniquely present in the hands, feet, or certain joints, or may be generalized to the entire body or large portion of the body. It seems an odd thing to believe someone can suffer pain and not readily know it, but don't we often believe we are sitting in a quiet room only to realize that this is not the case once the air-conditioning stops and the fan noise ceases.

Background pain is often mild, but can also be severe in some individuals. It may have a diurnal rhythm where the pain worsens during the afternoon or perhaps makes restful sleep difficult at night. Traditionally, anti-convulsion medications have been effective in reducing or controlling this type of pain, but they are insufficient for more acute pain.

Periodic episodes of severe pain and burning may also occur. This pain may last from minutes to hours but also may seem like endless days or even weeks. This pain can be extremely intense and completely debilitating. Eating and drinking may not only be difficult, but it may even be avoided because it leads to needing to frequent the bathroom, which in turn causes increased pain because of bowel movements. The burning sensation accompanying hand and foot pain can feel as if the extremities are in a steam-cooker. Pain may radiate up the arms and legs and may feel as if it has settled in the bones. Avoiding what causes the onset of these painful episodes may help, but unfortunately this is not always possible.

While relief may be gained from prescription pain medications, at times the extreme pain of Fabry disease goes beyond the ability even of powerful narcotic drugs. Patients continue to suffer in agony until the right medication or combination of medications is found.

Experiencing pain crises leaves patients in a weakened state that may take days and even months to achieve some degree of recovery. For many patients, these episodes of pain are more frequent in adolescence and early adulthood, but this is by no means true of all patients. Some patients may believe that they are getting better because the occurrence of these pain crises has diminished, only to develop renal, cardiac or cerebral vascular events later in life.

To complicate matters associated with the sensitivity to temperature change, fever, and physical exertion, Fabry patients often suffer anhidrosis or hypohidrosis, although in some hyperhidrosis may also be a complaint. Because of this inability to perspire adequately (or at all), family and teachers should be made aware that dangerous overheating can occur. Children commonly become very red in the face, and the hands and feet may begin to burn. This can frequently cause young patients with Fabry disease to fall behind their peers specifically in warm weather or when required to engage in physically demanding activities. Providing shade and keeping water nearby can be crucial. Wetting the hands, arms, face and feet to accelerate cooling can provide much needed relief.

Fortunately, air-conditioning is available in many homes and cars to provide comfortable temperatures during the hot summer months. When participating in activities outside, learning to stay cool can be helpful. There are a number of products on the market to help, from small fans with a mist of water to cooling vests. Simple things like eating ice chips, dressing in layers, wearing light-colored clothes or avoiding direct exposure to the sun are other measures one can take.

For those who are able to perspire adequately and handle warm temperatures, or when temperatures are cooler, patients may still have difficulty with physical exertion. Exercise intolerance can leave patients short of breath and exhausted well before healthy people in similar situations. This may become obvious in school-aged children as they try to keep up with peers in physical education class or in extracurricular sport activities. Even social events such as a school dance can pose difficulties because of the necessity for more frequent rest breaks. Making sure the school staff is aware of these limitations can be important. It may be best to let the child set his/her own pace. In some cases a medical exemption from physical education class may be necessary.

Independent of exercise intolerance, a state of generalized fatigue or tiredness may develop in both adolescents and adults. Although it is usually not debilitating, this symptom can have a detrimental impact on quality of life and be difficult for others to understand or appreciate.

Gastrointestinal involvement can be a severe problem affecting many patients' lives. As with extremity pain, bouts of diarrhea, constipation, stomach pain and vomiting can be episodic or chronic. Care should be taken so Fabry-associated abdominal pain is not confused with more common ailments and *vice versa*. Diarrhea and stomach cramping are prevalent and debilitating gastrointestinal symptoms. Those who suffer from abdominal symptoms are often forced to plan their day around the location of the nearest restroom. Gastrointestinal symptoms frequently strike within 30–60 min after meals making social involvement with friends and family difficult. Episodes of diarrhea and vomiting resulting in 10–30 trips to the toilet per day are not only embarrassing, they can be physically exhausting and make regular school/work attendance impossible. Dietary factors can play a role, but unfortunately there is great variability between patients making a recommended diet complicated at best.

Many patients report that pain and gastrointestinal involvement are the two greatest factors impairing quality of life. These complications may cause patients to undergo numerous expensive and difficult tests in the search for the etiology. Some patients give up of finding an answer, resigning to the notion that this is just how life is. In fact, some young suffers may believe this is how it is for most people and wonder why they can't cope as well as their friends or unaffected family members. These very young patients may be very surprised to find out that the rest of the world does not share the same (gastrointestinal) difficulties.

You mean your hands and feet don't hurt and burn like they are on fire every time you run a temperature?

How can you stand to walk bare foot on this sidewalk? It burns my feet right through the soles of my shoes.

Why don't you get all sweaty like the rest of us? I don't know. I get so hot I just can't stand it, but my socks don't even get damp. I don't need to use antiperspirant either.

How can you eat that? It makes me sick every time I have some.

Most symptoms experienced by Fabry patients are also common to the general population, and thus are relatively non-specific. This contributes to a fairly high incidence of misdiagnosis, which causes delays in receiving proper treatment.

Misdiagnosis and delay can be an even bigger problem for females who inherit the mutated gene. Since Fabry is an X-linked disease, many in the medical community assume this is equalent to a recessive genetic trait. This has been a long-held view, believing females with Fabry disease were just 'carriers' and rarely affected. Recent research has largely dispelled this view by showing that the impact of Fabry disease can be just as severe among females as among males.

In general, females who inherit the mutated Fabry gene have a wider degree of variability of symptoms and often have a slightly later onset. Females may range from asymptomatic to exhibiting full-blown symptoms as well as random degrees of involvement. Symptoms expressed by all patients should be taken seriously regardless of gender. Females heterozygous for Fabry disease should be thought of as Fabry patients and treated likewise. Use of the term 'carrier' should be discontinued.

Outward signs of Fabry may not be pronounced, but when noticed can be telling. Angiokeratomas are the most readily visible, but due to their frequent 'bathing suit' distribution from the waist to groin, may not be noticed during a normal examination. This particular skin abnormality is not exclusive to Fabry disease sufferers, but, when brought to the attention of a dermatologist, may lead to a correct diagnosis. In most instances, angiokeratomas do not cause any significant problems; sometimes they can be removed with argon laser treatment. However, these small red to blue-black lesions have been known to be rather embarrassing for young men because of their rash-like appearance and location. In some instances, angiokeratomas may produce larger wart-like lesions. They can result in bleeding on towels, bedding and clothing, although this is usually minor. As with other signs and symptoms, not all Fabry sufferers have angiokeratomas.

The other visible signs of Fabry disease are normally seen only by an optometrist or ophthalmologist. The characteristic corneal opacity that forms on the surface of the eye can be seen during a slit-lamp examination. Fabry disease is one of a short list of causes for this finding, so, like dermatologists, optometrists are relatively good at referring potential Fabry patients for diagnosis. Other eye findings may result from the vascular involvement associated with Fabry such as torturous blood vessels in the retina. While Fabry may not result in noted vision problems, it may be possible in some cases.

Nephrology is another medical specialty that can help confirm a Fabry diagnosis. Excess levels of urinary protein and other signs of kidney disease are prominent features of Fabry disease. Even though Fabry may not be readily apparent as the cause for declining kidney function, a renal biopsy will often clarify the matter. If left untreated, most male patients with what is viewed as 'classic' Fabry will eventually progress to end-stage renal disease and kidney failure. Recent research has also brought to light the impact of renal involvement in the female patient population which is greater than previously believed (Fabry RADAR 2007: The Fabry Registry Aggregate Data Annual Report: Genzyme Corporation; 2007).

Kidney failure is a great and looming fear for many Fabry patients. The requirement for dialysis can place an enormous burden on the patient and family. Fortunately, many patients are able to receive a kidney transplant either via cadaver or live donor such as a family member. Uniformly, receiving a kidney transplant has been expressed by patients as a positive step even if the procedure itself may be viewed with apprehension.

Cardiac involvement can be a particularly troubling aspect for both males and females with Fabry disease. While the associated clinical findings may paint a particular picture, the realities of daily life can be frustrating in trying to adequately convey symptoms to a physician.

The transient nature of cardiac conductive abnormalities can be alarming, and in some cases very difficult to document. Spells of palpitations may be short-lived and can occur with atrial or ventricular tachycardia or other arrhythmias. Patients may be aware of these abnormal heart rhythms. They may be of brief duration or extend for hours before conversion back to a normal heart rhythm. Seeking medical attention for these arrhythmias can be a frustrating process since symptoms may resolve before reaching medical care.

Cardiac symptoms may occur in conjunction with a slowed heart rate resulting in shortness of breath, light-headedness, dizziness, and fainting. Eventually, implantation of a cardiac pacemaker or pacemaker-cardioverter defibrillator combination may be necessary. Left ventricular hypertrophy with reduced cardiac efficiency may also contribute to these symptoms. Mitral valve prolapse and additional complications of cardiac disease such as congestive heart failure can contribute to cause further impact. For patients who develop significant cardiac complications, the possibility of a heart attack is a significant concern.

Neurological events are another aspect of Fabry disease that can take a toll on the patient. They can be as simple and non-specific as frequent headaches to Transient Ischemic Attacks (TIAs), or strokes, the latter of which can of course be very alarming and serious events for patients and their families. While these cerebrovascular events are not normally associated with younger patients, they present another potentially debilitating aspect that can strike without warning. Anti-coagulant medications are helpful in attempting to prevent blood clots, which can be of significant concern for a condition that is known to cause narrowing of blood vessels due to glycosphingolipid accumulation in endothelial cells lining the vascular system.

Patients may also suffer complications resulting from peripheral neuropathy commonly seen in Fabry disease. Extremity pain is probably the most frequently experienced result, but patients may also develop some degree of temperature sensitivity. In particular cold temperatures may become especially difficult to tolerate and quite painful, but sensitivity to heat may also occur. In time, patients may also experience a loss in temperature and vibration sensation. In these instances, care may be needed to prevent burns or frost bite to the feet and hands.

Auditory involvement is noted in many Fabry sufferers. Tinnitus and high-frequency hearing loss are relatively common. In some instances, greater degrees of gradual bilateral hearing loss may occur. The development of reduced hearing may first be noticed by family members. Hearing aid use is helpful in compensating for the impact of reduced hearing.

Spells of dizziness, vertigo and nausea may also occur as the vestibular system can be affected in conjunction with hearing impairment. Episodes of extreme dizziness may range in duration from minutes to hours with repeated bouts of vomiting. These episodes can be extremely difficult for the patient to endure. In more severe cases of hearing impairment, the use of cochlear implants has proven successful with marked improvement in the patient's ability to hear. Instances of sudden deafness in one ear have also occurred in association with TIA.

Patients may develop pulmonary symptoms. A nagging cough may develop with a frequent and irritating need to clear the throat. A cough from seasonal allergies or a simple cold may take months to clear up. Some patients may progress to chronic bronchitis. Airway obstructions may also occur resulting in wheezing and shortness of breath. In some instances supplemental oxygen may be needed. These symptoms also contribute to fatigue and reduced general health.

Owing to the nature of vascular involvement associated with Fabry disease, sexual dysfunction may become an additional complication. This imposes yet another physical and emotional burden on patients.

The progressive and chronic nature of Fabry disease can significantly impact all aspects of a patient's life. The burden this condition may place on an individual's life should not be underestimated. Whether due to the condition itself or the associated disease burden, depression can present a considerable hurdle for any patients. Treatment and education about depression should be considered wherever appropriate. Many patients do not appreciate the impact depression can have on their health. Counseling and treatment may provide substantial benefit.

Potential contributors to depression are the psychosocial aspects of living with Fabry disease. This impact often starts in childhood. Not being able to keep up with one's peers may cause a young patient to feel set apart and not able to fit in or participate as desired. This could be at school or other activities. There seems to be no link between Fabry and any impaired academic ability, although sports and other physical activities certainly can be impacted. Some students may not be able to attend school regularly due to episodes of pain or gastrointestinal involvement.

Participation in school, social or family activities, and work can be hindered, leading to lowered self esteem. Isolation or withdraw can occur due to such factors as pain, diarrhea or vomiting shortly after meals, hearing impairment, heat intolerance, fatigue or even the fear of Fabry associated symptoms. These and other symptoms may contribute to a patient feeling alone. They may believe no one else suffers like this or can understand what they are going through. The rarity of Fabry disease and the current insufficient number of medical professionals that know of the condition may also contribute to feelings of isolation.

Feelings of guilt may be a substantial burden for some patients. An individual may feel guilty for passing Fabry disease on to a child or children. These feelings may weigh heavily on the parent-patient and can be long-lasting. Feelings of guilt may be true for both males and females, but seems to be a more difficult for female patients.

In an attempt to cope with symptoms of Fabry, some patients may look outside the normal realm of traditional medical intervention. The consumption of alcohol to ease pain may lead to the additional burden of alcohol addiction. The use of (medicinal) cannabis may be sought to moderate gastrointestinal problems, pain and other symptoms. These and other recreational drugs may contribute further to complicate factors affecting the medical management of the disease.

As may be expected, the impact of Fabry disease on all aspects of quality of life measures can be enormous. There are those fortunate enough to have very little impact on their daily functioning, but it may also range to moderate or severe impairment. Disability and dependency on government provided healthcare and disability income programs is a reality for many Fabry sufferers.

To help manage the burden of disease, an emotional support system can prove extremely important for a patient's well being and daily functioning. Understanding family or friends can help to meet this need. Educating the members of the support team about Fabry disease can prove crucial. People may be afraid of what they don't understand so encourage steps to get beyond this potential barrier. Providing educational materials or directing patients, care givers and family members to sources of these materials and additional support may help enhance care outcomes and assist in quality of life issues.

Fabry disease has had a long history where no specific treatment was available to address the underlying condition. Fortunately, that changed in 2001 for many countries in Europe and elsewhere in the world with the regulatory approval of the Enzyme Replacement Therapy (ERT) drugs Fabrazyme® and Replagal®. In 2003 the Food and Drug Administration granted approval for Fabrazyme® allowing United States physicians to join their foreign counterparts in treating Fabry disease patients with ERT. Now, as in the past, treatment requires the appropriate standard of care measures for all aspects of Fabry disease, along with ERT.

The complexity of Fabry disease often requires the involvement of many medical specialists. Communication between these specialist and involvement of the patient or care giver all working together as a health care team provides the most optimal environment for positive patient care.

While research has provided much information about this rare condition, Fabry is anything but a simple disease. To date no set rules have been developed to predict disease impact or patient outcome. There is great variability in signs and symptoms, which require each patient to be evaluated and treated on an individual bases to ensure optimal care.

A discussion of treatment for Fabry disease is not complete without the mention of drug cost. Enzyme replacement therapy is currently among the most expense drug treatment options in the world. Without a reimbursement mechanism in place the vast majority of patients will not be able to receive treatment for the underlying disease. Dealing with reimbursement issues places a further level of burden on the disease community.

Fabry disease is a complex condition that requires a multi-disciplinary approach to treat. The future for patients and their families is looking brighter as new challenges are being addressed. The goal of all parties involved should be targeted toward the best possible outcome for the Fabry disease patient.

Part I
Pre-clinical

Chapter 1
Molecular Genetics of Fabry Disease and Genotype–Phenotype Correlation

Andreas Gal

Abstract Alpha-galactosidase A, the enzyme deficient in Fabry disease, is a polypeptide of 429 amino acids encoded by the seven exons of the *GLA* gene. From the literature, a total of 599 *GLA* sequence changes, including 435 pathogenic point mutations (missense, nonsense, and splice site) and 150 disease causing 'short length' rearrangements (mainly deletions and duplications affecting less than 65 nucleotides) as well as 14 DNA polymorphisms were compiled. While no obvious mutation 'hot spots' for point mutations were detected, about 30% of the rearrangements occurred in exon 7, which accounts for only 22.6% of the coding region. The clinical phenotype in Fabry disease can be extremely variable, both in males and females, within the same family and among patients from unrelated families carrying the same mutation. Thus establishing genotype–phenotype correlations in Fabry disease is not straight forward and usually requires the analysis of large cohorts of probands. In addition to patients with the classic Fabry disease phenotype, a considerable number of patients have been described that presented with an 'oligosymptomatic' phenotype, occasionally called cardiac or renal forms. This attenuated phenotype is characterized by later onset and slower progression of the disease, the patients are older at the time of major organ failure, and show a longer survival. Results of the few studies reported to date suggest that the attenuated phenotype is more often seen in patients with missense mutations than in those carrying constitutional or functional null alleles. Thirty-three different missense mutations have been reported to date in patients with attenuated phenotypes. The great majority of the residues affected by these mutations seem to be partially, mostly, or completely buried in the 3D-crystallographic structure model of α-galactosidase A. About half of the variants represent conservative amino acid changes, and only about 25% of the residues are considered evolutionarily highly conserved. While during the past years some progress has been made in the analysis of the correlation between *GLA* mutations and the patients' phenotypes, there are only very few data on the phenotypic effect of other genes (so called modifiers) in patients with Fabry disease.

A. Gal (✉)
Institut für Humangenetik, Universitätsklinikum Hamburg-Eppendorf, Hamburg, Germany
e-mail: gal@uke.de

D. Elstein et al. (eds.), *Fabry Disease*, DOI 10.1007/978-90-481-9033-1_1,

Keywords DNA · Mutation · Polymorphisms · X-chromosomal inheritance

This chapter gives a short overview of the α-galactosidase A gene (*GLA*), mutated in Fabry disease, the sequence variants found in the gene in health and disease, and the correlation between genotype and phenotype.

1.1 The *GLA* Gene Encodes α-Galactosidase A

The *GLA* gene was mapped to the long arm of the X chromosome, in the region Xq22.1. It contains 7 exons ranging from 92 to 291 base pairs (bp) in length (Table 1.1). The coding region consists of 1,290 bp and encodes a polypeptide of 429 amino acids, with the first 31 residues representing a signal sequence. Human *GLA* is unusual in that it lacks a 3′-untranslated region and has the mRNA polyadenylation signal in the coding sequence.

Table 1.1 Size of the 7 human *GLA* exons and number of mutations detected

Exon	Coding sequence		Point mutations		Small rearrangements	
	Base pairs	%	*n*	%	*n*	%
1	194	15.0	57	13.9	18	12.0
2	175	13.6	53	13.0	15	10.0
3	178	13.8	57	14.0	16	10.7
4	92	7.1	22	5.4	7	4.7
5	162	12.6	70	17.2	22	14.7
6	198	15.3	85	20.8	26	17.3
7	291	22.6	64	15.7	46	30.6
Total	1,290	100	408	100	150	100

Note that splice site mutations and polymorphisms outside the coding sequence are intronic variants and therefore not included

1.1.1 General Classification and Nomenclature of Mutations

The term *mutation* denotes any permanent alteration of the genetic material, although, in daily practice, it is frequently (but incorrectly) associated exclusively with a disease. Mutations can be classified in a number of ways, for example disease causing alterations and nonpathogenic variants (polymorphisms). Mutations can be familial, i.e. transmitted from generation to generation within a family; de novo, variants first occurring in the index case in a family; or novel, if the sequence change has not been previously reported in the literature. The finding of the same mutation in two different, apparently unrelated patients may indicate either that the two individuals are (in fact distantly) related or that it is a recurrent mutation; that is, a change of the DNA that has already been documented but which has occurred at least twice independently due to de novo events. Mutations at CpG dinucleotides have been shown to account for the majority of recurrent point mutations seen in families with Fabry disease [1–6].

Establishing genotype–phenotype correlations in Fabry disease necessitates the analysis of large cohorts of probands and the availability of comprehensive clinical and genetic data. The prospect of a computer-based disease-specific database requires a standard nomenclature for describing mutations that allows uniform and unequivocal assignments of sequence variants. A standardized nomenclature is also essential for comparing the data obtained in various laboratories. Today, the majority of scientists working in the field agree upon the 'Nomenclature for the description of sequence variations' posted on the HGV (Human Genome Variation Society) web page (http://www.genomic.unimelb.edu.au/mdi/).

In general, the abbreviated names (acronyms) of human genes are written in italic capital letters to distinguish between the gene and its product (this latter is not written in italic). The description of any sequence change always starts with a lower-case letter indicating the type of sequence referred to; that is 'g' for genomic DNA, 'c' for coding DNA, and 'p' for protein. For DNA, the four capital letters A, C, G, and T, corresponding to the four nucleotides, are used, whereas to describe a change at the protein level, the three-letter amino acid code is preferred. The designation of nucleotide (DNA) changes begins with a number, whereas that for a protein begins with a letter (e.g. c.100C > T: cytosine is replaced by thymine at position 100; p.C100T (more correctly p.Cys100Thr): a missense mutation, cysteine is replaced by threonine). Positions of amino acids and nucleotides (coding DNA [cDNA]) are numbered starting, respectively, with the translation initiation codon and the nucleotide A of the ATG initiation triplet as number 1. For numbering nucleotides in introns, the last nucleotide of the preceding exon and a plus sign and the first nucleotide of the following exon and a minus sign is used at the beginning and at the end of the intron, respectively, for example c.639 + 1G > A or c.640–1G > T. In case of molecular rearrangements, instead of the earlier designation 'ins' (insertion) current nomenclature recommendation favours the term 'dup' (duplication) when the mutation creates a run of two or more bases (for a recent summary see [4]).

1.1.2 GLA Mutations in Fabry Disease

In this chapter, DNA mutations are described following the HGV recommendations and according to the *GLA* reference sequences GenBank U78027.1 (cDNA) or X14448.1 (genomic sequence). Figure 1.1 shows that a total of 599 *GLA* mutations were compiled from the literature. In agreement with earlier findings, 447 (~75%) of these changes are point mutations (435 pathogenic missense, nonsense, and splice site mutations, and 12 polymorphisms) and 152 (~25%) 'short length' rearrangements (mainly deletions and duplications affecting less than 65 nucleotides, 150 very probable disease causing mutations, and 2 polymorphisms). Large rearrangements involving one or more exons or the whole gene seem to be infrequent in patients with Fabry disease, accounting for only about 3% of all disease alleles (for a recent summary see [4], [5]). This low frequency is remarkable, especially in view of the fact that *GLA* is rich in *Alu*-repeats, highly abundant

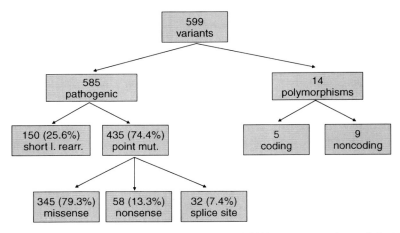

Fig. 1.1 Classification and distribution of 599 published DNA sequence variants of the human *GLA* gene (as of 30 June 2009). Short l. rear: short length rearrangements, mut.: mutation

sequence motifs frequently implicated in human diseases by predisposing to unequal recombinations.

Figures 1.2 and 1.3 show the distribution of the 345 very probable disease causing missense (Fig. 1.2) and 90 pathogenic nonsense and splice site (Fig. 1.3) point mutations, whereas Fig. 1.4 shows the distribution of the 150 pathogenic 'short length' rearrangements over the seven coding *GLA* exons. The mutations p.Leu166Gly (CTG>GGG), p.Ile219Asn (ATC>AAT), p.Gln280Ser (CAA>TCA), and p.Ile384Asn (ATC>AAT) are included in Fig. 1.2 although they are not typical point mutations as they derive from the simultaneous change of two nucleotides within the same codon. Although based on the number of mutations per nucleotide there is not an obvious mutation 'hot spot', there are some differences in the gross distribution of point mutations over the 1,290 bp *GLA* coding region (Table 1.1). For example, exons 5 and 6 together harbour 155 point mutations (missense, nonsense, and polymorphisms shown in Figs. 1.2 and 1.3 and Table 1.2), representing 38% of all coding region point mutations, whereas these two exons comprise only 27.9% (360 bp) of the total *GLA* coding sequence. Thus, the data show a somewhat higher frequency of point mutations in exons 5 and 6 compared to other *GLA* exons. Exon 4 harbours only 22 (5.4%) of all coding region point mutations, which is about 24% less than one would predict (29; 7.1%) in case of an even distribution of point mutations over the coding exons. Remarkably, about one-third (46; 30.6%) of the 150 small rearrangements in the coding region occurred in exon 7 (Fig. 1.4), which accounts for only 22.6% of the coding region, suggesting that this part of the gene is prone to rearrangements.

The disease causing effect of missense mutations is thought to be due primarily to the structural changes of the polypeptide caused by the amino acid replacement. However, both computer-based analysis and in vitro functional studies suggest that the pathology of such 'simple' mutations might occasionally be more complex. Indeed, some DNA changes thought to be missense mutations (e.g.

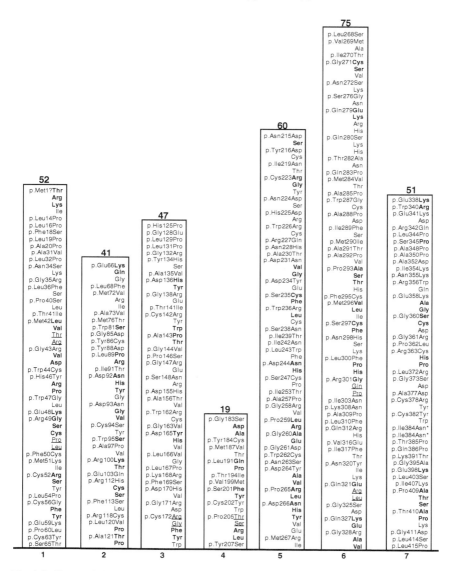

Fig. 1.2   Very probable disease causing missense point mutations of the human *GLA* gene grouped according to their position in exons 1–7 (as of 30 June 2009). Numbers on *top* of columns give the total number of mutations listed for the exon. If mutants result from different changes of the same nucleotide of a codon, variants are written in *bold* or are *underlined*. See also Fig. 1.3. *: changes of different nucleotides within the same codon result in the same mutation

p.Ser65Thr, p.Gly183Ser, p.Lys213Asn, or p.Met267Ile) seem to interfere with normal splicing of the *GLA* mRNA [7]. Similarly, two deep intronic point mutations (c.639 + 861C > T and c.639 + 919G > A) apparently result in α-galactosidase A deficiency by causing complex changes in the pattern of splicing [8, 9]. There are

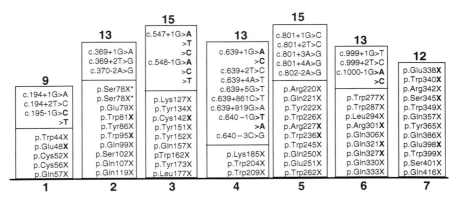

Fig. 1.3 Very probable disease causing point mutations of the human *GLA* gene that affect splice sites (*top part* of column) or result in premature termination of protein translation (nonsense mutations, *bottom*), grouped according to their positions in exons 1–7 (as of 30 June 2009). Numbers on *top* of columns give the total number of mutations listed. If mutants result from different changes of the same nucleotide of a codon, variants are written in *bold* or are *underlined*. See also Fig. 1.2*: changes of different nucleotides within the same codon result in the same mutation

a few reports of patients carrying two different, very probable disease-causing *GLA* mutations in *cis*, i.e. on the same allele, that are not due to a complex rearrangement, such as p.Glu66Gln + p.Arg112Cys, p.Leu89Arg + 1 bp deletion in codon 303, Ala143Thr + Gln312His, or Asp264Tyr + Val269Met. In contrast, about 2% of the patients carry a pathogenic *GLA* mutation and the not-disease-associated non-synonymous variant p.Asp313Tyr.

Table 1.2 shows a list of common *GLA* gene polymorphisms and rare non-pathogenic variants, including four missense changes. It has been suggested that some of the variants affect the expression of the *GLA* gene or the catalytic activity of the enzyme in vitro (for further details see Chapter 6). However, no experimentally validated data have been presented to date that any of the sequence changes listed in Table 1.2, alone or in combination, are disease causing.

1.1.3 De Novo Mutations

As expected for a X-chromosomal trait with reduced reproductive fitness of male patients and increased frequency of spontaneous (de novo) mutations, most of the patients/families with Fabry disease carry *GLA* mutations that occurred independently. Consequently, different patients/families show different mutations, i.e. the great majority of *GLA* mutations is unique ('private'). The proportion of de novo mutations in a given cohort of Fabry patients is unknown. In a recent survey of mutation data compiled from the literature, a minimum frequency of 3.3% of de novo mutations was calculated [4], which is similar to the figures 3–10% derived

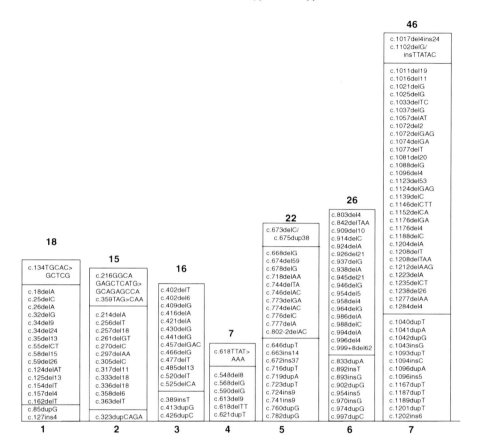

Fig. 1.4 Very probable disease causing short-length rearrangements affecting less than 65 base pairs of the human *GLA* gene grouped according to their positions in exons 1–7, including complex rearrangements (*top* of columns), deletions (*middle part*), and insertions/duplications (*bottom*) (as of 30 June 2009). For the sake of simplicity, for rearrangements affecting more than three nucleotides only the position of the first base is given

from theoretical considerations [10] and 8% found in an recent independent study [5]. However, these numbers may represent an underestimate of the natural variability of the *GLA* mutation spectrum, for in most cases, apparently unrelated patients carrying the same mutation have not been further examined (for example by haplotype analysis) to address the question of recurrent mutations. In any case, these data underline once more the importance of a professional genetic counselling of each newly diagnosed patient with Fabry disease with a thorough analysis of the family history for in 9 out of 10 such cases further undiagnosed family members should also be present.

Table 1.2 DNA polymorphisms of the human *GLA* gene

Position	Nucleotide change	Protein change
5'UTR	c.-30G > A	
	c.-12G > A	
	c.-10C > T	
Exon 2	c.305C > T	p.Ser102Leu
	c.369T > C	p.=
Intron 2	c.370-77_81del5	
Exon 3	c.376A > G	p.Ser126Gly
Intron 4	c.639 + 68A > G	
	c.640-201del6	
	c.640-146T > C	
	c.640-16A > G	
Exon 6	c.937G > T	p.Asp313Tyr
Intron 6	c.1000-22C > T	
Exon 7	c.1187T > A	p.Phe396Tyr

1.1.4 Molecular Genetic Bases of Fabry Disease in Females

In X-linked diseases, heterozygous females are commonly referred to as carriers, a term that describes solely the individual's genotype and, by definition, does not provide any information on the phenotype. Unlike many other X-chromosomal conditions, in which heterozygotes are usually free of disease, a large proportion of Fabry disease carriers presents with signs and symptoms of the disease commonly seen in male patients with the condition. Yet, in general, the onset of disease is later and the overall phenotype tends to be milder in females than in males. However, the phenotype of heterozygotes for Fabry disease can be very variable, ranging from no clinical manifestations to the rare cases presenting with classic Fabry disease. As the definitions 'X-linked recessive' or 'X-linked dominant' do not capture the wide spectrum of variable expression in heterozygotes in X-chromosomal conditions, Dobyns proposed, in a recent review, using only the term 'X-linked' trait [11].

Brouns et al. described the co-occurrence of Turner syndrome and Fabry disease in a severely affected female patient with two affected male siblings [12]. The majority of blood lymphocytes of this female patient were X monosomic (45,X), and, as expected, analysis of her peripheral blood DNA revealed the presence of the pathogenic familial p.Pro259Arg mutation in apparently homozygous state. The patient also had a low frequency mosaic in peripheral blood with a cell line in which a deletion of the short arm of the second X chromosome (46,X,del(X)(p11)) was seen. It is expected that the structurally aberrant X chromosome is preferentially inactivated, which makes the patient functionally hemizygous for the *GLA* mutation and explains her very severe Fabry phenotype. Rodriguez-Mari et al. reported the opposite situation, a female patient with a classical severe phenotype, who was homozygous for the familial p.Gln279Arg mutation [13].

1.2 Genotype–Phenotype Correlation

Analysis of genotype–phenotype correlations in Fabry disease is complicated by a number of factors. First, most of the changes of the *GLA* gene represent unique ('private') mutations; that is the number of patients carrying the same mutation is limited. Second, there is a high degree of clinical variability both among patients from the same family and the small number of unrelated patients carrying the same ('recurrent') mutation. Third, many of the clinical features of Fabry disease are frequently observed in the general population, making it difficult to pin down precisely the phenotypic features associated with the *GLA* mutations. Fourth, in an advanced stage of disease, part of the phenotype may be due to factors not directly related to *GLA* mutations. For example, it is possible that some of the symptoms are secondary and result from the general cellular dysfunction due to the slowly progressive and/or focal accumulation of the misfolded mutant protein [14]. Consequently, it is difficult to define genotype–phenotype relationship by studying individual probands or families. However, the analysis of large cohorts of patients has the potential to provide the necessary amount of information to address such questions. In order to minimize the influence of factors other than the *GLA* mutation, most of the studies include only male patients.

1.2.1 Classic Phenotype and GLA Mutations

Alleles with nonsense and splice-site mutations of *GLA* or out-of-frame short length rearrangements usually lead to a premature termination codon, thus a truncated and most likely non-functional enzyme is predicted. Furthermore, most of the mRNAs with a premature termination codon will not be translated and instead are rapidly eliminated by a protective molecular mechanism called nonsense mediated mRNA decay. Consequently, no product is made from these alleles (null alleles). Missense mutations may affect enzyme activity to very variable extent. Clearly, replacement of a residue in the enzyme active site, or that essential for proper three-dimensional protein folding, usually results in an enzyme protein that is completely inactive (functional null mutant). Matsuzawa et al. analysed the structure and function relationship (genotype–phenotype in broad sense) for a number of α-galactosidase A missense mutants with known enzymatic characteristics by producing computer models of the mutant proteins [15]. The data suggested that in the case of *GLA* missense mutations associated with the classic disease phenotype, a dysfunctional and unstable enzyme is predicted due to significant structural changes in functionally important regions. In contrast, mutations associated with an attenuated phenotype were usually located distant from the active site and resulted in small structural changes. Some of these enzyme variants (e.g. p.Met72Val, p.Gln279Glu and p.Met296Ile) had normal K_m and V_{max} values and showed residual catabolic activity, but were subject to post-translational inactivation and degradation.

Table 1.3 Genotype–phenotype correlations found in cohorts of patients with Fabry disease by three independent studies

References	No. of probands	Parameter chosen	Variable analysed	Findings
[16]	36 (k)	GLA missense mutations	α-galactosidase A activity	Higher in patients with cons. aa change than in those with noncons. substitution
[17]	31 (m)			
[18]	191 (m)	GLA missense mutations	Number of affected organs/organ systems	Increases more slowly with age for cons. than for noncons. aa change
[17]	49 (m)	α-galactosidase A activity	Onset of chronic renal insufficiency	Later in patients with residual activity than in those with no activity
[17]	22 (m)	GLA missense mutations	Frequency of chronic renal insufficiency	Lower in patients with cons. than in those with noncons. aa change
[17]	47 (m)	GLA missense mutations	Renal survival	Longer for patients with cons. than for those with noncons. aa change
[16]	36 (k)	No neuropathic pain	α-galactosidase A activity	Higher than in families with pain
[16]	15 (k)	Neuropathic pain	GLA missense mutation	No difference for cons. vs. noncons. aa change
[18]	191 (m)	GLA mutations	FOS-MSSI	No difference in scores if patients with missense mutations were compared to those with all other mutations
[18]	191 (m)	p.Asn215Ser	FOS-MSSI	Scores are lower (phenotype is less severe) than in patients with all other mutations

k: kindred, m: males, aa: amino acid, cons.: conservative, noncons.: nonconservative, FOS-MSSI: Fabry outcome study Mainz severity score index

Table 1.3 summarizes a number of conclusions drawn from three different studies analysing the relationship between GLA mutations and the severity of the patients' phenotypes with special emphasis on missense mutations [16–18]. It seems that the total number of affected organs/organ systems increases less rapidly with the age of the patient if the wild-type and mutant amino acids belong to the same group (conservative amino acid change) than if they do not (non-conservative amino acid replacement). However, if patients were grouped according to the type of mutation (missense vs. all other mutations), no significant difference was seen between the two patients' groups concerning the general severity of the disease measured by the MSSI (Mainz severity score index). The data of Branton et al. showed that, compared to patients carrying a non-conservative change, kidney pathology was less severe in patients with a conservative amino acid replacement, with lower frequency and later onset of chronic renal insufficiency, and longer renal survival [17].

1.2.2 Residual Enzyme Activity and Genotype–Phenotype Correlation

A missense mutation represents the smallest possible structural change of the polypeptide – the replacement of one amino acid by another one. This change may result in complete loss of catabolic activity of α-galactosidase A, or the enzyme may still be partially (or fully) active. As the presence or absence of largely diminished but still measurable activity of α-galactosidase A depends largely on the patients' genotype, residual activity can be used as a quantifiable intermediate marker to bridge the gap between the DNA-based individual genotypes and the highly variable clinical phenotype. Table 1.3 summarizes some observations on genotype and phenotype correlations made in patients with residual enzyme activity. In general, residual enzyme activity is associated with a less severe phenotype than that of patients showing no enzyme activity. Patients with residual enzyme activity exhibited a later onset of major organ involvement compared to individuals without residual enzyme activity. In addition, residual activity of the α-galactosidase A was higher in patients with a conservative amino acid replacement than in those with a non-conservative change. Patients with the p.Asn215Ser mutation, a variant with high residual activity, had less severe phenotypes than those carrying other *GLA* mutations. In patients with neuropathic pain, residual α-galactosidase A activity was found to be lower than in those with no pain, although the nature of the amino acid change (conservative vs. non-conservative) had no effect in this case.

The lack of a strong correlation between selected phenotypic features and the type of *GLA* mutations referred to here and earlier (see Section 1.2.1) may be due to the considerable functional heterogeneity of the mutations within the different groups as defined by the authors of the different studies, in particular in the case of missense variants. Indeed, some of the enzyme mutants with non-synonymous changes have no useful catabolic activity while others show high residual activity. Therefore, in a pilot study, we have tentatively classified a high number of *GLA* mutations according to their expected biological consequences. The first group consisted of all likely null alleles, constitutional or functional, that is nonsense mutations, splice site mutations, out-of-frame rearrangements, and missense mutations that alter residues of the active site or may grossly interfere with the proper folding of the protein (e.g. dimerisation, disulfide bonds or proline residues). Missense mutations associated with the attenuated phenotype (Section 1.2.3) formed the next group, whereas mutations that did not fit (yet) in either of the former two groups were put in the third category. It seems that the data set generated this way was more consistent and homogeneous, and, more importantly, allowed a stronger conclusion on the correlation between the genotype and a particular phenotypic feature than the one obtained by the analysis using the classical (descriptive) mutation types (unpublished results).

1.2.3 Molecular Genetics of the Variant Fabry Phenotypes

A considerable number of patients have been described, who had residual enzyme activity and presented with a variant phenotype – an attenuated ('oligosymptomatic') form of Fabry disease – occasionally called the cardiac or renal form. Table 1.4 lists selected features of 33 GLA missense mutations found in patients with attenuated phenotypes. It seems that parts of the α-galactosidase A molecule have enough structural freedom to accommodate the molecular alterations caused by these mutations without a complete loss of enzyme activity. Remarkably, some of these 'mild' mutations are clustered in exons 2 and 6 that harbour, respectively, eight and ten variants, equalling 54% of the mutations listed in Table 1.4 even though these two exons represent only 28.9% of the GLA coding region. Methionine-51 and asparagine-215 seem to be the only wild-type residues listed in Table 1.4 that are implicated in special functions of the mature enzyme. The latter is part of a specific site for N-glycosylation of the enzyme, whereas Met51 seems to interact with Trp47, a key residue in the active site, and is located on the dimer interface of α-galactosidase A.

Table 1.4 Human GLA missense mutations identified in Fabry disease patients presenting with variant phenotypes. Mutations are grouped according to the evolutionary conservation of the wild-type residue

Group of both AAs/type of AA change		Evolutionary conservation		BLOSUM 62 Score	3D posi-tion/putative function of AA
		Grade	AAs in related proteins		
Poorly conserved (≤60%)					
p.Ala20Pro	Neutr nonpol	3/12		−1	Signal seq.
p.Met51Ile	Neutr nonpol	4/13		1	Dimer interf.
p.Met51Lys	Noncons	4/13	2× Arg 1× His	−1	Dimer interf.
p.Met72Val	Neutr nonpol	7/14		1	Totally buried
p.Ala97Val	Neutr nonpol	5/13		0	Mostly buried
p.Arg112His	Charged	8/14	3× Lys	0	Mostly buried
p.Arg112Cys	Noncons	8/14		−3	Mostly buried
p.Asn215Ser	Neutr polar	8/14		1	Glycosylation
p.Ser247Cys	Noncons	3/14		−1	Buried
p.Val269Met	Neutr nonpol	6/14		1	Compl. buried
p.Phe273Leu	Neutr nonpol	8/14	5× Gly	0	N.d.
p.Gln279Lys	Noncons	8/14		1	N.d.
p.Gln279Glu	Noncons	8/14	5× Glu	2	Buried
p.Thr410Ala	Noncons	4/14		0	Buried
Conserved (61–89%)					
p.Ala73Val	Neutr nonpol	11/14		0	N.d.
p.Ile91Thr	Noncons	9/13		−1	Buried

Table 1.4 (continued)

Group of both AAs/type of AA change	Evolutionary conservation		BLOSUM 62 Score	3D posi-tion/putative function of AA
	Grade	AAs in related proteins		
p.Ala143Thr	Noncons	10/14	2× Ser	0	N.d.
p.Ser238Asn	Neutr polar	9/12		1	N.d.
p.Met296Ile	Neutr nonpol	10/14	2× Ile, 2× Leu	1	Compl. Buried
p.Met296Val	Neutr nonpol	10/14		1	Compl. Buried
p.Arg301Gln	Noncons	12/14		1	Part. buried
p.Arg301Gly	Noncons	12/14		−2	Part. buried
p.Gly328Arg	Noncons	11/14		−2	Buried
p.Gly373Asp	Noncons	10/14		−2	Buried
p.Gly395Ala	Neutr nonpol	9/14	2× Ala	0	N.d.
Highly conserved (≥90%)					
p.Asn34Ser	Neutr polar	12/12		1	Buried
p.Gly35Arg	Noncons	12/12		−2	N.d.
p.Met42Val	Neutr nonpol	13/13		1	Buried
p.Glu66Gln	Noncons	13/13		2	Mostly buried
p.Phe113Leu	Neutr nonpol	14/14		0	Compl. buried
p.Pro146Ser	Noncons	13/14		−1	N.d.
p.Pro259Leu	Neutr nonpol	13/14		−3	N.d.
p.Ile317Thr	Noncons	14/14		−1	Buried

Evolutionary conservation was analysed by comparing the amino acid composition of human α-galactosidase A to that of 14 eukaryotic orthologues using the *HomoloGene* program (details are freely available from the author). BLOSUM62 scores were taken from the table published by Henikoff and Henikoff [19]. '3D position/putative function of AA' were taken from the table published by Garman and Garboczi [20] and Garman [21]

AA: amino acid, compl.: completely, interf.: interface, N.d.: no data, neutr: neutral, noncons: nonconservative, nonpol: nonpolar, part.: partially, seq.: sequence

For a first analysis of the role of various factors in establishing a correlation between genotype and phenotype, four selected features of the corresponding residues were compiled in Table 1.4. These are: chemical nature of the amino acid change, evolutionary conservation of the wild-type residue, relative substitution probabilities of the amino acid pairs (wild-type vs. mutant) in very conserved regions of protein families, and likely position of the mutant residue in the 3D crystal structure. The analysis resulted in the following five major conclusions:

(i) The data show that, on one hand, half of the variants represent relatively minor alterations in the form of a conservative amino acid change, the substitution of an amino acid by another one with a side chain of similar chemical properties and, in the majority of cases, of similar size. On the other hand, as mentioned above, it seems that in some portions of the enzyme protein non-conservative amino acid changes are also tolerated and do not result in complete loss of catabolic activity.

(ii) We selected from the databases 14 eukaryotic α-galactosidase A orthologues and aligned their amino acid sequences. The grade of evolutionary conservation of the wild-type α-galactosidase A residues was assessed by comparing the sequences of the 14 orthologues to that of the human α-galactosidase A. This analysis showed that 14 (42.4%) of the 33 'mild' mutations affect residues classified by us as evolutionarily poorly conserved; that is, the residue was present only in 8 or less (≤60%) of the orthologues. Only eight (25%) of the 33 mutations change residues considered evolutionarily highly conserved; that is, present in ≥90% of the 14 eukaryotic orthologues analyzed.

(iii) Remarkably, in a number of cases, the residue of the human mutant (or a chemically related one) was found at the corresponding position of one or more of the orthologues (e.g. p.Phe273Leu, p.Gln279Glu or p.Met296Ile).

(iv) BLOSUM (BLOcks of Amino Acid SUbstitution Matrix) scores correspond to the likelihood that two different amino acids with a biological role appear at the same position in closely related sequences [19]. A positive score indicates a more likely substitution while a negative score is given to a less likely substitution. The average BLOSUM62 score of the 33 missense variants in Table 1.4 is close to 0 compared to −1.2 calculated for all other missense mutations listed in Fig. 1.2. The distribution of the individual scores of the 'mild' mutations is shifted to the right, towards the positive values, when compared to that of missense mutations associated with the classical phenotype of Fabry disease (Fig. 1.5). This finding is in line with the observation that, in the group of 'mild' mutations, the amino acid change has a less dramatic effect on the enzyme function.

(v) Based on the analysis of a three-dimensional model of the putative structure of α-galactosidase A, Garman and Garboczi [20] and Garman [21] classified the different *GLA* missense alleles into active site mutations, buried mutations, and 'others' (see Chapter 6). Missense mutations that are associated with the classic severe Fabry disease affect most often residues near the active site or disrupt the hydrophobic core of the enzyme. In contrast, most of the residues listed in Table 1.4 are classified as partially, mostly, or completely buried in the 3D crystallographic structure model of α-galactosidase A.

Although all variants listed in Table 1.4 were identified in patients with the attenuated phenotype, it is very likely that only a portion of these changes are truly 'mild' mutations (see Chapter 2). One should always keep in mind that clinical phenotypes in Fabry disease can be extremely variable, both in males and females. Indeed, several of the sequence changes listed in Table 1.4, such as p.Met51Lys, p.Arg112His, p.Arg112Cys, p.Phe113Leu, p.Ala268Val or p.Arg301Gln, have also been detected in patients with the classical phenotype [2, 22, 23]. Clearly, also in families with the above mentioned mutations, there is a continuous spectrum of disease severity and the patients with the attenuated phenotypes described may represent the extreme mild end of the largely variable clinical presentations. Similarly, the so-called cardiac or renal variants may in part reflect the large clinical heterogeneity in Fabry disease. Given the fact that Fabry disease is a progressive condition, patients

Fig. 1.5 Distributions (%) of the BLOSUM62 scores of the 33 missense mutants (*dotted line*) listed in Table 1.4 and all other missense mutations (*broken line*) of *GLA* compiled in Fig. 1.2

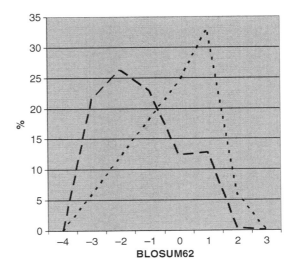

with the cardiac variant may develop later proteinuria, which is, by definition, an involvement of the renal system. Thus the term 'oligosymptomatic' reflects only an approximation at a given moment in time that may theoretically exist for any sign or symptom of the disease [14]. The situation might be different in the case of the p.Asn215Ser mutation. This variant has been found consistently in patients with the attenuated phenotype, and was detected only in a single patient with the classic phenotype but no kidney involvement [22]. Clearly, this latter patient might carry a second *GLA* mutation that escaped detection, or *GLA*-related or -unrelated genetic modifiers that could explain his unexpectedly severe phenotype.

While during the past years some progress has been made in the analysis of the correlation between *GLA* mutations and the patients' phenotypes, there are only very few data on the phenotypic effect of other genes in patients with Fabry disease (for a recent report of the author's group see [24]). Thus it remains a challenge for the future to identify more *GLA*-unrelated genetic modifiers which, together with epigenetic and non-genetic factors, constitute the genetic palette, and further define the hues and shades of the clinical phenotype of patients with Fabry disease.

References

In the past years, several papers have been published on various aspects of Fabry disease including the *GLA* gene and its mutations. In order to avoid redundancy, the number of references has been kept to a minimum in this chapter. References to individual mutations are available on request from the author.

1. Eng CM, Niehaus DJ, Enriquez AL et al (1994) Fabry disease: twenty-three mutations including sense and antisense CpG alterations and identification of a deletional hot-spot in the α-galactosidase A gene. Hum Mol Genet 3(10):1795–1799

2. Ashton-Prolla P, Tong B, Shabbeer J, Astrin KH, Eng CM, Desnick RJ (2000) Fabry disease: twenty-two novel mutations in the α-galactosidase A gene and genotype/phenotype correlations in severely and mildly affected hemizygotes and heterozygotes. J Invest Med 48(4):227–235

3. Shabbeer J, Yasuda M, Luca E, Desnick RJ (2002) Fabry disease: 45 novel mutations in the α-galactosidase A gene causing the classical phenotype. Mol Genet Metab 76:23–30

4. Gal A, Schäfer E, Rohard I (2006) The genetic basis of Fabry disease. In: Mehta A, Beck M, Sunder-Plassmann G (eds) Fabry disease: perspectives from 5 years of FOS. Oxford PharmaGenesis, Oxford, pp 323–330

5. Shabbeer J, Yasuda M, Benson SD, Desnick RJ (2006) Fabry disease: identification of 50 novel α-galactosidase A mutations causing the classic phenotype and three-dimensional structural analysis of 29 missense mutations. Hum Genomics 2(5):297–309

6. Eng CM, Ashley GA, Burgert TS, Enriquez AL, D'Souza M, Desnick RJ (1997) Fabry disease: thirty-five mutations in the α-galactosidase A gene in patients with classic and variant phenotypes. Mol Med 3(3):174–182

7. Lai LW, Whitehair O, Wu M-J, O'Meara M, Lien Y-H H (2003) Analysis of splice-site mutations of the α-galactosidase A gene in Fabry disease. Clin Genet 63:476–482

8. Ishii S, Nakao S, Minamikawa-Tachino R, Desnick RJ, Fan JQ (2002) Alternative splicing in the α-galactosidase A gene: increased exon inclusion results in the Fabry cardiac phenotype. Am J Hum Genet 70:994–1002

9. Filoni C, Caciotti A, Carraresi L et al (2008) Unbalanced GLA mRNAs ratio quantified by real-time PCR in Fabry patients' fibroblasts results in Fabry disease. Eur J Hum Genet 16(11):1311–1317

10. Schäfer E, Baron K, Widmer U et al (2005) Thirty-four novel mutations of the GLA gene in 121 patients with Fabry disease. Hum Mutat 25(4):412

11. Dobyns WB (2006) The pattern of inheritance of X-linked traits is not dominant or recessive, just X-linked. Acta Paediatr 95(Suppl 451):11–15

12. Brouns R, Eyskens F, de Boeck K et al (2009) Fabry disease in a patient with Turner syndrome. J Inherit Metab Dis. Short report #162. doi 10.1007/s10545-009-1035–x

13. Rodríguez-Marí A, Coll MJ, Chabás A (2003) Molecular analysis in Fabry disease in Spain: fifteen novel GLA mutations and identification of a homozygous female. Hum Mutat 22(3):258

14. Ries M, Gal A (2006) Genotype–phenotype correlation in Fabry disease. In: Mehta A, Beck M, Sunder-Plassmann G (eds) Fabry disease: perspectives from 5 years of FOS. Oxford PharmaGenesis, Oxford, pp 331–336

15. Matsuzawa F, Akikawa S, Doi H, Okumiya T, Sakuraba H (2005) Fabry disease: correlation between structural changes in α-galactosidase, and clinical and biochemical phenotypes. Hum Genet 117(4):317–328

16. Altarescu GM, Goldfarb LG, Park K-Y et al (2001) Identification of fifteen novel mutations and genotype – phenotype relationship in Fabry disease. Clin Genet 60:46–51

17. Branton MH, Schiffmann R, Sabnis SG et al (2002) Natural history of Fabry disease. Influence of α-galactosidase A activity and genetic mutations on clinical course. Medicine 81(2):122–138

18. Schäfer E, Mehta A, Gal A (2005) Genotype and phenotype in Fabry disease: analysis of the Fabry outcome survey. Acta Paediatr 94(Suppl 447):87–92

19. Henikoff JG, Henikoff S (1996) Blocks database and its applications. Methods Enzymol 266:88–105

20. Garman SC, Garboczi DN (2004) The molecular defect leading to Fabry disease: structure of human α-galactosidase. J Mol Biol 337:319–335

21. Garman SC (2007) Structure-function relationships in α-galactosidase A. Acta Paediatr 96(Suppl 455):6–16

22. Germain DP, Shabbeer J, Cotigny S, Desnick RJ (2002) Fabry disease: twenty novel α-galactosidase A mutations and genotype–phenotype correlations in classical and variant phenotypes. Mol Med 8(6):306–312

23. Davies JP, Winchester BG, Malcolm S (1993) Mutation analysis in patients with the typical form of Anderson – Fabry disease. Hum Mol Genet 2(7):1051–1053

24. Rohard I, Schaefer E, Kampmann C, Beck M, Gal A (2008) Association between polymorphisms of endothelial nitric oxide synthase gene (NOS3) and left posterior wall thickness (LPWT) of the heart in Fabry disease. J Inherit Metab Dis. Short report #122. doi 10.1007/s10545-008-0920–z

Chapter 2
The Structure of Human α-Galactosidase A and Implications for Fabry Disease

Abigail I. Guce and Scott C. Garman

Abstaract The three-dimensional structure of human α-galactosidase A has been determined by x-ray crystallography, revealing the molecular and mechanistic basis for the defects leading to Fabry disease. The structure showed that the active site of the enzyme is formed from the C-terminal ends of seven beta strands in the first domain, a $(\beta/\alpha)_8$ barrel. The structure of the complex of α-galactosidase A with ligand bound shows that the enzyme makes specific contacts with every functional group on the ligand. The enzyme uses a double displacement reaction mechanism to cleave terminal α-galactosides off of the substrate. Mapping the mutations that lead to Fabry disease onto the structure reveals three groups of mutations: those that perturb the active site of the enzyme, those that affect the hydrophobic core of the protein, and those that have other effects on the structure. Most of the mutations that lead to disease alter the hydrophobic core of α-galactosidase A, thus Fabry disease is usually caused by misfolding of the mutant polypeptide.

Keywords Crystal structure · Enzyme mechanism · Ligand binding · Reaction mechanism · X-ray crystallography

2.1 Overview of the Structure

The three-dimensional structure of human α-galactosidase A was determined by x-ray crystallography in 2004 [1], revealing the locations of the atoms in the glycoprotein. The crystal structure showed a homodimeric molecule with each monomer containing two domains. The N-terminal domain is a classic $(\beta/\alpha)_8$ barrel, and the C-terminal domain contains eight antiparallel β strands packed into a β sandwich (Fig. 2.1). Residues 32–328 comprise the N-terminal domain, and residues 329–421

S.C. Garman (✉)
Department of Chemistry, University of Massachusetts, Amherst, MA, USA; Department of Biochemistry & Molecular Biology, University of Massachusetts, Amherst, MA, USA
e-mail: garman@biochem.umass.edu

D. Elstein et al. (eds.), *Fabry Disease*, DOI 10.1007/978-90-481-9033-1_2,
© Springer Science+Business Media B.V. 2010

Fig. 2.1 Overview of the α-galactosidase A dimer. The α-galactosidase A polypeptide trace is shown with a rainbow from *blue* at the N-terminus to *red* at the C-terminus. N-linked carbohydrates are shown as bonds, and the galactose ligand is shown as spheres, marking the active site in the first domain

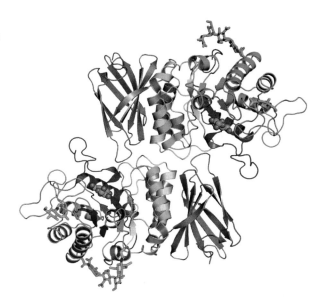

fold into the C-terminal antiparallel β domain. The C-terminal residues 421–429 are disordered in most crystal structures, and the 31-residue signal sequence is removed during the folding of the protein in the endoplasmic reticulum. The lozenge-shaped dimer has overall dimensions of approximately 75 × 75 × 50 Å.

The N-terminal domain contains the active site, which is located at the C-terminal end of β strands β1–β7, near the center of the β barrel. The active site appears as a small depression on the surface of the molecule. The function of the C-terminal domain is unclear, but it is conserved in all members of the family, including α-galactosidases from rice and from *Trichoderma reesei* [2, 3]. The interface between the N- and C-terminal domains of human α-galactosidase A is extensive, burying 2,500 Å^2 of surface area, including many hydrophobic interactions. The dimer interface is also extensive, with 2,200 Å^2 of buried surface area.

Three N-linked carbohydrates are found on the surface of the molecule, away from the location of the active site and away from the dimer interface. The carbohydrate residues attach to aspartic acid residues N139, N192, and N215 and extend from the surface of the molecule. N-linked carbohydrates are critical for the correct folding and trafficking of the molecule in the cell [4–6]. The N-linked carbohydrates are highly heterogeneous in composition, as judged from the distribution of carbohydrates on the recombinant glycoproteins used in enzyme replacement therapies [7]. The N139 site contains complex carbohydrate with two to four branches and from zero to four sialic acid residues per chain. The N192 and N215 carbohydrates are mixtures of complex, hybrid, and oligomannose glycoforms, each with variable amounts of phosphorylation and sialylation [7]. Assuming independence of the three N-linked glycosylation sites, the recombinant enzymes used in enzyme replacement therapies represent approximately 500 and 1,300 different glycoforms.

Fig. 2.2 The electrostatic surface of α-Galactosidase A. The α-galactosidase A dimer surface is shown colored by electrostatics as calculated by the program CCP4mg. The dimer is colored by electrostatic potential, from -10 $k_B T/e$ (*red*) to $+10$ $k_B T/e$ (*blue*), with the galactose ligand colored *green* and the N-linked carbohydrates *yellow*. The overall dimer is markedly negatively charged, consistent with a molecule that is most stable in the low pH of the lysosome

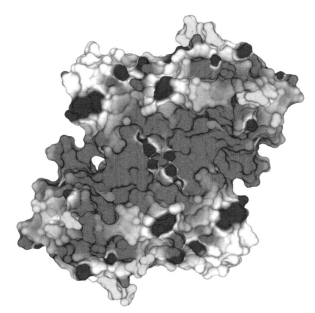

The dimer has a pronounced negative charge, with 22 more acidic residues than basic residues in the polypeptide sequence. This results in a dimer with a highly negative electrostatic potential surface at neutral pH (Fig. 2.2). With the large excess of acidic residues over basic residues, the α-galactosidase A protein has a pronounced negative charge at neutral pH and little net charge at lysosomal pH. The calculated isoelectric point of the mature polypeptide is 5.2, and because of the negative charges on the carbohydrate, the glycoprotein migrates at approximately pH 4.5 on an isoelectric focusing gel [7].

2.2 Active Site and Ligand Binding

The correct function of α-galactosidase A requires the enzyme to discriminate between α-galactosides and the many other saccharides in the lysosome. The enzyme manages this by folding into a three dimensional fold that gathers 15 residues into an active site configuration specific for α-galactosides (Fig. 2.3). The active site is formed from the side chain residues of W47, D92, D93, Y134, C142, K168, D170, C172, E203, L206, Y207, R227, D231, D266, and M267. C142 and C172 make a disulfide bond. The two active sites in the dimer are separated by approximately 50 Å.

A number of crystal structures of human α-galactosidase A have now been determined, revealing details of ligand binding interactions [1, 8]. The cocrystal structures of human α-galactosidase A with the catalytic product α-galactose bound reveal that the enzyme makes contacts to each functional group on the ligand (Fig. 2.3). When galactose monosaccharide (an equilibrium mixture of α

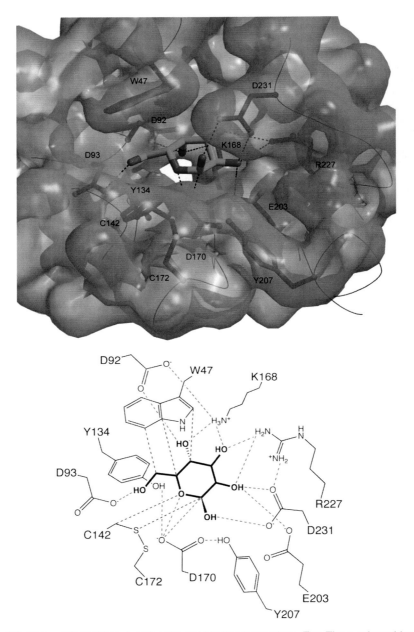

Fig. 2.3 The α-galactosidase A active site and binding interactions. *Top*: The α-galactosidase A active site is shown with a galactose ligand (*green*) bound. The surface indicates the complementary shapes of the protein and the ligand in the active site. The residues in active site are labeled, and interactions between the protein and the ligand are shown as *dashed lines*. *Bottom*: The interactions between the protein and the α-galactose ligand are detailed. *Red dashed lines* represent hydrogen bonds, and *blue dashed lines* represent van der Waals interactions. Note that the protein makes contacts to every functional group on the ligand

and β anomers) is soaked into crystals of human α-galactosidase A, only the α anomer appears in the active site. In contrast, the rice and *Trichoderma reesei* α-galactosidase active sites are able to accommodate both the α and β anomers of galactose [2, 3]. In human α-galactosidase A, Y207 (one of three active site residues not conserved in the rice and *Trichoderma reesei* α-galactosidase sequences) sterically occludes binding of β-galactose.

The chemical chaperone 1-deoxygalactonojirimycin (DGJ) was originally modeled into the binding site of human α-galactosidase A [9]; later a crystal structure of the complex was determined [8]. DGJ, an iminosugar analog of galactose, has identical binding interactions to the protein as galactose does. Thus the chemical chaperone acts as a competitive inhibitor of the α-galactosidase A enzyme. The binding of DGJ presumably helps stabilize the folded conformation of wild type and mutant α-galactosidase A glycoproteins, allowing for more efficient delivery of the enzyme to the lysosome.

2.3 Catalytic Mechanism

The α-galactosidase A enzyme uses a double displacement reaction mechanism [10], where two consecutive nucleophilic attacks on the anomeric carbon of the substrate lead to breakage of the glycosidic linkage with overall retention of the anomer in the product. This double displacement mechanism requires two carboxylates, one acting as a nucleophile and one acting as an acid and then a base over the course of the reaction mechanism. In human α-galactosidase A, the catalytic nucleophile is D170 and the catalytic acid/base is D231 [10a]. The double displacement reaction mechanism can be broken down into discrete steps (Fig. 2.4). First, the D170

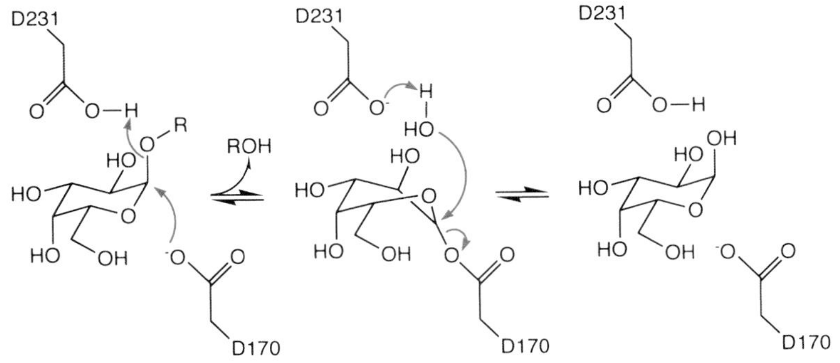

Fig. 2.4 The α-galactosidase A catalytic mechanism. α-Galactosidase A uses a double displacement reaction mechanism, where the substrate undergoes two successive nucleophilic attacks on the same chiral carbon. First, D170 makes a nucleophilic attack on C1 of the substrate, breaking the glycosidic linkage and generating a covalent intermediate. Second, a water molecule (deprotonated by D231) makes a nucleophilic attack on the same carbon, breaking the covalent bond between the enzyme and ligand and generating the product of the reaction, α-galactose. When the product diffuses from the active site, the enzyme is ready for another cycle of catalysis

nucleophile attacks C1 of the substrate, breaking the glycosidic linkage (assisted by the donation of a proton by D231). This results in a covalent glycosyl-enzyme intermediate, and the free portion of the cleaved product diffuses away. Second, D231, acting as a base, deprotonates a water molecule, which attacks C1 of the glycosyl-enzyme intermediate, breaking the bond between the protein and the sugar and generating α-galactose as the catalytic product. Finally, the α-galactose product diffuses out of the active site, regenerating the empty enzyme for another catalytic cycle.

2.4 Fabry Disease Mutations

Fabry disease phenotypes fall into three general classifications, depending on the degree of residual enzymatic activity. The classical or severe phenotype leads to dysfunction in multiple organ systems (including the skin, eyes, heart, kidneys), while two other milder phenotypes (which typically show some residual enzymatic activity) have symptoms restricted to the heart and kidney respectively. The structure of the human α-galactosidase A glycoprotein allows for some degree of personalized medicine in Fabry disease, where a patient's treatment might be chosen in light of the individual's α-galactosidase A gene sequence. Using the database of mutations identified in Fabry patients, it may be possible to predict the course and severity of the disease depending on the specific mutation in the α-galactosidase A gene sequence.

There have been a large number of mutations identified in Fabry disease patients. As of 2009, the database of missense and nonsense mutations in Fabry disease contains 257 missense and 43 nonsense mutations. The effect of those mutations on the α-galactosidase A glycoprotein is summarized in Table 2.1. The full database of mutations is considerably larger, because it includes insertions and deletions that lead to frame shifts, mutations that lead to splice defects, and mutations in the promoter region of the gene, but in this chapter, we address only the mutations that affect the structure of the protein.

Table 2.1 α-Galactosidase A protein mutants in Fabry disease

Wild type protein sequence		Fabry disease sequence: severe/ (variant)	Importance in α-galactosidase A	Side chain accessible surface area (Å^2)	Mutation category	References
1	M	I	AUG start		Other	[11]
		T				[12]
		R				[13]
14	L	P	In signal sequence		Other	[14]
16	L	P	In signal sequence		Other	[15]
19	L	P	In signal sequence		Other	[16]
20	A	(P)	In signal sequence		Other	[17]
31	A	V	In signal sequence		Other	[12]
32	L	P	Signal sequence cleavage site	5.7	Other	[18]
34	N	S	H-bond to N224	1.5	Buried	[19]

Table 2.1 (continued)

Wild type protein sequence		Fabry disease sequence: severe/ (variant)	Importance in α-galactosidase A	Side chain accessible surface area (Å^2)	Mutation category	References
35	G	R	G phi/psi, R collides with N192 carbohydrate	8.3	Other	[20]
40	P	S		0.0	Buried	[21]
		L				[22]
42	M	V	No room for beta branch	0.8	Buried	[23]
		T				[13]
		L				[24]
43	G	D	No room for side chain	0.0	Buried	[25]
		R				[26]
		V				[13]
44	W	X	Stop	0.0	Other	[27]
46	H	R	Next to W47 in the active site	0.0	Buried	[12]
		Y				[28]
47	W	L	Active site residue	2.6	Active	[29]
		G				[28]
48	E	K	H-bond to main chain E48 and N272	0.0	Other	[30]
49	R	L	Located on dimer interface	2.0	Buried	[20]
		S				[23]
		P				[28]
		G				[26]
50	F	C	Buried in hydrophobic pocket	0.7	Buried	[13]
51	M	K	Contacts to active site W47 and dimer interface	10.1	Active	[31]
		I				[32]
52	C	S	Disulfide required near the active site	12.0	Other	[33]
		R				[11]
		X	Stop			[34]
56	C	G	Disulfide bond	13.2	Other	[19]
		F				[33]
		Y				[23]
		X	Stop			[35]
59	E	K	Ion pairs across dimer interface to H406	7.6	Other	[33]
63	C	Y	Disulfide bond	0.7	Other	[36]
65	S	T	Near disulfide bond	3.5	Buried	[37]
66	E	Q	Partially buried in ion pair	3.3	Buried	[38]
		K				[36]
		G				[32]
68	L	F	Buried in hydrophobic pocket	0.2	Buried	[13]
72	M	V	Totally buried	0.0	Buried	[39]
		R				[40]
		I				[26]
73	A	V	Totally buried	0.0	Buried	[32]
78	S	X	Stop	21.7	Other	[41]
79	E	X	Stop	13.2	Other	[42]
81	W	X	Stop	0.1	Other	[43]
		S	Buried in hydrophobic pocket		Buried	[30]
85	G	D	Restricted phi/psi in turn	7.3	Other	[18]
86	Y	C	H-bond to main chain L311	0.0	Other	[12]
		X	Stop			[44]
88	Y	D	Buried in hydrophobic pocket, initiates β2	3.8	Buried	[29]
89	L	R	Buried in hydrophobic pocket	0.0	Buried	[43]
		P				[12]

Table 2.1 (continued)

Wild type protein sequence		Fabry disease sequence: severe/ (variant)	Importance in α-galactosidase A	Side chain accessible surface area (Å^2)	Mutation category	References
91	I	(T)	Buried in hydrophobic pocket	0.0	Buried	[12]
92	D	H	Active site residue	0.0	Active	[23]
		Y				[12]
		N				[31]
93	D	G	Active site residue	0.0	Active	[23]
		N				[35]
94	C	Y	Disulfide bond	0.0	Other	[12]
		S				[28]
95	W	S	Buried in hydrophobic pocket	0.0	Buried	[22]
		X	Stop		Other	[30]
97	A	V	Mostly buried in turns, no room for larger side chain	4.7	Buried	[12]
		P				[45]
99	Q	X	Stop	27.0	Other	[43]
100	R	K	Ion pairs to D155, stacked on Y151	2.5	Other	[43]
		T				[12]
103	E	Q	Totally exposed	18.9	–	[36]
107	Q	X	Stop	12.9	Other	[23]
112	R	C	Mostly buried, guanidium group in ion pair	2.2	Other	[38]
		(H)				[43]
		S				[35]
113	F	(L)	Completely buried in packed hydrophobic core	0.0	Buried	[12]
		S				[28]
118	R	C	Totally exposed	13.3	–	[32]
119	Q	X	Stop	17.6	Other	[23]
121	A	P	Buried, little room for large side chain	0.1	Buried	[46]
128	G	E	Restricted phi/psi in turn	8.2	Other	[11]
129	L	P	Buried, located between α4 and β4	0.0	Buried	[47]
131	L	P	Completely buried	0.0	Buried	[43]
132	G	R	No room for side chain	0.0	Buried	[13]
134	Y	S	Active site residue	0.0	Active	[12]
		X	Stop			[22]
135	A	V	Buried in a hydrophobic pocket	0.1	Buried	[35]
136	D	H	Buried	0.0	Buried	[31]
138	G	R	Buried, no room for side chain	0.0	Buried	[12]
		E				[26]
141	T	I	H-bond with D93	0.0	Active	[13]
142	C	Y	Active site residue, disulfide bond	3.9	Active	[48]
		R				[34]
		X	Stop			[34]
		W				[36]
143	A	P	Larger side chain disrupts C52–C94 disulfide	5.2	Other	[43]
		T				[12]
144	G	V	In turn, G restricted phi/psi	7.9	Other	[43]
146	P	(S)	Partially buried in hydrophobic pocket	3.0	Other	[49]
147	G	R	Only able to accommodate a small side chain	1.3	Buried	[36]
148	S	R	H-bond to D155, little room for large side chain	0.0	Buried	[12]

Table 2.1   (continued)

Wild type protein sequence		Fabry disease sequence: severe/ (variant)	Importance in α-galactosidase A	Side chain accessible surface area (Å²)	Mutation category	References
		N				[22]
151	Y	X	Stop	10.8	Other	[35]
152	Y	X	Stop	1.7	Other	[13]
155	D	H	H-bond to Y100	0.0	Buried	[50]
156	A	T	Buried, no room for larger side chain	0.0	Buried	[43]
		V				[48]
157	Q	X	Stop	15.0	Exposed	[43]
162	W	R	Mostly buried in hydrophobic pocket	4.2	Buried	[19]
		C				[51]
		X	Stop			[52]
163	G	V	In turn, restricted phi/psi	1.0	Other	[12]
165	D	V	Buried ion pair to H125	2.1	Buried	[20]
166	L	V	Buried, little room for branch at beta carbon	1.0	Buried	[48]
167	L	P	Buried in hydrophobic pocket	0.1	Buried	[53]
168	K	R	Active site residue	1.9	Active	[13]
169	F	S	Buried in hydrophobic pocket	0.0	Buried	[29]
170	D	V	Active site mutation, nucleophile	0.0	Active	[12]
		H				[30]
171	G	D	No room for larger side chain	0.0	Buried	[35]
		R				[50]
172	C	Y	Active site residue, disulfide bond	11.7	Active	[43]
		R				[22]
		F				[31]
		G				[54]
		W				[36]
177	L	X	Stop	12.0	Other	[35]
183	G	D	Buried, no room for side chain	0.3	Buried	[34]
		S				[13]
187	M	V	Totally buried, no room for branched beta carbon	0.0	Buried	[22]
191	L	P	Buried in hydrophobic pocket	1.3	Buried	[29]
		Q				[31]
194	T	I	Little room for longer side chain	0.4	Buried	[36]
199	V	M	Buried, little room for longer side chain	0.3	Buried	[13]
201	S	F	Buried, no room for larger side chain	2.4	Buried	[35]
202	C	W	Disulfide bond	0.0	Other	[49]
		Y				[12]
204	W	X	Stop	0.1	Other	[22]
205	P	T	Buried hydrophobic residue	0.0	Buried	[11]
		R				[13]
		L				[36]
207	Y	S	Active site residue, H-bond to D170	5.5	Active	[13]
215	N	(S)	Mutation disrupts N-linked glycosylation	12.0	Other	[55]
216	Y	D	Buried hydrophobic residue	1.1	Buried	[12]
220	R	X	Stop	7.0	Other	[56]
221	Q	X	Stop	17.1	Other	[13]

Table 2.1 (continued)

Wild type protein sequence		Fabry disease sequence: severe/ (variant)	Importance in α-galactosidase A	Side chain accessible surface area (Å^2)	Mutation category	References
222	Y	X	Stop	4.7	Other	[57]
223	C	G	Disulfide bond	0.0	Other	[58]
		R				[13]
		Y				[13]
224	N	D	Buried H-bonding network to N34	0.0	Other	[41]
		S				[22]
225	H	R	Buried H-bonding to T41, S201, and H225	0.0	Other	[59]
226	W	X	Stop	0.0	Other	[20]
		R	Buried in hydrophobic pocket		Buried	[22]
		C				[30]
227	R	Q	Active site residue	0.2	Active	[19]
		X	Stop			[55]
230	A	T	Affects critical D231 in active site	45.4	Active	[22]
231	D	N	Active site residue	9.2	Active	[60]
234	D	Y	H-bond network to main chain D234, F273 and G274	0.1	Other	[13]
		E				[35]
235	S	C	Initiates α6 helix	2.7	Buried	[34]
236	W	C	H-bond to E358	1.6	Other	[23]
		L				[34]
		X	Stop			[26]
239	I	T	Buried in hydrophobic pocket	0.0	Buried	[61]
242	I	N	Buried in hydrophobic pocket	0.3	Buried	[42]
243	L	F	Buried in hydrophobic pocket, no room for F	0.0	Buried	[26]
244	D	N	Ion pair to R356	12.4	Other	[43]
		H				[34]
245	W	X	Stop	3.6	Other	[26]
247	S	P	H-bond to Q330, no room for P	2.8	Buried	[31]
		C				[26]
250	Q	X	Stop	27.3	Other	[31]
257	A	P	No room for P	0.0	Buried	[29]
258	G	R	Buried, restricted phi/psi in turn	1.5	Buried	[28]
259	P	L	P259 and G260 form beta turn	10.5	Other	[34]
		R				[31]
260	G	A	Buried in turn, restricted phi/psi	0.0	Buried	[48]
261	G	D	Buried in turn, no room for side chain	0.0	Buried	[42]
262	W	C	Buried in a hydrophobic pocket, stack with P259	0.0	Buried	[36]
263	N	S	Buried H-bonding network to W226 and N228	1.3	Buried	[12]
264	D	V	Near active site residue	2.2	Active	[19]
		Y				[35]
265	P	R	Buried, little room for longer side chain	1.8	Buried	[51]
		L				[36]
266	D	V	Near active site residue	0.8	Active	[19]
		H				[22]
		N				[44]
		E				[26]
267	M	I	Buried, little room for branch at beta carbon	0.3	Buried	[34]

Table 2.1 (continued)

Wild type protein sequence		Fabry disease sequence: severe/ (variant)	Importance in α-galactosidase A	Side chain accessible surface area (Å²)	Mutation category	References
268	L	S	Buried hydrophobic residue	0.0	Buried	[36]
269	V	A	Completely buried	0.0	Buried	[55]
270	I	T	Buried hydrophobic residue	0.0	Buried	[36]
271	G	C	In turn, restricted phi/psi, no room for C side chain	3.3	Other	[13]
272	N	K	H-bond to E48, no room for K side chain	0.0	Other	[33]
276	S	N	H-bond to Q279 on dimer axis	0.9	Other	[36]
		G				[35]
277	W	X	Stop	6.6	Other	[34]
279	Q	(E)	H-bond to main chain G274 on dimer axis	0.2	Other	[38]
		H				[28]
		R				[30]
280	Q	H	Little room for larger side chain	5.0	Other	[28]
		K				[50]
282	T	N	H-bond to main chain N278	0.0	Other	[31]
284	M	T	Buried in hydrophobic pocket	0.3	Buried	[11]
285	A	P	Buried in hydrophobic pocket	0.0	Buried	[35]
287	W	X	Stop	0.0	Other	[55]
		G	Buried hydrophobic residue		Buried	[23]
		C				[22]
288	A	D	Buried in hydrophobic pocket on helix 7	0.9	Buried	[43]
		P				[13]
289	I	F	No room for F side chain	0.0	Buried	[34]
293	P	S	Buried	0.0	Buried	[29]
		A				[13]
294	L	X	Stop	0.4	Other	[28]
296	M	(V)	Completely buried in a hydrophobic pocket	0.0	Buried	[62]
		(I)				[17]
297	S	F	No room for F side chain	0.0	Buried	[19]
		C				[26]
298	N	K	H-bond to active site W47 and to I270 main chain	0.0	Active	[11]
		H				[23]
		S				[12]
300	L	H	No room for aromatic side chain	0.0	Buried	[36]
		F				[35]
301	R	(Q)	Partially buried, ion pair to D299	4.1	Other	[27]
		X	Stop			[43]
		P				[31]
		G				[63]
303	I	N	Partially buried in hydrophobic pocket	1.7	Buried	[13]
310	L	F	Domain interface	0.2	Buried	[64]
313	D	Y	Domain interface, little room for Y side chain	7.3	Buried	[19]
316	V	E	Domain interface helix	0.1	Buried	[36]
317	I	T	Buried in a hydrophobic pocket	2.4	Buried	[13]
		N				[36]
320	N	K	H-bond to Q321 and main chain W287	0.2	Other	[48]

Table 2.1 (continued)

Wild type protein sequence		Fabry disease sequence: severe/ (variant)	Importance in α-galactosidase A	Side chain accessible surface area (Å²)	Mutation category	References
		Y				[22]
		I				[36]
321	Q	E	H-bond network to N320 and T39	7.0	Other	[34]
		X	Stop			[36]
325	G	D	No room for D side chain	0.4	Buried	[36]
327	Q	K	H-bond to N263	0.3	Other	[55]
		E				[36]
328	G	R	No room for side chain	0.2	Buried	[38]
		A				[19]
		V				[35]
330	Q	X	Stop	3.8	Other	[50]
333	Q	X	Stop	18.2	Other	[46]
338	E	K	H-bond to R356 and Q330	1.0	Other	[35]
		X	Stop			[35]
340	W	X	Stop	0.1	Other	[19]
		R	Buried at the domain interface		Buried	[23]
341	E	K	H-bond to F329 and main chain G373	0.1	Other	[65]
		D				[13]
342	R	X	Stop	0.0	Other	[55]
		Q	Guanidium group in H-bond network			[49]
344	L	P	Buried in domain interface	1.3	Buried	[36]
345	S	P	Linker between β10 and β11, totally exposed	16.5	Other	[36]
349	W	X	Stop	2.2	Other	[31]
350	A	P	Buried, domain interface	0.0	Buried	[36]
352	A	D	Buried, domain interface	0.0	Buried	[53]
355	N	K	H-bond with R363	0.1	Other	[26]
356	R	W	Ion pair with D244 of N term domain	5.0	Other	[66]
357	Q	X	Stop	8.3	Other	[67]
358	E	K	Ion pair to K240 and H-bond to W236	4.6	Other	[67]
		G				[26]
360	G	S	G360 and G361 in a turn at dimer interface	0.4	Other	[50]
361	G	R	No room for larger side chain	3.7	Other	[26]
362	P	L	Initiates β12 strand between domain interface	12.1	Other	[13]
363	R	H	Guanidinium packs on F337	5.3	Other	[29]
		C				[13]
365	Y	X	Stop	3.9	Other	[68]
373	G	S	Buried, no room for side chain	0.0	Buried	[48]
		D				[69]
377	A	D	Buried in hydrophobic pocket	0.1	Buried	[28]
378	C	Y	Disulfide bond	0.0	Other	[34]
382	C	W	Disulfide bond	0.0	Other	[70]
		Y				[30]
383	F	(–)	Deletion shifts register of β13	7.2	Other	[71]
384	I	N	Buried in hydrophobic pocket	0.0	Buried	[13]
385	T	P	P kinks strand β13	6.6	Other	[13]
386	Q	X	Stop	0.3	Other	[12]
396	F	X	Stop	13.7	Other	[13]
398	E	X	Stop	21.5	Other	[19]

Table 2.1 (continued)

Wild type protein sequence		Fabry disease sequence: severe/ (variant)	Importance in α-galactosidase A	Side chain accessible surface area (Å²)	Mutation category	References
		K	Unknown		Exposed	[13]
399	W	X	Stop	10.5	Other	[12]
401	S	X	Stop	10.3	Other	[13]
404	R	(–)	Deletion shifts register of β15	20.3	Other	[19]
407	I	K	No room for long side chain	0.1	Buried	[30]
409	P	T	Buried, initiates strand β16	0.0	Buried	[28]
		A				[28]
		S				[26]
410	T	K	Buried, no room for K side chain	0.0	Buried	[31]
		(A)	A introduces hole into hydrophobic pocket		Buried	[57]
411	G	D	Buried, no room for D side chain	0.1	Buried	[41]
414	L	S	Domain interface	0.0	Buried	[30]
415	L	P	Buried, P kinks strand β16	0.0	Buried	[72]

The mutations in α-galactosidase A that perturb the structure of the protein can be grouped into three broad categories. First, there are mutations that compromise the active site of the enzyme, leading to loss of enzyme activity. Second, perturbations in the hydrophobic core of the protein lead to folding defects in the enzyme. This class comprises the largest group of mutations in Fabry disease, indicating that Fabry disease is usually a protein folding disease. The rest of the mutations are grouped into a third category, which includes mutations that lead to broken disulfide bonds, loss of N-linked glycosylation sites, mutations with no obvious explanation, and others. Figure 2.5 maps the mutations onto the structure, showing that most of

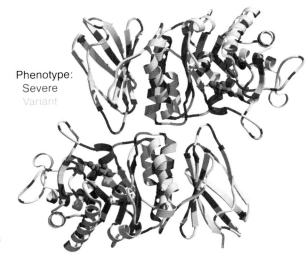

Fig. 2.5 Fabry disease mutations and the α-galactosidase A protein. The α-galactosidase A dimer is shown in ribbon form. Residues affected in the severe form of Fabry disease are colored *blue*, and those affected in the variant phenotypes of Fabry disease are colored *yellow*. Overall, more than half of the residues in the protein have been implicated in Fabry disease. The residues affected in the variant phenotypes tend to be more exposed than those found in the severe phenotype

Phenotype:
Severe
Variant

the molecular defects that lead to Fabry disease fall far from the active site of the enzyme. Over half of the residues in the mature protein are found mutated in the database of Fabry disease patients.

Fabry disease can serve as model for the entire family of lysosomal storage disorders because of the wealth of information available at the genetic, clinical, and structural levels. The extensive database of mutations identified in Fabry disease patients, combined with the three-dimensional structure of the glycoprotein, leads to a unique molecular understanding of the disease. Additionally, the family of lysosomal storage diseases have many similar traits, so better understanding of the molecular defects in Fabry disease will lead to better understanding of the entire family. Finally, the three-dimensional structure of α-galactosidase A shows that Fabry disease is typically a disease of protein misfolding, so it can serve as a model for other protein misfolding diseases, including Alzheimer's and Parkinson's diseases.

References

1. Garman SC, Garboczi DN (2004) The molecular defect leading to Fabry disease: structure of human α-galactosidase. J Mol Biol 337(2):319–335
2. Fujimoto Z, Kaneko S, Momma M, Kobayashi H, Mizuno H (2003) Crystal structure of rice α-galactosidase complexed with D-galactose. J Biol Chem 278(22):20313–20318
3. Golubev AM, Nagem RA, Brandao Neto JR, Neustroev KN, Eneyskaya EV, Kulminskaya AA et al (2004) Crystal structure of α-galactosidase from *Trichoderma reesei* and its complex with galactose: implications for catalytic mechanism. J Mol Biol 339(2):413–422
4. Chen Y, Jin M, Egborge T, Coppola G, Andre J, Calhoun DH (2000) Expression and characterization of glycosylated and catalytically active recombinant human α-galactosidase A produced in Pichia pastoris. Protein Expr Purif 20(3):472–484
5. Matsuura F, Ohta M, Ioannou YA, Desnick RJ (1998) Human α-galactosidase A: characterization of the N-linked oligosaccharides on the intracellular and secreted glycoforms overexpressed by Chinese hamster ovary cells. Glycobiology 8(4):329–339
6. Ioannou YA, Zeidner KM, Grace ME, Desnick RJ (1998) Human α-galactosidase A: glycosylation site 3 is essential for enzyme solubility. Biochem J 332:789–797
7. Lee K, Jin X, Zhang K, Copertino L, Andrews L, Baker-Malcolm J et al (2003) A biochemical and pharmacological comparison of enzyme replacement therapies for the glycolipid storage disorder Fabry disease. Glycobiology 13(4):305–313
8. Lieberman RL, D'Aquino JA, Ringe D, Petsko GA (2009) The effects of pH and iminosugar pharmacological chaperones on lysosomal glycosidase structure and stability. Biochemistry 48(22):4816–4827
9. Ishii S, Chang HH, Kawasaki K, Yasuda K, Wu HL, Garman SC et al (2007) Mutant α-galactosidase A enzymes identified in Fabry disease patients with residual enzyme activity: biochemical characterization and restoration of normal intracellular processing by 1-deoxygalactonojirimycin. Biochem J 406(2):285–295
10. Koshland DE (1953) Stereochemistry and the mechanism of enzymatic reactions. Biol Rev Cambridge Philos Soc 28:416–436
10a. Guce AI, Clark NE, Salgado EN, Vanern DR, Kulminskaya AA, Brumer H 3rd, Garman SC (2010) Catalytic mechanism of human α-galactosidase. J Biol Chem 285(6):3625–3632
11. Blanch LC, Meaney C, Morris CP (1996) A sensitive mutation screening strategy for Fabry disease: detection of nine mutations in the α-galactosidase A gene. Hum Mutat 8(1):38–43

12. Eng CM, Ashley GA, Burgert TS, Enriquez AL, D'Souza M, Desnick RJ (1997) Fabry disease: thirty-five mutations in the α-galactosidase A gene in patients with classic and variant phenotypes. Mol Med 3(3):174–182
13. Shabbeer J, Yasuda M, Luca E, Desnick RJ (2002) Fabry disease: 45 novel mutations in the α-galactosidase A gene causing the classical phenotype. Mol Genet Metab 76(1):23–30
14. Tse KC, Chan KW, Tin VP, Yip PS, Tang S, Li FK et al (2003) Clinical features and genetic analysis of a Chinese kindred with Fabry's disease. Nephrol Dial Transplant 18(1): 182–186
15. Garzuly F, Marodi L, Erdos M, Grubits J, Varga Z, Gelpi E et al (2005) Megadolichobasilar anomaly with thrombosis in a family with Fabry's disease and a novel mutation in the α-galactosidase A gene. Brain 128(Pt 9):2078–2083
16. Teraguchi M, Tanaka A, Akiola K, Lan HT, Nishi Y, Yamano T, Yoshikawa J (2004) Fabry disease female proband with clinical manifestations similar to hypertrophic cardiomyopathy. Jpn Heart J 45(4):685–689
17. Nakao S, Takenaka T, Maeda M, Kodama C, Tanaka A, Tahara M et al (1995) An atypical variant of Fabry's disease in men with left ventricular hypertrophy. N Engl J Med 333(5): 288–293
18. Madsen KM, Hasholt L, Sorensen SA, Fermer ML, Dahl N (1995) Two novel mutations (L32P) and (G85N) among five different missense mutations in six Danish families with Fabry's disease. Hum Mutat 5(3):277–278
19. Eng CM, Resnick-Silverman LA, Niehaus DJ, Astrin KH, Desnick RJ (1993) Nature and frequency of mutations in the α-galactosidase A gene that cause Fabry disease. Am J Hum Genet 53(6):1186–1197
20. Davies J, Christomanou H, Winchester B, Malcolm S (1994) Detection of 8 new mutations in the α-galactosidase A gene in Fabry disease. Hum Mol Genet 3(4):667–669
21. Koide T, Ishiura M, Iwai K, Inoue M, Kaneda Y, Okada Y et al (1990) A case of Fabry's disease in a patient with no α-galactosidase A activity caused by a single amino acid substitution of Pro-40 by Ser. FEBS Lett 259(2):353–356
22. Ashton-Prolla P, Tong B, Shabbeer J, Astrin KH, Eng CM, Desnick RJ (2000) Fabry disease: twenty-two novel mutations in the α-galactosidase A gene and genotype/phenotype correlations in severely and mildly affected hemizygotes and heterozygotes. J Investig Med 48(4):227–235
23. Davies JP, Eng CM, Hill JA, Malcolm S, MacDermot K, Winchester B et al (1996) Fabry disease: fourteen α-galactosidase A mutations in unrelated families from the United Kingdom and other European countries. Eur J Hum Genet 4(4):219–224
24. Rosenthal D, Lien YH, Lager D, Lai LW, Shang S, Leung N et al (2004) A novel α-galactosidase A mutant (M42L) identified in a renal variant of Fabry disease. Am J Kidney Dis 44(5):e85–e89
25. Iga MI, Okayama A, Matsuyama M, Sasaki T, Murai K, Hashida S, Morishita K, Tsubouchi H (2001) Disease: Fabry disease. Hum Genet 109:126
26. Germain DP, Shabbeer J, Cotigny S, Desnick RJ (2002) Fabry disease: twenty novel α-galactosidase A mutations and genotype-phenotype correlations in classical and variant phenotypes. Mol Med 8(6):306–312
27. Sakuraba H, Oshima A, Fukuhara Y, Shimmoto M, Nagao Y, Bishop DF et al (1990) Identification of point mutations in the α-galactosidase A gene in classical and atypical hemizygotes with Fabry disease. Am J Hum Genet 47(5):784–789
28. Blaydon D, Hill J, Winchester B (2001) Fabry disease: 20 novel GLA mutations in 35 families. Hum Mutat 18(5):459
29. Cooper A, Cooper JA, Wraith JE (2000) Human gene mutations in GLA. Hum Genet 107(5):535–536
30. Rodriquez-Mari A, Coll MJ, Chabas A (2003) Molecular analysis in Fabry disease in Spain: fifteen novel GLA mutations and identification of a homozygous female. Hum Mutat 22(3):258

31. Ashley GA, Shabbeer J, Yasuda M, Eng CM, Desnick RJ (2001) Fabry disease: twenty novel α-galactosidase A mutations causing the classical phenotype. J Hum Genet 46(4): 192–196

32. Spada M, Pagliardini S, Yasuda M, Tukel T, Thiagarajan G, Sakuraba H et al (2006) High incidence of later-onset fabry disease revealed by newborn screening. Am J Hum Genet 79(1):31–40

33. Eng CM, Niehaus DJ, Enriquez AL, Burgert TS, Ludman MD, Desnick RJ (1994) Fabry disease: twenty-three mutations including sense and antisense CpG alterations and identification of a deletional hot-spot in the α-galactosidase A gene. Hum Mol Genet 3(10): 1795–1799

34. Topaloglu AK, Ashley GA, Tong B, Shabbeer J, Astrin KH, Eng CM et al (1999) Twenty novel mutations in the α-galactosidase A gene causing Fabry disease. Mol Med 5(12):806–811

35. Shabbeer J, Robinson M, Desnick RJ (2005) Detection of α-galactosidase A mutations causing Fabry disease by denaturing high performance liquid chromatography. Hum Mutat 25(3):299–305

36. Schafer E, Baron K, Widmer U, Deegan P, Neumann HP, Sunder-Plassmann G et al (2005) Thirty-four novel mutations of the GLA gene in 121 patients with Fabry disease. Hum Mutat 25(4):412

37. Chen C-H, Shyu P-W, Wu S-J, Sheu S-S, Desnick RJ, Hsiao K-J (1997) Identification of a novel point mutation (S65T) in α-galactosidase A gene in Chinese patients with Fabry disease. Hum Mutat 11:328–330

38. Ishii S, Sakuraba H, Suzuki Y (1992) Point mutations in the upstream region of the α-galactosidase A gene exon 6 in an atypical variant of Fabry disease. Hum Genet 89(1):29–32

39. Okumiya T, Kawamura O, Itoh K, Kase R, Ishii S, Kamei S et al (1998) Novel missense mutation (M72V) of α-galactosidase gene and its expression product in an atypical Fabry hemizygote. Hum Mutat (Suppl 1):S213–S216

40. Slee PH, van Boven LJ, Slee DS (2000) Fabry disease: data from four families. Ned Tijdschr Geneeskd 144(50):2412–2415

41. Guffon N, Froissart R, Chevalier-Porst F, Maire I (1998) Mutation analysis in 11 French patients with Fabry disease. Hum Mutat (Suppl 1):S288–S290

42. Takata T, Okumiya T, Hayashibe H, Shimmoto M, Kase R, Itoh K et al (1997) Screening and detection of gene mutations in Japanese patients with Fabry disease by non-radioactive single-stranded conformation polymorphism analysis. Brain Dev 19(2):111–116

43. Eng C, Smith DP, Mulligan LM, Nagai MA, Healey CS, Ponder MA et al (1994) Point mutation within the tyrosine kinase domain of the RET proto-oncogene in multiple endocrine neoplasia type 2B and related sporadic tumours. Hum Mol Genet 3(2):237–241

44. Lee JK, Kim GH, Kim JS, Kim KK, Lee MC, Yoo HW (2000) Identification of four novel mutations in five unrelated Korean families with Fabry disease. Clin Genet 58(3): 228–233

45. Kimura K, Sato-Matsumura KC, Nakamura H, Onodera Y, Morita K, Enami N et al (2002) A novel A97P amino acid substitution in α-galactosidase A leads to a classical Fabry disease with cardiac manifestations. Br J Dermatol 147:545–548

46. Lorenz M, Hauser AC, Puspok-Schwarz M, Kotanko P, Arias I, Zodl H et al (2003) Anderson-Fabry disease in Austria. Wien Klin Wochenschr 115(7–8):235–240

47. Whybra C, Kampmann C, Willers I, Davies J, Winchester B, Kriegsmann J et al (2001) Anderson-Fabry disease: clinical manifestations of disease in female heterozygotes. J Inherit Metab Dis 24(7):715–724

48. Okumiya T, Ishii S, Kase R, Kamei S, Sakuraba H, Suzuki Y (1995) α-galactosidase gene mutations in Fabry disease: heterogeneous expressions of mutant enzyme proteins. Hum Genet 95(5):557–561

49. Ploos van Amstel JK, Jansen RPM, de Jong JGN, Hamel BCJ, Wevers RA (1994) Six novel mutations in the α-galactosidase A gene in families with Fabry disease. Hum Mol Genet 3(3):503–505

50. Dobrovolny R, Dvorakova L, Ledvinova J, Magage S, Bultas J, Lubanda JC et al (2005) Relationship between X-inactivation and clinical involvement in Fabry heterozygotes. Eleven novel mutations in the α-galactosidase A gene in the Czech and Slovak population. J Mol Med 83(8):647–654

51. Germain D, Biasotto M, Tosi M, Meo T, Kahn A, Poenaru L (1996) Fluorescence-assisted mismatch analysis (FAMA) for exhaustive screening of the α-galactosidase A gene and detection of carriers in Fabry disease. Hum Genet 98(6):719–726

52. Rosenberg KM, Schiffman R, Kaneski C, Brady RO, Sørensen SA, Hasholt L (2000) Five novel mutations in fourteen patients with Fabry disease. Hum Mutat 15(2):207–208

53. Morrone A, Cavicchi C, Bardelli T, Antuzzi D, Parini R, Di Rocco M et al (2003) Fabry disease: molecular studies in Italian patients and X inactivation analysis in manifesting carriers. J Med Genet 40(8):e103

54. Yasuda M, Shabbeer J, Benson SD, Maire I, Burnett RM, Desnick RJ (2003) Fabry disease: characterization of α-galactosidase A double mutations and the D313Y plasma enzyme pseudodeficiency allele. Hum Mutat 22(6):486–492

55. Davies JP, Winchester BG, Malcolm S (1993) Mutation analysis in patients with the typical form of Anderson-Fabry disease. Hum Mol Genet 2(7):1051–1053

56. Meaney C, Blanch LC, Morris CP (1994) A nonsense mutation (R220X) in the α-galactosidase A gene detected in a female carrier of Fabry disease. Hum Mol Genet 3(6):1019–1020

57. Yang CC, Lai LW, Whitehair O, Hwu WL, Chiang SC, Lien YH (2003) Two novel mutations in the α-galactosidase A gene in Chinese patients with Fabry disease. Clin Genet 63(3):205–209

58. Germain DP, Poenaru L (1999) Fabry disease: identification of novel α-galactosidase A mutations and molecular carrier detection by use of fluorescent chemical cleavage of mismatches. Biochem Biophys Res Commun 257(3):708–713

59. Politei JM, Pagano MA, Dubrovsky A, Pereira F, Matte U, Burin M et al (2005) Neuropathic pain in a young female patient with Fabry's disease: a new mutation of the α-galactosidase A gene. Rev Neurol 41(8):506–507

60. Redonnet-Vernhet I, Ploos van Amstel JK, Jansen RP, Wevers RA, Salvayre R, Levade T (1996) Uneven X inactivation in a female monozygotic twin pair with Fabry disease and discordant expression of a novel mutation in the α-galactosidase A gene. J Med Genet 33(8):682–688

61. Kotanko P, Kramar R, Devrnja D, Paschke E, Voigtlander T, Auinger M et al (2004) Results of a nationwide screening for Anderson-Fabry disease among dialysis patients. J Am Soc Nephrol 15(5):1323–1329

62. von Scheidt W, Eng CM, Fitzmaurice TF, Erdmann E, Hübner G, Olsen EGJ et al (1991) An atypical variant of Fabry's disease with manifestations confined to the myocardium. N Engl J Med 324(6):395–399

63. Lai L, O'Meara M, Lien YH (2001) Disease: Fabry disease. Hum Genet 109:468–469

64. Calado J, Dickson J, Rueff J (2004) Disease: Fabry disease. Hum Genet 115:347–356

65. Beyer EM, Karpova EA, Udalova OV, Ploos van Amstel JK, van Diggelen OP, Tsvetkova IV (1999) The multiple cases of Fabry disease in a Russian family caused by an E341K amino acid substitution in the α-galactosidase A. Clin Chim Acta 280(1–2):81–89

66. Bernstein HS, Bishop DF, Astrin KH, Kornreich R, Eng CM, Sakuraba H et al (1989) Fabry disease: six gene rearrangements and an exonic point mutation in the α-galactosidase gene. J Clin Invest 83(4):1390–1399

67. Miyazaki T, Kajita M, Ohmori S, Mizutani N, Niwa T, Murata Y et al (1998) A novel mutation (E358K) in the α-galactosidase A gene detected in a Japanese family with Fabry disease. Hum Mutat (Suppl 1):S139–S140

68. Miyamura N, Araki E, Matsuda K, Yoshimura R, Furukawa N, Tsuruzoe K et al (1996) A carboxy-terminal truncation of human α-galactosidase A in a heterozygous female with Fabry disease and modification of the enzymatic activity by the carboxy-terminal domain. Increased,

reduced, or absent enzyme activity depending on number of amino acid residues deleted. J Clin Invest 98(8):1809–1817

69. Germain DP, Salard D, Fellmann F, Azibi K, Caillaud C, Bernard MC et al (2001) Identification of a novel de novo mutation (G373D) in the α-galactosidase A gene (GLA) in a patient affected with Fabry disease. Hum Mutat 17(4):353

70. Galanos J, Nicholls K, Grigg L, Kiers L, Crawford A, Becker G (2002) Clinical features of Fabry's disease in Australian patients. Intern Med J 32(12):575–584

71. Cariolou MA, Christodoulides M, Manoli P, Kokkofitou A, Tsambaos D (1996) Novel trinucleotide deletion in Fabry's disease. Hum Genet 97:468

72. Serebrinsky GP, Pascucelli V, Politei JM (2006) Gene symbol: GLA. Disease: Fabry disease. Hum Genet 119(3):361

Chapter 3
Subcellular, Cellular and Organ Pathology of Fabry Disease

Milan Elleder

Current knowledge, novel views, and challenges

Abstract Survey of the known structural alterations is presented at the subcellular, cellular and organ levels with an attempt to correlate them with the primary enzyme catalytic defect and with pathways representing the main substrate influx into the deficient lysosomal system; the latter of which has turned out to be largely unknown. All these structural changes are presented as a basis of the known functional sequels responsible for the altered biology of the storage lysosomal system and of storage affected cells and which, ultimately, lead to cell death, and organ destruction and failure. Cell types expressing lysosomal storage are listed, some of which are less well known, while others are suggested as candidates for future studies.

Keywords Fabry disease · α galactose lipid conjugates · Lipid storage · Storage lysosome · Cell pathology · Organ pathology

3.1 Biological Introduction to Structural Findings (Biological Background of the Storage)

Pathology of Fabry disease unravels the degree of lysosomal turnover of a-Gal substrates in individual cell types. In *terms of biochemistry* the substrates are represented by α galactose-sphingolipid conjugates:

M. Elleder (✉)
First Faculty of Medicine, Institute of Inherited Metabolic Disorders, Charles University, Prague, Czech Republic
e-mail: melleder@cesnet.cz

Fabry disease (alpha galactosidase deficiency) unlike other lysosomal enzymopathies is unique as it lacks a (lethal) infantile form.

D. Elstein et al. (eds.), *Fabry Disease*, DOI 10.1007/978-90-481-9033-1_3,
© Springer Science+Business Media B.V. 2010

(i) *major substrate* which belongs to the glycolipid *globo-series* is represented by globotriaosylceramide (Gb3Cer), also known as membrane antigen CD77 [1]. It may be either a final synthetic product or as a transient product of degradation of globoside (Gb4Cer). However, both are well-known components of cell membranes and knowledge of their turnover in various cell types may thus be of great importance for understanding tissue storage patterns in a-Gal deficiency (for details see chapter Biochemistry).

(ii) *minor substrates* are represented by *digalactosyl ceramide* and *blood group B* glycolipids, the latter especially in secretory states. Storage of blood group B lipids has been demonstrated [2, 3] but represents only a minor storage component. Patients with this biological background do not seem to be at greater risk of a more serious disease course [4]. However, representative cohorts of patients with blood group B (both secretors and non-secretors) have, so far, not been studied, at either clinical or cellular levels (see also Section 3.4.7).

Though major substrates of α-galactosidase are glycosphingolipids, there are also glycoproteins bearing oligosaccharide chains with an alpha-galactosyl moiety (blood group B, P1 antigen, etc.). This currently enigmatic category of substrates should be kept in mind with regard to studies showing unexplainable lucent storage lysosomes, suggesting the possibility of non-lipid substrate accumulation (Sections 3.2.1.2 and 3.4.2).

In terms of molecular cell biology, the knowledge of substrate pathways is relatively limited. What remains to be clarified are all the pathways through which the substrates are delivered to the lysosomal compartment for degradation. The only pathway which has been defined is from the extracellular space, represented by (i) endocytosis of Gb3Cer transported by plasma lipoproteins and (ii) phagocytosis of RBC rich in globosides, as reviewed [5, 6]. However, storage across the spectrum of different cell types, including secretory cells, can hardly be explained this way. Nothing is known about intracellular sources (i.e. cell membrane, and intracellular membranes through the known types of auto-phagocytosis) [7, 8]. Thus, it may be important to know the relationships between these processes, which may differ in different cell types and even in different conditions of a given cell type.

3.2 Storage Lysosome and Storage Cell in a-Gal Deficiency

3.2.1 Storage Lysosome

3.2.1.1 Histochemistry and Biochemistry of Stored Lipids

Accumulated polar glycolipids are PAS-positive, neutral, and birefringent (i.e. present in the form of liquid crystals, which can be rather unstable in cryostat sections). Lipids can be detected using lectins [9] or verotoxin [10]. Excellent in situ detection is possible using commercially available monoclonal antibodies against Gb3Cer (Fig. 3.1). Extra situ detection is performed using both traditional biochemical and novel molecular analyses (TLC, Tandem Mass Spectrometry). The bulk of the lipid is extractible with a sequence of organic solvents [11] (for

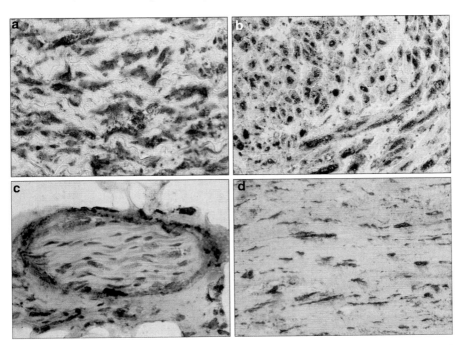

Fig. 3.1 Immunohistochemical detection of stored Gb3Cer in samples of FD. (**a**) lamina media of mammary artery (VSMC); (**b**) heart auricle (cardiomyocytes); (**c**) peripheral nerve (perineurium), (**d**) mitral valve (fibroblasts). Cryostat sections. Bioptic (**a, b, d**) and post mortem (**c**). In all cases the staining was abolished by lipid pre-extraction (objectives **a, c, d** 40×, **b** 20×)

exceptions see Fig. 3.2). This allows it to be easily distinguished from residual autofluorescent bodies (see below) which are frequently co-deposited with the stored lipids (see below). Relationships between lipid and ceroid are demonstrated in (Fig. 3.2).

3.2.1.2 Ultrastructure

It reflects the biophysical nature of the stored lipid, i.e. its polar nature and tendency to aggregate into higher order membranous structures, either classical concentric or, more often, parallel (zebra-like), with various degrees of packing. Atypical variants of stored lipid ultrastructure have been described, taking the form of short crescent-shaped stacks of membranes, mutually intersecting at their ends, and often intermixed with linearly arranged membranes (Fig. 3.3b, c). Their lipid nature has been demonstrated but any relationship to blood group B glycolipid has been ruled out [12, 13]. The reason for the atypical arrangement is thus unexplained (increased proportion of diagalactosylceramide? lysoGb3Cer?). The ultrastructure of storage lysosomes may be significantly modified by simultaneous deposition of ceroid (see below). Lucent variants of storage lysosomes are known (Fig. 3.3d, Section 3.4.2).

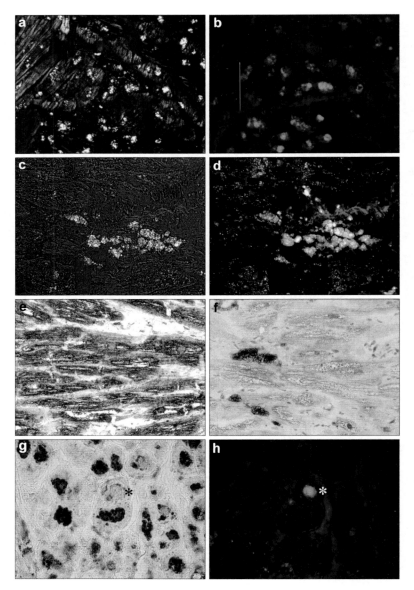

Fig. 3.2 Lipid vs. lipofuscin/ceroid in storage. (**a–d**) Unstained cryostat sections of the heart showing participation of autofluorescent ceroid/lipofuscin in lipid storage. In each case (**a–d**) single sections were analyzed using birefringence (**a, c**) demonstrating stored lipid and then autofluorescence (**b, d**). Note that both lipid and ceroid/lipofuscin are present in identical cells. (**e–f**) Gb3 immunostaining demonstrates presence of extraction-resistant, firmly found Gb3 in macrophages in the heart in contrast to extraction-sensitive Gb3 in cardiomyocytes. (**e–f**) Cryostat section immunostained for Gb3 and examined for autofluorescence; showing ceroid/lipofuscin accumulation in cardiocytes with the exception of one showing by extensive accumulation of ceroid/lipofuscin (*asterisk*). Autofluorescence in other cardiomyocytes is blocked by lipid immunostaining (obj. **a, b** 40×; **c–f** 20×; **g, h** 60×)

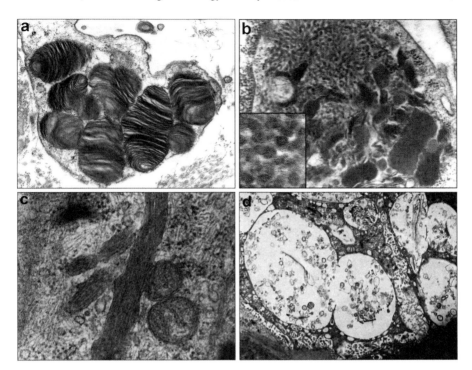

Fig. 3.3 Ultrastructural patterns of the stored lipids. (**a**) typical and (**b**), (**c**) atypical. For details see text. (**d**) demonstrates expanded lysosome in a sweat gland epithelium with minimum of lipid corresponding structures (magn. **a** 20,000×, **b** 30,000×, insert 240,000×, **c** 50,000×, **d** 4,600×)

3.2.1.3 Autofluorescent Residual Bodies

Profound alteration of storage lysosomes in long-standing storage leads to ceroid-lipofuscin deposition together with stored lipids during the storage process. According to the current view of lipopigments classification [14], in some cell types, this could lead to co-existence of induced ceroid-type with already present age pigment (lipofuscin) a situation typical in cardiomyocytes. The deposition of the latter can be inhibited by the lysosomal storage process itself. Induced ceroid deposition, still unexplained at molecular and cell levels, has very important practical implications. (i) Ceroid deposition may interfere with in situ detection of lipid storage. Undoubtedly, many reports of positive staining with Sudan Black, are the result, perhaps exclusively, of induced ceroid, which can be easily identified using autofluorescence. (ii) Ceroid deposition may significantly modify the ultrastructure of the storage lysosome (Fig. 3.4). Ultrastructural studies of delipidized tissue samples may provide detailed information. (iii) In advanced stage of storage ceroid may be the main accumulated component leaving the stored lipid barely detectable (Fig. 3.2g, h). Ceroid deposition could decrease efficacy of ERT and other therapies, since it is considered to be irreversible. The relatively high tendency toward ceroid

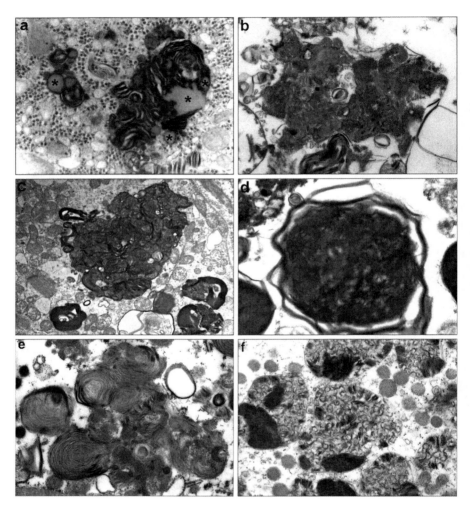

Fig. 3.4 Storage lysosome ultrastructure modified by simultaneous ceroid/lipofuscin accumulation. (**a**) portions corresponding to classic lipofuscin (age pigment) are marked by *asterisks* (liver); (**b–e**) (heart) lipid membranous pattern is profoundly modified by dense or hemidense amorphous components; (**f**) non-lipid membranes strongly resembles curvilinear profiles deposited in neuronal ceroid-lipofuscinoses (magn. **a, b, d, e, f** 20,000×, **c** 4,600×)

deposition in FD is evidenced by the fact that FD is a solely adult-type lipid storage disorder, indicating that it is a slowly progressive condition. Moreover, ceroid storage is expressed mostly by cell types with long life span (SMC) or by post-mitotic cells (cardiomyocytes). Curiously enough, our cases reveal that podocytes, which are considered to be post-mitotic, display minimum ceroid deposition (Section 3.4.4).

3.2.1.4 Biology of the Storage Lysosome

Most of the present knowledge is represented by classical biochemical data providing information on the qualitative and quantitative aspects of the storage process. Data which would characterize the biology of the storage lysosome itself and its difference from normal lysosomal compartments are virtually missing, leading to the following questions: (i) how is the storage lysosome integrated into the cell biology of the affected cell, especially in long-standing storage in cells with long life-spans or in post-mitotic cells? (ii) Is the turnover of its membrane components and lysosomal enzymes altered? (iii) Is membrane dynamics of the storage compartment known to be of remarkable degree in wild type cells [15] inhibited? (iv) How is regulated the tendency to fusion with other storage lysosomes? (v) Its possible role in exocytosis, auto-phagocytosis, or its relation to exosome dynamics, is virtually unknown.

3.2.1.5 Integrity of the Limiting Membrane of the Storage Lysosome

It is often remarked, in ultrastructural reports, that some of the storage deposits are not membrane-bound. The extreme in this sense was a detailed study of the heart and kidney in FD which showed the absence of a limiting membrane around storage deposits in the former, but its presence around the latter [16]. Thus, the integrity of storage lysosomes is still an open question. Its loss would lead to dispersion of stored compartmentalized glycolipids throughout the cytoplasm which could trigger a series of downstream events with great potential to influence cell biology in both positive and negative ways, including focal cytoplasmic degradation (see also Section 3.4.1).

Loss of the lysosomal limiting membrane system in a programmed manner should be considered in explaining the cataract of the ocular lens (Section 3.4.8)

3.2.1.6 Shape of the Storage Lysosome

The common shape is rounded, reflecting expansion in three dimensions. Multiple storage lysosomes displaying varying degrees of fusion can lead to sizable vacuoles. The central part of the voluminous lysosomes is either lucent or filled with condensed, densely-packed concentric membranes (Fig. 3.5a, b). This suggests significant lysosomal fusion which represents part of the progression of the storage process; the biological consequences of this await elucidation. The tendency toward fusion differs in various cell types. Exceptionally, the storage compartment can display needle-like or slender fusiform configurations, as seen in sweat gland epithelium (Fig. 3.5c, d) suggesting unstable dynamic shape.

It is reasonable to assume that less storage-affected cells retain the capacity to restart the biogenesis of new lysosomal/endosomal system ready to exert its function and to realize the process of autophagocytosis. The former should be advantageous for ERT. If this capacity is retained in cells in advanced stage of storage transformation cannot be answered (see also below). Our studies at the cell level strongly

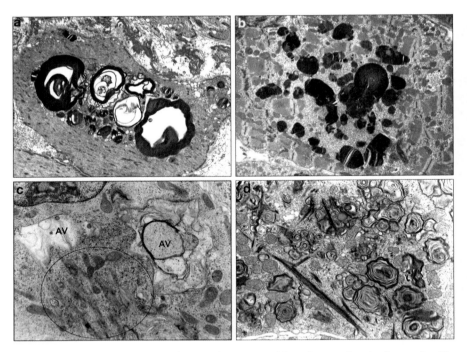

Fig. 3.5 (**a, b**) show size diversity of storage lysosomes with tendency to fuse leading to sizeable structures with different degrees of compaction of the lipid membranes; (**c**) elongated oval storage lysosomes (*circled area*); (**d**) needle-like storage compartments in skin eccrine gland (AV denotes autophagy like vacuoles) (magn. **a** 3,000×, **b** 3,500×, **c** 13,000×, **d** 10,000×)

suggest ineffectivity of ERT in advanced stage of storage in FD hemizygotes and thus concept of enzyme replacement therapy was recommended to be changed for enzyme preventive therapy [11].

3.2.2 Storage Cell–Cell with Altered Biology (Not Only in Fabry Disease)

Storage cells have been defined, so far, mainly morphologically: as cells with expanded and functionally compromised lysosomal systems. The spectrum of sequelae at all levels (structural, functional, and biochemical) is covered here under the multi-disciplinary heading of 'biological.' Altered biology of the storage cell is responsible for organ pathology and pathophysiology and thus for the phenotype of FD. It represents an ever-expanding field in molecular cell pathology of FD. Available details will be given under organ pathology. Briefly, it includes cytokine production, altered turnover of extracellular matrix (including basement membranes), cardiocyte hypertrophy (Section 3.4.3), and interference with secretion (Sections 3.4.2 and 3.4.5). Other pathologies are defined at the biochemical and molecular levels; these include, just to mention a few, induction of oxidative stress by Gb3 storage in EC [17], reduced activities of respiratory chain enzymes in FD fibroblasts [18], altered processing of constitutively secreted proteins [19], ectopic intracellular increase of the stored substrate [20, 21], induction of dipeptidyl peptidase IV in renal glomeruli [22] and possibly altered autophagy [23].

In summary; there is induction of novel functions, with broad effects on the one hand and loss of functions leading to loss of storage cell integrity on the other hand. The cumulative result is responsible for the progression of the clinical phenotype. This occurs in certain cell types, namely those that cannot be effectively replaced and are sentenced to cumulate all the negative consequences, and thus to cell death.

Cell death precipitated by storage in FD has been described in vascular smooth muscle cells (Section 3.4.1), cardiocytes (Section 3.4.3), and podocytes (Section 3.4.4). Whether it is apoptosis cannot be convincingly concluded. Recent studies indicate it may be in play in storage cardiomyocytes (Section 3.4.3). Replacement of damaged postmitotic cells or cells with very low regeneration potential is impossible or ineffective. Cell death of other cell types may be easily compensated through cell regeneration. Nothing is known about cell death, and altered turnover in endothelial cells. It is reasonable to suppose the blood serum levels of some of the biomarkers of the disease, e.g. Gb3Cer and its lysoderivative [24] may reflect the degree of cell damage and loss in the storage cell population either due to storage induced premature cell death or by spontaneous attrition in storage expressing clones. Besides storage the only known factor responsible for cell death in FD is ischemic necrosis caused by arterial dysfunction (Sections 3.4.5 and 3.4.8).

Dynamics of storage within a given clone is difficult to asses as most of the storage affected cells do not belong to a classical well defined clones based on stem cell of the adult type. Nevertheless the situation in the stratified epithelia suggests there may be significant tendency to storage in the progenitors situated in the basal layer without any substantial increase, or with decrease in the next cell generations (dilution of the storage compartment by cytokinesis?) (Sections 3.4.2 and 3.4.8).

The evolution of cell pathology in human FD contrasts with the relatively benign course seen in the mouse model, suggesting a species-specific reaction of cells to lysosomal storage in a-Gal deficiency [25].

3.3 Cell Types Expressing Storage in a-Gal Deficiency

Endothelium. Storage in blood vessel endothelium (Fig. 3.6a) is an integral part of the classic Fabry disease phenotype complex. The main pathway of critical substrate influx is considered to be endocytosis of Gb3 in serum lipoproteins [6]; links to transcytosis remain to be defined [26]. Conversion of EC (endothelial cells) to storage cells has been shown to lead to induction of oxidative stress [17] and increased Gb3 in caveolin-associated endothelial plasma membrane fractions [20]. EC storage predisposes vessels to thromboses [27] and to endothelial dysfunction [28, 29]. Increased levels of endothelial microparticles, reversible after ERT, have also been

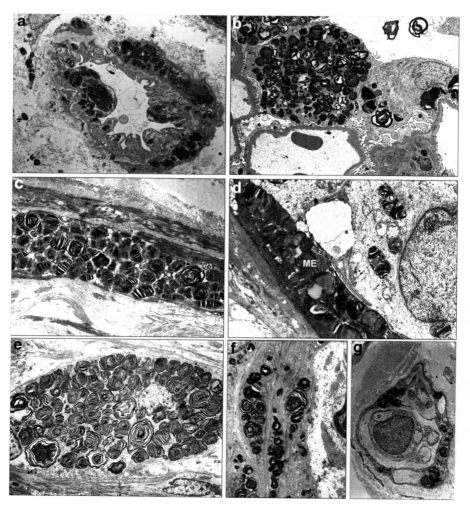

Fig. 3.6 Group of cell types known to express the highest degree of storage in a-Gal deficiency. (**a**) complex capillary endothelium-pericyte; (**b**) glomerular podocyte; (**c**) smooth muscle cell; (**d**) myoepithelial cell in a sweat gland; (**e**) peripheral neuron, here in the bronchial wall; perineurial cells in large (**f**) and terminal (**g**) nerve fibres (magn. **a** 4,000×, **b, c, g** 4,000×, **d** 10,000×, **f** 3,000×)

described [30]. On the other hand, signs of EC damage in FD has been ascribed to renal insufficiency rather than to lysosomal storage [31]. Nothing is known of the altered life span of storage EC and of their turnover. Storage of lipid can be accompanied by ceroid induction (personal observation). What remains to be established is the situation in alveolar capillary endothelium; the recent, unpublished observations, showed the absence of storage (Section 3.4.6). Sinusoidal endothelium displays minimum storage or is unaffected [26], the only exception being splenic sinus endothelium, which expresses a high degree of storage [32]. For storage in lymphatic endothelium see Section 3.4.1.

Perivascular (pericapillary) cells – pericytes and podocytes. Both belong to the standard type of storage cells in a-Gal deficiency (Fig. 3.6a, b). Their well-known predisposition to storage is unexplained in terms of molecular biology. With regard to pericytes, it might be their close association and interaction with endothelial cells [33]. Analogous perivascular cells in brain capillary networks have never been described to express storage. Podocyte biology is characterized by its almost fixed post-mitotic state [34]. Nothing is known about the turnover of the α-galactose-sphingolipid conjugates in this cell type.

Smooth muscle cells (SMC) belong to cell types that express high-level storage and thus represent, together with cardiomyocytes and podocytes, prototypes of storage cells in a-Gal deficiency. All observations support this as a feature of all members of the SMC family (Fig. 3.6c). Highest storage intensity has been repeatedly described in vascular and bronchial SMC, less intensity in esophageal and intestinal SMC as well as the SMC of the muscular layers of ureter, urinary bladder, seminal vesicles, prostate, and arrector pilorum muscles in the skin. The most serious sequelae of storage have been described in VSMC (vascular smooth muscle cells) (see Section 3.4.1). Impaired pupillary constriction with pilocarpine [35] suggests storage in the sphincter pupillae muscle. Storage has also been described in ciliary smooth muscle [36]. On the contrary uterine and uterine tube SMC were uniformly free of storage in a surgical specimen from a female patient. The absence contrasted with presence of storage in VSMC in the specimen (unpublished observation). This, so far unique, observation suggests the potential influence of estrogen and should attract interest to this group of SMC in female Fabry patients. As for the myoepithelial cells of skin eccrine glands, they also frequently display lysosomal storage (Fig. 3.6d). Nothing definite can be said about myofibroblasts and myoepitheloid cells of the renal juxtaglomerular apparatus.

Heart. Cardiomyocytes are well-known to exhibit a high degree of storage with profound sequelae. Details are given in Section 3.4.3.

The neuronal system displays differential expression of lysosomal storage. Peripheral neurons are regularly affected irrespective of the site, with foamy transformation of their perikarya. Storage in nerve processes is regularly expressed by cells of the perineurium along the entire length of the nerve fiber (Fig. 3.6e–g). Storage in central neurons is summarized in Section 3.4.5. Ceroid accumulation is a regular part of the storage process and frequently attains high levels so that the lipid may be in minority or undetectable (Section 3.2).

Fibroblasts (dermal and other locations) display various degrees of storage. Fibroblasts in skin (except those around hair follicles) and especially those in heart valves (Fig. 3.7a, b) were frequently seen to express high storage degree (Section 3.4.3). However, their function does not seem to be compromised as there is no evidence of defective healing and fibrin organization processes in FD. Fibroblasts engaged in thrombus organization in coronary arteries did not display detectable storage (personal observation). Storage in corneal keratocytes was recorded inconstantly (Section 3.4.8). Modified liver intralobular fibroblasts, known as Ito cell

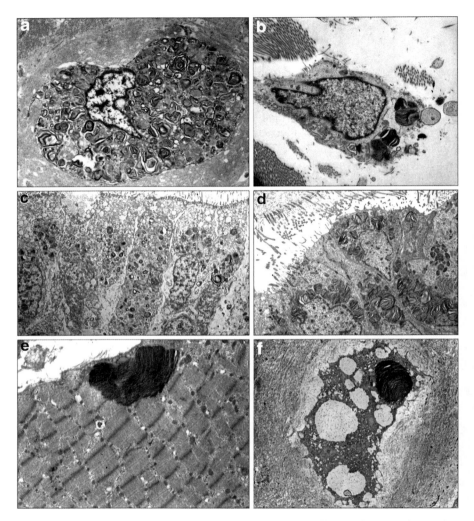

Fig. 3.7 Demonstration of other cell types affected by storage in aGal deficiency. (**a**) heart valve fibroblast; (**b**) dermal fibroblast; (**c**) bronchial epithelium; (**d**) uterine tube epithelium; (**e**) skeletal muscle; (**f**) chondrocyte in bronchial cartilage; (magn. **a** 4,000×, **b** 6,000×, **c** 3,000×, **d** 3,000×, **e** 6,000×, **f** 2,500×)

were described to express storage (Section 3.4.7). As for other mesenchymal cells, storage has been observed in chondrocytes (Fig. 3.7f) and regularly in adipocytes (unpublished).

Ciliary bronchial epithelium displays high levels of storage, maximally at the apical region (Section 3.4.6) [37, 38]. This author has made similar observations (Fig. 3.7c). *Ciliary epithelium in the uterine tube* was found to display comparable degrees of storage (unpublished) (Fig. 3.7d). Prominent storage in *epididymal epithelium* has been repeatedly described [26, 39].

Squamous epithelium has only rarely been described to display storage, limited to the basal layer [40]. Storage was observed in the conjunctival epithelium and corneal epithelium (Section 3.4.8). *Urothelial epithelium* has been found to express storage (unique unpublished observation).

Secretory cells with regulated types of secretion. Discrete storage has been found in *mucinous cells of the gastric mucosa* (unpublished), in Brunner duodenal glands [41] and in goblet cells in both conjunctival epithelium [42] and respiratory epithelium (personal observation). Storage involvement of the oral and ocular glands should be predicted based on clinical observations [35, 43]. Storage in *skin sweat glands* is well-known and can attain high levels (Section 3.4.2). The *exocrine pancreas* can be severely affected (Section 3.4.7).

Endocrine glands. There are rare reports of acromegaly in Fabry patients [44], but no storage has been demonstrated histologically, only acidophil hyperplasia [45]. Subclinical storage in the adenohypophysis has been described through detailed analysis of postmortem specimens [46, 47]. Prominent, albeit subclinical, storage in sustentacular and secretory cells in the adenohypophysis were been found during the autopsy of a male patient with FD (unpublished observation). Storage has also been described in Leydig cells [26, 39, 48]. Recently we observed variable degrees of lysosomal storage in endocrine cells of the human gastric mucosa (Section 3.4.7).

Skeletal muscles express an incomparably low degree of storage, which presents as individual storage lysosomes (Fig. 3.7e) which are unlikely to significantly influence the biology of the muscle fiber syncycium [49]. Skeletal myopathy has never been described in FD. There was a single reported case of rhabdomyolysis in FD [50].

These findings, interesting from the theoretical point of view, suggest prominent involvement of various epithelial cells, namely those with regulated exocytosis. However, storage does not seem to interfere significantly with cell function. A reasonable explanation is that these cells are easily replaced by regeneration and hence the organ escapes serious involvement.

Macrophages. Despite large amounts of red blood cell globoside, storage is not excessive and never attains high levels. In lymph nodes and in the peripheral lymphatic tissue generally, storage macrophages are present in both lymphatic follicles and the red pulp of the spleen [32], however, they do not resemble typical expanded storage populations, as seen in other LSDs which are significantly manifested in macrophages (Gaucher, Niemann Pick diseases). Therefore, splenomegaly is not part of the FD clinical picture; if present it is an exceptional finding associated with a co-morbidity that significantly affects organ enlargement [48]. Nevertheless, increases in serum chitotriosidase activity in FD points to storage activation of macrophages that is reversible with ERT [51]. Lymph node enlargement is unusual but has been noted in the literature [52]. Macrophage lipid scavenging activity in atherosclerotic lesions is retained and results in apolar lipid accumulation dominating over Gb3 storage, which is often undetectable (personal observation). Langerhans epidermal cells are free of storage (personal observation).

Lysosome related organelle system. There are no convincing signs of storage modification in granules of this system.

3.4 Organ Pathology

The clinical phenotype of human FD is given mainly by storage involvement and subsequent regression of post-mitotic cells or cells of clones with long life-spans and very low regeneration capacity. Vascular dysfunction may cause significant damage to various organs especially the brain.

3.4.1 Pathology of Blood and Lymphatic Vessels

3.4.1.1 Pathology of Blood Vessels

Pathology of vessels is an integral part of a-Gal deficiency. It reflects high expression of storage in both endothelial and smooth muscle cells. It presents as micro-angiopathy (involving the terminal parts of the vascular network) and macro-angiopathy reflecting involvement of elastic and muscular arteries. In terms of pathophysiology, it is a combination of EC and VSMC dysfunction.

Endothelial storage tends to be generalized. The endothelial cells display lysosomal storage of various degrees, ranging from individual storage lysosomes to massive lysosomal system expansion. There are no significant signs of endothelial cells hypertrophy or activation of apical or basal pole membranes. Frequently there is multiplication of basal membranes which contrasts with deficient basement membranes seen in angiokeratoma (Fig. 3.8a–c). Differences between various types of endothelia and current knowledge on EC dysfunction are mentioned in Section 3.3.

Vascular smooth muscle cell (VSMC) storage is generalized. Storage in SMC is generally of a high degree, transforming the SMC into storage cells. Storage may progress to focal cytoplasmic necrosis, characterized by a breakdown that is limited to the cytoplasm occupied by the storage compartment. The next stage is necrosis of the entire sarcoplasm. This is accompanied by densification of the cell, loss of stored lipids, and progressive disappearance of storage lysosomes (Fig. 3.8d–f), including loss of the membrane components and luminal enzyme markers. Defects of elastic lamellae and fibrosis (Fig. 3.9) are common. Calcification may also occur [26] (Fig. 3.8 g).

The spectrum of sequelae of VSMC storage differs considerably and ranges from thinning and distension of the arterial wall due to VSMC regression (in one of our female patients a coronary artery wall was revealed to be paper thin) to progressive fibrous thickening mainly of the intimal layer. The intimal cell population (fibroblasts or myofibroblasts) need not express significant storage. Lumen narrowing in smaller arteries (arterioles) can occur, but dilation can also take place. Direct inspection of the ocular vascular system has demonstrated the spectrum of possible changes (dilatations, microaneurysms, thromboses, and tortuosity) in both arteries and veins. The spectrum of arterial changes in FD has been described in several papers [26, 45, 53, 54].

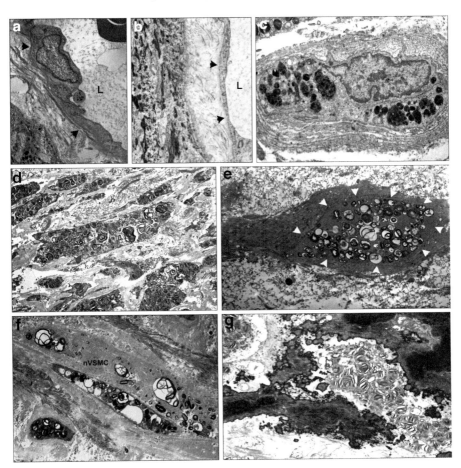

Fig. 3.8 (**a, b**) selected portions of angiokeratoma showing reduced or barely recognizable basement membrane (*arrowheads*); L denotes for lumen; (**c**) storage capillary endothelial cells with multiple thin basement membranes; (**d**) VSMC with prominent storage in media of a muscular artery; (**e**) VSMC with large cytoplasmic focus of lysosomal storage. The whole area (marked by *arrowheads*) underwent densification and delineation from the rest of the sarcoplasm; (**f**) complete necrosis of VSMC (marked with nVSMC) with marked reduction of storage lysosomes and densification of the sarcoplasm with loss of all cytoplasmic details (compare with Fig. 3.9); (**g**) media of a muscular artery with storage in VSMC and extensive fibrosis and calcification in the wall (magn. **a** 4,000×, **b** 6,000×, **c** 1,500×, **d** 3,000×, **e** 3,500×, **f** 3,000×, **g** 3,000×)

Several clinical studies described tendency toward increased intima-medial thickening reflecting increased fibrosis of the arterial wall unrelated to atherosclerotic process [55–57]; however, not all observations have been confirmed [58].

It is not an exaggeration to say that the structural integrity of the vessel wall in FD depends, to a considerable degree, on the status of the VSM, which represents the

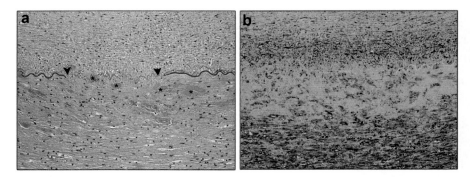

Fig. 3.9 Renal artery. (**a**) defect in internal elastic membrane (between *arrows*) with homogenized dense necrotic VSMC in the vicinity (*asterisks*) HE stain; (**b**) analogous part showing necrotic VSMC deficient in smooth muscle actin (obj. **a, b** 20×)

biological center of the vessel wall. Since the VSMC system represents a biological entity interconnected by a system of gap junctions, similar to other smooth muscle populations [59], it may be interesting to note the extend to which this interconnection is altered in FD. What is entirely unknown is the status of vasa vasorum, which may influence local progression of the vascular wall pathology and its predisposition to atherosclerosis.

Arterial dysfunction and the associated consequences in the brain and heart have been described [60–66].

Predisposition of the Fabry lysosomal arteriopathy to atherosclerosis is accepted in some studies [5, 67]. Severe atherosclerosis has been observed in both ERT-untreated FD [68] and ERT treated male patients [69]. On the other hand, resistance to atherosclerosis has been described in a cohort of Fabry patients [70]. Atherosclerotic lesions can be localized, reflecting restricted damage [71] (and our unpublished observations). Severe coronary symptoms have been described without signs of atherosclerosis [64, 72].

3.4.1.2 Pathology of Lymphatic Vessels and Lymph Nodes

Lymphatic drainage is frequently disturbed in FD as suggested by frequent observations of lymphedema [73]. Storage in cutaneous lymphatic endothelium has also been described [12]. We have observed this repeatedly in skin biopsies of Fabry patients (Fig. 3.10); however, how this interferes with lymphatic drainage is not clear. Severe dysfunction of the cutaneous lymphatic network has been demonstrated by microfluorescence, microlymphography, and lymphatic pressure measurements which showed severe structural and functional changes [74]. The absence of cutaneous lymphatic collectors in the lower limbs has been described in a male Fabry patient with lymphedema [74].

Blockade of regional *lymph nodes* may be responsible, but adequate knowledge about their microstructure is lacking. Infiltration with foamy histiocytes has been

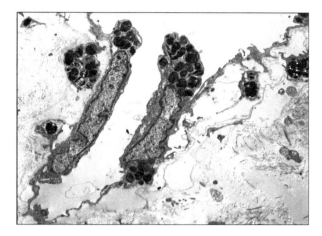

Fig. 3.10   Storage in endothelial cells of a dermal lymphatic capillary (magn. 4,000×)

described in the past [75], but generally lymph nodes are not significantly affected sites; although exceptions have been described; they were characterized by lymphadenopathy and fever, and resembled lymphoma. Histology of the lymph node was considered compatible with FD [52].

Nothing is known about the status of lymphatic vessels in other organs and about the possible negative consequences, especially in organs with intense lymphatic drainage, e.g. intestinal villi. Whether storage in cutaneous lymphatic endothelium reflects storage in lymphatic endothelium generally cannot yet be answered. It may be useful to compare extracutaneous lymph vessel status, using EM, in patients with lymphedema. There is only one report describing alteration (nonspecific?) of intestinal lymphatic vessels [76]. Storage related dysfunction of the cutaneous lymphatic system is most probably triggered and kept by gravitational-dependent mechanisms.

3.4.2 Pathology of the Skin

Storage in blood capillaries is expressed in the endothelium and elements of the vessel wall (pericytes and smooth muscle cells) and in eccrine sweat glands with varying degrees of intensity (Fig. 3.11b–d). The latter were reported to be affected (both myoepithelial and epithelial cells of the secretory coils or excretory tubules) [77–79]. The storage ultrastructure corresponds to the classic concentric membranous pattern in rounded lysosomes (Section 3.2). There are exceptions represented by needle-like lipid storage subcompartments (Fig. 3.5d) or by clear storage vacuoles repeatedly described in hemizygotes [78, 80] (Figs. 3.3d and 3.11f). An explanation for the latter finding is still missing. Could it be a theoretical non-lipid substrate (see Section 3.2), or lysosomal expansion due to an osmotic imbalance, or

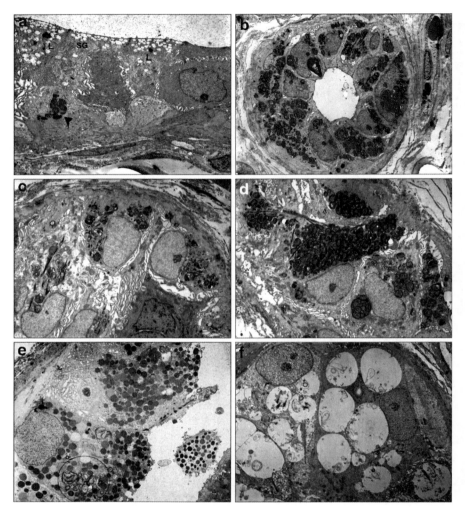

Fig. 3.11 Skin eccrine glands. (**a**) a case showing the absence of storage in epithelium containing only lipofuscin (L) and secretory granules (SG). Lysosomal storage is present only in the myoepithelial cell (*arrowhead – lower left quadrant*); (**b–d** a case with storage in the epithelium and myoepithelium either diffuse uniform (**b**) or of variable degrees (**c, d**); (**e**) another case with a number of secretory granules of variable internal density and with a small area of lipid storage (*circled area – lower left quadrant*); (**f**) voluminous lysosomes with minimum lipid membranes inside in another epithelial cell of the same secretory coil (magn. **a** 2,000×, **b** 1,500×, **c–e** 2,000×, **f** 1,500×)

does it represent an additional lysosomal load of degradable substrates and therefore a reversible phenomenon? In some of our cases (unpublished) sweat eccrine glands are free of any storage and harbor age pigment in amounts proportional to the age of the patient. Storage in myoepithelial cells have been observed independently of storage in epithelial cells (Fig. 3.11a). Storage may be accompanied by prominent basement membrane thickening around the secretory coils. Fusion of lipid rich lysosomes with clear secretory granules have also been described [77]. Could this lead to Gb3 translocation into sweat?

A well-known symptom in FD is hypo- or anhidrosis, the mechanism of which has still not been convincingly explained (Section 3.4.5). What is missing is a study specifying the relationship between anhidrosis and the dynamics of sweat secretory granule exocytosis and lysosomal storage which would answer the following: (i) Is anhidrosis due to sweat secretory granule retention caused by the absence of the exocytosis triggering stimulus and their degradation by autophagocytosis (lysosomal load by degradable substrates)? (ii) Does lysosomal storage interfere with biogenesis of secretory granules? (iii) What is the explanation for the absence of lysosomal storage in sweat glands in some FD patients? and (iv) is there myoepithelial cell dysfunction (i.e. altered expulsion of the secreted substance)? It is worth mentioning that a common early symptom of FD is hyperhidrosis [81].

Storage has been observed in the matrix of hair follicle bulbs, the arrector pilorum muscles [11, 82], and basal keratinocytes [40]. Storage process in dermal structures has been described in a number of publications [12, 79, 83]. As for nerves in the skin, see Section 3.4.5. Storage in lymphatic endothelium was mentioned above (Section 3.4.1), similarly as storage in dermal fibroblasts (Section 3.3).

In organ-restricted variants (cardiac -; renal-) storage in the skin region may be entirely missing or significantly less expressed.

Angiokeratoma (AK). Dozens of years of clinical and histopathological experience has perfected our knowledge of AK distribution and histological structure [12]. However, in terms of pathophysiology, explanations are still missing. AK is defined as a teleangiectatic lesion of the capillaries in the upper dermis covered by a hyperkeratotic epidermis and surrounded by epidermal 'collars.' It has been frequently described in the bucal mucosa [43]. There is nothing analogous anywhere in the capillary network of the rest of the body. Because AK is in the subgroup of lysosomal storage disorders (LSD) that manifest in endothelium [84], it is reasonable to assume their development is linked to lysosomal storage in endothelial cells. However, AK in FD is identical to Fordyce type AK [85] and there are cases of both individual and disseminated angiokeratoma without any linkage to LSD [86]. Whether there is a common pathway leading to the evolution of AK in LSD-associated vs. LSD-unassociated cannot be answered presently. The unique detailed ultrastructural observations of AK in FD, described to date [12, 26], show endothelial lysosomal storage, absence of pericytes, and deficient basement membranes (Fig. 3.8a, b). It is generally accepted that AK is a localized expression of generalized blood capillary storage, i.e. the absence of AK can never be taken to mean the absence of skin storage in FD.

AK has been described in female Fabry patients [87–90]. In one of them [90], lucent lysosomes dominated in endothelial cells. In female patients, AK should manifest storage, and thus be of help in diagnosing borderline heterozygous states with inconclusive α-Gal activity, provided AK is not of the LSD-unassociated type.

3.4.3 Pathology of the Heart

Biological background. Heart involvement is an integral part of a-Gal deficiency. However, the biological background is not entirely clear. Nothing is known about possible globo-series lipid turnover in cardiocytes. The possible extracellular source of lipid substrates (delivered by endocytosis) presently appears to be the main source of substrate for cardiomyocyte lysosomes. The predisposition of cardiocytes toward storage is increased by their post-mitotic state. In other words, they cannot be spontaneously replaced by new cardiocyte generation and the presence of stem cells in the human heart is still debatable [91–93]. According to storage expression (see below), both conductive and contractile cardiocytes should have high a-Gal substrate turnover. Cardiologic follow-ups of Fabry patients disclosed peculiar sensitivity of the posterolateral wall of the left ventricle to storage processes which remains to be explained. It indicates the existence of different biological conditions associated with cardiocytes along cardiac contractile fibers.

Storage process and its sequelae. Storage affects both the contractile and conductive systems of the heart. Gradual expansion of the lysosomal system by undegraded substrate leads to distension of the lysosomal system, which expands from the typical perinuclear area deeper into the sarcoplasm. There is always remarkable variability in the size of storage lysosomes; ranging from discrete (<500 nm in diameter) to 4–5 µm in diameter. The storage areas are well demonstrated by both luminal (Fig. 3.12e) and membrane lysosomal markers. Ceroid deposition (see Section 3.2) is consistently present; often as multiple discrete autofluorescent granules mixed with larger globules, the latter resembling age pigment (Fig. 3.12d); ceroid participation may modify the ultrastructure (see Section 3.2). Progression of storage interferes with the biology of affected cardiomyocytes through mechanisms that are not well understood, leading usually to cardiac hypertrophy which is a common reaction to a variety of metabolic disorders affecting the heart [94]. Interference with OXFOS in storage-affected cardiomyocytes has been recently suggested as a possible mechanism responsible for starting the hypertrophy process. Extra-cardial circulating growth promoting factor has also been proposed as another factor [55]. Cardiomyocyte hypertrophy is represented by widening of the sarcoplasm caused by sarcomer enlargement and by enlarged hyperchromic nuclei, sometimes double (Fig. 3.12a, b). The latter reflects tetraploid DNA content in the absence of cytokinesis. Disarray and branching of fibers may also be present (Fig. 3.12b). Heart weight may exceed 1,000 g. Weight increase is mainly due to the process of hypertrophy, partly to the expanded lysosomal system (weight of the stored lipid itself in negligible [95]). Further progression of storage leads to cardiomyocyte degeneration, easily demonstrated using standard EM (Fig. 3.13a–c). Frequently there are changes in the inner mitochondrial membrane structure and entrapment of mitochondria inbetween the aggregated storage lysosomes (Fig. 3.13c). Fibrillolysis has been described [96], and is assumed to lead to increased cardiomyocytes stiffness, further contributing to diastolic dysfunction. The number of endocrine granules in atrial cardiomyocytes has not been found to be decreased (unpublished). Some of the damaged cardiocytes can be invaded by

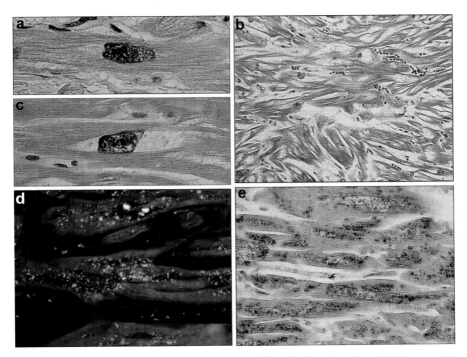

Fig. 3.12 Heart. (**a, c**) hypertrophic cardiomyocytes with typically enlarged nuclei; (**b**) area with fiber branching and disarray; (**d**) paraffin section (unstained) with autofluorescent ceroid/lipofuscin granules dispersed in the lysosomal storage area; (**e**) prominent immunohistochemical signal for cathepsin D in the cardiomyocyte storage area (obj. **a–e** 40×)

macrophages scavenging the interior of the damaged sarcoplasm being exposed to non-degradable stored lipid and ceroid-lipofuscin. It strongly resembles the phenomenon of myocytolysis following individual cell necrosis [97]. We have seen the intracellular invasion repeatedly (Fig. 3.14a–d). Signs of cardiomyocyte apoptosis have been described [98].

Fibrosis is a common phenomenon accompanying cardiac fiber hypertrophy either in mild diffuse forms, as described in cardiac hypertrophy processes [99–102], or as a focal reparative reaction following muscle fiber necrosis. Such reactive, massive fibrosis is a frequent finding in the posterolateral wall of the left ventricle, demonstrable with gadolinium enhancement CMR [103–105].

Conductive system. Involvement of the heart's conductive system is a common manifestation of Fabry cardiomyopathy [106]; involvement by lysosomal storage has also been described [107]. Becker et al. [108] demonstrated storage involvement along the whole conductive system, i.e. in cells of sinoatrial and atrioventricular nodes as well as in the His bundle and its branches. Others have described mild storage in the cells of the atrioventricular node [109]. No further details concerning their participation in hypertrophy in conjunction with contractile cardiomyocytes

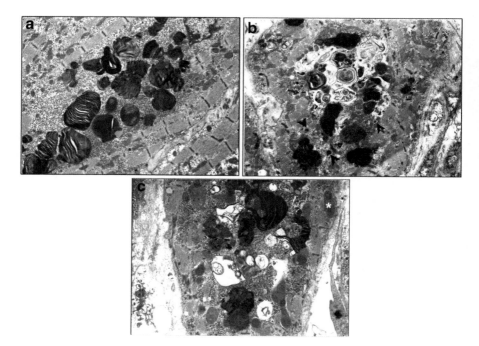

Fig. 3.13 Atrial cardiomyocytes; (**a**) storage area in cardiomyocyte without any signs of cellular alteration, (**b, c**) with apparent cellular alterations. Abnormal mitochondrion (in **c** *upper right quadrant*) is marked by *asterisk*, secretory granules (atrial natriuretic peptide) in **b** marked with *arrowheads* (*lower left* and *lower right quadrant*) (magn. **a, b** 4,000×, **c** 6,000×)

or concerning functional alteration, regression, or necrosis of the conductive cardiocytes are available. Therefore, interpretation of EEG changes (shortening or prolongation of the PR interval, supraventricular arrhythmias or even atrioventricular or bundle branch blocks) are not possible. It is worth mentioning that Purkynje cells were found to exhibit comparable degrees of polyploidy to normal cardiocytes in human hearts, which is contrary to nodal myocytes [110]. We observed storage, mild hypertrophy and degeneration of various degrees in Purkynje cells in His bundles (Fig. 3.15a–d).

Heart valves may express massive storage, sometimes accompanied by progressive fibrosis, leading to significant valve dysfunction which represents an additional burden on a storage-affected heart. Valve fibroblasts display intensive lysosomal lipid storage (Section 3.3). This could interfere with the degradation of all extracellular matrix components which would promote thickening of the valve. Since the tendency toward fibrosis is exceptional in FD in general, heart valve affection points to different turnover of the valvular EC matrix or to a different biochemical EC matrix composition, suggesting higher participation of α-Gal substrates. It is worth mentioning that individual heart valves may differ in the degree of their affection.

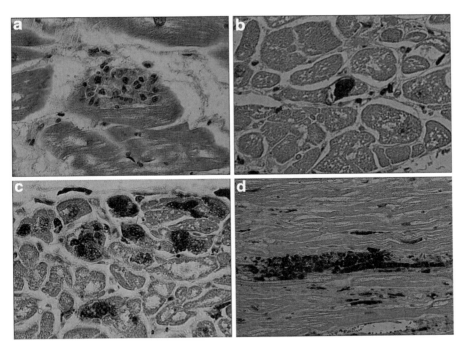

Fig. 3.14 Heart ventricle. Invasion of cardiocytes by macrophages resulting in intracellular myocytolysis. (**a**) HE stain; (**b–d**) CD68 immunostaining of macrophages (obj. **a, b, c** 60×, **d** 20×)

Pulmonary regurgitation [111], aortic regurgitation [112], mitral stenosis [113] or insufficiency [114] have all been described which indicate different local challenges for heart valve cellular populations. Usually, simple valvular thickening dominates [98]. As heart valve involvement is infrequent in FD [98, 106], the significant roles of other acquired factors must be considered.

Heart in female patients can be affected to a considerable degree [115]. The storage process has not been clinically demonstrated to be different from that in Fabry hemizygotes, i.e. heart hypertrophy is diffuse without any sign of mosaic-type involvement; it is only quantitatively less expressed [104, 116, 117]. Histologically the storage process in cardiomyocytes was of a mosaic type [118], resulting from X-inactivation in the heart. Despite this mosaic type of storage, there is no clinical evidence of regionally accentuated storage sequelae in female Fabry hearts. It is reasonable that the whole heart would react as a functional entity, since the signal for hypertrophy should affect all cardiomyocytes in all fibers irrespective of the pattern of the storage process.

In contrast to other organs, the heart is predisposed to storage and it can be the only organ affected [95, 119, 120]. The only exception is the renal variant of Fabry disease where storage is restricted to kidney cells [121].

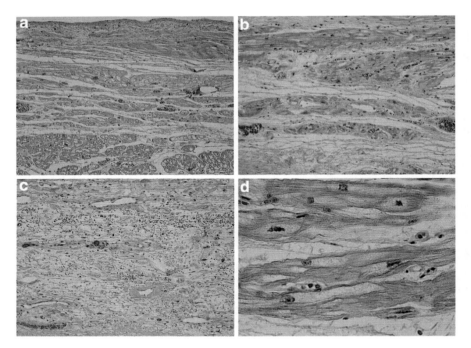

Fig. 3.15 Conductive system (His bundles) HE stain. Storage and signs of hypertrophy in Purkynje cells. Serious destruction of the bundle is apparent in **c**. (obj. **a–c** 10×, **d** 40×)

3.4.4 Pathology of the Kidney

Except for the ubiquitous vessels, there are two major sites of lysosomal storage in the kidney: – the glomeruli and the tubules (Fig. 3.16a). Storage in the *glomeruli* is mostly expressed in podocytes (Section 3.3, Fig. 3.1b), which are progressively transformed into the storage cells, with minimal induction of ceroid deposition (Fig. 3.16c, d). With progression of storage there is fusion of the pedicels. Transformation into storage cell is accompanied by induction of DPP IV activity [22]. Further progression of storage combined, probably, with storage-induced vascular dysfunction leads to podocyte degeneration and disappearance which leads to glomerular fibrosis, caused by mesangial cells production of EC matrix, and to gradual loss of filtration capacity [122, 123]. This corresponds to common mechanisms in glomerular pathology [124]. Endothelial cells and mesangial cells are much less affected than podocytes; the former even less so than their extra-renal counterparts. Glomerular storage may lead to a peculiar duplication of the capillary BM with deposition of membranous non-lipid material [125]. Nothing is known about storage in the juxtaglomerular (myoepitheloid) cells which display differentiation toward smooth muscle cells, well known to exhibit high tendency to storage (Section 3.3).

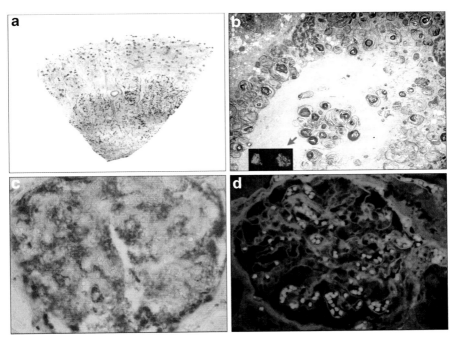

Fig. 3.16 Kidney in a florid lipid storage state. (**a**) Frozen section stained with PAS (scanned slide). Bulk of the positive staining is from the stored lipid. Note the stippling of the cortex from storage in glomeruli (see detail in **c**) and prominent tubular storage at the corticomedullary junction from storage in the Henle loop and collecting tubules. Cortical tubules are free of storage. (**b**) Medullary tubules with advanced stages of storage and desquamation of lipid loaded epithelia, which then pass into the urine and are responsible for liquid lipid crystals detectable either by birefringence (insert) or biochemically in the urinary sediment. (**c**) demonstrate prominent lipid storage in the glomerulus (PAS staining, frozen section); (**d**) paucity of autofluorescent ceroid (paraffin unstained section) in storage podocytes. (magn. **b** 2,000×, obj. **c, d** 40×)

Studies of *nephron* storage distribution in Fabry disease have been reviewed [19]. Briefly, peak storage is in the collecting ducts and loops of Henle. In both parts, expression is frequently variable, sometimes being expressed in only individual cells. Part of the tubular pathology shows signs of regeneration, suggesting increased cell turnover. Storage in the proximal part has been only rarely reported. It should be stressed that this part of the nephron is generally resistant to storage in other lysosomal storage disorders affecting the kidney, the only exception being disorders affecting the lysosomal organelle related system (quoted in Elleder [26]).

Renal tubular dysfunction in Fabry disease has been described in the past [126], but has never attracted much attention. Nevertheless, tubular dysfunction has been described as dominating the early clinical course [127, 128]. Our recent study showed, for the first time, a biochemically defined change in the uromodulin producing segment of the nephron in FD and its positive response to enzyme replacement therapy [19].

All studies on the effect of ERT on kidney status in FD should explain: (i) if the enzyme passes through the glomerular basement membrane and is endocytosed across the apical pole of the tubular epithelium, (ii) or is taken up by the basal epithelial pole after unhindered free passage through the glomerular capillaries, (iii) if the applied enzyme is present in the urine and (iv) if it can degrade Gb3 after its release into the urine.

Urine in FD serves as important diagnostic sample of stored lipids [129] released from the desquamated storage epithelium (Fig. 3.16b).

3.4.5 Neuropathology

Clinically, the neurology of a-Gal deficiency is characterized by a tendency toward transient ischemic attacks and strokes at younger ages, and by peripheral nervous system dysfunction (peripheral sensitive and autonomic neuropathies). Both males and females are affected [130–132].

In terms of neuropathology, the neuronal system displays differential expression of storage in a-Gal deficiency. There are two extremes: one extreme being represented by the system of peripheral neurons in autonomic ganglia, which regularly display a high degree of storage (Fig. 3.6e) irrespective of the tissue; the same is true of neurons in posterior root ganglia [133, 134]. Storage in perineurial cells is found regularly (Section 3.3, Fig. 3.6f, g), the functional consequences of this is unknown. Well-known sensory neuropathy is related to abnormal discharges producing pain via storage-affected dorsal root neurons [135]. This correlates well with findings of exclusive, massive storage in dorsal root ganglia [133]. Sensory neuropathy is often combined with hypo- or anhidrosis and is explained by degeneration of small myelinated and unmyelinated nerve fibers and of small neurons in the affected dorsal root ganglia [133, 134]. Electrophysiological studies in a large cohort of FD patients showed higher vulnerability of small-diameter nerve fibers than of thickly myelinated fibers [136]. Loss of large myelinated nerve fibers and segmental demyelination were described without sensory neuropathy [137]. Anhidrosis has been linked to storage in sweat glands [138, 139], but it was present even in the absence of storage in sweat glands [140].

The other extreme is represented by cerebral and cerebellar cortical neurons, which have been repeatedly described as free of lysosomal storage. In other brain regions neuronal storage has been observed, albeit with a different expression [45, 54, 140–144]. Exact evaluation of the neurolysosomal storage must take into account high tendency to ceroid accumulation (Section 3.2.1.3) and distinguish it from lipid storage. The latter can be demonstrated using sensitive immunohistochemical detection [47]. There are reports of axonopathic leukoencephalopathy, probably of ischemic origin [54] With regard to retinal neurons, electron microscopy has failed to detect storage [145].

It is fair to conclude that neuronal involvement does not have a recognizable clinical correlate. It is generally accepted that most cerebral damage is of a vascular origin (Section 3.4.1) The only altered structure presently considered responsible

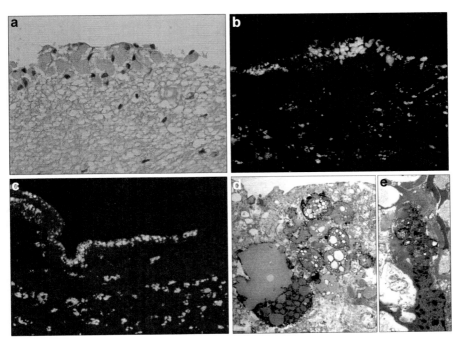

Fig. 3.17 Brain. (**a**) Ependym lining IIIrd ventricle. HE staining. Focal aggregation of highly granulated cells poor in cilia corresponding to tanycytes. The granules correspond to ceroid demonstrated by intensive autofluorescence either in both focally aggregated (**b**) and linearly arranged foci of ependymal cells (**c**) and in many subependymal cells. (**d, e**) Ultrastructure corresponds to large pleiomorphic lysosomal residual bodies free of recognizable lipid membranes (obj. **a** 40×, **b, c** 20×, magn. **d** 4,000×, **e** 4,500×)

for the neurology in a-Gal deficiency is therefore angiopathy with evidence of a genetic predisposition [146], and a possible pathogenic relationship to blood myeloperoxidase levels [147].

Beside neurons, storage has been described in *ependyme and in subependymal astrocytes* in certain regions [47] or in subependymal astrocytes only [140, 148, 149]. We observed (unpublished) mosaic type storage in the ependyme (tanycytes) and in nearby subependymal regions in an adult patient; storage was characterized by excessive lipofuscin accumulation (see Section 3.2) with questionable lipid storage (Fig. 3.17). This suggests a relationship to the system of adult neural stem cells [150].

Leptomeningeal storage. Leptomeningeal structures have received very little attention to date. Our studies have shown a constant presence of high degrees of storage in arachnothelial cells [151] (Fig. 3.18). Storage in arachnothelial cells has been described repeatedly in the past [142, 149, 152, 153]. These finding may explain signs of leptomeningeal irritation in FD.

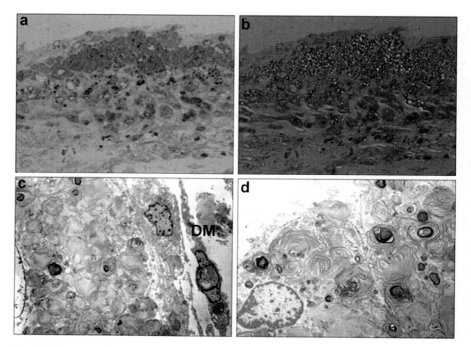

Fig. 3.18 Leptomeninx. Prominent storage in arachnotel. (**a, b**) semithin section stained with Toluidine blue; (**b**) the same section showing prominent birefringence of the stored lipid. 9**c, d**) ultrastructure of the arachnothelial cells; DM dura mater face (obj. **a, b** 40×, magn. **c** 2,000×, **d** 4,000×)

3.4.6 Pathology of the Lung

Clinically there are frequent symptoms of chronic airflow obstruction [38, 154–156]. The pathologic basis of lung dysfunction is predominantly due to storage

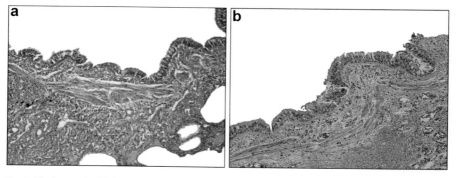

Fig. 3.19 Lung: (**a, b**) bronchial smooth muscle layer thicker in FD (**a**) than in controls (**b**) HE (obj. 20×)

in bronchial SMC (see Section 3.3) with a tendency toward storage-induced hypertrophy (Fig. 3.19). Respiratory epithelium (both ciliary and mucinous) express lysosomal storage (see Section 3.2). Bronchial vegetative neurons display prominent storage as part of the general involvement of the autonomic nervous system. Nerve fibers display storage in the perineurium (Section 3.4.5). We have seen storage in parts of the bronchial chondrocyte population as well (Fig. 3.7f). There is also an indication that type II pneumocytes belong on the list of storage-affected cells [41]. Storage in the pulmonary vasculature, in both pulmonary and bronchial arteries and veins, is identical to storage in extrapulmonary vessels (i.e. endothelium and medial SMC storage).

Regarding storage in pulmonary capillary endothelium, reports on this subject are extremely rare and incomplete. A single storage lysosome in a capillary has been reported [41]. Smith et al. described storage in pulmonary vessels but without specifying if alveolar capillaries were involved [157]. An unpublished study of the author showed an absence of storage in capillary endothelial cells in two cases of FD, one hemizygote, one heterozygote (Fig. 3.20). This points to absence of lysosomal turnover of α galactose-sphingolipid conjugates. Absence of alveolar EC storage corresponds to absence of any signs of altered alveocapillary gas exchange in FD patients.

The author is not aware of any reports on the microstructure of the bronchial endocrine system.

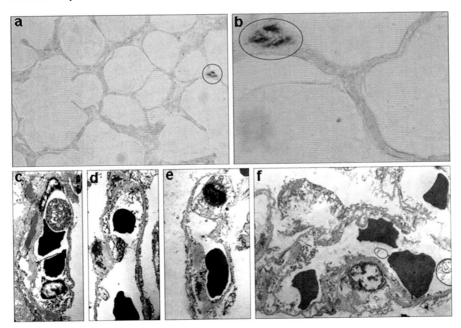

Fig. 3.20 Lung alveolar area. Hemizygous FD. (**a, b**) frozen section stained with PAS showing staining restricted to larger arterioles (encircled areas), alveolar capillaries are negative; (**c–f**) absence of storage in alveolar capillaries in electron microscope. (obj. **a** 10×, **b** 40×, magn. **c** 1,500×, **d** 1,000×, **e, f** 3,000×)

3.4.7 Pathology of the Gastrointestinal System

Liver storage is of a low degree and is manifested in hepatocytes (Fig. 3.21e). Storage in Kupffer cells is present but not excessive. Sinusoidal endothelium is generally free of storage [26, 46, 158, 159]. Low storage degree is seen in

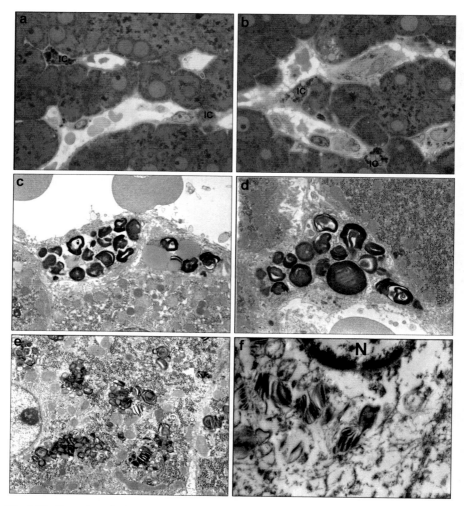

Fig. 3.21 Gastrointestinal tract. Liver. (**a–d**) Storage in Ito cells. (**a, b**) standard semithin sections stained with Toluidine blue. Ito cells are marked IC. Note indirect proportion between constitutional lipid droplets (lucent vacuoles) and storage lysosomes (deep blue granules). (**c, d**) Ultrastructural correlate of storing Ito cells with residual lipid droplets (**c**) or free of them (**d**). (**e**) Storage in hepatocytes in untreated male patient; (**f**) epithelial cell of portal bile ductule with discrete apical storage lysosomes. N nucleus (**a, b** oil immersion obj. 100×; **c, d** magn. 3,000×, **e** 4,000×, **f** 10,000×)

portal cholangioles (Fig. 3.21f). Variable degree of storage, indirectly proportional to accumulation of constitutional apolar lipid droplets, was seen in Ito cells [160] (Fig. 3.21a–d). This suggests tendency to partial depletion of carotenoids. Storage-based hepatopathy has never been described in FD.

Altered GIT function is now considered to be an integral part of the clinical picture in FD [161, 162]. Severe small and large bowel involvements have been described [163] with structural changes that are apparent on radiographs [164]. For further information see Kenshav [165].

Impaired autonomic function is considered to be responsible for GIT dysfunction [35]. This is supported by storage involvement of the intestinal neural system, which has been repeatedly described, and the SMC in the muscular layers [41, 166–168]. There is no evidence of storage in the peripheral endocrine system [41]. However, so far, no systematic search has been done. The author observed storage (unpublished) in the endocrine cells of the gastric mucosa (Fig. 3.22b). Similarly nothing is known about possible storage involvement of the rich lymphatic network in the gut, despite frequent reports of serious involvement of the dermal lymphatic vessels (see Section 3.4.1). FD has also numerous oral and craniofacial manifestations [43].

Pancreas. Involvement of the exocrine pancreas has been described repeatedly using EM but without any signs of pancreatic dysfunction [144]; in some cases even negative findings were reported [169]. It is again worth noting the report which described the accumulation of blood group B glycolipid, in addition to Gb3 and digalactosylceramide, in the pancreas (but not in other solid organs) of a patient with Fabry disease and type B blood [3]. We had an identical (unpublished) observation in an adult male patient, blood group B secretor (Fig. 3.22a). Therefore, pancreatic dysfunction might contribute to gastrointestinal dysfunction in Fabry patients. Positive responses to pancreatin [162] speak in favor of this.

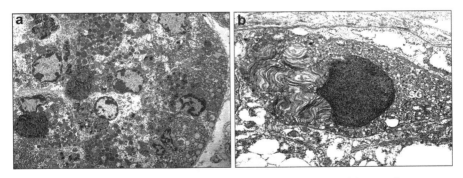

Fig. 3.22 (**a**) prominent storage in the secretory and centroacinar cells of the exocrine pancreas in a patient with B blood group (secretor). Lipid storage is accompanied by massive ceroid accumulation (1,000×). (**b**) Incidental observation in a gastric biopsy showing storage in an endocrine cell of the gastric mucosa (SG marks secretory granules – *middle right*) (5,000×)

3.4.8 Pathology of the Senses

3.4.8.1 Cochleovestibular Apparatus

Hearing loss is a frequent phenomenon in FD [170, 171]. Structural studies of the Corti apparatus are represented by a single report on histology, which showed degeneration with partial hair cell loss and reduction in the number of spiral ganglion cells [172]. No signs of lysosomal storage were reported. Generally the mechanism responsible is believed to be of vascular origin [173–175]. The vestibular apparatus, also frequently reported be involved [176, 177], did not display any pathology suggestive of lysosomal involvement [172]. Histology of the inner ear in the mouse model was found to be normal [178]. It is worth mentioning that the apical regions of vestibular hair cells type II and inner and outer hair cells in the organ of Corti are rich in lysosomes. Their involvement in lysosomal storage disorder is different [179–182]. In the mouse model for FD, neither functional nor histological differences were found [178].

3.4.8.2 Ocular Pathology

Storage in the eye is dominated by macroscopically defined whorl-like corneal opacities (cornea verticillata) and cataracts. Lysosomal storage is expressed in the corneal epithelium, which is maximal in the basal epithelial layer [36, 42, 145, 183–187] and has also been confirmed by in vivo confocal microscopy [188, 189]. Storage in the corneal epithelium is sometimes associated with a focal subepithelial ridge formed by a reduplicated Bowman's membrane (BM) containing amorphous dense material [187]. Changes in the BM have been either clearly identified [145, 183, 185, 189, 190] or not found at all [42, 183, 185, 186]. Changes at the level of the BM do not correlate with changes in the cornea verticillata and therefore cannot be considered to be responsible [185]. Storage in keratocytes has been found to be both present [36] and absent [42, 186, 187]. No storage has been observed in the corneal endothelium [187].

In the *ocular lens* storage is expressed in the *lens epithelium* but not in the lens fibers [36, 184]. The author confirms absence of structurally definable lipid storage in lens fibres (unpublished). Situation in the ocular lens can thus be summarized as presence of lysosomal storage in capsular epithelium representing the stem cell layer and its disappearance during the process of programmed profound simplification of the epithelial lens cytoplasm [191] within each clone (loss of nucleus and decompartmentalization of the cytoplasm without any loss of viability). It is reasonable to suppose the storage lipid must get into contact with the cytosolic compartment and probably interfere with its physical properties.

Conjunctival epithelium has been repeatedly described as expressing storage [42, 183, 192].

Storage has been observed in the pigmented epithelium of the iris and in the pigmented epithelium of the retina, but not in retinal neurons [145, 184]. Storage in the ocular vasculature is always present.

Acknowledgement Bulk of the studies was supported by a research project of the Ministry of Education Youth and Sports (Grant No. MSM 0021620806). Technical assistance in manuscript preparation by Eva Horáková, perfect laboratory work of Irena Knesplová, Marie Kolářová and Lenka Kryšpinová and are greatly appreciated. The author thanks also to Dr. Tom Secrest for language text editation

References

1. Maloney MD, Lingwood CA (1994) CD19 has a potential CD77 (globotriaosyl ceramide)-binding site with sequence similarity to verotoxin B-subunits: implications of molecular mimicry for B cell adhesion and enterohemorrhagic Escherichia coli pathogenesis. J Exp Med 180(1):191–201
2. Ledvinova J, Poupetova H, Hanackova A, Pisacka M, Elleder M (1997) Blood group B glycosphingolipids in alpha-galactosidase deficiency (Fabry disease): influence of secretor status. Biochim Biophys Acta 1345(2):180–187
3. Wherrett JR, Hakomori SI (1973) Characterization of a blood group B glycolipid, accumulating in the pancreas of a patient with Fabry's disease. J Biol Chem 248(9):3046–3051
4. Linthorst GE, Folman CC, Aerts JM, Hollak CE (2003) Blood group does not correlate with disease severity in patients with Fabry disease (alpha-galactosidase A deficiency). Blood Cells Mol Dis 31(3):324–326
5. Bodary PF, Shayman JA, Eitzman DT (2007) Alpha-galactosidase A in vascular disease. Trends Cardiovasc Med 17(4):129–133
6. Desnick RJ, Ioannou YA, Eng CM (2001) α-galactosidase A deficiency: Fabry disease. In: Scriver CR, Beaudet AL, Sly WS, Valle D (eds) The metabolic and molecular bases of inherited disease, 8th edn. McGraw-Hill, New York, pp 3733–3774
7. Cuervo AM (2004) Autophagy: many paths to the same end. Mol Cell Biochem 263(1–2):55–72
8. Maxfield FR, McGraw TE (2004) Endocytic recycling. Nat Rev Mol Cell Biol 5(2):121–132
9. Kanda A, Nakao S, Tsuyama S, Murata F, Kanzaki T (2000) Fabry disease: ultrastructural lectin histochemical analyses of lysosomal deposits. Virchows Arch 436(1):36–42
10. Zeidner KM, Desnick RJ, Ioannou YA (1999) Quantitative determination of globotriaosylceramide by immunodetection of glycolipid-bound recombinant verotoxin B subunit. Anal Biochem 267(1):104–113
11. Keslova-Veselikova J, Hulkova H, Dobrovolny R et al (2008) Replacement of alpha-galactosidase A in Fabry disease: effect on fibroblast cultures compared with biopsied tissues of treated patients. Virchows Arch 452(6):651–665
12. Dvorak AM, Cable WJ, Osage JE, Kolodny EH (1981) Diagnostic electron microscopy. II. Fabrys disease: use of biopsies from uninvolved skin. Acute and chronic changes involving the microvasculature and small unmyelinated nerves. In: Summers SC, Rosen PP (eds) Pathology annual. Appleton-Century-Crofts, New York, pp 139–158
13. Elleder M, Ledvinova J, Vosmik F, Zeman J, Stejskal D, Lageron A (1990) An atypical ultrastructural pattern in Fabry's disease: a study on its nature and incidence in 7 cases. Ultrastruct Pathol 14(6):467–474
14. Seehafer SS, Pearce DA (2006) You say lipofuscin, we say ceroid: defining autofluorescent storage material. Neurobiol Aging 27(4):576–588
15. Zhang M, Sun M, Dwyer NK et al (2003) Differential trafficking of the Niemann-Pick C1 and 2 proteins highlights distinct roles in late endocytic lipid trafficking. Acta Paediatr Suppl 92(443):63–73, discussion 45
16. Simon M, Frey H, Gruler H, Bultmann B (1990) Glycolipid storage material in Fabry's disease: a study by electron microscopy, freeze-fracture, and digital image analysis. J Struct Biol 103(1):40–47

17. Shen JS, Meng XL, Moore DF et al (2008) Globotriaosylceramide induces oxidative stress and up-regulates cell adhesion molecule expression in Fabry disease endothelial cells. Mol Genet Metab 95(3):163–168
18. Lucke T, Hoppner W, Schmidt E, Illsinger S, Das AM (2004) Fabry disease: reduced activities of respiratory chain enzymes with decreased levels of energy-rich phosphates in fibroblasts. Mol Genet Metab 82(1):93–97
19. Vylet'al P, Hulkova H, Zivna M et al (2008) Abnormal expression and processing of uromodulin in Fabry disease reflects tubular cell storage alteration and is reversible by enzyme replacement therapy. J Inherit Metab Dis 31(4):508–517
20. Shu L, Shayman JA (2007) Caveolin-associated accumulation of globotriaosylceramide in the vascular endothelium of alpha-galactosidase A null mice. J Biol Chem 282(29): 20960–20967
21. Thomaidis T, Relle M, Golbas M et al (2009) Downregulation of alpha-galactosidase A upregulates CD77: functional impact for Fabry nephropathy. Kidney Int 75(4):399–407
22. Elleder M, Stejskal J (1985) Induction of dipeptidylpeptidase IV activity in human renal glomeruli–a histochemical study. Acta Histochem 77(1):75–78
23. Settembre C, Fraldi A, Jahreiss L et al (2008) A block of autophagy in lysosomal storage disorders. Hum Mol Genet 17(1):119–129
24. Aerts JM, Groener JE, Kuiper S et al (2008) Elevated globotriaosylsphingosine is a hallmark of Fabry disease. Proc Natl Acad Sci USA 105(8):2812–2817
25. Ohshima T, Murray GJ, Swaim WD et al (1997) Alpha-Galactosidase A deficient mice: a model of Fabry disease. Proc Natl Acad Sci USA 94(6):2540–2544
26. Elleder M (2003) Sequelae of storage in Fabry disease–pathology and comparison with other lysosomal storage diseases. Acta Paediatr Suppl 92(443):46–53, discussion 45
27. Utsumi K, Yamamoto N, Kase R et al (1997) High incidence of thrombosis in Fabry's disease. Intern Med 36(5):327–329
28. Heare T, Alp NJ, Priestman DA et al (2007) Severe endothelial dysfunction in the aorta of a mouse model of Fabry disease; partial prevention by N-butyldeoxynojirimycin treatment. J Inherit Metab Dis 30(1):79–87
29. Park JL, Whitesall SE, D'Alecy LG, Shu L, Shayman JA (2008) Vascular dysfunction in the alpha-galactosidase A-knockout mouse is an endothelial cell-, plasma membrane-based defect. Clin Exp Pharmacol Physiol 35(10):1156–1163
30. Gelderman MP, Schiffmann R, Simak J (2007) Elevated endothelial microparticles in Fabry children decreased after enzyme replacement therapy. Arterioscler Thromb Vasc Biol 27(7):e138
31. Vedder AC, Biro E, Aerts JM, Nieuwland R, Sturk G, Hollak CE (2009) Plasma markers of coagulation and endothelial activation in Fabry disease: impact of renal impairment. Nephrol Dial Transplant 24(10):3074–3081
32. Elleder M (1994) The spleen and storage disorders. In: Cuschieri A, Forbes CD (eds) Disorders of the spleen, 1st edn. Blackwell Scientific Publications, Oxford, pp 151–190
33. Armulik A, Abramsson A, Betsholtz C (2005) Endothelial/pericyte interactions. Circ Res 97(6):512–523
34. Pavenstadt H, Kriz W, Kretzler M (2003) Cell biology of the glomerular podocyte. Physiol Rev 83(1):253–307
35. Cable WJ, Kolodny EH, Adams RD (1982) Fabry disease: impaired autonomic function. Neurology 32(5):498–502
36. Witschel H, Mathyl J (1969) Morphological bases of the specific ocular changes in Fabry's disease. Klin Monatsbl Augenheilkd 154(4):599–605
37. Kelly MM, Leigh R, McKenzie R, Kamada D, Ramsdale EH, Hargreave FE (2000) Induced sputum examination: diagnosis of pulmonary involvement in Fabry's disease. Thorax 55(8):720–721
38. Rosenberg DM, Ferrans VJ, Fulmer JD et al (1980) Chronic airflow obstruction in Fabry's disease. Am J Med 68(6):898–905

39. Nistal M, Paniagua R, Picazo ML (1983) Testicular and epididymal involvement in Fabry's disease. J Pathol 141(2):113–124
40. Kaesgen U, Goebel HH (1989) Intraepidermal morphologic manifestations in lysosomal diseases. Brain Dev 11(5):338–341
41. Bagdade JD, Parker F, Ways PO, Morgan TE, Lagunoff D, Eidelman S (1968) Fabry's disease. A correlative clinical, morphologic, and biochemical study. Lab Invest 18(6): 681–688
42. McCulloch C, Ghosh M (1984) Ultrastructural changes in the cornea and conjunctiva of aheterozygous woman with Fabry's disease. Can J Ophthalmol 19(4):192–198
43. Baccaglini L, Schiffmann R, Brennan MT, Lancaster HE Jr, Kulkarni AB, Brahim JS (2001) Oral and craniofacial findings in Fabry's disease: a report of 13 patients. Oral Surg Oral Med Oral Pathol Oral Radiol Endod 92(4):415–419
44. Tsukada N, Hanu N, Oguchi K, Yanagisawa N, Tsukagoshi H, Hattori H (1980) Fabry's disease with malocclusion and acromegalic-appearance: clinical and electromicroscopic studies (author's transl). No To Shinkei 32(3):311–319
45. Takao M, Mori T, Orikasa H et al (2007) Postmortem diagnosis of Fabry disease with acromegaly and a unique vasculopathy. Virchows Arch 451(3):721–727
46. Faraggiana T, Churg J, Grishman E et al (1981) Light- and electron-microscopic histochemistry of Fabry's disease. Am J Pathol 103(2):247–262
47. deVeber GA, Schwarting GA, Kolodny EH, Kowall NW (1992) Fabry disease: immunocytochemical characterization of neuronal involvement. Ann Neurol 31(4):409–415
48. Witschel H, Meyer W (1968) Fabry's diseae. Clinical and pathologic studies of a clinical case. Klin Wochenschr 46(6):305–311
49. Tome FM, Fardeau M, Lenoir G (1977) Ultrastructure of muscle and sensory nerve in Fabry's disease. Acta Neuropathol 38(3):187–194
50. Barba Romero M-A, Medrano Gonzales F, Gomez Garrido J, Gomez Merino E, Perez Martinez J, Blazquez Cabrera JA (2003) Fabry disease: exceptional cause of rhabdomyolysis? Acta Paediatr Suppl 443:101–102
51. Vedder AC, Cox-Brinkman J, Hollak CE et al (2006) Plasma chitotriosidase in male Fabry patients: a marker for monitoring lipid-laden macrophages and their correction by enzyme replacement therapy. Mol Genet Metab 89(3):239–244
52. Mayou SC, Kirby JD, Morgan SH (1989) Anderson-Fabry disease: an unusual presentation with lymphadenopathy. J R Soc Med 82(9):555–556
53. Garzuly F, Marodi L, Erdos M et al (2005) Megadolichobasilar anomaly with thrombosis in a family with Fabry's disease and a novel mutation in the alpha-galactosidase A gene. Brain 128(Pt 9):2078–2083
54. Okeda R, Nisihara M (2008) An autopsy case of Fabry disease with neuropathological investigation of the pathogenesis of associated dementia. Neuropathology 28(5): 532–540
55. Barbey F, Brakch N, Linhart A et al (2006) Cardiac and vascular hypertrophy in Fabry disease: evidence for a new mechanism independent of blood pressure and glycosphingolipid deposition. Arterioscler Thromb Vasc Biol 26(4):839–844
56. Boutouyrie P, Laurent S, Laloux B, Lidove O, Grunfeld JP, Germain DP (2002) Arterial remodelling in Fabry disease. Acta Paediatr Suppl 91(439):62–66
57. Kalliokoski RJ, Kalliokoski KK, Penttinen M et al (2006) Structural and functional changes in peripheral vasculature of Fabry patients. J Inherit Metab Dis 29(5):660–666
58. Moore DF, Altarescu G, Pursley R et al (2002) Arterial wall properties and Womersley flow in Fabry disease. BMC Cardiovasc Disord 2:1
59. Kentish JC, Ward JPT (2008) Smooth muscle and the cardiovascular and lymphatic systems. In: Standring S (ed) Grays anatomy the anatomical basis of clinical practice. Elsevier, London, pp 127–144
60. Altarescu G, Moore DF, Pursley R et al (2001) Enhanced endothelium-dependent vasodilation in Fabry disease. Stroke 32(7):1559–1562

61. Hilz MJ, Kolodny EH, Brys M, Stemper B, Haendl T, Marthol H (2004) Reduced cerebral blood flow velocity and impaired cerebral autoregulation in patients with Fabry disease. J Neurol 251(5):564–570

62. Kalliokoski RJ, Kalliokoski KK, Sundell J et al (2005) Impaired myocardial perfusion reserve but preserved peripheral endothelial function in patients with Fabry disease. J Inherit Metab Dis 28(4):563–573

63. Moore DF, Scott LT, Gladwin MT et al (2001) Regional cerebral hyperperfusion and nitric oxide pathway dysregulation in Fabry disease: reversal by enzyme replacement therapy. Circulation 104(13):1506–1512

64. Ogawa T, Kawai M, Matsui T et al (1996) Vasospastic angina in a patient with Fabry's disease who showed normal coronary angiographic findings. Jpn Circ J 60(5):315–318

65. Seino Y, Vyden JK, Philippart M, Rose HB, Nagasawa K (1983) Peripheral hemodynamics in patients with Fabry's disease. Am Heart J 105(5):783–787

66. Stemper B, Hilz MJ (2003) Postischemic cutaneous hyperperfusion in the presence of forearm hypoperfusion suggests sympathetic vasomotor dysfunction in Fabry disease. J Neurol 250(8):970–976

67. Moore DF, Kaneski CR, Askari H, Schiffmann R (2007) The cerebral vasculopathy of Fabry disease. J Neurol Sci 257(1–2):258–263

68. Shirai T, Ohtake T, Kimura M et al (2000) Atypical Fabry's disease presenting with cholesterol crystal embolization. Intern Med 39(8):646–649

69. Schiffmann R, Rapkiewicz A, Abu-Asab M et al (2006) Pathological findings in a patient with Fabry disease who died after 2.5 years of enzyme replacement. Virchows Arch 448(3):337–343

70. Vedder AC, Gerdes VE, Poorthuis BJ et al (2007) Failure to detect Fabry patients in a cohort of prematurely atherosclerotic males. J Inherit Metab Dis 30(6):988

71. Jardine DL, Fitzpatrick MA, Troughton WD, Tie AB (1994) Small bowel ischaemia in Fabry's disease. J Gastroenterol Hepatol 9(2):201–204

72. Fisher EA, Desnick RJ, Gordon RE, Eng CM, Griepp R, Goldman ME (1992) Fabry disease: an unusual cause of severe coronary disease in a young man. Ann Intern Med 117(3):221–223

73. Orteu CH, Jansen T, Lidove O et al (2007) Fabry disease and the skin: data from FOS, the Fabry outcome survey. Br J Dermatol 157(2):331–337

74. Amann-Vesti BR, Gitzelmann G, Widmer U, Bosshard NU, Steinmann B, Koppensteiner R (2003) Severe lymphatic microangiopathy in Fabry disease. Lymphat Res Biol 1(3):185–189

75. Wallace RD, Cooper WJ (1965) Angiokeratoma corporis diffusum universale (Fabry). Am J Med 39(4):656–661

76. Le Bodic MF, Le Bodic L, Buzelin F, Bureau B, Mussini-Montpellier J (1978) Vascular lesions of Fabry's disease. Optical, histochemical and ultrastructural studies. Ann Anat Pathol (Paris) 23(1):23–39

77. Kang WH, Chun SI, Lee S (1987) Generalized anhidrosis associated with Fabry's disease. J Am Acad Dermatol 17(5 Pt 2):883–887

78. Lao LM, Kumakiri M, Mima H et al (1998) The ultrastructural characteristics of eccrine sweat glands in a Fabry disease patient with hypohidrosis. J Dermatol Sci 18(2):109–117

79. Nakamura T, Kaneko H, Nishino I (1981) Angiokeratoma corporis diffusum (Fabry disease): ultrastructural studies of the skin. Acta Derm Venereol 61(1):37–41

80. Idoate MA, Pardo-Mindan FJ, Gonzalez Alamillo C (1992) Fabry's disease without angiokeratomas showing unusual eccrine gland vacuolation. J Pathol 167(1):65–68

81. Lidove O, Ramaswami U, Jaussaud R et al (2006) Hyperhidrosis: a new and often early symptom in Fabry disease. International experience and data from the Fabry Outcome Survey. Int J Clin Pract 60(9):1053–1059

82. Clarke JT, Knaack J, Crawhall JC, Wolfe LS (1971) Ceramide trihexosidosis (Fabry's disease) without skin lesions. N Engl J Med 284(5):233–235

83. Kanekura T, Fukushige T, Kanda A et al (2005) Immunoelectron-microscopic detection of globotriaosylceramide accumulated in the skin of patients with Fabry disease. Br J Dermatol 153(3):544–548

84. Kanitakis J, Allombert C, Doebelin B et al (2005) Fucosidosis with angiokeratoma. Immunohistochemical & electronmicroscopic study of a new case and literature review. J Cutan Pathol 32(7):506–511

85. Braverman IM, Ken-Yen A (1983) Ultrastructure and three-dimensional reconstruction of several macular and papular telangiectases. J Invest Dermatol 81(6):489–497

86. Kelly B, Kelly E (2006) Angiokeratoma corporis diffusum in a patient with no recognizable enzyme abnormalities. Arch Dermatol 142(5):615–618

87. Burda CD, Winder PR (1967) Angiokeratoma corporis diffusum universale (Fabry's disease) in female subjects. Am J Med 42(2):293–301

88. Handa Y, Yotsumoto S, Isobe E et al (2000) A case of symptomatic heterozygous female-Fabry's disease without detectable mutation in the alpha-galactosidase gene. Dermatology 200(3):262–265

89. Morais P, Santos AL, Baudrier T, Mota AV, Oliveira JP, Azevedo F (2008) Angiokeratomas of Fabry successfully treated with intense pulsed light. J Cosmet Laser Ther 10(4):218–222

90. Voglino A, Paradisi M, Dompe G, Onetti Muda A, Faraggiana T (1988) Angiokeratoma corporis diffusum (Fabry's disease) with unusual features in a female patient. Light-and electron-microscopic investigation. Am J Dermatopathol 10(4):343–348

91. Barile L, Messina E, Giacomello A, Marban E (2007) Endogenous cardiac stem cells. Prog Cardiovasc Dis 50(1):31–48

92. Liu J, Sluijter JP, Goumans MJ et al (2009) Cell therapy for myocardial regeneration. Curr Mol Med 9(3):287–298

93. Thijssen DH, Torella D, Hopman MT, Ellison GM (2009) The role of endothelial progenitor and cardiac stem cells in the cardiovascular adaptations to age and exercise. Front Biosci 14:4685–4702

94. Gilbert-Barness E (2004) Review: metabolic cardiomyopathy and conduction system defects in children. Ann Clin Lab Sci 34(1):15–34

95. Elleder M, Bradova V, Smid F et al (1990) Cardiocyte storage and hypertrophy as a sole manifestation of Fabry's disease. Report on a case simulating hypertrophic non-obstructive cardiomyopathy. Virchows Arch A Pathol Anat Histopathol 417(5):449–455

96. Chimenti C, Hamdani N, Boontje NM et al (2008) Myofilament degradation and dysfunction of human cardiomyocytes in Fabry disease. Am J Pathol 172(6):1482–1490

97. Davies MJ (1984) The cardiomyopathies: a review of terminology, pathology and pathogenesis. Histopathology 8(3):363–393

98. Sheppard MN, Cane P, Florio R et al (2009) A detailed pathologic examination of heart tissue from three older patients with Anderson-Fabry disease on enzyme replacement therapy. Cardiovasc Pathol

99. Bishop JE, Laurent GJ (1995) Collagen turnover and its regulation in the normal and hypertrophying heart. Eur Heart J 16(Suppl C):38–44

100. Pelouch V, Dixon IM, Golfman L, Beamish RE, Dhalla NS (1993) Role of extracellular matrix proteins in heart function. Mol Cell Biochem 129(2):101–120

101. Weber KT, Sun Y, Tyagi SC, Cleutjens JP (1994) Collagen network of the myocardium: function, structural remodeling and regulatory mechanisms. J Mol Cell Cardiol 26(3):279–292

102. Ikeda K, Tojo K, Udagawa T et al (2008) Cellular physiology of rat cardiac myocytes in cardiac fibrosis: in vitro simulation using the cardiac myocyte/cardiac non-myocyte co-culture system. Hypertens Res 31(4):693–706

103. Kawano M, Takenaka T, Otsuji Y et al (2007) Significance of asymmetric basal posterior wall thinning in patients with cardiac Fabry's disease. Am J Cardiol 99(2):261–263

104. Moon JC, Sachdev B, Elkington AG et al (2003) Gadolinium enhanced cardiovascular magnetic resonance in Anderson-Fabry disease. Evidence for a disease specific abnormality of the myocardial interstitium. Eur Heart J 24(23):2151–2155

105. Moon JC, Sheppard M, Reed E, Lee P, Elliott PM, Pennell DJ (2006) The histological basis of late gadolinium enhancement cardiovascular magnetic resonance in a patient with Anderson-Fabry disease. J Cardiovasc Magn Reson 8(3):479–482

106. Linhart A, Kampmann C, Zamorano JL et al (2007) Cardiac manifestations of Anderson-Fabry disease: results from the international Fabry outcome survey. Eur Heart J 28(10):1228–1235

107. Bannwart F (1982) Fabry's disease. Light and electron microscopic cardiac findings 12 years after successful kidney transplantation. Schweiz Med Wochenschr 112(48):1742–1747

108. Becker AE, Schoorl R, Balk AG, van der Heide RM (1975) Cardiac manifestations of Fabry's disease. Report of a case with mitral insufficiency and electrocardiographic evidence of myocardial infarction. Am J Cardiol 36(6):829–835

109. Ikari Y, Kuwako K, Yamaguchi T (1992) Fabry's disease with complete atrioventricular block: histological evidence of involvement of the conduction system. Br Heart J 68(3):323–325

110. Rumyantsev PP, Erokhina IL, Antipanova EM, Martynova MG (1990) DNA and sex chromatin content in nuclei of conductive system and working myocytes of normal and hypertrophied human heart. Acta Histochem Suppl 39:225–237

111. Matsui S, Murakami E, Takekoshi N, Hiramaru Y, Kin T (1977) Cardiac manifestations of Fabry's disease. Report of a case with pulmonary regurgitation diagnosed on the basis of endomyocardial biopsy findings. Jpn Circ J 41(9):1023–1036

112. Choi S, Seo H, Park M et al (2009) Fabry disease with aortic regurgitation. Ann Thorac Surg 87(2):625–628

113. Leder AA, Bosworth WC (1965) Angiokeratoma Corporis Diffusum Universale (Fabry's Disease) with Mitral Stenosis. Am J Med 38:814–819

114. Desnick RJ, Blieden LC, Sharp HL, Hofschire PJ, Moller JH (1976) Cardiac valvular anomalies in Fabry disease. Clinical, morphologic, and biochemical studies. Circulation 54(5):818–825

115. Ferrans VJ, Hibbs RG, Burda CD (1969) The heart in Fabry's disease. A histochemical and electron microscopic study. Am J Cardiol 24(1):95–110

116. Bass JL, Shrivastava S, Grabowski GA, Desnick RJ, Moller JH (1980) The M-mode echocardiogram in Fabry's disease. Am Heart J 100(6 Pt 1):807–812

117. Goldman ME, Cantor R, Schwartz MF, Baker M, Desnick RJ (1986) Echocardiographic abnormalities and disease severity in Fabry's disease. J Am Coll Cardiol 7(5):1157–1161

118. Chimenti C, Pieroni M, Morgante E et al (2004) Prevalence of Fabry disease in female patients with late-onset hypertrophic cardiomyopathy. Circulation 110(9):1047–1053

119. Ogawa K, Abe T, Yoshimura K, Nagashima K, Nagashima T (1985) Cardiac accumulation of trihexosylceramide in a case with amyotrophic lateral sclerosis. Jpn J Exp Med 55(3):123–127

120. von Scheidt W, Eng CM, Fitzmaurice TF et al (1991) An atypical variant of Fabry's disease with manifestations confined to the myocardium. N Engl J Med 324(6):395–399

121. Nakao S, Kodama C, Takenaka T et al (2003) Fabry disease: detection of undiagnosed hemodialysis patients and identification of a "renal variant" phenotype. Kidney Int 64(3):801–807

122. Alroy J, Sabnis S, Kopp JB (2002) Renal pathology in Fabry disease. J Am Soc Nephrol 13(Suppl 2):S134–S138

123. Gubler MC, Lenoir G, Grunfeld JP, Ulmann A, Droz D, Habib R (1978) Early renal changes in hemizygous and heterozygous patients with Fabry's disease. Kidney Int 13(3):223–235

124. Barisoni L, Schnaper HW, Kopp JB (2009) Advances in the biology and genetics of the podocytopathies: implications for diagnosis and therapy. Arch Pathol Lab Med 133(2):201–216

125. Fischer EG, Moore MJ, Lager DJ (2006) Fabry disease: a morphologic study of 11 cases. Mod Pathol 19(10):1295–1301

126. Pabico RC, Atancio BC, McKenna BA, Pamukcoglu T, Yodaiken R (1973) Renal pathologic lesions and functional alterations in a man with Fabry's disease. Am J Med 55(3):415–425

127. Parchoux B, Guibaud P, Maire I et al (1978) Fabry's disease. Initial nephrogenic diabetes insipidus in children. Pediatrie 33(8):757–765

128. Wornell P, Dyack S, Crocker J, Yu W, Acott P (2006) Fabry disease and nephrogenic diabetes insipidus. Pediatr Nephrol 21(8):1185–1188

129. Mills K, Morris P, Lee P et al (2005) Measurement of urinary CDH and CTH by tandem mass spectrometry in patients hemizygous and heterozygous for Fabry disease. J Inherit Metab Dis 28(1):35–48

130. Mitsias P, Levine SR (1996) Cerebrovascular complications of Fabry's disease. Ann Neurol 40(1):8–17

131. Nill M, Muller MJ, Beck M, Stoeter P, Fellgiebel A (2006) Pathophysiological aspects of brain structural disturbances in patients with Fabry disease: literature review. Fortschr Neurol Psychiatr 74(12):687–695

132. Fellgiebel A, Muller MJ, Ginsberg L (2006) CNS manifestations of Fabry's disease. Lancet Neurol 5(9):791–795

133. Gadoth N, Sandbank U (1983) Involvement of dorsal root ganglia in Fabry's disease. J Med Genet 20(4):309–312

134. Onishi A, Dyck PJ (1974) Loss of small peripheral sensory neurons in Fabry disease. Histologic and morphometric evaluation of cutaneous nerves, spinal ganglia, and posterior columns. Arch Neurol 31(2):120–127

135. Gemignani F, Marbini A, Bragaglia MM, Govoni E (1984) Pathological study of the sural nerve in Fabry's disease. Eur Neurol 23(3):173–181

136. Dutsch M, Marthol H, Stemper B, Brys M, Haendl T, Hilz MJ (2002) Small fiber dysfunction predominates in Fabry neuropathy. J Clin Neurophysiol 19(6):575–586

137. Vital A, Vital C, Maleville J (1984) Fabry's disease: an ultrastructural study of muscle and peripheral nerve. Clin Neuropathol 3(4):168–172

138. Fukuhara N, Suzuki M, Fujita N, Tsubaki T (1975) Fabry's disease on the mechanism of the peripheral nerve involvement. Acta Neuropathol 33(1):9–21

139. Cable WJ, Dvorak AM, Osage JE, Kolodny EH (1982) Fabry disease: significance of ultrastructural localization of lipid inclusions in dermal nerves. Neurology 32(4):347–353

140. Tabira T, Goto I, Kuroiwa Y, Kikuchi M (1974) Neuropathological and biochemical studies in Fabry's disease. Acta Neuropathol 30(4):345–354

141. Grunnet ML, Spilsbury PR (1973) The central nervous system in Fabry's disease. An ultrastructural study. Arch Neurol 28(4):231–234

142. Kaye EM, Kolodny EH, Logigian EL, Ullman MD (1988) Nervous system involvement in Fabry's disease: clinicopathological and biochemical correlation. Ann Neurol 23(5):505–509

143. Rahman AN, Lindenberg R (1963) The Neuropathology of hereditary dystopic lipidosis. Arch Neurol 9:373–385

144. Schibanoff JM, Kamoshita S, O'Brien JS (1969) Tissue distribution of glycosphingolipids in a case of Fabry's disease. J Lipid Res 10(5):515–520

145. Riegel EM, Pokorny KS, Friedman AH, Suhan J, Ritch RH, Desnick RJ (1982) Ocular pathology of Fabry's disease in a hemizygous male following renal transplantation. Surv Ophthalmol 26(5):247–252

146. Moore DF, Gelderman MP, Fuhrmann SR, Schiffmann R, Brady RO, Goldin E (2006) Fabry disease and vascular risk factors: future strategies for patient-based studies and the knockout murine model. Acta Paediatr Suppl 95(451):69–71

147. Kaneski CR, Moore DF, Ries M, Zirzow GC, Schiffmann R (2006) Myeloperoxidase predicts risk of vasculopathic events in hemizgygous males with Fabry disease. Neurology 67(11):2045–2047

148. Haebara H, Hasama F, Amano A (1975) Neural involvement in Fabrys disease. In: Körney S, Tariska S, Gosztonyi G (eds) 7th congress of neuropathology. Akadémici Kiadó, Budapest, pp 263–266

149. Sung JH, Hayano M, Mastri AR, Desnick R (1975) Neuropathology of Fabrys disease. In: Körney S, Tariska S, Gozstonyi G (eds) 7th congress of neuropathology. Akadémici Kiadó, Budapest

150. Mazurova Y, Rudolf E, Latr I, Osterreicher J (2006) Proliferation and differentiation of adult endogenous neural stem cells in response to neurodegenerative process within the striatum. Neurodegener Dis 3(1–2):12–18

151. Elleder M, Christomanou H, Kustermann-Kuhn B, Harzer K (1994) Leptomeningeal lipid storage patterns in Fabry disease. Acta Neuropathol 88(6):579–582

152. Lou HO, Reske-Nielsen E (1971) the central nervous system in Fabry's disease. A clinical, pathological, and biochemical investigation. Arch Neurol 25(4):351–359

153. Tagliavini F, Pietrini V, Gemignani F, Lechi A, Pallini R, Federico A (1982) Anderson-Fabry's disease: neuropathological and neurochemical investigation. Acta Neuropathol 56(2):93–98

154. Bartimmo EE Jr, Guisan M, Moser KM (1972) Pulmonary involvement in Fabry's disease: a reappraisal follow-up of a San Diego kindred and review of literature. Am J Med 53(6): 755–764

155. Brown LK, Miller A, Bhuptani A et al (1997) Pulmonary involvement in Fabry disease. Am J Respir Crit Care Med 155(3):1004–1010

156. Magage S, Lubanda JC, Susa Z et al (2007) Natural history of the respiratory involvement in Anderson-Fabry disease. J Inherit Metab Dis 30(5):790–799

157. Smith P, Heath D, Rodgers B, Helliwell T (1991) Pulmonary vasculature in Fabry's disease. Histopathology 19(6):567–569

158. Elleder M (1985) Fabry's disease: absence of storage as a feature of liver sinus endothelium. Acta Histochem 77(1):33–36

159. Meuwissen SG, Dingemans KP, Strijland A, Tager JM, Ooms BC (1982) Ultrastructural and biochemical liver analyses in Fabry's disease. Hepatology 2(2):263–268

160. Prasad R (2008) Abdominal viscera liver. In: Standring S (ed) Grays anatomy the anatomocal basis of clinical practice, 40th edn. Churchill Livingstone, Elsevier, London, pp 1163–1176

161. Roland D, Dehout F, van Maldergem L (2003) Fabry disease – gastrointestinal symptoms, renal aspects, neurological and ocular manifestations. Acta Paediatrica Suppl 443:110–115

162. Goodwin SE, Richfield L, Milligan A, Mehta A (2003) Gastrointestinal symptoms in patients with Fabry disease and their response to pancreatin supplements. Acta Paediatr Suppl 443:110–115

163. Flynn DM, Lake BD, Boothby CB, Young EP (1972) Gut lesions in Fabry's disease without a rash. Arch Dis Child 47(251):26–33

164. Rowe JW, Gilliam JI, Warthin TA (1974) Intestinal manifestations of Fabry's disease. Ann Intern Med 81(5):628–631

165. Keshav S (2006) Gastrointestinal manifestations of Fabry disease. In: Mehta A, Beck M, Sunder-Plassmann G (eds) Fabry diseas Perspectives from 5 years of FOS, 1st edn. Oxford Pharma Genesis Ltd, Oxford, pp 271–279

166. Jack CI, Morris AI, Nasmyth DG, Carroll N (1991) Colonic involvement in Fabry's disease. Postgrad Med J 67(788):584–585

167. O'Brien BD, Shnitka TK, McDougall R et al (1982) Pathophysiologic and ultrastructural basis for intestinal symptoms in Fabry's disease. Gastroenterology 82(5 Pt 1):957–962

168. Sheth KJ, Werlin SL, Freeman ME, Hodach AE (1981) Gastrointestinal structure and function in Fabry's disease. Am J Gastroenterol 76(3):246–251

169. Roth J, Roth H (1978) Electron microscopic observations in internal organs in morbus Fabry (author's transl). Virchows Arch A Pathol Anat Histol 378(1):75–90

170. Hegemann S, Hajioff D, Conti G et al (2006) Hearing loss in Fabry disease: data from the Fabry Outcome Survey. Eur J Clin Invest 36(9):654–662

171. Keilmann A (2003) Inner ear function in children with Fabry disease. Acta Paediatr Suppl 92(443):31–32, discussion 27
172. Schachern PA, Shea DA, Paparella MM, Yoon TH (1989) Otologic histopathology of Fabry's disease. Ann Otol Rhinol Laryngol 98(5 Pt 1):359–363
173. Sergi B, Conti G (2007) Hearing loss in a family affected by Fabry disease. J Inherit MetabDis 30(3):370–374
174. Malinvaud D, Lecanu JB, Halimi P, Avan P, Bonfils P (2006) Tinnitus and cerebellar developmental venous anomaly. Arch Otolaryngol Head Neck Surg 132(5):550–553
175. Ries M, Kim HJ, Zalewski CK et al (2007) Neuropathic and cerebrovascular correlates of hearing loss in Fabry disease. Brain 130(Pt 1):143–150
176. Conti G, Sergi B (2003) Auditory and vestibular findings in Fabry disease: a study of hemizygous males and heterozygous females. Acta Paediatr Suppl 92(443):33–37, discussion 27
177. Palla A, Widmer U, Straumann D (2003) Head-impulse testing in Fabry disease–vestibular function in male and female patients. Acta Paediatr Suppl 92(443):38–42, discussion 27
178. Noben-Trauth K, Neely H, Brady RO (2007) Normal hearing in alpha-galactosidase A-deficient mice, the mouse model for Fabry disease. Hear Res 234(1–2):10–14
179. Guo YK, Xie DH, Yang XM (2005) Morphological and functional alterations of ear in lysosomal neuraminidase gene deficient mouse. Zhonghua Er Bi Yan Hou Tou Jing Wai Ke Za Zhi 40(11):824–829
180. Coenen R, Gieselmann V, Lullmann-Rauch R (2001) Morphological alterations in the inner ear of the arylsulfatase A-deficient mouse. Acta Neuropathol 101(5):491–498
181. Schachern PA, Cureoglu S, Tsuprun V, Paparella MM, Whitley CB (2007) Age-related functional and histopathological changes of the ear in the MPS I mouse. Int J Pediatr Otorhinolaryngol 71(2):197–203
182. Elleder M, Voldrich L, Ulehlova L, Dimitt S, Armstrong D (1988) Light and electron microscopic appearance of the inner ear in juvenile ceroid lipofuscinosis (CL). Pathol Res Pract 183(3):301–307
183. Macrae WG, Ghosh M, McCulloch C (1985) Corneal changes in Fabry's disease: a clinicopathologic case report of a heterozygote. Ophthalmic Paediatr Genet 5(3):185–190
184. Font RL, Fine BS (1972) Ocular pathology in Fabry's disease. Histochemical and electron microscopic observations. Am J Ophthalmol 73(3):419–430
185. Tripathi RC, Ashton N (1976) Application of electron microscopy to the study of ocular inborn errors of metabolism. Birth Defects Orig Artic Ser 12(3):69–104
186. Francois J, Hanssens M, Teuchy H (1978) Corneal ultrastructural changes in Fabry's disease. Ophthalmologica 176(6):313–330
187. Weingeist TA, Blodi FC (1971) Fabry's disease: ocular findings in a female carrier. A light and electron microscopy study. Arch Ophthalmol 85(2):169–176
188. Falke K, Buttner A, Schittkowski M et al (2009) The microstructure of cornea verticillata in Fabry disease and amiodarone-induced keratopathy: a confocal laser-scanning microscopy study. Graefes Arch Clin Exp Ophthalmol 247(4):523–534
189. Mastropasqua L, Nubile M, Lanzini M, Carpineto P, Toto L, Ciancaglini M (2006) Corneal and conjunctival manifestations in Fabry disease: in vivo confocal microscopy study. Am J Ophthalmol 141(4):709–718
190. Hirano K, Murata K, Miyagawa A et al (2001) Histopathologic findings of cornea verticillata in a woman heterozygous for Fabry's disease. Cornea 20(2):233–236
191. Standring S (2008) The eye. In: Standring S (ed) Grays anatomy, 40th edn. Elsevier, London, pp 675–703
192. Libert J, Tondeur M, Van Hoof F (1976) The use of conjunctival biopsy and enzyme analysis in tears for the diagnosis of homozygotes and heterozygotes with Fabry disease. Birth Defects Orig Artic Ser 12(3):221–239

Chapter 4
Biochemistry of Fabry Disease

Martin Hřebíček and Jana Ledvinová

Abstract Fabry disease is a sphingolipid storage disorder resulting from a deficiency of the lysosomal hydrolase, α-galactosidase A. The deficiency leads to lysosomal accumulation of α-galactosidase A substrates, neutral glycosphingolipids with terminal α-galactosyl moieties, in multiple tissues. Globotriaosylceramide (Gb3Cer, CD77), the critical substrate of α-galactosidase A, is involved in cell signaling and associates itself with lipid rafts in the plasma membrane, where it also functions as a receptor for the Shiga-like toxins of *E. Coli*. Possible roles of Gb3Cer accumulation in the pathogenesis of Fabry disease, as well as biochemistry and function of minor α-galactosidase A substrates are discussed. There are two human lysosomal enzymes with the ability to hydrolyze substrates with terminal α-galactose, α-galactosidase A and α-*N*-acetylgalactosaminidase (NAGA). Both enzymes are active in vitro against saccharide, glycolipid and artificial substrates. α-*N*-acetylgalactosaminidase's primary function appears to be hydrolysis of acetylated oligosaccharides and glycopeptides, while α-galactosidase A is the enzyme responsible for degradation of glycolipid substrates. α-Galactosidase A requires an activator protein, saposin B, for its activity in vivo. Properties of the above proteins and the biochemistry of their deficiencies in humans are also addressed.

Keywords Fabry disease · α-galactosidase A · Globotriaosylceramide · Glycosphingolipids · Saposin B

4.1 Introduction

The catabolism of sphingolipids, a class of lipids with a complex structure and important biological functions, is ensured by their sequential degradation by a series of hydrolases found within lysosomes. Hereditary deficiencies of non-redundant

M. Hřebíček (✉)
First Faculty of Medicine, Institute of Inherited Metabolic Disorders, Charles University, Prague and General University Hospital, Prague, Czech Republic
e-mail: martin.hrebicek@lf1.cuni.cz

D. Elstein et al. (eds.), *Fabry Disease*, DOI 10.1007/978-90-481-9033-1_4,
© Springer Science+Business Media B.V. 2010

lysosomal hydrolases result in human disorders with variable clinical presentations linked to the accumulation of substrates of the deficient hydrolase within the lysosomes. Fabry disease is a sphingolipid storage disorder resulting from a deficiency of the lysosomal hydrolase, α-galactosidase A. The key topics discussed in this chapter are the biochemistry of α-galactosidase A, metabolism of its predominant substrates, glycosphingolipids with a terminal α-galactose, under physiological conditions and in Fabry disease.

Fabry disease is an X-linked disorder and both sexes are clinically affected. There are, however, significant differences between hemizygous males and heterozygous females not only in the clinical presentation but also in residual enzyme activities, metabolite levels, and other biochemical parameters. The symptoms of the disease and the cellular pathology are clearly associated with the storage of glycosphingolipids, but the molecular mechanism by which the storage leads to cellular damage remained unknown for a long time. Only recent advances have suggested the role these compounds may play in the pathogenesis of Fabry disease.

4.2 Sphingolipids and Their Physiological Importance

Sphingolipids are a complex class of lipids with a hydrophobic ceramide (N-acylsphingosine) as the key sphingolipid structure. The molecule is composed of a long-chain sphingoid base and an amide-linked fatty acid, the diversity of which makes the lipid part very heterogeneous.

The polar head-groups of the sphingolipids are either phosphocholine attached to ceramide in a molecule of sphingomyelin or a carbohydrate chain composed of one or more monosacharides bound typically by a glycosidic linkage. Carbohydrate chains can be sialylated or sulphated to give rise to a group of acidic glycosphingolipids, gangliosides, and sulphatides.

The simplest glycosphingolipid in the majority of eukaryotic cells is glucosylceramide (GlcCer, Glcβ1-1′Cer) from which more complex glycosphingolipids are derived via stepwise elongation of the oligosaccharide chain. In the first step, the addition of β-linked galactose gives lactosylceramide (LacCer, Galβ1-4GlcβCer). Further extensions give rise to different core structures of glycosphingolipids (Table 4.1), which can be tissue specific [1]. For example, the neolacto-series is typical for hematopoietic cells, the lacto-series for secretory organs, the globo-series for erythrocytes and kidney cells, and the ganglio-series predominates in nervous tissue. This diversity is related to differences in function of individual glycosphingolipids [1].

Although the majority of complex glycosphingolipids in higher animals are built on GlcCer, some cells also synthesize galactosylceramide (GalCer, Galβ1-1′Cer) which can be further sulphated to sulphatide. Both galactolipids are characteristic lipid components of myelin sheaths but their saccharide part is seldom extended [1]. Therefore the gala-series is quite rare.

Table 4.1   The major root structures of vertebrate glycosphingolipids

Type of series	Core structure
Globo-	**GalNAc(β1→3)Gal(α1→4)Gal** (β1→4)Glc(β1→1′)Cer
Isoglobo-	GalNAc(β1→3)Gal(α1→3)Gal(β1→4)Glc(β1→1′)Cer
Lacto-	**Gal(β1→3)GlcNAc** (β1→3)Gal(β1→4)Glc(β1→1′)Cer
Neolacto-	Gal(β1→4)GlcNAc (β1→3)Gal(β1→4)Glc(β1→1′)Cer
Ganglio-	Gal(β1→3)GalNAc (β1→4)Gal(β1→4)Glc(β1→1′)Cer
Gala-	Gal(α1→4)Gal (β1→1′)Cer

Note: Key structures characteristic for each series are underlined
'Lacto' does not refer to lactose
Root oligosaccharides of glycosphingolipid predominant in human tissues are
bolded

Detailed information on sphingolipid structures can be found on websites such as www.lipidmap.org, http://www.lipidlibrary.co.uk, www.cyberlipid.org, and www.chem.qmul.ac.uk/iupac/misc/glylp.html.

The biological functions of glycosphingolipids are related to the enormous diversity of structures in both parts of the molecule i.e. the hydrophobic ceramide and hydrophilic saccharide chain. According to their biophysical properties they form rather rigid structures in cell membranes but their structural variety allows numerous specific interactions (e.g. lipid-lipid, lipid-protein, and carbohydrate-carbohydrate). The location of cellular sphingolipids is predominantly on the outer leaflet of the plasma membrane and the luminal surface of intracellular vesicles and compartments. Because of their saturated nature and their potential for hydrogen bonding and dipolar interactions they tend to form membrane microdomains or rafts together with cholesterol and specific proteins (e.g. GPI-anchored proteins). While the existence of these structures continues to be discussed, other evidence suggests that these specific membrane domains are engaged in many cellular functions e.g. sorting processes, signaling, cell-cell recognition, and other types of interactions, the mechanisms of which are not entirely understood [2–5].

Sphingolipids are bioactive mediators in cell signaling. Their participation in this process by interactions with extra- and intracellular targets has been extensively studied. Among numerous bioactive sphingolipids, those best characterized as signaling molecules are ceramide, sphingosine, sphingosine-1-phosphate (S-1-P), and ceramide-1-phosphate. The crosstalk between these compounds defines important physiological processes, including regulation of cell growth and survival [6–8].

Gb3Cer, the critical substrate in Fabry disease, participates in a variety of cellular processes. This glycolipid is designated the P[k] antigen from blood group P antigens [9]. It has also been called CD77, a marker associated with Burkitt's lymphoma and a differentiation antigen of germinal center B-lymphocytes [10–12]. CD77 is involved in cellular signaling in CD19-mediated cell adhesion and interferon-alpha-induced growth inhibition and apoptosis [12–16]. The exact molecular mechanisms of these interactions and the molecular partners of Gb3Cer (CD77) in the hematopoietic system are still unknown.

Gb3Cer associates strongly with lipid rafts in the plasma membrane where it serves as a specific receptor for the Shiga-like toxin family of certain strains of *E. coli*. Binding of the toxin B-subunit by toxin-sensitive cells results in endocytosis and trafficking of the toxin/Gb3Cer complex by retrograde transport through the Golgi complex to the endoplasmic reticulum, followed by translocation into the cytosol and to the nuclear membrane where subunit A exerts its toxic function by inhibiting protein synthesis [17, 18].

Because Gb3Cer has been found to be over-expressed in some types of tumors, e.g. ovarian tumors resistant to chemotherapy [19, 20], targeting of the non-toxic verotoxin B subunit to receptor positive cells offers an alternative approach to cancer therapy [17, 21].

4.3 Pathobiochemistry of Glycosphingolipid Substrates of α-Galactosidase A

Deficiency of α-galactosidase A activity in Fabry disease leads to lysosomal accumulation of neutral glycosphingolipids with terminal α-galactosyl moieties in cells throughout the body. Their structures are shown in Fig. 4.1.

Lipid deposits are present primarily in the kidneys, cardiac myocytes, lungs, ganglion cells, blood vessels, especially in vascular endothelial and smooth muscle cells, and in the cornea of Fabry patients. The major non-degraded substrate is globotriaosylceramide (GbOse3Cer or Gb3Cer, also referred to as Gb3, GL-3, CTH, ceramide trihexoside, P^k antigen, and CD77 antigen). Its concentration can exceed normal level from ten to several hundred times in different organs of Fabry patients (Fig. 4.2). The accumulated glycosphingolipids originate from the metabolic turnover of membrane glycosphingolipids that are

Globotriaosylceramide, Gb_3Cer (oligosaccharide globo-series):
Gal(α1→4)Gal(β1→4)Glc(β1→1')Cer,

Digalactosylceramide, Ga_2Cer (oligosaccharide gala-series):
Gal(α1→4)Gal(β1→1')Cer,

Blood group B glycolipids, e.g. hexaglycosylceramide B-6-2 (neolacto-series)*:
Gal(α1→3)[Fucα1→2]Gal(β1→4)GlcNAc(β1→3)Gal(β1→4)Glc(β1→1')Cer,
IV^2-α-fucosyl-IV^3-galactosylneolactotetraosylceramide

P1 antigen (neolacto-series):
Gal(α1→4)Gal(β1→4)GlcNAc(β1→3)Gal(β1→4)Glc(β1→1')Cer,
IV^2-α-galactosylneolactotetraosylceramide

Fig. 4.1 The structures of glycolipid substrates of α-galactosidase A
*the same blood group B determinant is carried by the core structure of the lacto-series (e.g. B-6-1), see Table 4.1

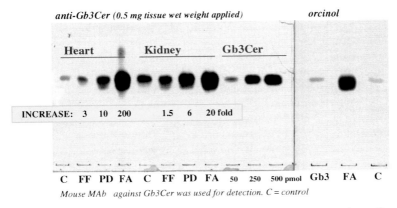

Fig. 4.2 Progress of Gb3Cer storage with age of patients. C = newborn control, age 2 months; FF = Fabry male fetus, 18 weeks; PD = prosaposin deficiency, age 4 months; FA = Fabry male patient, age 44 years, Gb3 = Gb3Cer standard. Immunodetection of Gb3Cer (*left part* of chromatogram) was performed on Polygram Sil G sheets (Macherey-Nagel, Dueren, Germany) using mouse monoclonal antibodies to Gb3Cer (Seikagaku, Japan) as described [22]. Binding of primary antibodies was detected using a Universal DAKO LSAB peroxidase kit (DAKO, Glostrup, Denmark). Chromatograms were evaluated densitometrically using a Camag TLC Scanner II (Cats3) (Camag Scientific, Muttenz, Switzerland) in reflection mode and quantitation was based on comparison with known amounts of glycolipid standards applied to the same chromatogram. *Right part* of chromatogram was stained by orcinol

present in large amounts in the kidneys, liver, vascular endothelium, lungs, and erythrocytes.

Globoside (globotetraosylceramide, Gb4Cer), a Gb3Cer precursor along the degradation pathway and an abundant glycolipid in cell membranes of different tissues, is believed to be the major contributor to the Gb3Cer load (e.g. in the kidneys). As a major glycolipid in erythrocytes, which have a rapid turnover, Gb4Cer was thought to be considerable source of Gb3Cer in the circulation [23]. In vivo metabolic studies on a porcine model with [14C]glucose showed that approximately 80% of the plasma Gb4Cer pool is derived from glycosphingolipids of senescent erythrocytes and 20% comes from synthesis in hepatocytes (and bone marrow) [23, 24]. However, tandem mass spectrometry (MS/MS) analysis of Gb3Cer isoforms has shown differences between erythrocytes with C24:0 and C24:1 as the predominant Gb3Cer species and plasma, where C16:0 is the predominant form [25, 26]. The ratio of C16:0–C24:0 species increases only very slightly in the plasma of Fabry patients, suggesting that the majority of the Gb3Cer may come from other sources, e.g. turnover of other cell types, excretion from secondary lysosomes of various cells, or biosynthesis.

It has been estimated that about 25% of plasma glycosphingolipids are newly synthesized each day [24] and turnover time for human plasma glycosphingolipids is from 4 to 8 days with a turnover rate of 1–6 μmol/day [27]. Plasma glycosphingolipids originating from both synthesis and degradation are transported by LDL and HDL lipoproteins [28] and can be reversibly exchanged between lipoprotein fractions [29]. Delivery to cells occurs through receptor binding or receptor-independent mechanisms [30]. In Fabry patients, a 3–5 fold increase in Gb3Cer plasma levels has been observed, but distribution between the major lipoprotein fractions was similar to controls and without any physical destabilization of the lipoprotein particles [31, 32]. Hypothetically, Gb3Cer transported in lipoprotein complexes in the circulation may be taken up by vascular endothelial and smooth-muscle cells via LDL-receptor-mediated endocytosis and contribute to its progressive accumulation in vessel cells, which can lead to vascular degeneration. On the other hand, small amounts of Gb3Cer may be released into the plasma and associate with lipoproteins and be subsequently cleared by the liver [23].

Study of pathogenic role of Gb3Cer accumulation in vascular endothelial cells of Fabry patients revealed evidence of activation of multiple specific endothelial markers [33], induction of oxidative stress, and up-regulation of adhesion molecules in vascular endothelium [34]. Recent studies, on a mouse model of Fabry disease, have suggested that production of vasoactive cycloxygenase (COX) derived products (from increased COX1 and COX2 activity localized in the endothelium) contributes to Fabry vasculopathy [35, 36]. Also, decreased nitric oxide (NO) bioavailability in aortic endothelial cells has been shown [37]. These findings could be a starting point for future investigation of interactions, which accelerate development of vascular complication in Fabry patients.

Recently, dramatically increased levels of globotriaosylsphingosine (lyso-Gb3Cer), a deacylated derivative of globotriaosylceramide (Fig. 4.3), has been reported in the plasma of Fabry patients and of Fabry mice [38]. This compound is suspected to contribute to disease presentation by induction of smooth muscle cell manifestation, probably via interference in signal transduction. Its origin is not clear – it could be formed biosynthetically through sequential glycosylation of sphingoid bases or alternatively by deacylation of Gb3Cer through an unknown sphingolipid deacylase. Although this compound can serve as a very useful marker for

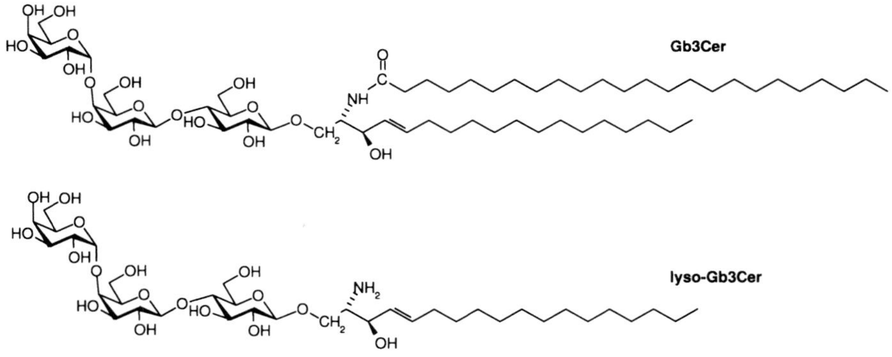

Fig. 4.3 Structures of globotriaosylceramide and its deacylated derivative, lyso-globotriaosylceramide

diagnosis and for treatment monitoring, the elucidation of its origin and function requires further studies.

High quantities of Gb3Cer are excreted in the urine of Fabry males with classical phenotype but also in the urine of some female heterozygotes. Its major origin is the exfoliated lipid-laden distal tubular cells of the kidney, which can serve as a 'non-direct kidney biopsy' for laboratory diagnosis [39, 40]. It is worth mentioning that the defect in the degradation of the Gb3Cer oligosaccharide chain, secondarily influences the composition of the ceramide part of the molecule, which is extremely heterogeneous due to the diversity of the fatty acids and sphingoid bases. Resolution of molecular species of Gb3Cer using MS/MS has revealed significant changes with an increased proportion of the C24:0 family in the plasma and urine of patients with Fabry disease [25, 41–43]. This effect is most pronounced in urine where the glycosphingolipid profile is considered to be mostly of renal origin [39, 44, 45], possibly with a small contribution from the plasma, in cases with a kidney barrier defect [46]. The same shift in urinary Gb3Cer isoforms has also been observed – and together with quantitative changes in Gb3Cer – in saposin B and prosaposin deficiencies [47, 48]. The shift can be considered a characteristic feature of defective Gb3Cer degradation. Although the metabolic basis of this phenomenon is not clear, the profile of urinary Gb3Cer isoforms can serve as a useful diagnostic marker.

In addition to Gb3Cer there are other minor substrates of α-galactosidase A with different cellular expressions and with different oligosaccharide root structures (Table 4.1). These include galabiosylceramide (digalactosylceramide, GaOse2Cer or Ga2Cer), P1 antigen, and blood group B glycolipids (Fig. 4.1) in patients with blood group B or AB.

Occurrence of galabiosylceramide is tissue specific and is confined to the kidney, heart, pancreas, lungs, and ganglia where increased levels, in Fabry patients, have been detected [23]. Also, the load of blood group B antigens is much lower than that of Gb3Cer and probably does not markedly influence the cell pathology [49]. Accumulation of B-6-2 and B-6-1 glycosphingolipids was originally found in the pancreas of Fabry patient with blood group B [50] and later on in the tonsils and urinary sediments of Fabry patients with blood group B and AB [51]. Besides erythrocyte membranes, antigens of ABO(H) system are present in body secretions and many tissues including the pancreas, small intestine, blood vessels, kidneys, and epidermal cells; either in glycolipid or glycoprotein forms. Expression in tissues of entodermal origin (e.g. gastrointestinal, respiratory, and urinary epithelium) also depends on the secretor status of the individual [52]. Hypothetically, blood group B Fabry patients, especially those with secretor status, may have a greater substrate burden and more severe clinical phenotype than patients with blood group A or O. This issue has not been yet resolved since little clinical data on Fabry patients with blood group B and AB has been evaluated [45, 49, 53]. Therefore further extensive studies would be beneficial to more precisely evaluate the possible contribution of these substrates to the disease burden.

Another critical substrate, substance P1 (Fig. 4.1), belongs to the P blood group antigens [9, 54]. This antigen is present in minute amounts on the plasma membrane of erythrocytes, but also on different leukocyte populations, thrombocytes, fibroblasts, and the endothelial and smooth muscle cells of the digestive and urogenital system [9]. However its accumulation in Fabry individuals has not been reported [23] and P1 antigen is not considered a significant risk factor [49].

Isoglobostructures, which also carry an α-galactosyl unit may represent a potential substrate pool for α-galactosidase A, but their presence in humans is still controversial [55–57]. But even if present in minute amounts, their contribution to storage would be negligible.

4.4 Biosynthesis, Degradation and Trafficking of Sphingolipids Involved in Pathology of Fabry Disease

In general, basic processes leading to the formation of glycosphingolipid molecules include the following events: de novo biosynthesis in the endoplasmic reticulum (ER) and Golgi apparatus and vesicular sorting to the plasma membrane (about 35%), metabolic recycling of fragments from lysosomal sphingolipid degradation i.e. salvage pathway (about 58%), and direct glycosylation after sorting from endosomes to the Golgi apparatus (about 7%) [58, 59]. This estimation is approximate and depends in large part on the type of cells involved and on different stimuli [59].

Sphingolipid synthesis happens in two compartments, the ER and the Golgi complex. Biosynthesis of glycosphingolipids starts with the formation of ceramide to which saccharide units are added in a stepwise fashion. Ceramide is synthesized on the cytoplasmic side of the ER and is then transferred by the vesicular transport to the Golgi apparatus for synthesis of GlcCer or by a non-vesicular pathway, using ceramide transfer protein (CERT), for biosynthesis of sphingomyelin [60–63].

Synthesis of glucosylceramide (GlcCer) – a key precursor of the majority of the glycosphingolipid series, takes place on the cytosolic face of the Golgi complex through the action of glucosylceramide synthase [64], which transfers a glucose residue from a UDP-glucose to the 1-position of the ceramide in the β-glycosidic linkage [65, 66]. The next reaction, catalyzed by lactosylceramide synthase, is the addition of galactose from a UDP-galactose donor to GlcCer in the lumen of the trans-Golgi complex [67]. Recently, the FFAP2 (four-phosphate adaptor protein 2) protein transporter was reported to be an important mediator of the non-vesicular transport of GlcCer from its site of synthesis to its site of translocation [68]. This is probably accomplished by FAPP2-mediated retrograde transport of newly synthesized GlcCer to the ER, translocation across the membrane, and transport into the Golgi lumen along secretory pathway for additional glycosylation steps [62, 69–71]. After biosynthesis, complex glycosphingolipids reach the plasma membrane through vesicular transport [62, 63].

Further glycosylation steps are catalyzed by glycosyltransferases with different specificities and result in the formation of complex glycosphingolipid structures (see Table 4.1) [72]. Some transferases also act on glycoproteins so that the same oligosaccharide structures are carried by both lipids and proteins. Typical examples include the ABO(H) blood group antigens and the P1 antigen, which exist in both glycosphingolipid and glycoprotein forms [9, 52, 54].

The key enzyme initiating the synthesis of Gb3Cer, through the addition of $\alpha1,4$-galactose to lactosylceramide, is Gb3/CD77 synthase ($\alpha1,4$-galactosyltransferase, P^k transferase, [$\alpha1,4$Gal-T]). This enzyme also uses galactosylceramide as an acceptor [73, 74]. Studies using the mouse model have shown that the Gb3/CD77 synthase was expressed mainly in the kidneys and lungs, and moderately in the heart, spleen, stomach, and testis, which corresponds, approximately, with the expression of Gb3/CD77 lipid products. The expression pattern is, with some exceptions, similar to that seen in human tissues [74, 75].

Synthesis of glycosphingolipids with terminal α-galactose from the neolacto- and lacto-series, P1, and blood group B antigens also starts from lactosylceramide. The P1 antigen is synthesized by the addition of a terminal $\alpha1,4$-galactose to a paragloboside precursor (lactoneotetraosylceramide) in a step catalyzed by P1 transferase. There is still little information about this enzyme, but studies with cloned Gb3/CD77 synthase have suggested, in contrast to previous reports [23, 73, 74], that the genes for P1 and Gb3/CD77 synthases could be identical [76].

The blood B glycan determinant is formed by $\alpha1,3$-galactosyltransferase ($\alpha1$-3GalT, B-transferase) encoded by the B allele at the *ABO* locus. B-transferase as well as A-transferase are highly specific towards the sugar acceptor, i.e. the enzymes react exclusively with those glycoconjugates carrying the terminal fucose group (H antigen, Fuc$\alpha1$-2Gal$\beta1$-4GlcNAc-). The so-called B-like structure (Gal$\alpha1$-3Gal$\beta1$-4GlcNAc), synthesized by a different $\alpha1$-3GalT, is widely expressed in mammals but absent in Old World monkeys, apes, and humans. There is a significant similarity between the nucleotide sequence of the gene encoding animal $\alpha1$-3GalT and the human *ABO* gene, which suggests that they are derived from a common ancestral gene [52, 54]. In human sera, naturally occurring antibodies against α-galactosylceramide (α-GalCer), and even more complex epitops with terminal Gal$\alpha1$-3Gal$\beta1$- sequence, are regularly found, probably due to immunization through exposure to microbial species. This constitutes a major barrier in xenotransplantation in humans [52, 54, 77].

This problem is also connected with the presence or absence of lipids of the isoglobo-series in humans, since results from some studies have been rather contradictory [55, 57]. Isoglobotriaosylceramide (iGb3Cer; Gal$\alpha1$-3Gal$\beta1$-4GlcβCer) was originally proposed as an endogenous natural killer T (NKT) cell activator of an invariant T-cell receptor via CD1d, a lipid presenting molecule [78]. However, recent work from the Christiansen group [79] has demonstrated that spliced isoglobotriaosyl synthase mRNA was not detected in human tissues because of a nonfunctional gene and that chimeric enzyme did not synthesize any product. Therefore, they concluded that iGb3Cer is unlikely to represent a primary natural endogenous ligand for NKT cells in humans. The structure of mouse CD1d-iGb3Cer complex has been determined by x-ray crystallography; structure-based models have predicted binding of both iGb3Cer and other ligands to a semi-invariant V$\alpha14$ T cell receptor for NKT-cell activation [80].

The degradation of glycosphingolipids occurs in the lysosomal compartment via a stepwise cleavage of monosaccharide units starting at the non-reducing end of the saccharide chain. The reactions are catalyzed by exoglycosidases with acidic pH optima. Glycosphingolipids, as plasma membrane components, reach lysosomes by endocytic membrane flow [81]. This process starts with the formation of invaginated vesicles containing glycosphingolipids together with other membrane components. They reach the lumen of endosomes as intra-endosomal vesicles or aggregates. After fusion with primary lysosomes, glycosphingolipids on the surface of small intra-lysosomal vesicles expose their oligosaccharide chains to the soluble glycohydrolases in the lysosol [63, 81]. However, in vivo degradation of glycosphingolipids with short carbohydrate chains with less then four monosaccharides depends critically on the coordinated action of lysosomal hydrolases and protein activators in the presence of negatively charged lipids (bis-(monoacylglycero)-phosphate, BMP) [82]. Protein activators, as detergents, enable lipid solubilization and subsequent selective degradation of hydrophobic membrane glycosphingolipids. Mutations causing deficiency of either the lysosomal enzymes or the cooperating protein activators lead to lysosomal storage and sphingolipid storage disease [82–85].

4.5 Human α-Galactosidases: α-Galactosidase A and B

Early studies have shown that there were two human α-galactosidase forms: α-galactosidase A, which is deficient in patients with Fabry disease [86], and α-galactosidase B, which occurred at normal or slightly elevated levels in these patients [87]. α-Galactosidase B activity usually comprised up to 20–25% of the total α-galactosidase activity in crude human tissue homogenates or in body fluids [88–90] and because of similar properties, including almost identical molecular weights and the ability to hydrolyze substrates with terminal α-galactose, was considered an isoenzyme of α-galactosidase A. Both enzymes were purified to homogeneity from human tissues [91–93] and it was demonstrated that α-galactosidase B possesses both α-*N*-acetylgalactosaminidase and α-galactosidase activities [94, 95]. Accordingly, the term α-galactosidase B was abandoned in favor of α-*N*-acetylgalactosaminidase (NAGA, EC 3.2.1.49), while α-galactosidase A retained its original name (GLA, EC 3.2.1.22).

   Both enzymes were active in vitro against saccharide, glycolipid, and artificial substrates containing terminal non-reducing α-galactose, while only NAGA was able to cleave glycosides with terminal α-N-acetylgalactosamine residues. Hydrolysis of the glycolipid substrates in vitro required detergent, sodium taurocholate, at milimolar concentrations, to solubilize the glycolipids in an aqueous reaction environment [92, 93]. When the genes for GLA and NAGA were cloned, it was noted that they apparently arose from a duplication of an ancestral gene and the function of their products later diverged [96]. Of note, the genome of the nematode *C. elegans* contains only one gene orthologous to both human GLA and NAGA and the phylogenetic evidence suggests that it evolved from the GLA/NAGA ancestral gene before the duplication event, which resulted in separate NAGA and GLA genes in higher metazoans. The enzyme encoded by the gene hydrolyzes both acetylated and unacetylated substrates [97].

Enzymes that cleave glycosidic bonds (glycosidases) fall into two categories. Glycosidases that lead to products that have the same stereochemistry as the substrates are called *retaining,* while *non-retaining* glycosidases lead to inversion of the anomeric configuration in the product (for instance, alpha to beta) [98]. Both GLA and NAGA are retaining glycosidases and the products of reactions catalyzed by them emerge in the alpha conformation. The structure of GLA and its catalytic mechanism is the subject of a separate chapter in this book.

4.6 α-Galactosidase A (GLA)

GLA specifically recognizes substrates with terminal α-galactose; it is not able to catalyze hydrolysis of substrates with terminal α-N-acetylgalactosamine residues or galactose in the β-conformation. Purified human GLA has been shown to catalyze the hydrolysis of glycolipids, galabiosylceramide, and globotriaosylceramide, and the corresponding water-soluble saccharides, as well as artificial substrates with terminal α-galactose [93]. The pH optimum for all substrates is acidic – for hydrolysis of glycosphingolipids it was 4.1 with K_m 0.31 ± 0.05 mmol/l for galabiosylceramide and 0.18 ± 0.02 mmol/l for globotriaosylceramide, while hydrolysis of artificial substrate 4-MU-α-galactopyranoside was optimal at pH 4.6 with a K_m 2.8 ± 0.2 mmol/l. The observed low K_m for glycosphingolipid substrates, most probably, reflects a strong electrostatic interaction between GLA and anionic glycolipid-taurocholate mixed micelles, rather than the affinity of the enzyme for these substrates [93].

Recently it has been shown that lyso-Gb3Cer can act as a substrate for GLA, but its in vitro enzymatic conversion to lactosylsphingosine was at least 50-fold less efficient compared to Gb3Cer [38].

Measurement of GLA activity in cells or body fluids is commonly performed with synthetic substrates in the presence of N-acetylgalactosamine, which selectively inhibits the α-galactosidase activity of NAGA without influencing the activity of GLA [99]. The assay employing the fluorescent substrate 4-MU-α-galactopyranoside is sensitive and commonly used for diagnostics.

Gel filtration and native and denaturing electrophoresis studies [91, 93] have suggested that GLA is a dimer and its glycosylated monomer unit has a molecular weight of 49 kDa. This was later confirmed through determination of the three-dimensional structure of GLA by x-ray crystallography [100].

N-linked carbohydrates account for 5–15% of the GLA mass [101]. Multiple forms of the mature enzyme with observed differences in molecular mass and isoelectric points, are due to variable glycosylation [91]. Human GLA forms isolated from different tissues had their isoelectric points in the range 4.2–5.2, the lowest pI was from GLA isolated from plasma (pI = 4.2). pI differences were mainly due to the sialic acid content, as different GLA forms, partially deglycosylated by neuraminidase, appeared as a single band with pI = 5.2 [91] on isoelectric focusing.

Glycosylation of GLA has been studied in greatest detail in the recombinant human enzyme expressed in CHO cells. There are three N-glycosylation sites (Asn-139, Asn-192, and Asn-215) occupied by complex, high-mannose, and hybrid-type oligosaccharide chains, respectively, per monomer of GLA. The high mannose-type oligosaccharide chains contain two phosphomonoester bonds – presumably mannose-6-phosphate groups. Glycosylation site 3 (Asn-215) is essential for enzyme solubility and its exit fom the ER [102]. Asn-215 mutated to serine (N215S), which results in abolition of the corresponding N-glycosylation site, was observed in a subset of males affected with the cardiac variant phenotype of Fabry disease [103]. Patients carrying this mutation have no detectable GLA activity in plasma and 3–10% of the normal activity in tissues, findings that correspond well with properties of the mutant enzyme observed in vitro. No O-linked oligosaccharides were found in GLA [102].

There were significant differences in glycoforms isolated from intracellular and secreted recombinant human GLA produced in CHO cells. The chains identified in intracellular form were over 90% high mannose and only 8% complex-type oligosaccharides. The oligosaccharide species found in the secreted form are much more variable, containing high mannose (63%), complex (30%), and hybrid (5%) chains [101]. The high content of sialylated complex oligosaccharides in the GLA from human plasma and the prevalence of high mannose oligosaccharides in GLA from tissues, strongly suggests a similarity to the glycoforms observed in secreted and lysosomal forms of recombinant GLA expressed in CHO cells. In CHO cells over-expressing recombinant human GLA, about 65% is secreted [104]. It has been suggested that the glycoforms observed in intracellular GLA may be the result of trimming of the oligosaccharides within the lysosome.

As the majority of luminal lysosomal enzymes, GLA is targeted to lysosomes by the mannose-6 phosphate signal, which is created during the passage of the enzyme through the ER and Golgi apparatus. In human fibroblasts, GLA is synthesized as a phosphorylated 50.5 kDa precursor and over the course of several days is processed via several intermediates to the mature lysosomal form of 46 kDa [105]. The mature GLA subunit consists of 398 amino-acid residues; the leader peptide for translocation into the ER has 31 residues. The secreted enzyme has an apparent molecular mass of 52 kDa. GLA transport to lysosomes depends on the mannose-6-phosphate signal; in I-cell disease cells, which lack the enzyme necessary for formation of the mannose-6-phosphate group and in cells treated with NH_4Cl, GLA is secreted. Also, the internalization of human GLA into cultured skin fibroblasts is inhibited by mannose-6-phosphate added to the culture medium or by treatment of the enzyme with acid phosphatase [106, 107].

A number of substrate analogues including competitive inhibitors of GLA have been described. Some of them could be used as pharmacological chaperones for mutant GLAs and are discussed elsewhere in this book.

4.7 Mutant α-Galactosidases A

Classically affected hemizygous males usually have undetectable GLA activities both in tissues and plasma when measured using the common assays employing synthetic substrates [99]. Hemizygotes with clinically milder atypical variants of Fabry disease have activities in the range 5–35% of controls and patients may not have all the classical symptoms – often they present with later-onset cardiomyopathy or renal disease; the phenotypes are also known as cardiac and renal forms, respectively. Clearly, there is a correlation between residual enzyme activity and the severity of the clinical manifestation; severe deficiency of GLA is associated with the classic presentation, while Fabry patients with higher residual activities are likely to have milder phenotypes with later-onset forms [23]. The majority of classically affected males have no detectable cross-reacting material with anti-GLA antibodies [23, 90, 108].

Several studies [109–111] examined the properties of mutant GLAs from patients with atypical and mild classical presentations and found that a large proportion of these mutant enzymes retain partial or even full degradative capacity, but have defective conformational stability. Their thermal stability is often decreased, especially at neutral pH, which is characteristic of the ER and the Golgi compartments. Such improperly folded enzymes are regularly retained in the ER and are subject to ERAD (ER-associated degradation). Active-site chaperones, such as 1-deoxygalactonojirimycin (DGJ), can help the enzyme to attain the proper conformation and stabilize it, prevent excessive degradation by ERAD, and reach the lysosome [112]; all of which is discussed in detail in another chapter in this book.

Properties of mutant GLAs have important consequences for diagnostic measurements of activity and may lead to discordant findings when the activity is measured in plasma and cells, including pseudodeficiencies [113, 114]. The following examples is an incomplete list of variant GLAs with interesting biochemical properties.

Hemizygotes carrying the N215S [103], a common allele associated with the cardiac variant form, have very low or undetectable GLA activity in plasma and urine and 3–10% of normal activity in tissues. The mutation abolishes the third N-glycosylation site of GLA as discussed above [102]. Storage of non-degraded GSL substrates is restricted to the heart [115].

Kobayashi and coworkers [116] described a patient with a variant phenotype, who had a complete deficiency of GLA activity when measured with synthetic substrate, but displayed residual activity with the natural substrate.

The rare D313Y allele has about 60% of wild-type GLA activity in cells but is unstable at the neutral pH, which leads to its pseudodeficiency in plasma. The substitution was found in Fabry patients, but only in combination with another mutation on the same allele, and is considered non-pathogenic [113, 116, 117]. Another patient with GLA pseudodeficiency was described by Bach and coworkers [114]. The 51 year old patient, without any sign of Fabry disease and without increased excretion of Gb3Cer in the urine, had 10% of normal GLA activity in cultured skin fibroblasts. The mutant enzyme had a five times higher K_m and increased stability.

The gene for GLA is located on chromosome X and is subject to X inactivation [23]. The expression of GLA from wild-type and mutant alleles in tissues of heterozygous females depends on the degree of inactivation of each allele. Heterozygous females tend to have intermediate activities of GLA [99], but the activities often overlap the normal range, as detailed elsewhere in this book.

4.8 Saposin B

In vivo hydrolytic activity of GLA against glycosphingolipids is accelerated by saposin B, a small (11 kDa) thermostable glycosylated enzymatically inactive activator glycoprotein [118]. Saposin B is required for degradation of sulfatide by arylsulfatase A and for hydrolysis of globotriaosylceramide and digalactosylceramide by GLA. Patients with deficiency of saposin B present clinically with a variant form of metachromatic leukodystrophy of varying severity [85, 119–121]. The glycolipids elevated in the urine of Sap B deficient patients include both arylsulfatase A and GLA substrates: sulfatide, globotriaosylceramide, and digalactosylceramide [122, 123]. In prosaposin deficiency, the gene defect affects the function of all four saposins (saposins A, B, C, and D) and causes accumulation of multiple sphingolipids including Gb3Cer, which leads to complex sphingolipidosis, with early fatal consequences [48, 22, 124, 125]. A comparison between the catabolic potential of cells with α-galactosidase A and prosaposin deficiencies loaded with [H^3]Gb4Cer is shown in Fig. 4.4. In addition to its role as an activator in degradation of glycolipids, saposin B and other saposins participate in the presentation of lipid antigens by loading of them onto CD1d molecules [127].

Mature saposin B is a glycoprotein with 80 amino-acids residues and one N-linked N-glycosylation site. It was proposed that saposin B lifts single glycolipid molecules from membranes and the resulting water-soluble complexes are accessible to enzymes in the lysosomal lumen [85]. This model is strongly supported by the shell-like three-dimensional structure of the saposin B dimer, which has a hydrophobic lipid-binding pocket formed by two V-shaped saposin B monomers [128]. The pocket encloses the hydrophobic ceramide moiety of glycolipids while the polar head is exposed to the enzymes. Two conformations have been described; the open form was proposed to participate in membrane pertubation, changing into the closed form upon extraction of the lipid from the membrane [128, 129]. Saposin B is considered to be a broad-specificity activator protein and it has been shown that it binds, in vitro, a range of lipid substrates [130, 131].

Saposins (A, B, C, and D) are derived from the proteolytic processing of the precursor protein, prosaposin; they are necessary for hydrolysis of glycolipids with short glycan chains by lysosomal luminal hydrolases [85]. They also act as lipid-binding proteins. Saposins belong to the family of saposin-like proteins or SAPLIPS, whose members exhibit lipid-binding, membrane-perturbing or membrane-perforating properties and have diverse functions within the cells. SAPLIPS share the same three-dimensional protein fold [132].

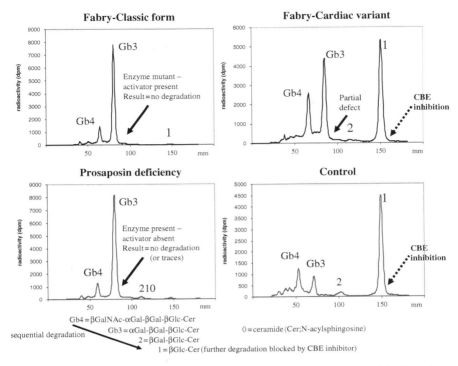

Fig. 4.4 Degradation of [^{3}H]Gb3Cer labeled on ceramide and formation of tritiated products in cultured fibroblasts of patients with classic Fabry disease and the cardiac variant compared with prosaposin deficiency. Cells were fed 4 days with [^{3}H]Gb4Cer (peak Gb4), precursor of the critical substrate [^{3}H]Gb3Cer (peak Gb3) that was formed in lysosomes by the action of β-hexosaminidase. In the next step, α-galactosidase A degraded [^{3}H]Gb3Cer to LacCer (peak 2) in control cells and, to a certain extent, also in fibroblasts from the cardiac variant of Fabry disease (17% residual activity in vitro). Degradation continued with β-galactosidase and formation of GlcCer (peak 1). The next enzyme on the pathway, β-glucocerebrosidase, was inhibited by conduritol B-epoxide (CBE) giving a clear background and without products of resynthesis. Thus GlcCer (peak 1) with contribution of LacCer (peak 2) represented all products of Gb3Cer degradation and reflected degradation capacity of α-galactosidase A. Notice that mutation of the enzyme protein had the same effect on Gb3Cer degradation as non-functional Sap B. On the other hand, comparison of fibroblast degradation capacity of mild Fabry cardiac variant and the classic form showed relatively high potential of the cells of the former to catabolize Gb3Cer. For details of procedure see [126]. Briefly: At the end of loading experiment, cells were harvested, lipids extracted with chloroform-methanol (2:1 v/v) and separated on HPTLC silica gel plates. Radioactivity of individual glycosphingolipids on the chromatogram was measured using radioscanner RITA (Raytest Isotopenmessgerate GmBH, Germany)

4.9 α-*N*-Acetylgalactosaminidase (NAGA)

NAGA has the ability to hydrolyze substrates with either terminal α-galactose or α-*N*-acetylgalactosamine residues. o-NP-α-*N*-acetylgalactosamine competitively inhibits hydrolysis of 4-MU-α-galactopyranoside by purified NAGA, showing that both acetylated and unacetylated substrates compete for the same active site. Both activities were precipitated by an antibody against NAGA. While the apparent K_m for glycolipid substrates are 5–10 times lower than those with water-soluble substrates, the low values obtained for glycolipids probably reflect an electrostatic interaction of the detergent/glycolipid mixed micelles rather than an affinity for the substrate. The apparent V_{max} values for the glycolipids were 50–100 times lower than those with the water-soluble substrates. The enzyme was also 2–5 times more active against acetylated substrates, suggesting that NAGAs primary function is degradation of acetylated oligosaccharides and glycopeptides [92].

NAGA hydrolyzes various α-galactosides including glycolipids in vitro (although with a high K_m), but it is apparently unable to fully compensate for GLA deficiency in Fabry patients, if at all. Glycolipid loading experiments in GLA deficient fibroblasts (including cell lines later shown to be carrying apparently null mutations) showed average residual degradative capacity for Gb3Cer of about 15% of that in wild-type cells [126]. Arguably the strongest evidence for the physiological substrates of NAGA and GLA is provided by their human deficient states. The deficiency of NAGA in humans (Schindler's disease) causes an autosomal recessive disorder commonly considered to be a glycoproteinosis, since the dominant accumulated substances are N- and O-linked glycopeptides. There are neutral glycosphingolipids with α-N-acetylgalactosaminyl residues in the humans, the blood group A glycosphingolipids (in the mouse that also includes the Forssmann antigen, which appears to be present only in traces in humans, if at all), but overt storage of these glycolipids has not been detected in limited samples from the clinically most severe type I patients [133]. NAGA deficient cells do not degrade major blood group A glycolipid A-6-2 [134] and it cannot be excluded that glycolipid storage contributes to the disease burden in these patients. Of note, morphological findings vary dramatically between the severe (type I) form, and forms with later onsets, adult (type II), and intermediate (type III) forms. In type I, the neuropathology is dominated by neuroaxonal dystrophy, but there are no apparent signs of lysosomal pathology, which is present in the type II although signs of neuronaxonal dystrophy are absent [133]. It has been hypothesized that type I patients, who all come from one family, may have another disease causing neuroaxonal dystrophy in addition to NAGA deficiency [135]; however, this question remains unanswered in the literature available to us.

4.10 Other Findings

An interesting observation was made by Vyleťal and co-workers, who noted abnormal expression and processing of uromodulin (Tamm-Horsfall protein) in the kidneys of Fabry patients. Fabry patients showed reduced uromodulin expression, its aberrant proteolytic processing, and decreased urinary excretion. The abnormal findings were more prominent in areas affected by storage and the above changes were reversed by enzyme replacement therapy. Since the lack of uromodulin is associated with impairment of tubular functions, it cannot be excluded that the abnormal expression of uromodulin in Fabry patients can contribute to tubular damage [136].

4.11 Conclusion

The study of biochemical changes in Fabry subjects has led to a better understanding of glycosphingolipid metabolism in man and to the discovery of the enzyme deficiency causing the disease – this enabled reliable diagnostics including prenatal testing and played an important role in the discovery of the GLA gene. A detailed knowledge of the biochemistry of wild-type and mutant GLAs has been instrumental in the development of enzyme substitution therapy, chaperone therapy, and other therapeutic approaches currently in use or in testing.

Acknowledgment We thank Dr. Klaus Harzer and Dr. František Šmíd for critically commenting on the manuscript. The support of the Ministry of Education, Youth, and Sports of the Czech Republic (Grant No. MSM 0021620806) is gratefully acknowledged.

References

1. Schnaar R, Suzuki A, Stanley P (2009) Glycosphingolipids. In: Varki A, Cummings R, Esko J, Freeze H, Stanley P, Bertozzi C, Hart G, Etzler M (eds) Essentials of glycobiology, 2nd edn. CSHL Press America, Plainview. Available from http://www.ncbi.nlm.nih.gov/bookshelf/br.fcgi?book=glyco2
2. Hannun YA, Obeid LM (2008) Principles of bioactive lipid signalling: lessons from sphingolipids. Nat Rev Mol Cell Biol 9(2):139–150
3. Hoetzl S, Sprong H, van Meer G (2007) The way we view cellular (glyco)sphingolipids. J Neurochem 103(Suppl 1):3–13
4. Prinetti A, Loberto N, Chigorno V, Sonnino S (2009) Glycosphingolipid behaviour in complex membranes. Biochim Biophys Acta 1788(1):184–193
5. van Meer G, Voelker DR, Feigenson GW (2008) Membrane lipids: where they are and how they behave. Nat Rev Mol Cell Biol 9(2):112–124
6. Chalfant CE, Spiegel S (2005) Sphingosine 1-phosphate and ceramide 1-phosphate: expanding roles in cell signaling. J Cell Sci 118(Pt 20):4605–4612
7. Hait NC, Oskeritzian CA, Paugh SW, Milstien S, Spiegel S (2006) Sphingosine kinases, sphingosine 1-phosphate, apoptosis and diseases. Biochim Biophys Acta 1758(12):2016–2026
8. Lebman DA, Spiegel S (2008) Cross-talk at the crossroads of sphingosine-1-phosphate, growth factors, and cytokine signaling. J Lipid Res 49(7):1388–1394
9. Schenkel-Brunner H (2000) Human blood groups. Chemical and biochemical basis of antigen specificity, 2nd edn. Springer, Wien, pp 273–303
10. Taga S, Carlier K, Mishal Z, Capoulade C, Mangeney M, Lécluse Y et al (1997) Intracellular signaling events in CD77-mediated apoptosis of Burkitt's lymphoma cells. Blood 90(7):2757–2767
11. Wiels J, Holmes EH, Cochran N, Tursz T, Hakomori S (1984) Enzymatic and organizational difference in expression of a Burkitt lymphoma-associated antigen (globotriaosylceramide) in Burkitt lymphoma and lymphoblastoid cell lines. J Biol Chem 259(23):14783–14787
12. Wiels J (2000) CD77. J Biol Regul Homeost Agents 14(4):288–289

13. George T, Boyd B, Price M, Lingwood C, Maloney M (2001) MHC class II proteins contain a potential binding site for the verotoxin receptor glycolipid CD77. Cell Mol Biol (Noisy-le-grand) 47(7):1179–1185

14. Khine AA, Firtel M, Lingwood CA (1998) CD77-dependent retrograde transport of CD19 to the nuclear membrane: functional relationship between CD77 and CD19 during germinal center B-cell apoptosis. J Cell Physiol 176(2):281–292

15. Maloney MD, Lingwood CA (1994) CD19 has a potential CD77 (globotriaosyl ceramide)-binding site with sequence similarity to verotoxin B-subunits: implications of molecular mimicry for B cell adhesion and enterohemorrhagic Escherichia coli pathogenesis. J Exp Med 180(1):191–201

16. Mori T, Kiyokawa N, Katagiri YU, Taguchi T, Suzuki T, Sekino T et al (2000) Globotriaosyl ceramide (CD77/Gb3) in the glycolipid-enriched membrane domain participates in B-cell receptor-mediated apoptosis by regulating lyn kinase activity in human B cells. Exp Hematol 28(11):1260–1268

17. Lingwood CA (1996) Role of verotoxin receptors in pathogenesis. Trends Microbiol 4(4):147–153

18. Müthing J, Schweppe CH, Karch H, Friedrich AW (2009) Shiga toxins, glycosphingolipid diversity, and endothelial cell injury. Thromb Haemost 101(2):252–264

19. Lingwood CA, Khine AA, Arab S (1998) Globotriaosyl ceramide (Gb3) expression in human tumour cells: intracellular trafficking defines a new retrograde transport pathway from the cell surface to the nucleus, which correlates with sensitivity to verotoxin. Acta Biochim Pol 45(2):351–359

20. Lingwood CA (1998) Oligosaccharide receptors for bacteria: a view to a kill. Curr Opin Chem Biol 2(6):695–700

21. Johansson D, Kosovac E, Moharer J, Ljuslinder I, Brännström T, Johansson A et al (2009) Expression of verotoxin-1 receptor Gb3 in breast cancer tissue and verotoxin-1 signal transduction to apoptosis. BMC Cancer 9:67

22. Hulková H, Cervenková M, Ledvinová J, Tocháčková M, Hrebícek M, Poupetová H et al (2001) A novel mutation in the coding region of the prosaposin gene leads to a complete deficiency of prosaposin and saposins, and is associated with a complex sphingolipidosis dominated by lactosylceramide accumulation. Hum Mol Genet 10(9):927–940

23. Desnick R, Ioannou Y, Eng C (2001) Alpha-galactosidase A deficiency: Fabry disease. In: Scriver C, Beaudet A, Sly W, Valle D (eds) The metabolic and molecular bases of inherited disease, 8th edn. McGraw-Hill, New York, pp 3733–3774

24. Dawson G, Sweeley CC (1970) In vivo studies on glycosphingolipid metabolism in porcine blood. J Biol Chem 245(2):410–416

25. Mills K, Johnson A, Winchester B (2002) Synthesis of novel internal standards for the quantitative determination of plasma ceramide trihexoside in Fabry disease by tandem mass spectrometry. FEBS Lett 515(1–3):171–176

26. Young E, Mills K, Morris P, Vellodi A, Lee P, Waldek S et al (2005) Is globotriaosylceramide a useful biomarker in Fabry disease? Acta Paediatr Suppl 94(447):51–54, discussion 37–8

27. Vance DE, Krivit W, Sweeley CC (1975) Metabolism of neutral glycosphingolipids in plasma of a normal human and a patient with Fabry's disease. J Biol Chem 250(20):8119–8125

28. Dawson G, Kruski AW, Scanu AM (1976) Distribution of glycosphingolipids in the serum lipoproteins of normal human subjects and patients with hypo- and hyperlipidemias. J Lipid Res 17(2):125–131

29. Loeb JA, Dawson G (1982) Reversible exchange of glycosphingolipids between human high and low density lipoproteins. J Biol Chem 257(20):11982–11987

30. Chatterjee S, Kwiterovich POJ (1984) Glycosphingolipids and plasma lipoproteins: a review. Can J Biochem Cell Biol 62(6):385–397

31. Clarke JT, Stoltz JM, Mulcahey MR (1976) Neutral glycosphingolipids of serum lipoproteins in Fabry's disease. Biochim Biophys Acta 431(2):317–325
32. Clarke JT (1981) The glycosphingolipids of human plasma lipoproteins. Can J Biochem 59(6):412–417
33. DeGraba T, Azhar S, Dignat-George F, Brown E, Boutière B, Altarescu G et al (2000) Profile of endothelial and leukocyte activation in Fabry patients. Ann Neurol 47(2):229–233
34. Shen J, Meng X, Moore DF, Quirk JM, Shayman JA, Schiffmann R et al (2008) Globotriaosylceramide induces oxidative stress and up-regulates cell adhesion molecule expression in Fabry disease endothelial cells. Mol Genet Metab 95(3):163–168
35. Park JL, Whitesall SE, D'Alecy LG, Shu L, Shayman JA (2008) Vascular dysfunction in the alpha-galactosidase A-knockout mouse is an endothelial cell-, plasma membrane-based defect. Clin Exp Pharmacol Physiol 35(10):1156–1163
36. Park JL, Shu L, Shayman JA (2009) Differential involvement of COX1 and COX2 in the vasculopathy associated with the alpha-galactosidase A-knockout mouse. Am J Physiol Heart Circ Physiol 296(4):H1133–H1140
37. Shu L, Park JL, Byun J, Pennathur S, Kollmeyer J, Shayman JA (2009) Decreased nitric oxide bioavailability in a mouse model of Fabry disease. J Am Soc Nephrol 20(9): 1975–1985
38. Aerts JM, Groener JE, Kuiper S, Donker-Koopman WE, Strijland A, Ottenhoff R et al (2008) Elevated globotriaosylsphingosine is a hallmark of Fabry disease. Proc Natl Acad Sci USA 105(8):2812–2817
39. Desnick RJ, Dawson G, Desnick SJ, Sweeley CC, Krivit W (1971) Diagnosis of glycosphingolipidoses by urinary-sediment analysis. N Engl J Med 284(14):739–744
40. Chatterjee S, Gupta P, Pyeritz RE, Kwiterovich POJ (1984) Immunohistochemical localization of glycosphingolipid in urinary renal tubular cells in Fabry's disease. Am J Clin Pathol 82(1):24–28
41. Fauler G, Rechberger GN, Devrnja D, Erwa W, Plecko B, Kotanko P et al (2005) Rapid determination of urinary globotriaosylceramide isoform profiles by electrospray ionization mass spectrometry using stearoyl-d35-globotriaosylceramide as internal standard. Rapid Commun Mass Spectrom 19(11):1499–1506
42. Fuller M, Sharp PC, Rozaklis T, Whitfield PD, Blacklock D, Hopwood JJ et al (2005) Urinary lipid profiling for the identification of fabry hemizygotes and heterozygotes. Clin Chem 51(4):688–694
43. Kitagawa T, Ishige N, Suzuki K, Owada M, Ohashi T, Kobayashi M et al (2005) Non-invasive screening method for Fabry disease by measuring globotriaosylceramide in whole urine samples using tandem mass spectrometry. Mol Genet Metab 85(3): 196–202
44. Chatterjee S, Clarke KS, Kwiterovich POJ (1986) Uptake and metabolism of lactosylceramide on low density lipoproteins in cultured proximal tubular cells from normal and familial hypercholesterolemic homozygotes. J Biol Chem 261(29):13480–13486
45. Pastores GM, Lien YH (2002) Biochemical and molecular genetic basis of Fabry disease. J Am Soc Nephrol 13(Suppl 2):S130–S133
46. Touboul D, Roy S, Germain DP, Baillet A, Brion F, Prognon P et al (2005) Fast fingerprinting by MALDI-TOF mass spectrometry of urinary sediment glycosphingolipids in Fabry disease. Anal Bioanal Chem 382(5):1209–1216
47. Kuchar L, Hlavata J, Asfaw B, Ledvinova J (2008) MS/MS sphingolipid profilig-useful diagnostic tool in disorders with Gb3Cer and sulphatide storage. J Inherit Metab Dis 31(Suppl 1):107
48. Kuchar L, Ledvinová J, Hrebícek M, Mysková H, Dvoráková L, Berná L et al (2009) Prosaposin deficiency and saposin B deficiency (activator-deficient metachromatic leukodystrophy): report on two patients detected by analysis of urinary sphingolipids and carrying novel PSAP gene mutations. Am J Med Genet A 149A(4):613–621

49. Linthorst GE, Folman CC, Aerts JMFG, Hollak CEM (2003) Blood group does not correlate with disease severity in patients with Fabry disease (alpha-galactosidase A deficiency). Blood Cells Mol Dis 31(3):324–326

50. Wherrett JR, Hakomori SI (1973) Characterization of a blood group B glycolipid, accumulating in the pancreas of a patient with Fabry's disease. J Biol Chem 248(9):3046–3051

51. Ledvinová J, Poupetová H, Hanácková A, Písacka M, Elleder M (1997) Blood group B glycosphingolipids in alpha-galactosidase deficiency (Fabry disease): influence of secretor status. Biochim Biophys Acta 1345(2):180–187

52. Schenkel-Brunner H (2000) Human blood groups: chemical and biochemical basis of antigen specificity, 2nd edn. Springer, Wien, pp 54–183

53. Mills K, Vellodi A, Morris P, Cooper D, Morris M, Young E et al (2004) Monitoring the clinical and biochemical response to enzyme replacement therapy in three children with Fabry disease. Eur J Pediatr 163(10):595–603

54. Stanley P, Cummings R (2009) Structures common to different glycans. In: Varki A, Cummings R, Esko J, Freeze H, Stanley P, Bertozzi C, Hart G, Etzler M (eds) Essentials of glycobiology, 2nd edn. CSHL Press America, Plainview. Available from http://www.ncbi. nlm.nih.gov/bookshelf/br.fcgi?book=glyco2

55. Li Y, Teneberg S, Thapa P, Bendelac A, Levery SB, Zhou D (2008) Sensitive detection of isoglobo and globo series tetraglycosylceramides in human thymus by ion trap mass spectrometry. Glycobiology 18(2):158–165

56. Salio M, Speak AO, Shepherd D, Polzella P, Illarionov PA, Veerapen N et al (2007) Modulation of human natural killer T cell ligands on TLR-mediated antigen-presenting cell activation. Proc Natl Acad Sci USA 104(51):20490–20495

57. Speak AO, Salio M, Neville DCA, Fontaine J, Priestman DA, Platt N et al (2007) Implications for invariant natural killer T cell ligands due to the restricted presence of isoglobotrihexosylceramide in mammals. Proc Natl Acad Sci USA 104(14):5971–5976

58. Tettamanti G, Bassi R, Viani P, Riboni L (2003) Salvage pathways in glycosphingolipid metabolism. Biochimie 85(3–4):423–437

59. Tettamanti G (2004) Ganglioside/glycosphingolipid turnover: new concepts. Glycoconj J 20(5):301–317

60. Futerman AH (2006) Intracellular trafficking of sphingolipids: relationship to biosynthesis. Biochim Biophys Acta 1758(12):1885–1892

61. Hanada K, Kumagai K, Yasuda S, Miura Y, Kawano M, Fukasawa M et al (2003) Molecular machinery for non-vesicular trafficking of ceramide. Nature 426(6968):803–809

62. Neumann S, van Meer G (2008) Sphingolipid management by an orchestra of lipid transfer proteins. Biol Chem 389(11):1349–1360

63. Schulze H, Kolter T, Sandhoff K (2009) Principles of lysosomal membrane degradation: cellular topology and biochemistry of lysosomal lipid degradation. Biochim Biophys Acta 1793(4):674–683

64. Ichikawa S, Sakiyama H, Suzuki G, Hidari KI, Hirabayashi Y (1996) Expression cloning of a cDNA for human ceramide glucosyltransferase that catalyzes the first glycosylation step of glycosphingolipid synthesis. Proc Natl Acad Sci USA 93(22):12654

65. Futerman AH, Pagano RE (1991) Determination of the intracellular sites and topology of glucosylceramide synthesis in rat liver. Biochem J 280(Pt 2):295–302

66. Jeckel D, Karrenbauer A, Burger KN, van Meer G, Wieland F (1992) Glucosylceramide is synthesized at the cytosolic surface of various Golgi subfractions. J Cell Biol 117(2): 259–267

67. Nomura T, Takizawa M, Aoki J, Arai H, Inoue K, Wakisaka E et al (1998) Purification, cDNA cloning, and expression of UDP-Gal: glucosylceramide beta-1,4-galactosyltransferase from rat brain. J Biol Chem 273(22):13570–13577

68. D'Angelo G, Polishchuk E, Di Tullio G, Santoro M, Di Campli A, Godi A et al (2007) Glycosphingolipid synthesis requires FAPP2 transfer of glucosylceramide. Nature 449(7158):62–67

69. Futerman AH (2007) Cell biology: taxi service for lipids. Nature 449(7158):35–37
70. Halter D, Neumann S, van Dijk SM, Wolthoorn J, de Mazière AM, Vieira OV et al (2007) Pre- and post-Golgi translocation of glucosylceramide in glycosphingolipid synthesis. J Cell Biol 179(1):101–115
71. Yamaji T, Kumagai K, Tomishige N, Hanada K (2008) Two sphingolipid transfer proteins, CERT and FAPP2: their roles in sphingolipid metabolism. IUBMB Life 60(8):511–518
72. Maccioni HJF, Giraudo CG, Daniotti JL (2002) Understanding the stepwise synthesis of glycolipids. Neurochem Res 27(7–8):629–636
73. Furukawa K, Iwamura K, Uchikawa M, Sojka BN, Wiels J, Okajima T et al (2000) Molecular basis for the p phenotype. Identification of distinct and multiple mutations in the alpha 1,4-galactosyltransferase gene in Swedish and Japanese individuals. J Biol Chem 275(48):37752–37756
74. Kojima Y, Fukumoto S, Furukawa K, Okajima T, Wiels J, Yokoyama K et al (2000) Molecular cloning of globotriaosylceramide/CD77 synthase, a glycosyltransferase that initiates the synthesis of globo series glycosphingolipids. J Biol Chem 275(20): 15152–15156
75. Fujii Y, Numata S, Nakamura Y, Honda T, Furukawa K, Urano T et al (2005) Murine glyco-syltransferases responsible for the expression of globo-series glycolipids: cDNA structures, mRNA expression, and distribution of their products. Glycobiology 15(12):1257–1267
76. Iwamura K, Furukawa K, Uchikawa M, Sojka BN, Kojima Y, Wiels J et al (2003) The blood group P1 synthase gene is identical to the Gb3/CD77 synthase gene. A clue to the solution of the P1/P2/p puzzle. J Biol Chem 278(45):44429–44438
77. Duk M, Westerlind U, Norberg T, Pazynina G, Bovin NN, Lisowska E (2003) Specificity of human anti-NOR antibodies, a distinct species of "natural" anti-alpha-galactosyl antibodies. Glycobiology 13(4):279–284
78. Zhou D, Mattner J, Cantu C III, Schrantz N, Yin N, Gao Y et al (2004) Lysosomal glycosphingolipid recognition by NKT cells. Science 306(5702):1786–1789
79. Christiansen D, Milland J, Mouhtouris E, Vaughan H, Pellicci DG, McConville MJ et al (2008) Humans lack iGb3 due to the absence of functional iGb3-synthase: implications for NKT cell development and transplantation. PLoS Biol 6(7):e172
80. Zajonc DM, Savage PB, Bendelac A, Wilson IA, Teyton L (2008) Crystal structures of mouse CD1d-iGb3 complex and its cognate Valpha14 T cell receptor suggest a model for dual recognition of foreign and self glycolipids. J Mol Biol 377(4):1104–1116
81. Kolter T, Sandhoff K (2006) Sphingolipid metabolism diseases. Biochim Biophys Acta 1758(12):2057–2079
82. Kolter T, Sandhoff K (2005) Principles of lysosomal membrane digestion: stimulation of sphingolipid degradation by sphingolipid activator proteins and anionic lysosomal lipids. Annu Rev Cell Dev Biol 21:81–103
83. Harzer K, Paton BC, Poulos A, Kustermann-Kuhn B, Roggendorf W, Grisar T et al (1989) Sphingolipid activator protein deficiency in a 16-week-old atypical Gaucher disease patient and his fetal sibling: biochemical signs of combined sphingolipidoses. Eur J Pediatr 149(1):31–39
84. Remmel N, Locatelli-Hoops S, Breiden B, Schwarzmann G, Sandhoff K (2007) Saposin B mobilizes lipids from cholesterol-poor and bis(monoacylglycero)phosphate-rich membranes at acidic pH. Unglycosylated patient variant saposin B lacks lipid-extraction capacity. FEBS J 274(13):3405–3420
85. Sandhoff K, Kolter T, Harzer K (2001) Sphingolipid activator proteins. In: Scriver C, Beaudet A, Sly W, Valle D (eds) The metabolic and molecular bases of inherited disease, 8th edn. McGraw-Hill, New York, pp 3371–3388
86. Kint JA (1970) Fabry's disease: alpha-galactosidase deficiency. Science 167(922): 1268–1269
87. Kint JA (1971) On the existence and the enzymic interconversion of the isozymes of alpha-galactosidase in human organs. Arch Int Physiol Biochim 79(3):633–634

88. Beutler E, Kuhl W (1972) Biochemical and electrophoretic studies of -galactosidase in normal man, in patients with Fabry's disease, and in Equidae. Am J Hum Genet 24(3):237–249

89. Desnick RJ, Allen KY, Desnick SJ, Raman MK, Bernlohr RW, Krivit W (1973) Fabry's disease: enzymatic diagnosis of hemizygotes and heterozygotes. Alpha-galactosidase activities in plasma, serum, urine, and leukocytes. J Lab Clin Med 81(2):157–171

90. Rietra PJ, Van den Bergh FA, Tager JM (1975) Properties of the residual alpha-galactosidase activity in the tissues of a Fabry hemizygote. Clin Chim Acta 62(3):401–413

91. Bishop DF, Desnick RJ (1981) Affinity purification of alpha-galactosidase A from human spleen, placenta, and plasma with elimination of pyrogen contamination. Properties of the purified splenic enzyme compared to other forms. J Biol Chem 256(3):1307–1316

92. Dean KJ, Sweeley CC (1979) Studies on human liver alpha-galactosidases. II. Purification and enzymatic properties of alpha-galactosidase B (alpha-N-acetylgalactosaminidase). J Biol Chem 254(20):10001–10005

93. Dean KJ, Sweeley CC (1979) Studies on human liver alpha-galactosidases. I. Purification of alpha-galactosidase A and its enzymatic properties with glycolipid and oligosaccharide substrates. J Biol Chem 254(20):9994–10000

94. Dean KJ, Sung SS, Sweeley CC (1977) The identification of alpha-galactosidase B from human liver as an alpha-N-acetylgalactosaminidase. Biochem Biophys Res Commun 77(4):1411–1417

95. Schram AW, Hamers MN, Tager JM (1977) The identity of alpha-galactosidase B from human liver. Biochim Biophys Acta 482(1):138–144

96. Wang AM, Bishop DF, Desnick RJ (1990) Human alpha-N-acetylgalactosaminidase-molecular cloning, nucleotide sequence, and expression of a full-length cDNA. Homology with human alpha-galactosidase A suggests evolution from a common ancestral gene. J Biol Chem 265(35):21859–21866

97. Hujová J, Sikora J, Dobrovolný R, Poupetová H, Ledvinová J, Kostrouchová M et al (2005) Characterization of gana-1, a Caenorhabditis elegans gene encoding a single ortholog of vertebrate alpha-galactosidase and alpha-N-acetylgalactosaminidase. BMC Cell Biol 6(1):5

98. Henrissat B, Davies G (1997) Structural and sequence-based classification of glycoside hydrolases. Curr Opin Struct Biol 7(5):637–644

99. Mayes JS, Scheerer JB, Sifers RN, Donaldson ML (1981) Differential assay for lysosomal alpha-galactosidases in human tissues and its application to Fabry's disease. Clin Chim Acta 112(2):247–251

100. Garman SC, Garboczi DN (2002) Structural basis of Fabry disease. Mol Genet Metab 77(1–2):3–11

101. Matsuura F, Ohta M, Ioannou YA, Desnick RJ (1998) Human alpha-galactosidase A: characterization of the N-linked oligosaccharides on the intracellular and secreted glycoforms overexpressed by Chinese hamster ovary cells. Glycobiology 8(4):329–339

102. Ioannou YA, Zeidner KM, Grace ME, Desnick RJ (1998) Human alpha-galactosidase A: glycosylation site 3 is essential for enzyme solubility. Biochem J 332(Pt 3):789–797

103. Eng CM, Resnick-Silverman LA, Niehaus DJ, Astrin KH, Desnick RJ (1993) Nature and frequency of mutations in the alpha-galactosidase A gene that cause Fabry disease. Am J Hum Genet 53(6):1186–1197

104. Ioannou YA, Bishop DF, Desnick RJ (1992) Overexpression of human alpha-galactosidase A results in its intracellular aggregation, crystallization in lysosomes, and selective secretion. J Cell Biol 119(5):1137–1150

105. Lemansky P, Bishop DF, Desnick RJ, Hasilik A, von Figura K (1987) Synthesis and processing of alpha-galactosidase A in human fibroblasts. Evidence for different mutations in Fabry disease. J Biol Chem 262(5):2062–2065

106. Keslová-Veselíková J, Hůlková H, Dobrovolný R, Asfaw B, Poupetová H, Berná L et al (2008) Replacement of alpha-galactosidase A in Fabry disease: effect on fibroblast cultures compared with biopsied tissues of treated patients. Virchows Arch 452(6):651–665

107. Mayes JS, Cray EL, Dell VA, Scheerer JB, Sifers RN (1982) Endocytosis of lysosomal alpha-galactosidase A by cultured fibroblasts from patients with Fabry disease. Am J Hum Genet 34(4):602–610
108. Beutler E, Kuhl W (1972) Purification and properties of human alpha-galactosidases. J Biol Chem 247(22):7195–7200
109. Ishii S, Chang H, Kawasaki K, Yasuda K, Wu H, Garman SC et al (2007) Mutant alpha-galactosidase A enzymes identified in Fabry disease patients with residual enzyme activity: biochemical characterization and restoration of normal intracellular processing by 1-deoxygalactonojirimycin. Biochem J 406(2):285–295
110. Ishii S, Kase R, Sakuraba H, Suzuki Y (1993) Characterization of a mutant alpha-galactosidase gene product for the late-onset cardiac form of Fabry disease. Biochem Biophys Res Commun 197(3):1585–1589
111. Kase R, Bierfreund U, Klein A, Kolter T, Utsumi K, Itoha K et al (2000) Characterization of two alpha-galactosidase mutants (Q279E and R301Q) found in an atypical variant of Fabry disease. Biochim Biophys Acta 1501(2–3):227–235
112. Fan J, Ishii S (2007) Active-site-specific chaperone therapy for Fabry disease. Yin and Yang of enzyme inhibitors. FEBS J 274(19):4962–4971
113. Froissart R, Guffon N, Vanier MT, Desnick RJ, Maire I (2003) Fabry disease: D313Y is an alpha-galactosidase A sequence variant that causes pseudodeficient activity in plasma. Mol Genet Metab 80(3):307–314
114. Bach G, Rosenmann E, Karni A, Cohen T (1982) Pseudodeficiency of alpha-galactosidase A. Clin Genet 21(1):59–64
115. Elleder M, Bradová V, Smíd F, Budsínský M, Harzer K, Kustermann-Kuhn B et al (1990) Cardiocyte storage and hypertrophy as a sole manifestation of Fabry's disease. Report on a case simulating hypertrophic non-obstructive cardiomyopathy. Virchows Arch A Pathol Anat Histopathol 417(5):449–455
116. Kobayashi T, Kira J, Shinnoh N, Goto I, Kuroiwa Y (1985) Fabry's disease with partially deficient hydrolysis of ceramide trihexoside. J Neurol Sci 67(2):179–185
117. Yasuda M, Shabbeer J, Benson SD, Maire I, Burnett RM, Desnick RJ (2003) Fabry disease: characterization of alpha-galactosidase A double mutations and the D313Y plasma enzyme pseudodeficiency allele. Hum Mutat 22(6):486–492
118. Kase R, Bierfreund U, Klein A, Kolter T, Itoh K, Suzuki M et al (1996) Only sphingolipid activator protein B (SAP-B or saposin B) stimulates the degradation of globotriaosylceramide by recombinant human lysosomal alpha-galactosidase in a detergent-free liposomal system. FEBS Lett 393(1):74–76
119. Hahn AF, Gordon BA, Hinton GG, Gilbert JJ (1982) A variant form of metachromatic leukodystrophy without arylsulfatase deficiency. Ann Neurol 12(1):33–36
120. Schlote W, Harzer K, Christomanou H, Paton BC, Kustermann-Kuhn B, Schmid B et al (1991) Sphingolipid activator protein 1 deficiency in metachromatic leucodystrophy with normal arylsulphatase A activity. A clinical, morphological, biochemical, and immunological study. Eur J Pediatr 150(8):584–591
121. Shapiro LJ, Aleck KA, Kaback MM, Itabashi H, Desnick RJ, Brand N et al (1979) Metachromatic leukodystrophy without arylsulfatase A deficiency. Pediatr Res 13(10):1179–1181
122. Henseler M, Klein A, Reber M, Vanier MT, Landrieu P, Sandhoff K (1996) Analysis of a splice-site mutation in the sap-precursor gene of a patient with metachromatic leukodystrophy. Am J Hum Genet 58(1):65–74
123. Li SC, Kihara H, Serizawa S, Li YT, Fluharty AL, Mayes JS et al (1985) Activator protein required for the enzymatic hydrolysis of cerebroside sulfate. Deficiency in urine of patients affected with cerebroside sulfatase activator deficiency and identity with activators for the enzymatic hydrolysis of GM1 ganglioside and globotriaosylceramide. J Biol Chem 260(3):1867–1871

124. Bradová V, Smíd F, Ulrich-Bott B, Roggendorf W, Paton BC, Harzer K (1993) Prosaposin deficiency: further characterization of the sphingolipid activator protein-deficient sibs. Multiple glycolipid elevations (including lactosylceramidosis), partial enzyme deficiencies and ultrastructure of the skin in this generalized sphingolipid storage disease. Hum Genet 92(2):143–152

125. Schnabel D, Schröder M, Fürst W, Klein A, Hurwitz R, Zenk T et al (1992) Simultaneous deficiency of sphingolipid activator proteins 1 and 2 is caused by a mutation in the initiation codon of their common gene. J Biol Chem 267(5):3312–3315

126. Asfaw B, Ledvinová J, Dobrovolny R, Bakker HD, Desnick RJ, van Diggelen OP et al (2002) Defects in degradation of blood group A and B glycosphingolipids in Schindler and Fabry diseases. J Lipid Res 43(7):1096–1104

127. Yuan W, Qi X, Tsang P, Kang S, Illarionov PA, Besra GS et al (2007) Saposin B is the dominant saposin that facilitates lipid binding to human CD1d molecules. Proc Natl Acad Sci USA 104(13):5551–5556

128. Ahn VE, Faull KF, Whitelegge JP, Fluharty AL, Prive GG (2003) Crystal structure of saposin B reveals a dimeric shell for lipid binding. Proc Natl Acad Sci USA 100(1):38–43

129. Stokeley D, Bemporad D, Gavaghan D, Sansom MSP (2007) Conformational dynamics of a lipid-interacting protein: MD simulations of saposin B. Biochemistry 46(47):13573–13580

130. Li SC, Sonnino S, Tettamanti G, Li YT (1988) Characterization of a nonspecific activator protein for the enzymatic hydrolysis of glycolipids. J Biol Chem 263(14):6588–6591

131. Vogel A, Schwarzmann G, Sandhoff K (1991) Glycosphingolipid specificity of the human sulfatide activator protein. Eur J Biochem 200(2):591–597

132. Bruhn H (2005) A short guided tour through functional and structural features of saposin-like proteins. Biochem J 389(Pt 2):249–257

133. Desnick R, Schindler D (2001) Alpha-N-Acetylgalactosaminidase deficiency: Schindler disease. In: Scriver C, Beaudet A, Sly W, Valle D (eds) The metabolic and molecular bases of inherited disease, 8th edn. McGraw-Hill, New York, pp 3483–3505

134. Asfaw B, Schindler D, Ledvinová J, Cerný B, Smíd F, Conzelmann E (1998) Degradation of blood group A glycolipid A-6-2 by normal and mutant human skin fibroblasts. J Lipid Res 39(9):1768–1780

135. Bakker HD, de Sonnaville ML, Vreken P, Abeling NG, Groener JE, Keulemans JL et al (2001) Human alpha-N-acetylgalactosaminidase (alpha-NAGA) deficiency: no association with neuroaxonal dystrophy? Eur J Hum Genet 9(2):91–96

136. Vyletal P, Hulková H, Zivná M, Berna L, Novak P, Elleder M et al (2008) Abnormal expression and processing of uromodulin in Fabry disease reflects tubular cell storage alteration and is reversible by enzyme replacement therapy. J Inherit Metab Dis 31(4):508–517

Chapter 5
Clinically Relevant Examples of Genotype–Phenotype Correlation

Gheona Altarescu

Abstract Although Fabry disease is a rare lysosomal storage disorder, intensive research has been performed in the last decade in order to elucidate the pathogenesis, underlying mechanisms and the best treatment for this disorder. Despite this, the motto '10 years 10 doctors' is still the reality mainly because of the difficulty to correlate between different signs and symptoms in one rare disease. Furthermore, there is no good correlation between phenotype-genotype and it is difficult if not impossible to predict which genotype will develop into a complete or partial Fabry phenotype and which females will remain asymptomatic and which will develop symptoms. This chapter will focus on describing the efforts that have been made over the years in order to try to correlate genotypes with specific phenotypes as well as modifier genes that might help predicting future symptoms of patients with Fabry disease.

Keywords Phenotype · Genotype · Modifier genes · Polymorphisms

5.1 Introduction: Genotyping

The α-galactosidase A gene (GLA)-(OMIM No. 300644) is located on Xq22.1 [1] and it is 12-kb long encompassing seven exons. GLA encodes for a 429 amino acid precursor protein that is processed to 370 amino acid glycoprotein functioning as a homodimer [2]. Based on The Human Gene Mutation Database at the Institute of Medical Genetics in Cardiff (http://www.hgmd.cf.ac.uk/ac/index.php), there are currently 431 mutations described. Of those, 295 are missense/nonsense type mutations, 66 small deletions, 12 large deletions, 21 splice defects, 3 complex rearrangements, and one is a large insertion. The reason for this relatively large number of different mutations in the GLA gene is not known. One might speculate that

G. Altarescu (✉)
Medical Genetics Institute, Shaare Zedek Medical Center, Jerusalem, Israel
e-mail: gheona@szmc.org.il

D. Elstein et al. (eds.), *Fabry Disease*, DOI 10.1007/978-90-481-9033-1_5,
© Springer Science+Business Media B.V. 2010

having the Fabry trait presents a selective advantage such as resistance to certain types of bacterial infections, in particular those that express the *Escherichia coli* shiga-like toxin verotoxin [3]. While the diagnosis of Fabry disease, once suspected, can be easily made in male patients by an enzymatic a-Gal A assay in plasma, leukocytes, or cultured fibroblasts, it often fails to distinguish Fabry heterozygotes with high residual enzyme activity from normal individuals with low enzyme activity. No single protocol to date is capable of detecting all GLA mutations, due to the extreme variability in the germline mutations, ranging from large deletions encompassing the entire gene and its flanking regions, to single base-pair substitutions. The Multiplex Ligation-dependent Probe Amplification (MLPA) is a recent technique that can easily detect these rearrangements and, hence, would be well suited for routine detection of deletions and duplications [4–6]. In the study by Schirinzi et al. [6] two novel different deletions were detected using MLPA assay on two Fabry patients although both were mutation negative by sequencing analysis. These data suggest that this type of screening should be systematically included in genetic testing surveys of patients with Fabry disease.

5.2 Genetic Misdiagnosis and Phenotypic Presentation

We would like to draw attention to the fact that sometimes even genetic diagnosis can be misleading. Recently there were reported results of biochemical and sequence analysis with quantification, by real-time PCR, of alternatively spliced GLA mRNAs in five male Fabry patients [7, 8]. In the study by Filoni et al. [7], the standard genomic DNA protocols based on sequencing analysis failed to identify any mutation in a 62-year-old male patient with a very low a-galactosidase A activity and a classical Fabry disease phenotype. Also, the standard genomic DNA analysis did not identify any mutation in this patient's 64-year-old sister, who had suffered since youth from acroparesthesias and abdominal pain but presented with a-galactosidase A activity within the normal range.

Because of this singular condition, studies of GLA mRNAs of fibroblasts using absolute real-time RT-PCR quantification might be required in cases in which a mutation can not be found. In the paper by Ishii et al. [9] an impressive reduction in predominant lysosomal GLA transcripts was detected in a patient with cardiac Fabry disease and residual enzyme activity of 9% of normal but no mutation found in the exons of the gene sequenced; in contrast, the alternatively spliced GLA mRNAs were dramatically over-expressed, suggesting a transcription regulation defect. The subsequent mRNAs sequence analysis showed the absence of any reported mutation; genomic DNA sequence analysis identified a new intronic mutation, g.9273C4T, located 5 nucleotides upstream of the alternative 30 splicing junction. This genetic lesion, absent in the normal population, was also identified in the patient's affected sister. These findings strongly suggest a correlation between the new intronic mutation and the unbalanced a-galactosidase A mRNAs ratio, which could therefore be responsible for the reduced enzyme activity that causes the Fabry disease. On the basis of such considerations, and taking advantage of real time RT-PCR analysis we have recently developed, studies at the transcriptome level should be included in the routine molecular investigation when DNA standard protocols fail to identify any genetic lesion.

5.3 Modifier Genes: Cerebral Lesions

Due to the lack of correlation between genotype and phenotype, several modifier genes were analyzed and correlation with various symptoms of Fabry disease was attempted. Since not all patients with Fabry disease develop cerebral lesions, it is important to identify potential genetic modifiers of this process. In a prospective observational study we evaluated 57 consecutive Fabry hemizygous male patients for brain FLAIR MRI lesions [10]. The authors found that the-174 G/C of IL6 polymorphism of interleukin 6 (IL-6), the G894T polymorphism of endothelial nitric oxide synthase (eNOS), the factor V G1691A mutation as well as the G79A and the A-13G polymorphisms of protein Z were significantly associated with cerebral lesions, but not the prothrombin G20210A variant and the methylenetetrahydrofolate reductase (MTHFR) C677T variant. A clear relationship between a number of pro-thrombotic gene polymorphisms and the presumptive ischemic small-vessel cerebral lesions in Fabry disease [10] was found. Subsequently, an interaction was found between the factor VG1691A mutation of endothelial nitric oxide synthase and α-galactosidase A deficiency in mouse models [11]. α-Galactosidase A deficiency markedly increased tissue fibrin deposition in mice carrying the factor V G1691A mutation compared with factor V G1691A mutation alone.

5.4 Modifier Genes: Vasculopathy

Recently, patients with polymorphisms of eNOS described above were found to have higher left ventricular posterior wall thickness – linking genetic modifiers to a cardiac biomarker in Fabry disease [12]. These findings suggest that endogenous proteins may modulate Fabry cerebral vasculopathy and will potentially allow the prospective identification of patients who are most at risk for developing these complications. Such complications are likely to be associated with a concomitant increase in oxidative stress and accelerated atherosclerosis, especially in genotypically susceptible individuals

A common mutation correlated with cardiac involvement is N215S. This mutation affects a highly conserved, functional N-glycosylation consensus site of GALA [13, 14]. However, it has also been reported before in one patient with a long history of renal disease [15]. Regarding this latter finding, Erdos et al. [16] reported three Fabry patients presented with renal involvement and bearing the mutation N215S. In addition, analysis of gDNA and cDNA in one female of this family disclosed homozygosity for the N215S mutation

5.5 Modifier Genes: Cardiac Left Ventricular Hypertrophy

Hypertrophic cardiomyopathy measured by left posterior wall thickness (LPWT) of the heart, represents a major component of Fabry disease morbidity in adult patients. Endothelium-derived nitric oxide (eNO), produced by eNO synthase (eNOS), is a key regulator of vessel wall function and cardiovascular homeostasis. The effect of the polymorphisms c.894G > T (p.Glu298Asp) in exon 7 and the 27 bp tandem repeat (VNTR; allele a: 4 and allele b: 5 repeats) in intron 4 of the NOS3 gene, encoding eNOS, was analyzed on the LPWT of 102 patients with Fabry disease. In the cohort of 46 male patients, LPWT mean value of the group with *GG* genotype at position c.894 was smaller by 1 mm than that of *(GT + TT)* ($p = 0.058$). LPWT of patients with *bb* was thicker by 1.4 mm than that of *(ab + aa)* ($p = 0.022$). This has led to the possibility of an association between polymorphisms of endothelial nitric oxide synthase gene (NOS3) and LPWT of the heart in Fabry disease [12].

Vitamin D receptor (VDR) polymorphisms have been also correlated with Fabry disease as modifier genes. VDR polymorphisms, TaqI, ApaI, FokI, and BsmI have been analyzed in patients with Fabry disease and associated with a disease-specific severity score, the Mainz Severity Score Index (MSSI). A protective effect of the TaqI *tt* genotype was found so that there were significantly lower median scores in clinical categories in patients with the *tt* genotype vs. those with the *TT* genotype. Multivariate models of haplotypes with MSSI scores reveal that *T-A-f-B* and *t-A-F-B* haplotypes of (TaqI, ApaI, FokI, and BsmI) VDR gene polymorphisms were significantly associated with variation in the Fabry cardiac phenotype [17].

5.6 Summary: Epigenetic Genotype–Phenotype Correlations

Thus, recent inquiry into genetic modifiers that are epigenetic effectors for specific signs in the normal population and that are common among patients with Fabry disease have shown correlations that might be predictive. This implies that there is value in ascertaining and assessing epigenetic modifiers that may impact the Fabry phenotype. However, what is most interesting is the possibility that the effect of these modifier genes is not exactly that which is seen in normal populations, i.e., there may be a differential effect in Fabry disease that is not necessarily equivalent to what would be predicted from other populations.

References

1. Bishop DF, Kornreich R, Desnick RJ (1988) Structural organization of the human alpha-galactosidase A gene: further evidence for the absence of a 3' untranslated region. Proc Natl Acad Sci USA 85:3903–3907
2. Garman SC, Garboczi DN (2004) The molecular defect leading to Fabry disease: structure of human alpha-galactosidase. J Mol Biol 337:319–335

3. Cilmi SA, Karalius BJ, Choy W, Smith RN, Butterton JR (2006) Fabry disease in mice protects against lethal disease caused by Shiga toxin-expressing enterohemorrhagic Escherichia coli. J Infect Dis 194:1135–1140
4. Hartmann C, John AL, Klaes R et al (2004) Large BRCA1 gene deletions are found in 3% of German high-risk breast cancer families. Hum Mutat 24:534
5. Schouten JP, McElgunn CJ, Waaijer R, Wijnenburg DZ, Diepvens F, Pals G (2002) Relative quantification of 40 nucleic acid sequences by multiplex ligation dependent probe amplification. Nucleic Acids Res 30:e57
6. Schirinzi A, Centra M, Prattichizzo C et al (2008) Identification of GLA gene deletions in Fabry patients by Multiplex Ligation-dependent Probe Amplification (MLPA). Mol Genet Metab 94:382–385
7. Filoni C, Caciotti A, Carraresi L et al (2008) Unbalanced GLA mRNAs ratio quantified by real-time PCR in Fabry patients' fibroblasts results in Fabry disease. Eur J Hum Genet 16:1311–1317
8. Fervenza FC, Torra R, Lager DJ (2008) Fabry disease: an under-recognized cause of proteinuria. Kidney Int 73:1193–1199
9. Ishii S, Nakao S, Minamikawa-Tachino R et al (2002) Alternative splicing in the alpha-galactosidase A gene: increased exon inclusion results in the Fabry cardiac phenotype. Am J Hum Genet 70:994–1002
10. Altarescu G, Moore DF, Schiffmann R (2005) Effect of genetic modifiers on cerebral lesions in Fabry disease. Neurology 64:2148–2150
11. Shen Y, Bodary PF, Vargas FB et al (2006) Alpha-galactosidase A deficiency leads to increased tissue fibrin deposition and thrombosis in mice homozygous for the factor V Leiden mutation. Stroke 37:1106–1108
12. Rohard I, Schaefer E, Kampmann C, Beck M, Gal A (2008) Association between polymorphisms of endothelial nitric oxide synthase gene (NOS3) and left posterior wall thickness (LPWT) of the heart in Fabry disease. J Inherit Metab Dis
13. Blaydon D, Hill J, Winchester B (2001) Fabry disease: 20 novel GLA mutations in 35 families. Hum Mutat 18:459
14. Eng CM, Resnick-Silverman LA, Niehaus DJ, Astrin KH, Desnick RJ (1993) Nature and frequency of mutations in the alpha-galactosidase A gene that cause Fabry disease. Am J Hum Genet 53:1186–1197
15. Bekri B, Enica A, Ghafari T et al (2005) Fabry disease in patients with end-stage renal failure: the potential benefits of screening. Nephron Clin Pract 101:33–38
16. Eldos M, Nemeth K, Toth B et al (2008) Novel sequence variants of the a-galactosidase A gene in patients with Fabry disease. Mol Genet Metab 95:224–228
17. Teitcher M, Weinerman S, Whybra C et al (2008) Genetic polymorphisms of vitamin D receptor (VDR) in Fabry disease. Genetica 134:377–383

Chapter 6
Laboratory Diagnosis of Fabry Disease

Bryan Winchester and Elisabeth Young

Abstract The definitive diagnosis of Fabry disease in male patients is normally made by demonstrating a deficiency of α-galactosidase A in a blood sample, which may be white blood cells, plasma/serum or a dried blood spot. The diagnosis is confirmed by mutational analysis. The enzymatic assay is unreliable for detecting female carriers, who can only be diagnosed reliably by mutational analysis. The measurement of the storage products, globotriaosylceramide (Gb$_3$) in plasma and urine or globotriaosylsphingosine (lyso-Gb$_3$) in plasma can often provide support for a diagnosis and is useful for monitoring treatment. Methods for mass or high-risk screening have been developed based on measuring the α-galactosidase A activity and/or protein in dried blood spots or the storage products in urine collected on filter paper. In the future the detection of mutations in the α-galactosidase A using high-throughput methods for analysing DNA might be the first step rather than a confirmatory one in the diagnosis of Fabry disease.

Keywords Diagnosis of Fabry disease · α-galactosidase A · Heterozygote detection · Dried blood spots · Screening

6.1 Introduction

A recent survey of a large cohort of Fabry patients revealed that the average age of diagnosis was 25.7 $\pm$ 15.3 and 31.3 $\pm$ 17.4 years for male and female patients, respectively, with an average delay between onset of symptoms and diagnosis of ~12 years for both groups [1] Once there is a clinical suspicion of Fabry disease, the definitive diagnosis in male patients is usually made by demonstrating a deficiency of the lysosomal enzyme, α-galactosidase A, in a blood sample [2–9], which

B. Winchester (✉)
Biochemistry Research Group, UCL Institute of Child Health at Great Ormond Street Hospital, University College London, London, UK
e-mail: b.winchester@ich.ucl.ac.uk

D. Elstein et al. (eds.), *Fabry Disease*, DOI 10.1007/978-90-481-9033-1_6,
© Springer Science+Business Media B.V. 2010

may be white blood cells, plasma /serum [2–4] or a dried blood spot [10]. A deficiency of α-galactosidase A can also be demonstrated in cultured fibroblasts, tears, lymphoblasts, urine and other tissues [5]. Confirmation of the diagnosis is made by detection of a disease-causing mutation in the *GLA* gene. Female heterozygotes cannot be diagnosed reliably by measurement of the α-galactosidase A activity because of random inactivation of the X-chromosome in the cells of the sample [3–5]. Mutation analysis is necessary for the detection of heterozygotes [4, 5]. The measurement of the storage products, globotriaosylceramide (Gb3) in plasma [11] or urine [12] and globotriaosylsphingosine (lyso-Gb3) in plasma [13] can provide supporting evidence for the diagnosis and is useful for monitoring treatment [12, 14]. The advent of enzyme replacement therapy (ERT) [15, 16] has emphasised the importance of early diagnosis, even newborn screening for Fabry disease. Methods for screening based on analysing the α-galactosidase A in dried blood spots [8] and the urinary storage products collected on filter paper [17] have been developed for mass and high-risk screening for Fabry disease.

6.2 Enzymatic Diagnosis Using Plasma/Serum or Leukocytes

6.2.1 Practical Aspects

α-Galactosidase A activity can be measured reliably in plasma/serum and leukocytes using the synthetic substrate, 4-methylumbelliferyl–α-D-galactopyranoside, at pH 4.6 [2–4]. *N*-acetylgalactosamine is added to the reaction mixture to inhibit α-*N*-acetylgalactosaminidase (also called α-galactosidase B) [18], which can account for up to 20% of the total α-galactosidase activity in plasma and 5–10% of the α-galactosidase activity in leukocytes using this synthetic substrate. Other factors that can affect the activity include pH, temperature, endogenous inhibitors, anticoagulants and erythrocyte contamination [3, 4]. These factors have been taken into account in the development of standard assay procedures and the establishment of reference ranges. The assay using plasma/serum is carried out at 30°C to minimise denaturation and to ensure a measurable rate of hydrolysis. A strong acetate buffer is needed to maintain the pH during the incubation because of the buffering capacity of plasma/serum. There is no significant difference between the activities measured in serum and in plasma collected in tubes containing the anticoagulants, ethylenediamine tetraacetic acid, heparin, or acid-citrate dextrose. However, substances such as haemoglobin released from erythrocytes, can quench the fluorescence of the product, 4-methylumbelliferone. To overcome this problem a separate 4-methylumbelliferone standard, standard blank and substrate blank, including plasma/serum are set up for each sample assayed. The readings for the blanks may vary considerably amongst samples. Lipaemic plasma is another potential problem because the suspended lipids may not be cleared by the stopping reagent and may affect the fluorescence. The assay with leukocytes is carried out at 37°C. Quenching can also be a problem in the leukocyte assay unless a haemolysis step is included in the preparation of the leukocytes to remove contaminating erythrocytes. Another lysosomal enzyme should always be assayed to test the viability of the sample e.g. β-hexosaminidase in plasma/serum or β-galactosidase in leukocytes.

6.2.2 α-Galactosidase A Activity in Plasma/Serum and Leukocytes

Male patients with the classic presentation generally have very low or undetectable activity in plasma/serum (Fig. 6.1) and leukocytes (Fig. 6.2). The diagnosis should always be confirmed by mutation analysis. The levels of the storage products in urine or plasma are elevated in most patients with the classic phenotype and this can be used to support the diagnosis (see below). Some patients with a milder form of the classic phenotype have low levels of residual activity. Higher residual activity is often found in atypical male patients, who do not show the classic phenotype and have later onset of symptoms [4, 5, 19, 20], including the 'cardiac' [21] and 'renal' variants [22, 23]. This higher residual activity is usually associated with particular mutations e.g. N215S, R301Q. Male patients with an atypical clinical presentation and residual α-galactosidase activity should be investigated thoroughly by characterisation of the residual activity, complete sequencing of the *GLA* gene and measurement of the storage products in urine or plasma before a definitive diagnosis is made.

The α-galactosidase activity in affected females ranges from the low level found in affected males to well within the normal range (Figs. 6.1 and 6.2), with about 30% of female carriers having a normal level of α-galactosidase activity [5]. Therefore,

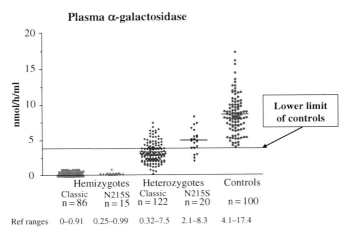

Fig. 6.1 Levels of plasma α-galactosidase in male hemizygotes, female heterozygotes and in healthy control individuals. *n* = number of subjects (reproduced from Beck [1] with permission from Oxford PharmaGenesis Ltd)

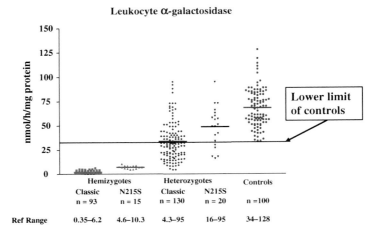

Fig. 6.2 Levels of leukocyte α-galactosidase in male hemizygotes, female heterozygotes and in healthy control individuals. n = number of subjects (reproduced from Beck [1] with permission from Oxford PharmaGenesis Ltd)

a normal α-galactosidase activity does not necessarily contradict a suspected clinical diagnosis in a female. Although many heterozygotes do have decreased activity in plasma/serum and leukocytes, it must be emphasised that many heterozygotes cannot be detected reliably by enzymology. Carrier identification is based on the detection of a proven disease-causing mutation in the *GLA* gene. Measurement of the storage products in urine or plasma can sometimes provide supporting evidence for the diagnosis (see below). It is assumed that the level of α-galactosidase activity A activity in leukocytes from heterozygotes reflects the patterns of X-inactivation in the cells in the sample. It has been proposed that X-inactivation may be a major factor determining the severity of clinical involvement in Fabry heterozygotes because a statistically significant difference was found between the severity score values of heterozygotes with random and non-random X-chromosome inactivation [24]. In contrast evidence has been obtained that heterozygotes show random X -inactivation and that the occurrence and severity of disease manifestations in the majority of Fabry heterozygotes are not related to skewed X-inactivation [25]. The observation that older obligate heterozygotes often have α-galactosidase A activities towards the top of the heterozygote range has been attributed to reactivation of the inactivated X-chromosome with ageing [5].

6.3 The Role of DNA Analysis in the Diagnosis of Fabry Disease

6.3.1 Identification of Mutations

The *GLA* gene, which is located at Xq22.1, has been fully characterised, [see Chapter 6; 5, 26, 27]. Over 470 disease-causing mutations are recorded in the Human Gene Mutation Database (Cardiff, UK; http://www.hgmd.cf.ac.uk/ac/

gene.php?gene=GLA). A variety of experimental procedures can be used to identify mutations in the GLA gene, depending on the nature of the mutation [4, 5].

Single base changes and small deletions and insertions account for a majority (>90%) of the mutations in the *GLA* gene. They can be detected by amplification of the exons and flanking regions by PCR followed by detection of sequence changes by various mutation-screening methods. The exons in the *GLA* gene range in size from 92 to 291 bp in length, which makes them amenable to amplification by PCR. The mutation screening methods include single-strand conformation polymorphism analysis [28], chemical cleavage of mismatches with fluorescent detection [29], and denaturing high performance liquid chromatography (DHPLC) [30]. The amplified exons plus flanking regions that contain sequence changes are then sequenced to identify the mutation precisely. The most reliable way to identify novel and known single base changes and small deletions and insertions is to sequence the entire coding sequence and flanking regions in both directions [31]. The process of sequencing multiple samples by the Sanger dideoxy method has been automated. Known single-point and small deletions can also be detected by a rapid, fluorophore probe-based technique that does not require gel electrophoresis [32]. Another approach to the rapid identification of known mutations in individuals and populations is the use of disease-specific chips or microarrays [33], which has been pioneered in the cancer field. A programme to develop chips for lysosomal storage diseases, including Fabry disease, is being carried out at Birmingham Childrens' Hospital, UK.

Large gene rearrangements, which only account for 3–4% of the mutations, can be detected by Southern blot hybridisation using full-length cDNA as the probe [34] or by multiplex PCR of the gene in 4 fragments [35]. It is difficult to detect deletions of one or more exons or the entire gene, especially in heterozygous females. Such mutations can be identified using *M*ultiplex *L*igation-dependent *P*robe *A*mplification (MLPA) [36] and it has been suggested that the MLPA test should be included routinely in the genetic analysis of Fabry patients [36].

If a mutation is not found in the exonic or flanking regions and there is not a large gene rearrangement, the possibility of a splice site mutation (~5% of known mutations) should be investigated by the use of the reverse-transcriptase polymerase chain reaction (RT-PCR) [37] or real-time PCR [38] to analyse total RNA. This is important because an alternatively spliced α-galactosidase A transcript is expressed at a level of 1–10% in normal tissues. A deficiency of α-galactosidase A activity may result from disturbing the balance between the normal and alternative transcripts. It has also been suggested that real-time PCR is included routinely in the genetic analysis of Fabry patients [38]. The RNA of symptomatic female patients, who have been reported not to have a detectable mutation in the coding region, should be analysed [39].

Various tests have been developed to detect specific mutations. If the mutation alters an existing restriction enzyme site in the genomic DNA, the mutation can be detected by re-amplification of the DNA fragment and digestion with the enzyme. If the mutation does not alter a restriction site, a restriction site can be created using a primer containing an altered base (amplification-created restriction site) [28]. DHPLC analysis can also be used to detect specific mutations rapidly

[29]. Direct sequencing of the appropriate amplified fragment in both directions has become a feasible strategy with the development of rapid and sensitive automated sequencers.

6.3.2 Effect of Genetic Variation on the Diagnosis of Fabry Disease

As with many other genes, polymorphisms in the *GLA* gene that increase or decrease the α-galactosidase A activity can complicate the diagnosis of Fabry disease. Three polymorphisms, g.1150G>A, g.1168G>A, g.1170C>T, in the untranslated sequence before the initiation sequence in the first exon have a combined frequency of 10% [40]. The g.1150A allele of the g.1150G>A polymorphism, which is found in 0.5% of normal individuals, gives rise to a 3-fold increase in plasma α-galactosidase A activity in hemizygotes [41]. This is attributed to transcriptional upregulation of gene expression due to interference with the binding of negatively acting transcription factor. In contrast the g.1170T allele polymorphism is associated with lower α-galactosidase A expression [42, 43]. This polymorphism is also located in a putative binding site for another transcription regulatory protein [41].

Sequence variants that affect the α-galactosidase activity are also found in the coding region. The polymorphism D313Y, which has approximately 60% of wild-type activity in vitro and decreased activity at neutral pH, leads to low plasma α-galactosidase activity but it is not disease causing [44, 45]. It has an incidence of 0.45% in normal X-chromosomes and has been found in combination with several disease-causing missense mutations. The existence of pseudodeficiency alleles necessitates the complete sequencing of the *GLA* gene in the index case of newly diagnosed families with Fabry disease. Any novel missense mutations should be expressed in vitro and the biosynthesis and kinetic and physicochemical properties of the mutant enzyme investigated to ascertain whether the mutation is likely to be disease-causing [20].

6.3.3 Confirmation of Diagnosis, Detection of Carriers and Genetic Counselling

The detection of a disease-causing mutation in the *GLA* gene is now considered an integral step in the diagnosis of Fabry disease in both male and female patients [4–9] It is essential for the confirmation of Fabry disease in a hemizygote and is the only reliable method for detecting manifesting females and obligate carriers. Although there are some recurrent mutations most are private to a family. Once the mutation in the index case has been identified and shown to be potentially disease-causing, a specific test for its detection is developed for the study of family members. Female carriers and affected and pre-symptomatic male patients can be identified and appropriate genetic counselling offered. A study of the family pedigrees of Fabry patients in the USA found that on average five family members were diagnosed with Fabry disease for every proband [46]. Another study that targeted screening of patients with appropriate symptoms identified approximately 5% of the patients as having Fabry disease and subsequent family studies detected 70 patients altogether in six families [47].

6.4 The Role of Measurement of Storage Products in Diagnosis

The deficiency of α-galactosidase A in Fabry diseases leads to the progressive accumulation within lysosomes of glycosphingolipids with terminal α-galactosyl residues. This occurs predominantly in the endothelial, perithelial, and smooth muscle cells of blood vessels but deposition also occurs in many other cell types. The levels of storage products in the urine and plasma are also elevated in most but not all patients with Fabry disease. The demonstration of an increase in the levels of the storage products in urine and /or plasma is very useful in making a diagnosis in many cases and for monitoring treatment. The predominant storage product in Fabry disease is globotriaosylceramide (Gb$_3$) [Gal(α1->4)Gal(β1->4)Glc(β1->1')Cer], which is also called CTH or GL-3 [4, 5]. Other storage products include galabiosylceramide (Ga$_2$ or CDH) [Gal(α1->4)Gal(β1->1')Cer], which is less widely distributed than Gb$_3$ and the blood group B and B$_1$ antigenic glycosphingolipids, the occurrence of which depend on the blood group and secretor status of the patient [48, 49]. All of these neutral glycolipids consist of families of isoforms due to heterogeneity in the fatty acid component of the ceramide [50]. Recently deacylated globotriaosylceramide, globotriaosylsphingosine or lysoGb$_3$, has been shown to be elevated in the plasma of male patients and symptomatic female patients [13].

α-Galactosidase A requires saposin B to hydrolyse its natural substrates in vivo [51, 52] but a detergent such as taurocholate can substitute in vitro. The enzyme does not require a detergent to hydrolyse the synthetic substrate in aqueous solution. Patients with a genetic deficiency of saposin B have normal α-galactosidase A activity with the synthetic substrate but the major lipids that accumulate are sulphatides with lesser accumulation of Gb$_3$. The patients present predominantly with the symptoms of late infantile or juvenile onset metachromatic leukodystrophy [53]. A deficiency of prosaposin the precursor of saposin B also leads to disruption of the turnover of Gb$_3$ along with many other glycolipids [54, 55]. The clinical presentation of these patients, a full glycolipid profile and normal α-galactosidase A activity should ensure that a detected elevation of Gb$_3$ is not interpreted as Fabry disease.

6.4.1 Methodology

Many methods have been used to measure glycosphingolipids in plasma and urine including HPLC and various forms of mass spectrometry (see 4 for summary). Small amounts of non-derivatised neutral and acidic glycosphingolipids, including the isoforms due to heterogeneity in the sphingosine and fatty acid components, can be readily detected by tandem mass spectrometry. However until recently it was diffi-cult to quantify the amounts present. This problem has been overcome by synthesis of novel internal standards, such as C-17-Gb$_3$ [11], [d$_4$]C16- and [d$_{47}$]C24-isoforms of Gb$_3$ and Ga$_2$ [56] and [d$_{35}$]C18-Gb$_3$ [57]. Improvements in the extraction of the glycosphingolipids from plasma and urine and the development of on-line purifi-cation procedures have also been made. Reliable measurements of urinary storage products can be obtained without separating the urinary sediment and supernatant either by sonicating whole urine [14] or by diluting urine [12]. Non-derivatised Gb$_3$ and other storage products can now be measured rapidly and quantitatively in urine and plasma by liquid chromatography coupled to electrospray ionisation tandem mass spectrometry in a semi-automated procedure [11, 12, 57]. By using the mass spectrometer in the multiple reaction monitoring mode, it is possible to measure the concentrations of the individual isoforms of a glycosphingolipid and to obtain its total concentration by summation of the concentrations of the individual isoforms [11, 12, 14, 50, 57–59]. The profiles of the isoforms of the storage products may also be informative in diagnosis and prognosis. An alternative way to determine Gb$_3$ in urine is to incubate urinary sediment with recombinant α-galactosidase A and to measure the released galactose by an enzymatic method [60]. The values obtained by this method, which does not require expensive equipment, correlate well with those obtained by HPLC.

There has been considerable discussion as to whether to relate the concentrations of urinary glycosphingolipids to creatinine, phosphatidyl choline, sphingomyelin or volume of urine [61, 62]. However, it has been shown that Gb$_3$/creatinine ratios closely match Gb$_3$/sphingomyelin [50] and Gb$_3$/phosphatidylcholine ratios [63]. As Gb3 and creatinine ratio can be measured simultaneously in a single analysis, the Gb$_3$/creatinine ratio is frequently used. Age-matched controls must be used and the values in babies need careful interpretation.

6.4.2 Gb3 in Plasma

The concentrations of total Gb$_3$ in plasma in male hemizygotes with the classic phe-notype, hemizygotes with N215S mutation, female heterozygotes associated with the classic phenotype in their male relatives, heterozygotes with the N215S muta-tion and healthy control individuals were determined using C-17-Gb$_3$ as the internal standard [4, 58] (Fig. 6.3 and Table 6.1). Gb$_3$ was elevated in 44/48 of the males with classic phenotype but not in four mildly affected patients. One of these patients was asymptomatic and had the F169S mutation, although his cousin had died of renal failure. Another had been classified as a 'renal' variant. Of the nine boys in this group, with ages ranging from 6 to 17 years, eight had an elevated Gb$_3$ level. The exception was 16-year old with an I317T mutation. Gb$_3$ was not elevated in the male patients with the N215S mutation. In contrast only 42% of the female heterozygotes with 'classic' mutations had elevated Gb$_3$ levels. Interestingly one of the four het-erozygotes with the N215S mutation had an elevated level of Gb$_3$. Similar results

Fig. 6.3 Levels of plasma globotriaosylceramide (Gb3) in male hemizygotes, female heterozygotes and in healthy control individuals. n = number of subjects (reproduced from Beck [1] with permission from Oxford PharmaGenesis Ltd)

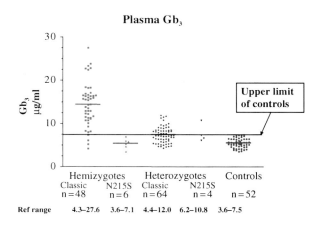

Table 6.1 Percentage of patients with an elevated level of Gb3 in plasma and urine

	Hemizygotes		Heterozygotes	
	Classic	N215S	Classic	N215S
Plasma	44/48	0/6	27/64	1/40
	92%	0%	42%	25%
Urine	56/56	4/10	96/105	0/8
	100%	40%	91.4%	0%

have been obtained by other groups and in on-going studies from our group [4, 5, 12]. Although the levels of Gb3 in plasma do not correlate with the severity of the disease in hemizygotes or heterozygotes [58, 64, 65], they are useful in supporting a diagnosis and particularly for monitoring treatment [12, 14, 57–59, 63, 66].

6.4.3 LysoGb3 in Plasma

LysoGb3 can be determined quantitatively in plasma by HPLC using an external standard of authentic lysoGb3 [13]. It is probably present from an early age in the plasma of male patients. The level of lysoGb3 increases steadily in the plasma of female patients and shows a weak correlation with disease progression. LysoGb3 was below the level of detection (10 nM) in unaffected males, an asymptomatic female and her unaffected siblings. Although the concentration of lysoGb3 ($\sim$0.2–0.4 μM) in the plasma of male patients is 20–30 times lower than that of Gb3, the relative increase in concentration between patients and unaffected males is very much greater than for Gb3, increasing the discrimination between patients and non-patients. The level of lysoGb3 in urine has not been reported presumably because it is not present in urine or the concentration is below the limit of detection. Currently lysoGb3 is measured by HPLC but it is readily detectable by mass spectrometry [11]. The determination of lysoGb3 is likely to prove to be a very valuable new tool for diagnosing and monitoring Fabry disease.

6.4.4 Gb₃ and Ga₂ in Urine

The levels of Gb₃ in whole urine and urinary sediments have been determined in many studies [4, 12, 50, 57–59, 63, 67] In our study using liquid chromatography coupled to electrospray ionisation tandem mass spectrometry and the C-17-Gb₃ internal standard, all the classic male patients and four out of 10 of the male patients with the N215S mutation had elevated levels of urinary Gb₃ [4, 50, 58] (Fig. 6.4, Table 6.1). The proportion (91%) of the heterozygotes with 'classic' mutations

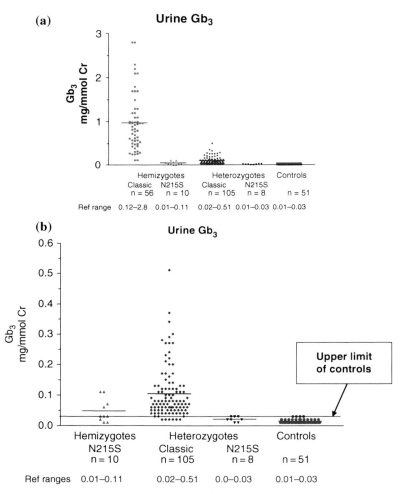

Fig. 6.4 Levels of urinary globotriaosylceramide (Gb₃) (**a**) male hemizygotes, female heterozygotes and healthy control individuals, and (**b**) N215S hemizygotes, classic heterozygotes and healthy control individuals. *n* = number of subjects (reproduced from Beck [1] with permission from Oxford PharmaGenesis Ltd)

with elevated urinary Gb_3 was higher than the proportion (42%) with elevated plasma Gb_3. All but one of the carriers with a normal level of urinary Gb_3 was symptomatic. All eight heterozygotes with the N215S mutation had a normal urinary Gb_3 level. Thus the urinary Gb_3 level is better at discriminating between patients and controls than the plasma Gb_3 level but it still does not detect many heterozygotes. This procedure is being used as a non-invasive method to screen school children in Tokyo for Fabry disease [59]. It is suggested that it will detect hemizygotic patients with the classic type and probably the renal variant of Fabry disease. To improve the detection of heterozygotes, the method has been modified to include measurement of urinary α-galactosidase A protein by an enzyme-linked immunoabsorbent assay (ELISA) [68]. Combining the two assays produced 96% sensitivity for heterozygote detection.

It has been reported that urinary Gb_3 levels do not correlate with the severity of disease manifestations [64, 65] but a recent report based on analysis of urine collected on filter paper indicates that there is a significant correlation between types of mutation and Gb_3/creatinine excretion [69].

Ga_2 (CDH) and Gb_3 can be measured together in a multiplex assay using tandem mass spectrometry [50]. A similar pattern of results was obtained for the level of Ga_2 in urine, except that a lower proportion (85%) of heterozygotes with classic mutations had elevated urinary Ga_2 compared with Gb_3. Combining the concentrations of Gb_3 and Ga_2 did not increase the discrimination between heterozygotes and controls. However the ratio of Ga_2 to Gb_3 was higher in heterozygotes than in hemizygotes.

To investigate whether the proportions of the isoforms (profiles) of the storage products might vary amongst patients, an extensive statistical analysis of the Gb_3 isoforms in plasma was carried out but no major trends were detected (upublished work). However, significant differences in the profiles Gb_3 and Ga_2 isoforms in urinary sediment were found amongst young, adult and atypical hemizygotes and heterozygotes using a combination of MALDI-TOF MS and tandem MS [67]. Isoform profiling may be useful in diagnosing and predicting the phenotype of patients. Profiling of urinary globotriaosylceramide isoforms has been carried out by electrospray ionization mass spectrometry using stearoyl-d_{35}-globotriaosylceramide as internal standard to attempt to identify heterozygotes [57]. In another study 29 urinary lipids were measured and ratios of the analytes calculated to try to find a parameter that identified Fabry hemizygotes and heterozygotes [70]. However none of the ratios completely identified heterozygotes but this approach might be useful for monitoring treatment in individual patients.

6.5 Prenatal Diagnosis

The α-galactosidase activity in fetal tissues reflects the genotype of the fetus [71] with deficient activity in Fabry hemizygotes and varying amounts in heterozygotes. Prenatal diagnosis of Fabry disease in a male fetus can be made directly in chorionic villi and in cultured chorionic villi cells [72] and cultured amniotic cells [73] by measuring α-galactosidase A activity and/or mutation analysis if the family mutation is known [74]. Fetal sex determination is performed e.g., by fluorescence in situ hybridisation (FISH) and subsequently chromosome analysis is carried out to support the diagnosis of an affected male. Heterozygous females can also be detected by mutation analysis of the fetus. However, the testing of female fetuses has not been offered widely because it is not possible to reliably predict the course and severity of disease in a female heterozygous for a particular mutation. Most, if not all, female heterozygotes will develop symptoms of Fabry disease [25]. Therefore it has been suggested that families should be counselled on this issue and that diagnosis of heterozygosity for Fabry disease in female fetuses should be offered if the parents demand the test [75]. However, with the advent of enzyme replacement therapy there are now very few requests for prenatal diagnosis of Fabry disease. Technically preimplantation diagnosis of Fabry disease by mutation analysis in blastomeres is feasible and has been performed but the results have not been published.

6.6 Mass and High-Risk Screening for Fabry Disease

The advent of enzyme replacement therapy has also emphasised the importance of early diagnosis, ideally newborn screening for Fabry disease [76]. Several procedures have been developed for screening for the lysosomal storage diseases, including Fabry disease, in the general and high-risk populations using blood or urine collected on filter paper [77]. Although mass screening for Fabry hemizygotes is technically feasible, the diagnosis of presymptomatic patients and patients with novel mutations poses many problems for geneticists and metabolic physicians [78, 79]. The detection of heterozygotes by screening is even more problematical because random X-inactivation affects the parameters measured in the tests and it is difficult to predict the phenotype from the genotype and biochemical parameters in newly diagnosed females.

6.6.1 Measurement of α-Galactosidase A Activity in Dried Blood Spots

A deficiency of α-galactosidase A activity can be demonstrated in the material eluted from a dried blood spot collected on a filter paper, using the conventional assay with the fluorigenic substrate [10]. The method of collection of the dried blood spot affects the values of α-galactosidase A activity and method-specific reference ranges need to be established [80]. Although classic hemizygotes are readily detected, only two thirds of carriers can be detected [81], as expected. The activity of β-glucuronidase is frequently activated in the blood of Fabry patients and it has been suggested that measurement of the ratio of α-galactosidase A to β-glucuronidase can improve the diagnostic specificity for female patients [82, 83]. The filter paper assay has been adapted for high-throughput using a 96-well microtitre plate for reading the fluorescence [84, 85]. When this procedure was applied to a newborn population of 37,104, twelve of the babies (0.03%) were found to have a deficiency of α-galactosidase A, giving an incidence for Fabry disease of 1 in ~3,100 [86]. Eleven of the twelve neonates had genotypes consistent with late-onset Fabry disease and only one had a mutation previously found in a patient with the classic phenotype. Undiagnosed family members were identified as a result of this work and therapy initiated. The incidence would have been 1 in ~4,600 if only known disease-causing mutations were included, with a ratio of later-onset to classic patients of 7:1. This study illustrates some of the ethical problems of newborn screening for a treatable later-onset disease: should screening take place soon after birth or in adulthood and when should treatment start? A similar trial using the same technology is taking place in Taiwan for both Fabry and Pompe disease [87]. Although the results for Fabry disease have not yet been published, affected infants and family members have been identified [87]. Enormously valuable experience about cut-off points, recall rates and the organisation of clinical support has been gained from this Pompe screening programme [88, 89]. The assay of α-galactosidase A in dried blood spots using the fluorigenic substrate has been incorporated into a routine diagnostic programme [90] and is being offered as an alternative to the conventional assay in leukocytes/plasma for routine diagnosis in several laboratories. It could also be applied to screening patients on dialysis for end-stage renal disease [91] and young male stroke patients [92] as long as the limitations on detection of heterozygotes and atypical hemizygtes are taken into account.

The α-galactosidase protein eluted from blood or plasma collected on filter paper can be immunoprecipitated and the protein concentration and α-galactosidase activity measured [93]. Fabry hemizygotes can be distinguished from controls in blood spots by this method but heterozygotes can only be differentiated by the additional measurement of saposin C, a marker of lysosomal hypertrophy.

Novel substrates and internal standards have recently been developed for the rapid and sensitive assay of lysosomal enzymes, including α-galactosidase A, in rehydrated dried blood spots, using electrospray tandem mass spectrometry [94]. The great advantage of this methodology is that the product of each specific enzyme assay has a different mass, permitting the simultaneous analysis or multiplexing of several assays by mass spectrometry. The substrate for each lysosomal enzyme is incubated separately with a rehydrated blood spot and then the reaction products are pooled and measured simultaneously by multiple-reaction monitoring of ion dissociations produced by electrospray ionization [95, 96]. The conditions for the multiplex assay of α-galactosidase A and four other lysosomal enzymes, which are deficient in lysosomal storage diseases for which there is treatment, have been optimized [97]. Pre-mixed samples of the novel substrates and internal standards for each assay and quality control samples have been produced to facilitate and standardise the assay [97, 98]. Using these conditions clear differentiation between the five activities in rehydrated blood spots from both adults and newborns from healthy individuals and patients was achieved, indicating the suitability of this methodology for high-throughput screening. The inclusion of an on-line trapping and clean-up step simplifies and speeds up the analysis of the multiplexed reaction mixtures [99]. Trials of screening for Fabry disease using this technology are in progress (Fig. 6.5) [76].

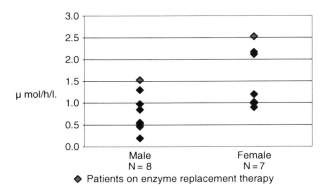

Fig. 6.5 α-Galactosidase A activity in dried blood spots from Fabry patients and a newborn population using the mass spectrometric assay. Levels in a newborn population. Males: 11.2 ± 6.4 S.D. μmol/h/l. Females: 11.7 ± 6.3 S.D. μmol/h/l. Unpublished data kindly provided by Dr. Olaf Bodamer, University of Salzburg, Austria

6.6.2 Screening for Fabry Disease by Measuring the Storage Products in Urine Collected on Filter Paper

Filter paper can also be used to collect and store urine for the analysis of storage products for screening for Fabry disease [17, 100]. Glycosphingolipids are extracted from the filter paper and total Gb_3 and creatinine determined simultaneously by liquid chromatography coupled to electrospray ionisation tandem mass spectrometry as described previously for whole urine [50]. The method was validated by studying the levels of urinary Gb_3/creatinine in children and adults with Fabry disease with different types of mutations [69]. The excretion of urinary Gb_3 was found to correlate well with sex and genotype and to fall on treatment. It has been proposed that this procedure could be the basis of a high-risk screening protocol for Fabry disease in adult patients with renal and vascular disease [101]. To assess the validity of this test for newborn screening for Fabry disease, the level of Gb_3/creatinine in the urine of healthy infants from birth to 6-months, was measured and reference ranges established at various postnatal ages, in male and female infants [102]. It was found that the urinary Gb_3/creatinine level varied markedly in newborns with both sex and postnatal age. In consequence it was concluded that screening for Fabry disease by measurement of urinary Gb_3 excretion is unlikely to be reliable before 30 days of age.

6.6.3 Protein Profiling

An alternative approach to screening for lysosomal storage diseases is to compare the lysosomal protein profiles for patients and healthy individuals [103]. Although the level of the protein defective in a particular LSD e.g. α-galacosidase A in Fabry disease will generally be decreased, the levels of other lysosomal proteins will be increased or decreased in response to the lysosomal hypertrophy. Therefore an abnormal lysosomal protein profile in a blood spot from a patient could be diagnostic for LSDs in general, a sub-group of LSDs e.g., the sphingolipidoses or a single disease, even if the disease-specific protein is not included in the profile. The concentration of lysosomal proteins released from dried blood spots can be measured accurately by immunoquantification using fluorescent microbead suspension array technology to give a protein profile. Currently 11 lysosomal proteins are being measured in a multiplex assay: nine lysosomal enzymes (including α-galacosidase A) and LAMP-1 and saposin C to normalise the samples in terms of lysosomal content. Most Fabry patients were identified by a marked deficiency of α-galactosidase A protein or by a profile of multiple lysosomal proteins. One newborn had a very high level of α-galactosidase A protein outside the reference range and also of iduronate 2-sulphatase (Hunter enzyme). Further work is being carried out to validate this procedure with a large number of normal and patient blood spots, including newborns. Algorithms are being developed to recognize disease-specific patterns. A comparative trial is being carried out of the protein profiling technology and the multiplex enzyme assay procedure based on novel substrates and mass spectrometry [104].

6.6.4 DNA from Bloodspots

Diagnosis of Fabry disease by analysis of DNA eluted from dried blood spots is an intriguing possibility for the future. This technology has been pioneered for the detection of viral infections in neonates e.g. HIV [105]. It is also being developed for newborn screening for more common genetic disorders such as cystic fibrosis [106] or in populations with a relatively high incidence of a particular disorder e.g., homocystinuria in Qatar [107]. Interestingly analysis of DNA from dried blood spots has been used to identify pseudodeficiency alleles in individuals detected with low α-glucosidase activity in a newborn screening programme for Pompe disease in Japan [108]. The ability to genotype potential patients rapidly using the original blood spots could have a big impact on confirmatory testing in newborn screening.

6.7 Conclusions

The methods being developed for screening for Fabry disease are equally applicable to routine diagnosis. It is anticipated that the use of dried blood spots and urine collected on filter paper will increase as the convenience of the material is appreciated and diagnostic laboratories adapt to the new technology. The development of cheaper, rapid, high-throughput methods for sequencing DNA [for review see 109] will revolutionise the diagnosis and genetic analysis of Fabry patients. Direct sequencing of the whole *GLA* gene from genomic DNA isolated from dried blood spots or buccal cells might be the first step in the laboratory diagnosis of Fabry disease. This will reveal potential disease-causing mutations and polymorphisms in the

GLA gene that might affect the severity and course of the disease in an individual. Polymorphisms or heterozygosity in secondary genes [9, 110] that can moderate Fabry disease could be identified by including these secondary genes on a Fabry disease-specific chip. This diagnostic information could then be used to plan the management of individual patients.

Acknowledgements We acknowledge the experience and dedication of our colleagues in the Enzyme Diagnostic Laboratory at Great Ormond Street Hospital, London, and in the research laboratories at the Institute of Child Health, particularly Dr. Kevin Mills, with whom we worked for many years and without whom this chapter could not have been written. We would also like to thank Dr. Olaf Bodamer for providing us with his unpublished data on the measurement of α-galactosidase activity in dried blood spots using a novel substrate and mass spectrometry.

References

1. Beck M (2006) Demographics of FOS – the Fabry Outcome Survey. In: Mehta A, Beck M, Sunder-Plassmann G (eds) Fabry disease: perspectives from 5 years of FOS. Pharmagenesis, Oxford, pp 155–161
2. Kint JA (1970) Fabry's disease: α-galactosidase deficiency. Science 167:1268–1269
3. Desnick RJ, Allen KY, Desnick SJ, Raman MK, Bernlohr RW, Krivit W (1973) Fabry's disease: enzymatic diagnosis of hemizygotes and heterozygotes. α-galactosidase activities in plasma, serum, urine and leukocytes. J Lab Clin Med 81:157–171
4. Winchester B, Young E (2006) Biochemical and genetic diagnosis of Fabry disease. In: Mehta A, Beck M, Sunder-Plassmann G (eds) Fabry disease: perspectives from 5 years of FOS. Pharmagenesis, Oxford, pp 169–181
5. Desnick RJ, Ioannou YA, Eng ME (2001) α-Galactosidase A deficiency: Fabry disease. In: Scriver CR, Beaudet AL, Sly D, Valle D (eds) The metabolic and molecular bases of inherited disease, vol 3, 8th edn. McGraw-Hill, New York, pp 3733–3774
6. Desnick RJ, Brady R, Barranger J, Collins AJ, Germain DP, Goldman M (2003) Fabry disease, an under-recognized multisystemic disorder: expert recommendations for diagnosis, management, and enzyme replacement therapy. Ann Intern Med 138(4):338–346
7. Caudron E, Sandrine R, Germain DP, Chaminade P, Prognon P (2007) Laboratory diagnosis of Fabry disease: historical perspectives and recent breakthroughs. Presse Med 36(Spec No 1):1S76–81
8. Zarate YA, Hopkin RJ (2008) Lysosomal storage disease 3:Fabry's disease. Lancet 372(9647):1427–1435
9. Schiffman R (2009) Fabry disease. Pharmacol Ther 122:65–77
10. Chamoles NA, Blanco M, Gaggioli D (2001) Fabry disease: enzymatic diagnosis in dried blood spots on filter paper. Clin Chim Acta 308(1–2):195–196
11. Mills K, Johnson A, Winchester B (2002) Synthesis of novel internal standards for the quantitative determination of plasma ceramide trihexoside in Fabry disease by tandem mass spectrometry. FEBS Lett 515(1–3):171–176
12. Boscaro F, Pieraccini G, la Marca G, Bartolucci G, Luceri C, Luceri F, Moneti G (2002) Rapid quantitation of globotriaosylceramide in human plasma and urine: a potential application for monitoring enzyme replacement therapy in Anderson-Fabry disease. Rapid Commun Mass Spectrom 16(16):1507–1514
13. Aerts JM, Groener JE, Kuiper S, Donker-Koopman WE, Strijland A, Ottenhoff R et al (2008) Elevated globotriaosylsphingosine is a hallmark of Fabry disease. Proc Natl Acad Sci (USA) 105(8):2812–2817
14. Mills K, Vellodi A, Morris P, Cooper D, Morris M, Young E, Winchester B (2004) Monitoring the clinical and biochemical response to enzyme replacement therapy in three children with Fabry disease. Eur J Pediatr 163(10):595–603

15. Schiffmann R, Kopp JB, Austin HA et al (2001) Enzyme replacement in Fabry disease: a randomised controlled trial. JAMA 285(21):2743–2749
16. Eng CM, Guffon N, Wilcox WR, Germain DP, Lee P, Waldek S et al (2001) Safety and efficacy of recombinant human alpha-galactosidase A replacement therapy in Fabry's disease. N Engl J Med 345(1):9–16
17. Auray-Blais C, Cyr D, Mills K, Giguere R, Drouin R (2007) Development of a filter paper method potentially applicable to mass and high-risk urinary screenings for Fabry disease. J Inherit Metab Dis 30(1):106
18. Mayes JS, Scheerer JB, Sifers RN, Donaldson ML (1981) Differential assay for lysosomal alpha-galactosidases in human tissues and its application to Fabry's disease. Clin Chim Acta 112(2):247–251
19. Bishop DF, Grabowski GA, Desnick RJ (1981) Fabry disease: an asymptomatic hemizygote with significant residual α-galactosidase A activity. Am J Hum Genet 33:71A
20. Ishii S, Chang HH, Kawasaki K, Yasuda K, Wu HL, Garman SC, Fan JQ (2007) Mutant alpha-galactosidase A enzymes identified in Fabry disease patients with residual enzyme activity: biochemical characterization and restoration of normal intracellular processing by 1-deoxygalactonojirimycin. Biochem J 406(2):285–295
21. Nakao S, Takenaka T, Maeda M, Kodama C, Tanaka A, Tahara M et al (1995) An atypical variant of Fabry's disease in men with left ventricular hypertrophy. N Engl J Med 333(5):288–293
22. Nakao S, Kodama C, Takenaka T, Tanaka A, Yasumoto Y, Yoshida A et al (2003) Fabry disease: detection of undiagnosed hemodialysis patients and identification of a 'renal variant' phenotype. Kidney Int 64(3):801–807
23. Branton MH, Schiffmann R, Sabnis SG, Murray GJ, Quirk JM, Altarescu G et al (2002) Natural history of Fabry renal disease: influence of alpha-galactosidase A activity and genetic mutations on clinical course. Medicine (Baltimore) 81(2):122–138
24. Dobrovolny R, Dvorakova L, Ledvinova J, Magage S, Bultas J, Lubanda JC et al (2005) Relationship between X-inactivation and clinical involvement in Fabry heterozygotes. Eleven novel mutations in the alpha-galactosidase A gene in the Czech and Slovak population. J Mol Med 83(8):647–654
25. Maier EM, Osterrieder S, Whybra C, Ries M, Gal A, Beck M et al (2006) Disease manifestations and X inactivation in heterozygous females with Fabry disease. Acta Paediatr Suppl 95(451):30–38
26. Bishop DF, Calhoun DH, Bernstein HS, Hantzopoulos P, Quinn M, Desnick RJ (1986) Human alpha-galactosidase A: nucleotide sequence of a cDNA clone encoding the mature enzyme. Proc Natl Acad Sci USA 83(13):4859–4863
27. Kornreich R, Desnick RJ, Bishop DF (1989) Nucleotide sequence of the human alpha-galactosidase A gene. Nucleic Acids Res 17(8):3301–3302
28. Blaydon D, Hill J, Winchester B (2001) Fabry disease: 20 novel GLA mutations in 35 families. Hum Mutat 18(5):459
29. Germain D, Biasotto M, Tosi M, Meo T, Kahn A, Poenaru L (1996) Fluorescence-assisted mismatch analysis (FAMA) for exhaustive screening of the alpha-galactosidase A gene and detection of carriers in Fabry disease. Hum Genet 98(6):719–726
30. Shabbeer J, Robinson M, Desnick RJ (2005) Detection of alpha-galactosidase A mutations causing Fabry disease by denaturing high performance liquid chromatography. Hum Mutat 25(3):299–305
31. Eng CM, Resnick-Silverman LA, Niehaus DJ, Astrin KH, Desnick RJ (1993) Nature and frequency of mutations in the alpha-galactosidase A gene that cause Fabry disease. Am J Hum Genet 53(6):1186–1197
32. Aoshima T, Sekido Y, Miyazaki T, Kajita M, Mimura S, Watanabe K et al (2000) Rapid detection of deletion mutations in inherited metabolic diseases by melting curve analysis with LightCycler. Clin Chem 46(1):119–122

33. Wu L, Williams PM, Koch W (2005) Clinical applications of microarray-based diagnostic tests. Biotechniques 39(10 Suppl):S577–S582

34. Bernstein HS, Bishop DF, Astrin KH, Kornreich R, Eng CM, Sakuraba H, Desnick RJ (1989) Fabry disease: six gene rearrangements and an exonic point mutation in the alpha-galactosidase gene. J Clin Invest 83(4):1390–1399

35. Kornreich R, Desnick RJ (1993) Fabry disease: detection of gene rearrangements in the human α-galactosidase gene by multiplex PCR amplification. Hum Mutat 2(2): 108–111

36. Schirinzi A, Centra M, Prattichizzo C, Gigante M, De Fabritiis M, Giancaspro V et al (2008) Identification of GLA gene deletions in Fabry patients by Multiplex Ligation-dependent Probe Amplification (MLPA). Mol Genet Metab 94(3):382–385

37. Ishii S, Nakao S, Minamikawa-Tachino R, Desnick RJ, Fan J-Q (2002) Alternative splicing in the α-galactosidase A gene: increased exon inclusion results in the Fabry cardiac phenotype. Am J Hum Genet 70(4):994–1002

38. Filoni C, Caciotti A, Carraresi L, Donati MA, Mignani R, Parini R et al (2008) Unbalanced GLA mRNAs ratio quantified by real-time PCR in Fabry patients' fibroblasts results in Fabry disease. Eur J Hum Genet 16(11):1311–1317

39. Handa Y, Yotsumoto S, Isobe E, Sai Y, Yoshii N, Nakao S et al (2000) A case of symptomatic heterozygous female Fabry's disease without detectable mutation in the alpha-galactosidase gene. Dermatology 200(3):262–265

40. Davies JP, Winchester BG, Malcolm S (1993) Sequence variations in the first exon of α-galactosidase A. J Med Genet 30(8):658–663

41. Fitzmaurice TF, Desnick RJ, Bishop DF (1997) Human α-galactosidase A: high plasma activity expressed by the 30G->A allele. J Inherit Metab Dis 20(5):643–657

42. Oliveira JP, Ferreira S, Barceló J, Gaspar P, Carvalho F, Sá Miranda MC, Månsson J-E (2008 Nov 3) Effect of single-nucleotide polymorphisms of the 5' untranslated region of the human alpha-galactosidase gene on enzyme activity, and their frequencies in Portuguese caucasians. J Inher Metab Dis Short Report 2008 #124 (Epub ahead of print)

43. Oliveira JP, Ferreira S, Reguenga C, Carvalho F, Månsson J-E (2008 Nov 3) The g.1170C>T polymorphism of the 5' untranslated region of the human alpha-galactosidase gene is associated with decreased enzyme expression – Evidence from a family study. J Inher Metab Dis Short Report 2008 #128 (Epub ahead of print)

44. Froissart R, Guffon N, Vanier MT, Desnick RJ, Maire I (2003) Fabry disease: D313Y is an alpha-galactosidase A sequence variant that causes pseudodeficient activity in plasma. Mol Genet Metab 80(3):307–314

45. Yasuda M, Shabbeer J, Benson SD, Maire I, Burnett RM, Desnick RJ (2003) Fabry disease: characterization of alpha-galactosidase A double mutations and the D313Y plasma enzyme pseudodeficiency allele. Hum Mutat 22(6):486–492

46. Laney DA, Fernhoff PM (2008) Diagnosis of Fabry disease via analysis of family history. J Genet Couns 17(1):79–83

47. Rozenfeld PA, Tarabuso A, Ebner R, Ramallo G, Fossati CA (2006) A successful approach for the detection of Fabry patients in Argentina. Clin Genet 69(4):344–348

48. Wherrett JR, Hakomori SI (1973) Characterization of a blood group B glycolipid, accumulating in the pancreas of a patient with Fabry's disease. J Biol Chem 248(9):3046–3051

49. Asfaw B, Ledvinova J, Dobrovolny R, Bakker HD, Desnick RJ, van Diggelen OP et al (2002) Defects in degradation of blood group A and B glycosphingolipids in Schindler and Fabry diseases. J Lipid Res 43(7):1096–1104

50. Mills K, Morris P, Lee P, Vellodi A, Waldek S, Young E et al (2005) Measurement of urinary CDH and CTH by tandem mass spectrometry in patients hemizygous and heterozygous for Fabry disease. J Inherit Metab Dis 28(1):35–48

51. Li SC, Kihara H, Serizawa S, Li YT, Fluharty AL, Mayes JS, Shapiro LJ (1985) Activator protein required for the enzymatic hydrolysis of cerebroside sulfate. Deficiency in urine if patients affected with cerebroside sulfatase activator deficiency and identity of activators

for the enzymatic hydrolysis of GM1 ganglioside and globotriaosylceramide. J Biol Chem 260(3):1867–1871

52. Kase R, Bierfreund U, Klein A, Kolter T, Itoh K, Suzuki M, Hashimoto Y, Sandhoff K, Sakuraba H (1996) Only sphingolipid protein B (SAP-B or saposin B) stimulates the degradation of globotriaosylceramide by recombinant human lysosomal alpha-galactosidase in a detergent-free liposomal system. FEBS Lett 393(1):74–76

53. Sandhoff K, Kolter T, Harzer K (2001) Sphingolipid activator proteins. In: Scriver CR, Beaudet AL, Sly D, Valle D (eds) The metabolic and molecular bases of inherited disease, vol 3, 8th edn. McGraw-Hill, New York, pp 3371–3388

54. Paton BC, Schmid B, Kustermann-Kuhn B, Poulos A, Harzer K (1992) Additional biochemical findings in a patient and fetal sibling with a genetic defect in the sphingolipid activator protein (SAP) precursor, prosaposin. Evidence for a deficiency in SAP-1 and for a normal lysosomal neuraminidase. Biochem J 285(2):481–488

55. Hulková H, Cervenková M, Ledvinová J, Tocháčková M, Hrebícek M, Poupetová H et al (2001) A novel mutation in the coding region of the prosaposin gene leads to a complete deficiency of prosaposin and saposins, and is associated with a complex sphingolipidosis dominated by lactosylceramide accumulation. Hum Mol Genet 10(9):927–940

56. Mills K, Eaton S, Ledger V, Young E, Winchester B (2005) The synthesis of internal standards for the quantitative determination of sphingolipids by tandem mass spectrometry. Rapid Commun Mass Spectrom 19(12):1739–1748

57. Fauler G, Rechberger GN, Devrnja D, Erwa W, Plecko B, Kotanko P et al (2005) Rapid determination of urinary globotriaosylceramide isoform profiles by electrospray ionization mass spectrometry using stearoyl-d35-globotriaosylceramide as internal standard. Rapid Commun Mass Spectrom 19(11):1499–1506

58. Young E, Mills K, Morris P, Vellodi A, Lee P, Waldek S, Winchester B (2005) Is globotriaosylceramide a useful biomarker in Fabry disease? Acta Paediatr Suppl 94(447):51–54

59. Kitagawa T, Ishige N, Suzuki K, Owada M, Ohashi T, Kobayashi M et al (2005) Non-invasive screening method for Fabry disease by measuring globotriaosylceramide in whole urine samples using tandem mass spectrometry. Mol Genet Metab 85(3):196–202

60. Rozenfeld PA, De Francesco NP, Borrajo GJC, Ceci R, Fossati CA (2009) An easy and sensitive method for determination of globotriaosylceramide (Gb3) from urinary sediment: utility for Fabry disease diagnosis and treatment monitoring. Clin Chim Acta 403(1–2): 194–197

61. Forni S, Fu X, Schiffmann R, Sweetman L (2009) Falsely elevated urinary Gb3 (globotriaosylceramide, CTH, GL3). Mol Genet Metab 97(1):91

62. Auray-Blais C, Millington DS, Barr C, Young SP, Mills K, Clarke JT (2009) Gb(3)/creatinine biomarkers for Fabry disease: Issues to consider. Mol Genet Metab 97(3):237

63. Whitfield PD, Calvin J, Hogg S, O'Driscoll E, Halsall D, Burling K et al (2005) Monitoring enzyme replacement therapy in Fabry disease–role of urine globotriaosylceramide. J Inherit Metab Dis 28(1):21–33

64. Vedder AC, Linthorst GE, van Breemen MJ, Groener JE, Bemelman FJ, Strijland A et al (2007) The Dutch Fabry cohort: diversity of clinical manifestations and Gb3 levels. J Inherit Metab Dis 30(1):68–78

65. Bekri S, Lidove O, Jaussaud R, Knebelmann B, Barbey F (2006) The role of ceramide trihexoside (globotriaosylceramide) in the diagnosis and follow-up of the efficacy of treatment of Fabry disease: a review of the literature. Cardiovasc Hematol Agents Med Chem 4(4):289–297

66. Roddy TP, Nelson BC, Sung CC, Araghi S, Wilkens D, Zhang XK et al (2005) Liquid chromatography-tandem mass spectrometry quantification of globotriaosylceramide in plasma for long-term monitoring of Fabry patients treated with enzyme replacement therapy. Clin Chem 51(1):237–240

67. Touboul D, Roy S, Germain DP, Baillet A, Brion F, Prognon P et al (2005) Fast fingerprinting by MALDI-TOF mass spectrometry of urinary sediment glycosphingolipids in Fabry disease. Anal Bioanal Chem 382(5):1209–1216

68. Kitagawa T, Suzuki K, Ishige N, Ohashi T, Kobayashi M, Eto Y et al (2008) Non-invasive high-risk screening for Fabry disease hemizygotes and heterozygotes. Pediatr Nephrol 23(9):1461–1471

69. Auray-Blais C, Cyr D, Ntwari A, West ML, Cox-Brinkman J, Bichet DG et al (2008) Urinary globotriaosylceramide excretion correlates with the genotype in children and adults with Fabry disease. Mol Genet Metab 93(3):331–340

70. Fuller M, Sharp PC, Rozaklis T, Whitfield PD, Blacklock D, Hopwood JJ et al (2005) Urinary lipid profiling for the identification of Fabry hemizygotes and heterozygotes. Clin Chem 51(4):688–694

71. Vedder AC, Strijland A, vd Bergh Weerman MA, Florquin S, Aerts JM, Hollak CE (2006) Manifestations of Fabry disease in placental tissue. J Inherit Metab Dis 29(1):106–111

72. Kleijer WJ, Hussaarts-Odijk LM, Sachs ES, Jahoda MG, Niermeijer MF (1987) Prenatal diagnosis of Fabry's disease by direct analysis of chorionic villi. Prenat Diagn 7(4):283–287

73. Brady RO, Uhlendorf BW, Jacobson CB (1971) Fabry's disease: antenatal detection. Science 172(979):174–175

74. Desnick RJ (2007) Prenatal diagnosis of Fabry disease. Prenat Diagn 27(8):693–694

75. Raas-Rothschild A, Lacombe D (2008) Fabry disease prenatal diagnosis. Prenat Diagn 28:268

76. Bodamer O (2008) Newborn screening in Fabry disease: What can be achieved by early diagnosis? Clin Ther 30(Suppl B):S41

77. Meikle PJ, Hopwod JJ (2005) Newborn screening for lysosomal disoders: current issues and approaches. Current Med Lit 5(30):41–48

78. Fletcher JM (2006) Screening for lysosomal storage disorders–a clinical perspective. J Inherit Metab Dis 29(2–3):405–408

79. Millington D (2008) Rapid and effective screening for lysosomal storage disease; How close are we? Clin Chem 54(10):1592–1594

80. Olivova P, van der Veen K, Cullen E, Rose M, Zhang XK, Sims KB et al (2009) Effect of sample collection on α-galactosidase A enzyme activity measurements in dried blood spots on filter paper. Clin Chim Acta 403(1–2):159–162

81. Linthorst GE, Vedder AC, Aerts JMFG, Hollak CEM (2005) Screening for Fabry disease using whole blood spots fails to identify one-third of female carriers. Clin Chim Acta 353:201–203

82. Lukacs Z, Keil A, Kohlschutter A, Beck M, Mengel E (2005) The ratio of alpha-galactosidase to beta–glucuronidase activities in dried blood for the identification of female Fabry disease patients. J Inherit Metab Dis 28(5):803–805

83. Lukacs Z, Hartung R, Beck M, Keil A, Mengel E (2007) Direct comparison of enzyme measurements from dried blood spots and leukocytes from male and female Fabry disease patients. J Inherit Metab Dis 30(4):614

84. Spada M, Pagliardini S (2002) Screening for Fabry disease in end-stage nephropathies. J Inherit Metab Dis 25(Suppl 1):113

85. Poeppl AG, Murray GJ, Medin JA (2005) Enhanced filter paper enzyme assay for high-throughput population screening for Fabry disease. Anal Biochem 337:161–163

86. Spada M, Pagliardini S, Yasuda M, Tukel T, Thiagarajan G, Sakuraba H, Ponzone A, Desnick RJ (2006) High incidence of later-onset Fabry disease revealed by newborn screening. Am J Hum Genet 79(1):31–40

87. Hwu W-L, Chien Y-H, Lee N-C (2008) Screening for Pompe disease and Fabry disease. Clin Ther 30(Suppl C):S77

88. Chien YH, Chiang SC, Zhang XK, Keutzer J, Lee NC, Huang AC et al (2008) Early detection of Pompe disease by newborn screening is feasible: results from the Taiwan screening program. Pediatrics 122(1):39–45

89. Kemper AR, Hwu WL, Lloyd-Puryear M, Kishnani PS (2007) Newborn screening for Pompe disease: synthesis of the evidence and development of screening recommendations. Pediatrics 120(5):1327–1334

90. Civallero G, Micheli K, De Mari J, Viapaina M, Burin M, Coelho JC, Giugliani R (2006) Twelve different enzyme assays on dried-blood filter paper samples for detection of patients with selected inherited lysosomal storage diseases. Clin Chim Acta 372:98–102

91. Kotanko P, Kramar R, Devrnja D, Paschke E, Voigtlander T, Auinger M et al (2004) Results of a nationwide screening for Anderson-Fabry disease among dialysis patients. J Am Soc Nephrol 15:1323–1329

92. Rolfs A, Bottcher T, Zschiesche M, Morris P, Winchester B, Bauer P et al (2005) Prevalence of Fabry disease in patients with cryptogenic stroke: a prospective study. Lancet 366(9499):1794–1796

93. Fuller M, Lovejoy M, Brooks DA, Harkin ML, Hopwood JJ, Meikle PJ (2004) Immunoquantification of α-galactosidase: evaluation for the diagnosis of Fabry disease. Clin Chem 50:1979–1985

94. Li Y, Scott CR, Chamoles NA, Ghavami A, Pinto BM, Turecek F, Gelb MH (2004) Direct multiplex assay of lysosomal enzymes in dried blood spots for newborn screening. Clin Chem 50:1785–1796

95. Gelb MH, Turecek F, Scott CR, Chamoles NA (2006) Direct multiplex assay of enzymes in dried blood spots by tandem mass spectrometry for the newborn screening of lysosomal storage disorders. J Inherit Metab Dis 29(2–3):397–404

96. Turecek F, Scott CR, Gelb MH (2007) Tandem mass spectrometry in the detection of inborn errors of metabolism for newborn screening. Methods Mol Biol 359:143–157

97. Zhang XK, Elbin CS, Chuang WL, Cooper SK, Marashio CA, Beauregard C, Keutzer JM (2008) Multiplex enzyme assay screening of dried blood spots for lysosomal storage disorders by using tandem mass spectrometry. Clin Chem 54(10):1725–1728

98. De Jesus VR, Zhang XK, Keutzer J, Bodamer O, Muhl A, Orsini JJ et al (2009) Development and evaluation of quality control dried blood spot materials in newborn screening for lysosomal storage diseases. Clin Chem 55(1):158–164

99. la Marca G, Casetta B, Malvagia S, Guerrini R, Zammarchi E (2009) New strategy for the screening of lysosomal storage disorders: the use of the online trapping-and-cleanup liquid chromatography/mass spectrometry. Anal Chem 81(15):6113–6121

100. Auray-Blais C, Cyr D, Drouin R (2007) Quebec neonatal mass urinary screening programme: From micromolecules to macromolecules. J Inherit Metab Dis 30(1):515–521

101. Auray-Blais C, Millington DS, Young SP, Clarke JT, Schiffmann R (2009) Proposed high-risk screening protocol for Fabry disease in patients with renal and vascular disease. J Inherit Metab Dis 32(2):303–308

102. Barr C, Clarke JT, Ntwari A, Drouin R, Auray-Blais C (2009) Fabry disease urinary globotriaosylceramide/creatinine biomarker evaluation by liquid chromatography-tandem mass spectrometry in healthy infants from birth to 6 months. Mol Genet Metab 97(3):237

103. Meikle PJ, Grasby DJ, Dean CJ, Lang DL, Bockmann M, Whittle AM et al (2006) Newborn screening for lysosomal storage disorders. Mol Genet Metab 88(4):307–314

104. Matern S (2008) Newborn screening for lysosomal storage diseases. Acta Paediatr 97:33–37

105. Stevens WS, Noble L, Berrie L, Sarang S, Scott LE (2009) Ultra-high throughput, automated nucleic acid detection of HIV for infant diagnosis using the GEN-PROBE APTIMA HIV-1 Screening Assay. J Clin Microbiol 47(8):2465–2469

106. Mérelle ME, Scheffer H, De Jong D, Dankert-Roelse JE (2006) Extended gene analysis can increase specificity of neonatal screening for cystic fibrosis. Acta Paediatr 95(11):1424–1428

107. Zschocke J, Kebbewar M, Gan-Schreier H, Fischer C, Fang-Hoffmann J, Wilrich J et al (2009) Molecular neonatal screening for homocystinuria in the Qatari population. Hum Mutat 30(6):1021–1022

108. Kumamoto S, Katafuchi T, Nakamura K, Endo F, Oda E, Okuyama T et al (2009) High frequency of acid alpha-glucosidase pseudodeficiency complicates newborn screening for

glycogen storage disease type II in the Japanese population. Mol Genet Metab 97(3): 190–195

109. Bentley DR, Balasubramanian S, Swerdlow HP, Smith GP, Milton J, Brown CG et al (2008) Accurate whole human genome sequencing using reversible terminator chemistry. Nature 456:53–59

110. Altarescu G, Moore DF, Schiffmann R (2005) Effect of genetic modifiers on cerebral lesions in Fabry disease. Neurology 64(12):2148–2150

Chapter 7
Biomarkers for Fabry Disease

Johannes M.F.G. Aerts

Abstract Biomarkers are surrogate markers of disease activity that may be helpful in the confirmation of a diagnosis and in clinical management. Biomarkers are usually chemical entities, ranging from simple metabolites to complex proteins and polynucleotides that can be measured in bodily fluids such as plasma or urine specimens. Metabolite and protein biomarkers have already been identified for the related lysosomal storage disorder Gaucher disease, and are presently used to support clinical decision making. The current status of biomarker identification and application for Fabry disease is described in this chapter. Attention is paid to metabolites (globotriaosylceramide and globotriaosylsphingosine) as well as the ongoing efforts to identify protein biomarkers. Present limitations in biomarkers are described and perspectives for further research are presented.

Keywords Fabry disease · Biomarker · Proteomics · Globotriaosylceramide · Globotriaosylsphingosine

7.1 Introduction

7.1.1 Molecular Basis of Fabry Disease

Fabry disease (OMIM 301500) is a lysosomal storage disorder resulting from deficient activity of the lysosomal hydrolase α-galactosidase A (EC 3.2.1.22) [1–3]. The α-galactosidase A gene (GLA), located on locus Xq22.1, contains seven exons and codes for a 429 amino acid precursor protein that is processed to 370 amino acid glycoprotein functioning as a homodimer [4–6]. Numerous mutations in the GLA gene have meanwhile been identified in connection to Fabry disease (see for a regularly updated overview http://www.hgmd.cf.ac.uk). The vast majority of these mutations are missense/nonsense type mutations, but also small and large deletions,

J.M.F.G. Aerts (✉)
Department of Medical Biochemistry, Academic Medical Center, University of Amsterdam, Amsterdam, The Netherlands
e-mail: j.m.aerts@amc.uva.nl

D. Elstein et al. (eds.), *Fabry Disease*, DOI 10.1007/978-90-481-9033-1_7,
© Springer Science+Business Media B.V. 2010

complex rearrangements, and one large insertion have been reported [7]. The identification of intronic mutations affecting splicing suggests that it may be also useful to include absolute real-time RT-PCR quantification of GLA transcripts in genetic diagnosis [8]. Unfortunately, the exact consequences at protein level of a large proportion of the identified missense mutations in the GLA gene are still not clear. Since the GLA gene is located on the X chromosome, all hemizygous males suffer from Fabry disease. Intriguingly, many female heterozygotes also display attenuated forms of the disease [9–14]. Female carriers of Fabry disease may ultimately develop symptoms similar to hemizygotes despite considerable amounts of circulating residual enzyme. This sharply contrasts with the general lack of symptoms among heterozygote carriers of another X-linked lysosomal hydrolase deficiency, Hunter disease.

The nature of mutations in the GLA gene, and the corresponding degree of residual α-galactosidase A activity, influences Fabry disease manifestation. In male patients with severe forms of Fabry disease there is usually a complete lack or severely reduced enzymatic activity. Relatively high residual enzyme activity is often noted in patients with a milder variant of Fabry disease with predominantly cardiac abnormalities, while having little or no kidney dysfunction and no painful acroparesthesia [15]. The onset of chronic renal insufficiency has been reported to be significantly delayed in Fabry patients with more than 1% residual enzyme activity [16]. However, there is also clear evidence for other modifiers beyond the GLA gene. Genotypes of polymorphisms G-174C of interleukin-6, G894T of endothelial nitric oxide synthase (eNOS), factor V G1691A mutation (factor V Leiden), and the A-13G and G79A of protein Z were all significantly associated with the presence of presumably ischemic cerebral lesions on brain MRI [17]. More recently it was also shown that two polymorphisms in the NOS3 gene, encoding endothelial eNOS, influence hypertrophic cardiomyopathy as measured by left posterior wall thickness of the heart [18].

Deficiency of α-Gal A results in accumulation of its glycosphingolipid substrates in lysosomes of endothelial, perithelial, and smooth muscle cells of the vascular system, as well as renal epithelial cells, myocardial cells, and cells of the autonomic nervous system [15]. The accumulating glycosphingolipids contain terminal α-galactosyl moieties, such as globotriaosylceramide (Gb3; also named ceramide-trihexoside: CTH); galabiosylceramide (Gb2); and, to a lesser extent, blood group B, B1, and P_1 antigens [19–21]. The prominent lysosomal storage of Gb3 in the endothelium is generally thought to cause a systemic vasculopathy with progressive renal insufficiency, cardiac involvement and CNS pathology in Fabry patients [1, 22].

7.1.2 Enzyme Replacement Therapy of Fabry Disease

Two different recombinant α-galactosidase A preparations are in use for the treatment of Fabry disease [23–25]. One enzyme is produced by Chinese hamster ovary (CHO) cells with classic recombinant technology (agalasidase β, Fabrazyme) and the other enzyme is produced by cultured human skin fibroblasts with an activated promoter of the α-gal A gene (agalasidase α, Replagal). Both recombinant enzymes are quite comparable in properties and differ only slightly in glycan composition [26]. The two enzyme preparations have independently been examined in clinical investigations and are both registered in Europe for the treatment of Fabry patients. Although both enzyme therapies were found to result in the desired clearance of globotriaosylceramide from the endothelium, the clinical effects are not as robust as anticipated. In some patients stabilization of renal function and improvement in cardiac hypertrophy occurs upon therapy, but a considerable number experiences progressive complications [27].

7.1.3 Heterogeneous Manifestation and Early Detection of Fabry Disease

The experience with enzyme replacement therapies so far has boosted the view that therapeutic intervention should preferably be undertaken at an early stage of Fabry disease, prior to any irreversible organ damage. Such early intervention depends on early identification of Fabry patients. Unfortunately, the early detection of Fabry patients based on clinical symptoms alone is seriously complicated by the fact that virtually all complications of Fabry disease are non-specific in nature and clinically indistinguishable from similar abnormalities that occur in the context of more common disorders in the general population. In addition there exists a remarkable heterogeneity in clinical manifestation of Fabry disease as been nicely pointed out by a number of recent studies on the natural course of the disorder [14, 22, 28, 29]. Currently it is generally accepted that Fabry disease in males exhibits a vast phenotypic spectrum. This diversity in clinical presentation holds even more for female carriers. Some females carrying Fabry disease remain asymptomatic throughout their entire life, whereas others manifest symptoms with a severity comparable to male patients. The observed residual enzyme activity in plasma or blood cells from female heterozygotes varies considerably due to random X-inactivation, ranging from normal to nearly completely absent, and is a poor predictor of the clinical course [30].

Given the importance of early detection of Fabry patients, numerous screening studies have been undertaken and are still ongoing. Some of the investigations rely on detection of abnormalities in the GLA gene. A serious complication in this connection is the present difficulty to distinguish whether some of the commonly encountered abnormalities in the GLA gene are truly disease-causing mutations or polymorphisms that are not obligate disease-causing [31]. Other screening procedures are based on the demonstration of reduced enzymatic activity in blood cells, plasma or dried blood spots. An associated limitation of such methods is the present inability to detect reliably female carriers and some atypically affected male hemizygotes. As an alternative screening method, it is presently also contemplated by Hopwood and colleagues to use quantification of α-Gal A protein with specific antibodies in analogy to screening for other lysosomal enzymopathies [32].

Because of the limitations of the present detection methods for Fabry patients, attention is paid to the identification of biomarkers that allow a solid confirmation of diagnosis as well as monitoring of disease manifestation and therapeutic correction. The current status of biomarkers for Fabry disease forms the topic of the remainder of this review.

7.2 Biomarkers

7.2.1 Definition

A biomarker is defined as an analyte that indicates the presence of a biological process, which is linked to clinical manifestations and outcome of a particular disease. An ideal biomarker provides indirect but ongoing determinations of disease activity. Potential clinical applications of biomarkers are found in improved diagnosis, monitoring of disease progression, and assessment of therapeutic correction.

7.2.2 Nature and Application of Biomarkers

Biomarkers are chemical entities, ranging from simple metabolites to complex proteins and polynucleotides. The use of biomarkers for clinical purposes is an ancient concept. Already in 1703, Herman Boerhaave, one of the founding fathers of modern medicine, stated: 'Chemistry is indispensable for medical science since it renders a spectrum of objective data and offers the most reliable methods for assessment'. To date biomarkers are already widely used in the clinical management of some conditions. An obvious example is the measurement of blood glucose and/or glycated haemoglobin in diabetic individuals. Biomarker assessments guide clinicians in decision making on initiation and optimization of therapeutic interventions. Among part of the medical community, there is some reluctance to accept the growing role of such markers in clinical management. There is a sound debate among advocates and opponents of the use of imaging and assessments of chemical structures to support clinical care. It is evident that proposed biomarkers should not be too hastily adopted in clinical decision making and that sound proof of their true value has to exist. Rigorous validation of the relationship between a proposed biomarker and disease activity and outcome is of key importance. Moreover, biomarkers should assist in, and not strictly direct, clinical management.

7.3 Nature, Discovery and Application of Biomarkers: Lessons from Gaucher Disease

7.3.1 Biomarkers of Gaucher Disease

The search for biomarkers of Fabry disease has very much been influenced by the already existing experience with a related lysosomal storage disorder, Gaucher disease [33]. The outcome of biomarker investigations for Gaucher disease is therefore here discussed firstly. It offers a splendid introduction on the nature, discovery and application of biomarkers for a lysosomal storage disease.

Gaucher disease is due to deficiency of the lysosomal hydrolase glucocerebrosidase (GBA1) [34, 35]. Deficient activity of glucocerebrosidase results in accumulation of its substrate glucosylceramide in lipid-laden macrophages in spleen, liver and bone. These typical storage cells, so-called Gaucher cells, underlie many of the visceral manifestations of the disorder [36, 37]. Gaucher disease has acted very much as the playground to develop new therapeutic interventions such as enzyme replacement therapy and substrate reduction therapy. The availability of these costly therapies for Gaucher disease prompted research regarding suitable biomarkers to monitor onset and progression of disease, as well as efficacy of therapeutic intervention [38]. Two different classes of chemical entities have been considered as potential biomarkers for Gaucher disease: metabolites and proteins stemming from storage cells.

7.3.2 Metabolite Biomarkers

Regarding metabolites as potential biomarkers for Gaucher disease, two distinct sets of glycosphingolipids have been extensively investigated: the primary storage lipid glucosylceramide and secondarily increased lipids. Already several decades ago, elevated concentrations of glucosylceramide have been detected in plasma of symptomatic Gaucher disease patients, as reviewed in [39]. Nevertheless, plasma glucosylceramide has not been commonly used as a biomarker for Gaucher disease [40]. The measurement of glucosylceramide has been tedious and the increases in lipid levels are not very pronounced in some Gaucher patients. Moreover, the exact relation between circulating glucosylceramide and storage cells in tissues of Gaucher patients is far from clear. Besides the elevated glucosylceramide, the plasma concentration of other lipids is also abnormal in symptomatic Gaucher patients. Most strikingly, the concentration of the ganglioside GM3 is also elevated in Gaucher plasma samples, almost to the same extent as glucosylceramide [41, 42]. Increases of GM3 have earlier also been noted in cells and spleens of Gaucher patients [43, 44]. The secondary elevation of GM3 may not be without consequences. Elevated glycosphingolipids like GM3 are thought to cause insulin resistance [45]. Indeed, a recent study revealed that Gaucher patients are insulin resistant without overt hyperglycaemia [46].

7.3.3 Protein Biomarkers

Regarding proteins as potential biomarkers for Gaucher disease, considerable attention has been paid to the identification of plasma markers for the macrophage-derived Gaucher cells. Abnormalities in plasma levels of tartrate-resistant acid phosphatase (TRAP), angiotensin-converting enzyme (ACE), hexosaminidase, ferritin, ApoE and lysozyme in serum or plasma samples of Gaucher patients had been documented for some time [39]. Later on, increased plasma levels of various cathepsins, among which cathepsin D, K and S, were reported for Gaucher patients [47]. All these proteins are known to be produced by macrophages. However, none of them appears to be a truly specific marker for pathological Gaucher cells and their levels in serum of symptomatic Gaucher patients show overlap with those observed in healthy subjects. Their use as biomarkers for Gaucher cells is therefore restricted.

7.3.3.1 Chitotriosidase

A breakthrough has been the serendipitous discovery in serum of symptomatic Gaucher patients of a thousand-fold increased capacity to degrade the fluorogenic substrate 4-methylumbelliferyl-chitotrioside [48]. The corresponding enzyme, named chitotriosidase, has been extensively characterized [49]. In situ hybridization and histochemistry of bone marrow aspirates and sections of spleens from Gaucher patients revealed that chitotriosidase is very specifically produced by storage cells. The levels of chitotriosidase and glucosylceramide, a measure for Gaucher cells, closely correlate in different sections of spleens from Gaucher patients. A relation between the total body burden on storage cells in Gaucher patients and their plasma chitotriosidase levels has been noted. The plasma chitotriosidase level does not reflect any particular clinical symptom of Gaucher disease, suggesting that it rather reflects the sum of secreted enzyme by Gaucher cells in various body locations. Plasma chitotriosidase can be determined by monitoring the hydrolysis of chito-oligosaccharides, or more conveniently that of the fluorogenic substrate 4-methylumbelliferyl-chitotrioside [48]. A far more convenient, sensitive and accurate detection is feasible by measuring the activity of chitotriosidase towards the recently designed fluorogenic substrate 4-methylumbelliferyl-deoxy-chitobioside [50, 51]. Interpretation of plasma chitotriosidase levels is intrinsically complicated by the common occurrence of a 24-bp duplication in the chitotriosidase gene, preventing the formation of chitotriosidase protein [52]. In most ethnic groups about 1 in every three individuals carries this abnormality and about 1 in every twenty individuals, including Gaucher patients, is homozygous for this trait. It should be mentioned that increased plasma chitotriosidase activity is not unique for Gaucher patients. Plasma chitotriosidase activity is increased, albeit much more modestly, in several lysosomal and non-lysosomal diseases such as sarcoidosis, visceral Leishmaniasis, leprosy, arthritis, multiple sclerosis, thalassemia, COPD, malaria and atherosclerosis [49].

7.3.3.2 PARC/CCL18 and MIP-1Beta

A subsequent search for other protein biomarkers led to the discovery of massive overproduction and secretion by Gaucher cells of the chemokine PARC/CCL18 [47, 53]. PARC/CCL18 can be reliably quantified by ELISA. Plasma PARC/CCL18 levels are 10–40-fold elevated in symptomatic Gaucher patients [53]. Due to its basic nature and small molecular mass PARC/CCL18 levels in urine are proportional to those in the circulation. Therefore, urinary PARC/CCL18 excretion offers insight in the body burden of Gaucher cells [54]. Measurement of plasma PARC/CCL18 has been found to yield an excellent additional tool to monitor changes in body burden of Gaucher cells. It is particularly useful for the evaluation of those patients that are chitotriosidase deficient. More recently, van Breemen and co-workers reported markedly elevated levels of the chemokines MIP-1α and MIP-1β in serum of symptomatic Gaucher patients [55]. Interestingly, these proteins were found to be produced by surrounding inflammatory spleen macrophages and not by mature Gaucher cells. A relation was observed between plasma MIP-1β and skeletal disease: stable high plasma MIP-1β levels despite prolonged enzyme replacement therapy were found to correlate with ongoing skeletal disease [55]. Clearly, rigorous analysis of a large cohort of Gaucher patients is required to establish the value of plasma MIP-1β as biomarker, especially its value as prognostic marker for skeletal response to therapy.

7.3.4 Proteomics Search for Novel Biomarkers

Attempts are still made to detect additional protein biomarkers for Gaucher disease. We and others have used analysis of gene expression in storage cells [47]. Another employed approach is based on proteomics, a thorough survey of total protein composition of bodily fluids, or cell and tissue specimens. Several mass spectrometry techniques have become available allowing accurate analysis of proteins, even in complex mixtures like plasma and urine samples. Meanwhile use has been made of a variety of proteomics methods to analyze plasma and spleen samples obtained from Gaucher patients. Firstly, two-dimensional gel electrophoresis followed by identification of proteins of interest using peptide mass finger printing led to identification of elevated levels of several cathepsins in spleens from Gaucher patients [56]. Analysis of plasma with this labour-intensive and relatively insensitive technique pointed out that samples from symptomatic Gaucher patients contain a large amount of cathepsins and other proteases. Next, we employed surface enhanced laser desorption/ionization time-of-fight mass spectrometry (SELDI-TOF MS) for the analysis of Gaucher plasma samples. In a fast and economic manner a subproteome of plasma can be obtained by SELDI-TOF MS. The analysis results in profiles of M/z (mass over charge) data reflecting different proteins. Discrimination models can be generated to distinguish between Gaucher patients and normal subjects based on their M/z data profiles, requiring a thorough statistical validation of discrimination models [57]. Double cross-validation showed that the sensitivity of the discrimination model is 89% and the specificity 90%. Interestingly, although the study revealed the presence of a very distinctive plasma subproteome in Gaucher patients, it rendered no exciting candidates for specific biomarkers. Upon analysis of the top 10 proteins contributing to the discrimination between the normal and Gaucher plasma subproteomes, it was found that they were all relatively small (molecular masses below 10,000 Da) degradation fragments of larger proteins, being up-regulated in Gaucher patients as a consequence of increased protease activity. More recently, a series of plasma specimens from type I Gaucher patients prior and after therapy were studied by a novel, label-free LC-MS approach, so-called LC-MSE [58]. This method allows identification and quantification of the more abundant plasma proteins. Comparison with the normal plasma profile revealed several protein abnormalities in symptomatic Gaucher patients, particularly in the complement and coagulation cascades. In hindsight this finding is not surprising since Gaucher patients show a low level of coagulation activation [39]. Reductions in apolipoproteins associated with HDL were also detected in plasma of Gaucher patients by LC-MSE, again consistent with earlier observations with conventional analyses [58]. LC-MSE is presently also used to study the proteome of laser capture dissected Gaucher cells from spleens of Gaucher patients. Preliminary analysis of the data reveals that some proteins already known to be strongly expressed by Gaucher cells are nicely detected and quantified. Moreover, a number of novel potential protein markers for the storage cells have been identified by the LC-MSE analysis. The findings are currently validated by independent techniques (ELISA, Western-Blots and RT-PCR) and it is investigated whether these proteins are also elevated in plasma of symptomatic Gaucher patients.

7.3.5 *Application of Biomarkers*

Some of the discovered biomarkers for Gaucher disease are already applied in the clinic. Plasma chitotriosidase measurement is nowadays commonly employed as a first screen in the diagnosis of Gaucher disease. Increasing plasma levels of chitotriosidase seem to reflect ongoing disease manifestation by the gradual accumulation of storage cells in the patient's body. In an attempt to assess the utility of plasma chitotriosidase activity measurement as a biomarker for treatment efficacy, Hollak and co-workers investigated the relationship between enzyme activity and clinical parameters [59]. In patients with high clinical severity scores, chitotriosidase levels were usually above 20,000 nmol/ml/h and always above 15,000 nmol/ml/h, whereas patients with less severe disease tended to have lower values. During enzyme supplementation therapy, the mean decrease in 12 months was 32% (range, 0–82%) and 78% of patients had a decrease of more than 15%. In six patients with a decrease in chitotriosidase activity of less than 15% the clinical response to treatment was inferior to that of other patients, with less reduction in organomegaly in four and bone problems in two patients. In addition, the chitotriosidase response was related to the severity of the disease; less reduction in plasma activity was seen in more severely affected individuals. On the basis of this investigation, it has been proposed that in patients in whom the initiation of treatment is questionable based solely on clinical parameters, a chitotriosidase activity above 15,000 nmol/ml/h may serve as an indicator of a high Gaucher cell burden and an indication for the initiation of treatment [59]. A reduction in chitotriosidase activity of less than 15% after 12 months of treatment, in combination with an insufficient response of at least one clinical parameter, should be a reason to consider dose increase. Furthermore, a sustained increase in chitotriosidase at any point during treatment should alert the physician to the possibility of clinical deterioration and the need for dose adjustment. A more recent retrospective analysis by Deegan and colleagues confirmed the value of the use of plasma chitotriosidase in Gaucher disease management and presented evidence for a comparable use of PARC/CCL18 [60].

7.4 Biomarkers for Fabry Disease

Following the successful biomarker discovery for Gaucher disease, attempts have been made to identify comparable metabolite and protein biomarkers for Fabry disease. The current situation regarding these two types of potential biomarkers is here separately discussed.

7.4.1 Lipid Abnormalities as Potential Biomarkers

For a long time the primary accumulating globoside Gb3 has been considered as a surrogate marker for Fabry disease. Reduction of Gb3 in tissue biopsies has actually served as criterion for the registration of agalsidase beta. The globoside Gb3 is not only elevated inside storage cells, but also present in abnormal high concentrations in bodily fluids like plasma and urine. It is very well documented that in symptomatic Fabry hemizygotes both plasma and urinary Gb3 are increased [1, 61]. Intriguingly, in female carriers of Fabry disease, the urinary Gb3 is generally increased, but plasma Gb3 levels tend to be in the normal range [14] Various methods have meanwhile been developed for the detection of Gb3. Mass spectrometry-based and HPLC-based procedures have become available allowing accurate quantification of the globoside [62–66]. It has to be stressed that demonstration of increased Gb3, either in plasma or urine, is of great value for diagnostic purposes. This particularly holds for putative Fabry females carrying a GLA mutation with unclear consequences. The presence of increased urinary globoside Gb3 in such cases supports the diagnosis of Fabry disease. It has been reported that urinary Gb3 levels correlate with the predicted severity of GLA mutations [67].

7.4.1.1 Gb3 as Biomarker

The value of plasma or urinary Gb3 as biomarker to monitor progression of Fabry disease is unfortunately questionable. In several investigations plasmaGb3 has been found to poorly reflect Fabry disease manifestation and therapeutic outcome [14, 68–70]. For example, in a recent survey of the Dutch cohort of Fabry patients, the elevated levels of Gb3 in plasma or urine did not correlate with overall severity of disease or specific Fabry-related symptoms. Although male patients with cerebral complications tended to show higher levels of plasma Gb3 compared to males without, the clinical value of urinary or plasma Gb3 as a surrogate marker for manifestation of Fabry disease seemed limited in this cross-sectional study [14]. Whether the monitoring of changes in Gb3 during longitudinal follow-up of enzyme replacement therapy, using 'hard end points' such as death, progression to end-stage renal disease or stroke, still needs to be firmly established.

The poor predictive value of plasma or urinary Gb3 levels for Fabry disease manifestation is not entirely surprising. Prominent Gb3 accumulation has been noted in placental tissue of a Fabry hemizygote [71, 72], a finding illustrating that onset of clinical complications occurs only after several years of lipid deposition. Gb3 accumulation apparently occurs in hemizygotes at or even before birth, long before any clinical symptoms are prominent. The same discrepancy between early storage of Gb3 and clinical symptoms is also noted in Fabry mice generated by disruption of the GLA gene [73]. Plasma Gb3 concentrations in some pre-symptomatic boys have been found to exceed those in symptomatic adult hemizygotes [14], The absence of infantile manifestations in Fabry patients completely lacking α-galactosidase A activity also indicates that Gb3 accumulation does not cause immediately, and may be even not directly, signs of disease. An investigation by Barbey and co-workers has provided evidence for the presence of an unidentified substance in plasma of symptomatic Fabry disease patients which stimulates proliferation of vascular smooth muscle cells and cardiomyocytes in vitro [74]. It is conceivable that this substance is a causative factor in the development of left ventricular hypertrophy and increased intima media thickness in Fabry patients [75–78]. Although Gb3 accumulation is clearly a prerequisite for manifestation of Fabry disease, all observations combined point to the existence of another factor in addition to Gb3 that triggers pathogenesis.

7.4.1.2 Globotriaosylsphingosine (LysoGb3)

The puzzling findings prompted us to re-examine Gb3 and its metabolites in Fabry patients [79]. During this investigation it was discovered that plasma of Fabry patients contains markedly increased concentrations of deacylated globotriaosylceramide, globotriaosylsphingosine (here abbreviated as lysoGb3). The relative increase in the plasma concentrations of the cationic amphiphilic lysoGb3 spectacularly exceeds that of Gb3 by more than an order of magnitude. High nanomolar lysoGb3 concentrations occur in plasma samples from symptomatic Fabry males. Also in the case of symptomatic Fabry females, clearly increased levels of lysoGb3 were detected whilst concomitantly Gb3 concentrations were in the high normal range [79] Thus, measurement of plasma lysoGb3 seems to offer a very useful diagnostic tool, particularly in the case of Fabry females.

LysoGb3 and Disease Manifestation

The relationship between plasma lysoGb3 concentrations and Fabry disease manifestations is presently investigated. It is already clear that in Fabry hemizygotes, both in man and mouse, plasma lysoGb3 is already increased at birth and consequently does not correlate strictly with symptoms [79]. In contrast, in the case of female hemizygotes, lysoGb3 is low at birth and increases gradually with age. Some degree of correlation of plasma lysoGb3 levels and disease manifestation seems to exist for female hemizygotes. Presently a large cohort of Fabry patients is being examined to establish the exact relation between plasma lysoGb3 and clinical symptoms. The preliminary results indicate that elevated plasma lysoGb3 can be best viewed as a risk factor in addition to age: the exposure time to high circulating lysoGb3 seems associated with clinical manifestations such as cerebral signs (Aerts and co-workers, publication in preparation).

A detrimental effect of prolonged exposure to high circulating lysoGb3 seems conceivable based on a number of observations. It has already been found that lysoGb3 at concentrations occurring in plasma of symptomatic Fabry patients is able to promote Gb3 storage in cultured cells [79]. The precise mechanism for this has yet to be established. Intriguingly, lysoGB3 was also found to induce proliferation of smooth muscle cells in vitro. This finding suggests a causative role of lysoGb3 in the pathogenesis of Fabry disease [79]. Preliminary investigations in Fabry mice have furthermore pointed out that the concentrations of lysoGb3 are particularly high in the liver and intestine. This observation has opened up a new hypothesis, coined 'the secret road'. Confronted with the inability to degrade Gb3, Fabry patients might adapt to this by exploiting an alternative road to get rid of the excessive lipid. The alternative pathway implies conversion of Gb3 to lysoGb3, transport of lysoGb3 to the liver and subsequent secretion from the body via bile. Such a rescue pathway would explain why Gb3 seems not to accumulate progressively with age in male Fabry patients. According to this hypothesis, formation of lysoGb3 would be a metabolic adaptation to the traffic jam caused by α-galactosidase A deficiency. An inevitable downside of the rescue pathway might however be that Fabry individuals are long term exposed to lysoGb3, causing changes in the vasculature and specific cells. It should be clear that this scenario is still entirely speculative. Studies are presently conducted in Fabry mice to test the challenging hypothesis. If excretion of lysoGb3 is indeed a major pathway in Fabry patients, one could try to pharmacologically promote this by increasing biliary secretion or reducing intestinal re-uptake of lysoGb3. Supporting the body in its attempt to remove lysoGb3 might be useful in addition to degrading stored Gb3 by enzyme therapy.

7.4.2 Protein Abnormalities as Potential Biomarkers

In symptomatic Fabry patients, abnormalities are encountered that point to a low grade inflammatory disorder [22]. Indeed, increased circulating levels of CRP, as well as the hydrolases myeloperoxidase, metalloproteinase 9, and chitotriosidase have been reported for symptomatic Fabry hemizygotes [80–82]. The abnormalities in the hydrolases, all produced by phagocytes, are not very striking and certainly not specific for Fabry disease. Since inflammation is not thought to be a major component of Fabry disease, the value of above mentioned hydrolases as biomarkers seems limited. Monitoring corrections induced by therapy in the levels of abnormal hydrolases may however be informative. For example, clear reductions were noted in elevated chitotriosidase in male Fabry patients during enzyme therapy and relapses following the induction of neutralizing antibodies against the therapeutic enzyme [81].

7.4.2.1 Markers of Endothelial Activation

The currently prevalent concept is that Fabry disease is a systemic vasculopathy due to Gb3 storage in endothelial cells. Considerable attention has therefore been focused on the identification of plasma protein abnormalities reflecting endothelial activation. Known plasma proteins reflecting endothelial activation have been considered as candidate biomarkers for Fabry disease. This has been further stimulated by various reports demonstrating disturbed vascular circulation and a prothrombotic state in Fabry disease [22, 83]. Reported have been for symptomatic Fabry patients increases in circulating soluble sICAM-1, sVCAM-1, P-selectin, PAI, and decreased thrombomodulin combined with increased monocyte CD11b expression, consistent with a prothrombotic state [84]. Clinical observations reveal a somewhat higher incidence of thrombosis in severely affected Fabry disease patients [85], and in mouse models [86, 87]. In addition, based upon case histories [88–90] and a study in mice [91], an association between α-galactosidase A deficiency and the early development of atherosclerosis has been suggested, though a more recent study revealed an increased carotid intima-media thickness in the absence of atherosclerosis in Fabry disease patients [78]. Laboratory investigations that have been performed to assess determinants of coagulation or activation of the endothelium in Fabry patients are not always in accordance. Only an elevated level of sVCAM-1 could be confirmed in another investigation [92]. In a very recent thorough study conducted with a large cohort of Fabry patients in the Academic Medical Center in Amsterdam, only minimal abnormalities in indicators of coagulation, fibrinolysis and platelet activation as well as endothelial activation were detected [93]. However, very severely affected patients with renal impairment formed an exception in this respect. The noted plasma abnormalities in these individuals might be ascribed to their renal insufficiency rather than the underlying disorder itself. Unfortunately, it has to be concluded that at present no known circulating marker for endothelial cell activation has been identified that can reliably serve as early biomarker for manifestation of Fabry disease.

7.4.2.2 Proteomics Investigations

Next to targeted analysis of plasma proteins already known to reflect endothelial activation, the search for protein biomarkers of Fabry disease has nowadays been extended to analysis of the entire plasma proteome. Moore and co-workers were the first to elegantly investigate plasma of children with Fabry disease prior and after ERT using tryptic digestion of plasma protein and differentially labelling peptides with stable isotopes, such that consistent mass differences are introduced into selected amino acid residues [94]. Peptides from samples pre- and post-therapy were then combined to reduce the risk of differential losses during subsequent separation and analysis. The mass differences introduced by the isotope tags could be resolved by mass spectrometry and the information used to identify the proteins of origin and define their relative abundance in the samples. The LC-MS analysis pointed out only modest therapy-induced changes in few proteins [94]. Most importantly, it stimulated the investigators to further analyze α-2-antiplasmin concentrations in Fabry patients using citrate-based plasma specimens and a chromogenic method. The mean level of α-2-antiplasmin in 34 Fabry patients aged 10–55 years was 85% vs. normal laboratory mean of 105; range 82–123%. Thirteen of 29 patients on ERT (45%), had below-normal α-2-antiplasmin levels, median 75%, range 63–80%. Because the low levels of α-2-antiplasmin were thought to result of overconsumption of this protein by plasmin, plasma samples in the patients with low or borderline α-2-antiplasmin for plasminogen. As expected, all patients with low α-2-antiplasmin levels also had below-normal plasminogen [94].

A systematic proteomics analysis of blood specimens from Fabry patients is also being conducted at the Academic Medical Center in Amsterdam (Aerts and co-workers, manuscript in preparation). In analogy to previous work on Gaucher disease, both SELDI-TOF MS and LC-MSE are used to analyze Fabry samples for abnormalities. Mass to charge (m/z) profiles of sera from symptomatic Fabry patients and control subjects were generated by SELDI-TOF MS and classified using bagging principal component discriminant analysis. In contrast to the situation for Gaucher disease, reliable distinction between Fabry patients and controls was not obtained (misclassification rate 0.425). Next, LC-MSE was used to study plasma samples of controls and untreated Fabry patients. A large number of plasma proteins was identified and quantified: 73 proteins in at least one third of the samples, and 43 proteins in every sample. In the case of symptomatic Fabry male hemizygotes, only significant reductions were noted for plasminogen, fibronectin and kininogen-1, and minor increases for alpha-2-macroglobulin, fibrinogen gamma chain, complement factor H, and complement C4-A. With the exception of plasminogen, no significant corrections in these proteins were detected following 18 months of enzyme therapy. Very mildly affected Fabry hemizygotes did not show clear abnormalities in the proteins mentioned above. Next, the LC MSE data were subjected to classification using bagging PCDA. Only 1 of 10 untreated Fabry patients, a mildly affected hemizygote, was misclassified as control. In conclusion, the extensive investigation of the plasma proteome of Fabry patients by SELDI-TOF MS or LC-MSE did not render a single biomarker. Only subtle changes in the plasma proteome of hemizygous or heterozygous Fabry patients were detected.

7.4.3 Urinary Protein Abnormalities

Progressive kidney dysfunction is nearly universal in male individuals with Fabry disease. The initial sign of nephropathy is proteinuria or microalbuminuria, which has been reported in affected male individuals as young as 16 year and is present in half of male individuals by age 35 year [16]. As in diabetic nephropathy, the degree of proteinuria is a major prognostic determinant for more rapidly progressive Fabry nephropathy, and may also directly contribute to the progression of renal disease. Very recently is has been reported that urinary uromodulin (UMOD) excretion is reduced in Fabry patients. Immunohistochemical analysis of the affected kidney revealed abnormal UMOD localization in the thick ascending limb of Henle's loop and the distal convoluted tubule, with UMOD expression inversely proportional to the degree of storage. It has been proposed that UMOD may act as biochemical marker of therapeutic response of the kidney to therapy [95].

7.4.4 Antibodies Towards Therapeutic Enzyme

It has been observed that male Fabry patients lacking endogenous enzyme may develop antibodies directed to the therapeutic recombinant enzymes [96, 97]. In our laboratory's experience these antibodies are generally neutralizing, i.e. able to inhibit α-Gal A in in vitro enzyme assays [96]. The consequences of these antibodies for therapeutic efficacy have not yet been firmly established. Although strictly speaking antibodies are not a biomarker, it may be nevertheless useful to monitor their presence regularly in male Fabry patients receiving enzyme replacement therapy.

7.5 Discussion and Conclusions

The searches for biomarkers of Gaucher disease have been extraordinary productive. Next to elevations in circulating glucosylceramide and gangliosides like GM3 in Gaucher patients, striking abnormalities in plasma concentrations of some proteins have been identified. For example, increases in chitotriosidase up to 10,000 fold above normal have been identified in some Gaucher patients. For some of these proteins, i.e. chitotriosidase and PARC/CCL18, it has been demonstrated that they stem from storage cells. The circulating levels of these proteins offer insight in the total burden of storage cells in Gaucher patients. Regular monitoring of chitotriosidase, or PARC/CCL18 in chitotriosidase-deficient individuals, with sensitive assays is widely applied in Gaucher clinics and assists in clinical decision making.

The outcome of investigations on biomarkers for Fabry disease has been comparatively disappointing. Accurate methods have been developed to quantify the primary storage lipid Gb3 in plasma and urine specimens. However, it is generally felt that measurement of plasma and urinary Gb3 is only useful for diagnostic purposes and offers no sensitive tool to monitor Fabry disease progression. An exciting new development has been the discovery of elevated lysoGb3 in Fabry patients. The water-soluble lysoglycosphingolipid can freely enter and leave cells, and most likely spreads throughout the body. Laboratory findings suggest that lysoGb3 may even play a role in the noted intima media thickening of vessels in Fabry patients and possibly also in cardiac hypertrophy. Systematic and solid investigations with large cohorts of Fabry patients have to reveal the true value of lysoGb3 as biomarker. In any case, the demonstration of increased plasma lysoGb3 in female heterozygotes offers an important additional diagnostic tool.

At present no reliable protein biomarker has been identified that allows robust monitoring of Fabry patients at an early stage of the disease. Extensive biomarker searches have not substantiated the current believe that marked activation of the endothelium is an early event in Fabry pathogenesis. Albeit activation of endothelial cells by Gb3 might still occur, it is apparently not always well measurable in the circulation with the available techniques. In mildly affected Fabry patients no striking abnormalities in known plasma markers of activated endothelium have been universally detected. This disappointing finding remains puzzling given the large number of reports substantiating abnormal behaviour of endothelial cells following Gb3 accumulation. NO synthesis is probably down regulated in Fabry disease [98]. It is likely that induction of reactive oxygen species (ROS) play a role in this down regulation [99]. Excess production of reactive oxygen species such as superoxide was demonstrated in FD patients [98]. The susceptibility of Fabry patients to alterations in NO regulation is illustrated by the detrimental effect of the presence of eNOS polymorphism, eNOSG894T that decreases NO synthesis [22].

A better understanding of the primary mechanism underlying vasculopathy in Fabry patients may help to initiate more targeted searches for early biomarkers. Controversy exists whether the storage in the endothelial cells and the prothrombotic state is the origin of arterial damage or whether smooth muscle cell proliferation in the arterial media layer is the initiating step in the cascade that leads to Fabry vasculopathy [74]. Interestingly, in an atypical Fabry hemizygote and a heterozygote, lipid storage was detected in smooth muscle, but endothelial cells were clear [89, 100]. Since residual enzyme activity was present in these cases, smooth muscle cells might be more prone to Gb3 storage than endothelial cells. More detailed proteomics analyses of plasma specimens of mildly affected Fabry patients may help to reach a better understanding of the pathophysiological mechanism underlying vasculopathy at an initial stage of Fabry disease.

In conclusion, ongoing fundamental and clinical research on biomarkers of Fabry disease is still warranted. The availability of biomarkers, comparable in quality to those for Gaucher disease, is urgently needed for detection of Fabry disease manifestation at an early stage and to assist decision making regarding initiation of invasive and costly therapeutic interventions.

References

1. Desnick RJ, Ioannou YA (2001) α-Galactosidase a deficiency. Fabry disease. In: Scriver CR, Beaudet AL, Sly WS, Valle D (eds) The metabolic and molecular bases of inherited disease, 8th edn. McGraw-Hill, New York, pp 3733–3774
2. Kint JA (1970) Fabry's disease: alpha-galactosidase deficiency. Science 167(922): 1268–1269

3. Brady RO, Gal AE, Bradley RM, Martensson E, Warshaw AL, Laster L (1967) Enzymatic defect in Fabry's disease. Ceramidetrihexosidase deficiency. N Engl J Med 276(21): 1163–1167

4. Hamers MN, Westerveld A, Khan M, Tager JM (1977) Characterization of alpha-galactosidase isoenzymes in normal and Fabry human-Chinese Hamster somatic cell hybrids. Hum Genet 36(3):289–297

5. Bishop DF, Kornreich R, Desnick RJ (1988) Structural organization of the human alpha-galactosidase A gene: further evidence for the absence of a 3' untranslated region. Proc Natl Acad Sci USA 85(11):3903–3907

6. Garman SC, Garboczi DN (2004) The molecular defect leading to Fabry disease: structure of human alpha-galactosidase. J Mol Biol 337(2):319–335

7. Shabbeer J, Yasuda M, Benson SD, Desnick RJ (2006) Fabry disease: identification of 50 novel alpha-galactosidase A mutations causing the classic phenotype and three-dimensional structural analysis of 29 missense mutations. Hum Genomics 2(5):297–309

8. Mignani R, Morrone A (2009) Is standard GLA gene mutation analysis definitive for the diagnosis of Fabry disease? Kidney Int 75(10):1115–1116

9. MacDermot KD, Holmes A, Miners AH (2001) Natural history of Fabry disease in affected males and obligate carrier females. J Inherit Metab Dis 24(Suppl 2):13–14

10. Whybra C, Kampmann C, Willers I et al (2001) Anderson-Fabry disease: clinical manifestations of disease in female heterozygotes. J Inherit Metab Dis 24(7):715–724

11. Gupta S, Ries M, Kotsopoulos S, Schiffmann R (2005) The relationship of vascular glycolipid storage to clinical manifestations of Fabry disease: a cross-sectional study of a large cohort of clinically affected heterozygous women. Medicine 84:261–268

12. Deegan PB, Baehner AF, Barba Romero MA et al (2006) Natural history of Fabry disease in females in the Fabry Outcome Survey. J Med Genet 43(4):347–352

13. Wang RY, Lelis A, Mirocha J, Wilcox WR (2007) Heterozygous Fabry women are not just carriers, but have a significant burden of disease and impaired quality of life. Genet Med 9(1):34–45

14. Vedder AC, Linthorst GE, van Breemen MJ et al (2007) The Dutch Fabry cohort: diversity of clinical manifestations and Gb3 levels. J Inherit Metab Dis 30(1):68–78

15. Desnick RJ, Ioannou YA (1996) α-Galactosidase a deficiency: Fabry disease. In: Scriver CR, Beaudet AL, Sly WS, Valle D (eds) The metabolic and molecular bases of inherited disease, 6th edn. McGraw-Hill, New York, pp 2741–2784

16. Branton MH, Schiffmann R, Sabnis SG et al (2002) Natural history of Fabry renal disease: influence of alpha-galactosidase A activity and genetic mutations on clinical course. Medicine (Baltimore) 81(2):122–138

17. Altarescu G, Moore DF, Schiffmann R (2005) Effect of genetic modifiers on cerebral lesions in Fabry disease. Neurology 64(12):2148–2150

18. Rohard I, Schaefer E, Kampmann C, Beck M, Gal A (2008 Oct 22) Association between polymorphisms of endothelial nitric oxide synthase gene (NOS3) and left posteriorwall thickness (LPWT) of the heart in Fabry disease. J Inherit Metab Dis (Epub ahead of print)

19. Sweeley CC, Klionsky B (1963) Fabry's disease: classification as a sphingolipidosis and partial characterization of a novel glycolipid. J Biol Chem 238:3148–3150

20. Mårtensson E (1966) Neutral glycolipids of human kidney isolation, identification, and fatty acid composition. Biochim Biophys Acta 116(2):296–308

21. Wherrett JR, Hakomori SI (1973) Characterization of a blood group B glycolipid, accumulating in the pancreas of a patient with Fabry's disease. J Biol Chem 24899:3046–3051

22. Schiffmann R (2009) Fabry disease. Pharmacol Ther 122(1):65–77

23. Brady RO, Tallman JF, Johnson WG et al (1973) Replacement therapy for inherited enzyme deficiency. Use of purified ceramidetrihexosidase in Fabry's disease. N Engl J Med 289(1):9–14

24. Schiffmann R, Kopp JB, Austin HA III et al (2001) Enzyme replacement therapy in Fabry disease: a randomized controlled trial. JAMA 285(21):2743–2749

25. Eng CM, Guffon N, Wilcox WR et al (2001) Safety and efficacy of recombinant human alpha-galactosidase A—replacement therapy in Fabry's disease. N Engl J Med 345(1):9–16

26. Blom D, Speijer D, Linthorst GE, Donker-Koopman WG, Strijland A, Aerts JM (2003) Recombinant enzyme therapy for Fabry disease: absence of editing of human alpha-galactosidase A mRNA. Am J Hum Genet 72(1):23–31

27. Vedder AC, Linthorst GE, Houge G et al (2007) Treatment of Fabry disease: outcome of a comparative trial with agalsidase alfa or beta at a dose of 0.2 mg/kg. PLoS ONE 2(7):e598

28. Mehta A, Ricci R, Widmer U et al (2004) Fabry disease defined: baseline clinical manifestations of 366 patients in the Fabry Outcome Survey. Eur J Clin Invest 34(3):236–242

29. Eng CM, Fletcher J, Wilcox WR et al (2007) Fabry disease: baseline medical characteristics of a cohort of 1765 males and females in the Fabry Registry. J Inherit Metab Dis 30(2): 184–192

30. Linthorst GE, Poorthuis BJ, Hollak CE (2008) Enzyme activity for determination of presence of Fabry disease in women results in 40% false-negative results. J Am Coll Cardiol 51(21):2082

31. Froissart R, Guffon N, Vanier MT, Desnick RJ, Maire I (2003) Fabry disease: D313Y is an alpha-galactosidase A sequence variant that causes pseudodeficient activity in plasma. Mol Genet Metab 80(3):307–314

32. Tan MA, Dean CJ, Hopwood JJ, Meikle PJ (2008) Diagnosis of metachromatic leukodystrophy by immune quantification of arylsulphatase A protein and activity in dried blood spots. Clin Chem 54(11):1925–1927

33. Beutler E, Grabowski GA (2001) Gaucher disease. In: Scriver CR, Sly WS, Valle D (eds) The metabolic and molecular bases of inherited disease, 8th edn. McGraw-Hill, New York, pp 3635–3668

34. Brady RO, Kanfer JN, Bradley RM, Shapiro D (1966) Demonstration of a deficiency of glucocerebroside-cleaving enzyme in Gaucher's disease. J Clin Invest 45:1112–1115

35. Patrick AD (1965) A deficiency of glucocerebrosidase in Gaucher's disease. Biochem J 97:17c–18c

36. Aerts JM, van Weely S, Boot R, Hollak CE, Tager JM (1993) Pathogenesis of lysosomal storage disorders as illustrated by Gaucher disease. J Inherit Met Dis 16:288–291

37. Boven LA, van Meurs M, Boot RG, Mehta A, Aerts JM, Laman JD (2004) Gaucher cells demonstrate a distinct macrophage phenotype and resemble alternatively activated macrophages. Am J Clin Pathol 122:359–369

38. Aerts JM, van Breemen MJ, Bussink AP et al (2008b) Biomarkers for lysosomal storage disorders: identification and application as exemplified by chitotriosidase in Gaucher disease. Acta Paediatr Suppl 97(457):7–14

39. Aerts JM, Hollak CE (1997) Plasma and metabolic abnormalities in Gaucher's disease. Baillieres Clin. Haematol 10:691–709

40. Meikle PJ, Whitfield PD, Rozaklis T et al (2008) Plasma lipids are altered in Gaucher disease: biochemical markers to evaluate therapeutic intervention. Blood Cells Mol Dis 40(3):420–427

41. Ghauharali-van der Vlugt K, Langeveld M, Poppema A et al (2008) Prominent increase in plasma ganglioside GM3 is associated with clinical manifestations of type I Gaucher disease. Clin Chim Acta 389(1–2):109–113

42. Hein LK, Meikle PJ, Hopwood JJ, Fuller M (2007) Secondary sphingolipid accumulation in a macrophage model of Gaucher disease. Mol Genet Metab 92(4):336–345

43. Saito M, Rosenberg A (1985) The fate of glucosylceramide (glucocerebroside) in genetically impaired (lysosomal beta-glucosidase deficient) Gaucher disease diploid human fibroblasts. J Biol Chem 260(4):2295–2300

44. Nilsson O, Svennerholm L (1982) Accumulation of glucosylceramide and glucosylsphingosine (psychosine) in cerebrum and cerebellum in infantile and juvenile Gaucher disease. J Neurochem 39(3):709–718

45. Aerts JM, Ottenhoff R, Powlson AS et al (2007) Pharmacological inhibition of glucosylceramide synthase enhances insulin sensitivity. Diabetes 56(5):1341–1349

46. Langeveld M, Ghauharali KJ, Sauerwein HP et al (2008) Type I Gaucher disease, a glycosphingolipid storage disorder, is associated with insulin resistance. J Clin Endocrinol Metab 93(3):845–851

47. Moran MT, Schofield JP, Hayman AR, Shi GP, Young E, Cox TM (2000) Pathologic gene expression in Gaucher disease: up-regulation of cysteine proteinases including osteoclastic cathepsin K. Blood 96(5):1969–1978

48. Hollak CE, van Weely S, van Oers MH, Aerts JM (1994) Marked elevation of plasma chitotriosidase activity. A novel hallmark of Gaucher disease. J Clin Invest 93(3):1288–1292

49. Bussink AP, van Eijk M, Renkema GH, Aerts JM, Boot RG (2006) The biology of the Gaucher cell: the cradle of human chitinases. Int Rev Cytol 252:71–128

50. Aguilera B, Ghauharali-van der Vlugt K, Helmond MT et al (2003) Transglycosidase activity of chitotriosidase: improved enzymatic assay for the human macrophage chitinase. J Biol Chem 278(42):40911–40916

51. Schoonhoven A, Rudensky B, Elstein D et al (2007) Monitoring of Gaucher patients with a novel chitotriosidase assay. Clin Chim Acta 381(2):136–139

52. Boot RG, Renkema GH, Verhoek M et al (1998) The human chitotriosidase gene. Nature of inherited enzyme deficiency. J Biol Chem 273(40):25680–25685

53. Boot RG, Verhoek M, de Fost M et al (2004) Marked elevation of the chemokine CCL18/PARC in Gaucher disease: a novel surrogate marker for assessing therapeutic intervention. Blood 103(1):33–39

54. Boot RG, Verhoek M, Langeveld M et al (2006) CCL18: a urinary marker of Gaucher cell burden in Gaucher patients. J Inherit Metab Dis 29(4):564–571

55. van Breemen MJ, de Fost M, Voerman JS et al (2007) Increased plasma macrophage inflammatory protein (MIP)-1alpha and MIP-1beta levels in type 1 Gaucher disease. Biochim Biophys Acta 1772(7):788–796

56. van Breemen MJ, Aerts JM, Sprenger RR, Speijer D (2008) Potential artefacts in proteome analysis of plasma of Gaucher patients due to protease abnormalities. Clin Chim Acta 396(1–2):26–32

57. Smit S, van Breemen MJ, Hoefsloot HC, Smilde AK, Aerts JM, de Koster CG (2007) Assessing the statistical validity of proteomics based biomarkers. Anal Chim Acta 592(2):210–217

58. Vissers JP, Langridge JI, Aerts JM (2007) Analysis and quantification of diagnostic serum markers and protein signatures for Gaucher disease. Mol Cell Proteomics 6(5):755–766

59. Hollak CE, Maas M, Aerts JM (2001) Clinically relevant therapeutic endpoints in type I Gaucher disease. J Inherit Metab Dis 24(Suppl 2):97–105

60. Deegan PB, Moran MT, McFarlane I et al (2005) Clinical evaluation of chemokine and enzymatic biomarkers of Gaucher disease. Blood Cells Mol Dis 35(2):259–267

61. Desnick RJ, Dawson G, Desnick SJ, Sweeley CC, Krivit W (1971) Diagnosis of glycosphingolipidoses by urinary-sediment analysis. N Engl J Med 284(14):739–744

62. Mills K, Vellodi A, Morris P et al (2004) Monitoring the clinical and biochemical response to enzyme replacement therapy in three children with Fabry disease. Eur J Pediatr 163(10):595–603

63. Fauler G, Rechberger GN, Devrnja D et al (2005) Rapid determination of urinary globotriaosylceramide isoform profiles by electrospray ionization mass spectrometry using stearoyl-d35-globotriaosylceramide as internal standard. Rapid Commun Mass Spectrom 19(11):1499–1506

64. Fuller M, Sharp PC, Rozaklis T et al (2005) Urinary lipid profiling for the identification of Fabry hemizygotes and heterozygotes. Clin Chem 51(4):688–694

65. Auray-Blais C, Cyr D, Mills K, Giguère R, Drouin R (2007) Development of a filter paper method potentially applicable to mass and high-risk urinary screenings for Fabry disease. J Inherit Metab Dis 30(1):106

66. Groener JE, Poorthuis BJ, Kuiper S, Helmond MT, Hollak CE, Aerts JM (2007) HPLC for simultaneous quantification of total ceramide, glucosylceramide, and ceramide trihexoside concentrations in plasma. Clin Chem 53(4):742–747

67. Auray-Blais C, Cyr D, Ntwari A et al (2008) Urinary globotriaosylceramide excretion correlates with the genotype in children and adults with Fabry disease. Mol Genet Metab 93(3):331–340

68. Young E, Mills K, Morris P et al (2005) Is globotriaosylceramide a useful biomarker in Fabry disease? Acta Paediatr Suppl 94(447):51–54

69. Whitfield PD, Calvin J, Hogg S et al (2005) Monitoring enzyme replacement therapy in Fabry disease–role of urine globotriaosylceramide. J Inherit Metab Dis 28(1):21–33

70. Bekri S, Lidove O, Jaussaud R, Knebelmann B, Barbey F (2006) The role of ceramide trihexoside (globotriaosylceramide) in the diagnosis and follow-up of the efficacy of treatment of Fabry disease: a review of the literature. Cardiovasc Hematol Agents Med Chem 4(4):289–297

71. Popli S, Leehey DJ, Molnar ZV, Nawab ZM, Ing TS (1990) Demonstration of Fabry's disease deposits in placenta. Am J Obstet Gynecol 162:464–465

72. Vedder AC, Strijland A, vd Bergh Weerman MA, Florquin S, Aerts JM, Hollak CE (2006) Manifestations of Fabry disease in placental tissue. J Inherit Metab Dis 29(1):106–111

73. Ohshima T, Murray GJ, Swaim WD et al (1997) alpha-Galactosidase A deficient mice: a model of Fabry disease. Proc Natl Acad Sci USA 94(6):2540–2544

74. Barbey F, Brakch N, Linhart A et al (2006) Cardiac and vascular hypertrophy in Fabry disease: evidence for a new mechanism independent of blood pressure and glycosphingolipid deposition. Arterioscler Thromb Vasc Biol 26(4):839–844

75. Boutouyrie P, Laurent S, Laloux B, Lidove O, Grunfeld JP, Germain DP (2002) Arterial remodelling in Fabry disease. Acta Paediatr Suppl 91(439):62–66

76. Barbey F, Brakch N, Linhart A et al (2006) Increased carotid intima-media thickness in the absence of atherosclerotic plaques in an adult population with Fabry disease. Acta Paediatr Suppl 95(451):63–68

77. Kalliokoski RJ, Kalliokoski KK, Penttinen M et al (2006) Structural and functional changes in peripheral vasculature of Fabry patients. J Inherit Metab Dis 29(5):660–666

78. Vedder AC, Gerdes VE, Poorthuis BJ et al (2007) Failure to detect Fabry patients in a cohort of prematurely atherosclerotic males. J Inherit Metab Dis 30(6):988

79. Aerts JM, Groener JE, Kuiper S et al (2008b) Elevated globotriaosylsphingosine is a hallmark of Fabry disease. Proc Natl Acad Sci USA 105(8):2812–2817

80. Kaneski CR, Moore DF, Ries M, Zirzow GC, Schiffmann R (2006) Myeloperoxidase predicts risk of vasculopathic events in hemizgygous males with Fabry disease. Neurology 67(11):2045–2047

81. Vedder AC, Cox-Brinkman J, Hollak CE et al (2006) Plasma chitotriosidase in male Fabry patients: a marker for monitoring lipid-laden macrophages and their correction by enzyme replacement therapy. Mol Genet Metab 89(3):239–244

82. Shah JS, Hughes DA, Tayebjee MH, MacFadyen RJ, Mehta AB, Elliott PM (2007) Extracellular matrix turnover and disease severity in Anderson-Fabry disease. J Inherit Metab Dis 30(1):88–95

83. Moore DF, Kaneski CR, Askari H, Schiffmann R (2007) The cerebral vasculopathy of Fabry disease. J Neurol Sci 257(1–2):258–263

84. DeGraba T, Azhar S, Dignat-George F et al (2000) Profile of endothelial and leukocyte activation in Fabry patients. Ann Neurol 47(2):229–233

85. Utsumi K, Yamamoto N, Kase R et al (1997) High incidence of thrombosis in Fabry's disease. Intern Med 36(5):327–329

86. Shen Y, Bodary PF, Vargas FB et al (2006) Alpha-galactosidase A deficiency leads to increased tissue fibrin deposition and thrombosis in mice homozygous for the factor V Leiden mutation. Stroke 37(4):1106–1108

87. Eitzman DT, Bodary PF, Shen Y et al (2003) Fabry disease in mice is associated with age-dependent susceptibility to vascular thrombosis. J Am Soc Nephrol 14(2):298–302

88. Diamantopoulos EJ, Andreadis EA, Vassilopoulos CV, Marakomichelakis GE (2002) Intermittent claudication unmasking underlying Fabry's disease. Int Angiol 21(2):201–203

89. Hůlková H, Ledvinová J, Pouptová H, Bultas J, Zeman J, Elleder M (1999) [Postmortem diagnosis of Fabry disease in a female heterozygote leading to the detection of undiagnosed manifest disease in the family]. Cas Lek Cesk 138(21):660–664

90. Schiffmann R, Rapkiewicz A, Abu-Asab M et al (2006) Pathological findings in a patient with Fabry disease who died after 2.5 years of enzyme replacement. Virchows Arch 448(3):337–343

91. Bodary PF, Shen Y, Vargas FB et al (2005) Alpha-galactosidase A deficiency accelerates atherosclerosis in mice with apolipoprotein E deficiency. Circulation 111(5):629–632

92. Demuth K, Germain DP (2002) Endothelial markers and homocysteine in patients with classic Fabry disease. Acta Paediatr Suppl 91(439):57–61

93. Vedder AC, Biró E, Aerts JM, Nieuwland R, Sturk G, Hollak CE (2009) Plasma markers of coagulation and endothelial activation in Fabry disease: impact of renal impairment. Nephrol Dial Transplant 24(10):3074–3081

94. Moore DF, Krokhin OV, Beavis RC et al (2007) Proteomics of specific treatment-related alterations in Fabry disease: a strategy to identify biological abnormalities. Proc Natl Acad Sci USA 104(8):2873–2878

95. Vylet'al P, Hůlková H, Zivná M et al (2008) Abnormal expression and processing of uromodulin in Fabry disease reflects tubular cell storage alteration and is reversible by enzyme replacement therapy. J Inherit Metab Dis 31(4):508–517

96. Linthorst GE, Hollak CE, Donker-Koopman WE, Strijland A, Aerts JM (2004) Enzyme therapy for Fabry disease: neutralizing antibodies toward agalsidase alpha and beta. Kidney Int 66:1589–1595

97. Ohashi T, Sakuma M, Kitagawa T, Suzuki K, Ishige N, Eto Y (2007) Influence of antibody formation on reduction of globotriaosylceramide (GL-3) in urine from Fabry patients during agalsidase beta therapy. Mol Genet Metab 92(3):271–273

98. Moore DF, Scott LT, Gladwin MT et al (2001) Regional cerebral hyperperfusion and nitric oxide pathway dysregulation in Fabry disease: reversal by enzyme replacement therapy. Circulation 104(13):1506–1512

99. Shen JS, Meng XL, Moore DF et al (2008) Globotriaosylceramide induces oxidative stress and up-regulates cell adhesion molecule expression in Fabry disease endothelial cells. Mol Genet Metab 95(3):163–168

100. Takenaka T, Teraguchi H, Yoshida A et al (2008) Terminal stage cardiac findings in patients with cardiac Fabry disease: an electrocardiographic, echocardiographic, and autopsy study. J Cardiol 51(1):50–59

Chapter 8
Fabry Disease Case Finding Studies in High-Risk Populations

Gere Sunder-Plassmann and Manuela Födinger

Abstract Because Fabry disease is medically important and effective interventions exist, an early diagnosis in symptomatic individuals would be desirable. However, the diagnosis is often delayed for several years after first symptoms have developed. One approach to overcome this clinical deficit is case finding studies among people with medical problems typically found in Fabry disease patients. During the last decade such studies revealed a surprising high prevalence of Fabry disease among patients with chronic kidney disease, heart disease, or stroke. Because specific treatment is available, several experts endorsed case finding studies in high risk populations within an organized frame or even routine testing of individuals with stroke, kidney- or heart disease. The methodologies recommended for case finding strategies include testing for enzyme activity in dried blood spots or examination of urine specimen for increased excretion of globotriaosylceramide. Together with newborn screening the results of large case finding studies among patients with stroke, left ventricular hypertrophy, or chronic kidney disease will allow for a better approximation of the true prevalence of the disease and will probably result in an improvement of clinical care of affected individuals.

Keywords Fabry disease · Chronic kidney disease · Dialysis · Transplantation · Stroke · Left ventricular hypertrophy · Epidemiology · Case finding

8.1 Introduction

Because Fabry disease frequently represents a diagnostic miracle for physicians and effective interventions exist, an early diagnosis would be desirable. However, the intermittent and transient characteristics of pain, the shortage of other more specific symptoms, the absence of physical findings, and a general lack of awareness of Fabry disease cause a diagnosis to be delayed for decades or even missed for the

G. Sunder-Plassmann (✉)
Division of Nephrology and Dialysis, Department of Medicine III, Medical University Vienna, Vienna, Austria
e-mail: gere.sunder-plassmann@meduniwien.ac.at

D. Elstein et al. (eds.), *Fabry Disease*, DOI 10.1007/978-90-481-9033-1_8,
© Springer Science+Business Media B.V. 2010

whole life [1]. One approach directed to overcome this clinical deficit are case find-ing studies among people with specific medical problems (in contrast to screening studies, that, by definition, are done in apparently well people [2]).

Following approval of enzyme replacement therapy for treatment of Fabry disease some 10 years ago the number of case finding studies among high risk pop-ulations including patients with chronic kidney disease, left ventricular hypertrophy or cryptogenic stroke has increased.

This article summarizes the most important results of Fabry disease case find-ing studies and provides a glimpse on laboratory methodologies suitable for case detection.

8.2 Kidney Disease

Patients on hemodialysis therapy represent a high-risk group for Fabry disease. Several case finding studies using currently available technology have revealed a considerably high prevalence of Fabry disease among this population (Table 8.1).

Three reports described the prevalence and outcome of Fabry disease among end-stage renal disease (ESRD) patients. In Europe [3] and in the US [4] the preva-lence of Fabry disease among patients on renal replacement therapy was 0.0188 (83/440,665 patients) and 0.0167 (42/250,352 patients), respectively. Interestingly, 12% of ESRD patients with Fabry disease were female in both registries. In the meantime several case finding studies among ESRD populations have shown a more than 10 times higher prevalence of Fabry disease as compared to the USRDS or EDTA-ERA registry (Table 8.1) [5, 6]. Most recently, Shah et al. found a prevalence of 0.085% (197/233,280) among US kidney transplant recipients [7]. In contrast, the first large case finding study among kidney transplant recipients revealed a prevalence of 0.383% [8], which was even somewhat higher as compared to the prevalence of Fabry disease among dialysis patients in the same country [5].

Because the prevalence of Fabry disease among chronic kidney disease (CKD) stage I–IV patients is not known a large multicenter case finding study was initiated in Austria in the year 2008. Patient enrollment is ongoing with a planned target of 5,000 patients (Anderson-Fabry Disease in Chronic Kidney Disease Patients Not on Renal Replacement Therapy (AFD-CKD); ClinicalTrials.Gov study identifier: NCT00728364).

8.3 Heart Disease

Cardiac disease causes substantial morbidity in men and women suffering from Fabry disease [9]. Some 15 years ago Nakao et al. were the first to examine the con-tribution of Fabry disease to left ventricular hypertrophy in an unselected population of patients referred to echocardiography. In this study, 7 of 230 male individuals (3%) presenting with a ventricular-septum or posterior wall-thickness of at least

Table 8.1 Overview of 18 case finding studies among patients with chronic kidney disease

References	Study population	Country	AGAL	N (all)	% (all)	N (males)	% (males)	N (females)	% (females)
Utsumi [33]	HD, PD	Japan	P	2/720	0.278	2/440	0.455	0/280	0.000
Desnick, Abstract, 2002 [34]	HD, PD, male	USA	P, L			9/1,903	0.473		
Spada, Abstract [35]	HD, PD, male	Italy	DBS			4/1,765	0.227		
Pagliardini, Abstract (2002)	ESRD, male	Europe	DBS			12/4,671	0.257		
Linthorst [36]	HD, PD male	Netherlands	WB			1/508	0.197		
Nakao [37]	HD, male	Japan	P			6/514	1.167		
Kotanko [5]	HD, PD	Austria	DBS	4/2,480	0.161	4/1,516	0.264	0/964	0.000
Rocha, Abstract (2004)	HD	Portugal	DBS	4/4,000	0.100	–	–		
Ichinose [38]	HD, male	Japan	P			1/450	0.222		
Bekri [39]	HD	France	L	1/106	0.943	1/59	1.695	0/47	0.000
Tanaka [40]	HD	Japan	P	4/696	0.575	4/401	0.998	1/295	0.339
Merta [6]	HD	Czech Republic	DBS	5/3,370	0.148	4/1,521	0.263	1/1,849	0.054
Maslauskien [41]	HD, male	Lithunia	DBS			0/536	0.000		
Terryn [42]	HD	Belgium	DBS	3/922	0.302	1/180	0.555	2/742	0.276
Andrade [43]	CKD, HD, PD, KTR, male	Canada	P			0/499	0.000		
Porsch [44]	HD, male	Brazil	DBS			2/558	0.358		
Rasaiah [45]	HD, PD	Canada	DBS	0/147	0.000	–	–		
De Schoenmakere [46]	KTR	Belgium	DBS	1/673					
Kleinert [8]	KTR, male	Austria	DBS, L			5/1,306	0.383		
Herrera, Abstract (2009)	HD	Spain	DBS	6/910		3/543		3/367	
Wallner, AFD-CKD, ongoing*	CKD w.o. RRT	Austria	Urine Gb3	5,000					

AGAL, alfa galactosidase A; HD, hemodialysis, PD, peritoneal dialysis, ESRD, end-stage renal disease, CKD, chronic kidney disease, KTR, kidney transplant recipients, RRT, renal replacement therapy; P, plasma, L, leukocyte, WB, whole blood, DBS, dried blood spot

*ClinicalTrials.gov identifier: NCT00728364

13 mm were diagnosed to suffer from Fabry disease. Two other studies among female or male individuals with unexplained hypertrophic cardiomyopathy revealed Fabry disease in 12% (4/34) and 3.9% (6/153; < 40 years of age: 1/74, > 40 years of age: 5/79) of patients [10, 11]. Other small studies failed to detect cases with Fabry disease: Ommen et al. did not find histopathology evidence for the presence of Fabry disease among 100 patients who underwent septal ablation for hypertrophic cardiomyopathy [12]. Similarly, Stöllberger et al. and Arad et al. did not find patients with Fabry disease among 26 individuals presenting with left ventricular hypertrabeculation/noncompaction [13] or among 75 with unexplained left ventricular hypertrophy [14]. More recently the largest study so far by Monserrat and colleagues studied 508 unrelated individuals with hypertrophic cardiomyopathy. They confirmed the diagnosis of Fabry disease in 5 of 15 patients with reduced plasma activity of alfa-galactosidase A (3/328 males, 0.9%; 2/180 females, 1.1%) [15]. Finally, Gaspar and colleagues reported preliminary results of a case finding study among patients with an interventricular septum thickness of ≥ 13 mm disclosing Fabry disease in 3 among 87 patients (2/43 males, 1/44 females) [16]. Furthermore, reports of heart transplantation in patients with Fabry disease provided the basis for a case finding study among male heart transplant recipients [17, 18]. This study, however, failed to establish a diagnosis of Fabry disease among several hundred male heart transplant recipients [19].

The ongoing Viennese Prevalence Study of Anderson-Fabry Disease (VIEPAF) is currently examining urine globotriaosylceramide excretion among 5,000 consecutive female and male individuals presenting with an interventricular wall thickness of ≥ 12 mm (ClinicalTrials.gov study identifier: NCT00871611). There is certainly no doubt that this largest study thus far will provide the best approximation of the true prevalence of Fabry disease among incident patients referred to a tertiary care echocardiography center presenting with left ventricular hypertrophy. Case finding studies in populations with heart disease are summarized in Table 8.2.

8.4 Stroke

Stroke is a common clinical manifestation of Fabry disease and occurs frequently before diagnosis and in the absence of other clinical events [20]. A recent analysis of 2,446 patients enrolled in the Fabry Registry showed 138 strokes among 86 males (6.9%) and 52 females (4.3%). Most patients had not experienced renal or cardiac events before their first stroke (70.9% of males and 76.9% of females). Interestingly, 50% of males and 38.3% of females experienced their first stroke before being diagnosed with Fabry disease [20]. Thus, young stroke patients are considered as a high-risk population for Fabry disease. Rolfs et al. previously identified roughly 4% of subjects with cryptogenic stroke to suffer from Fabry disease [21]. In contrast, the Middelheim Fabry Study was unable to find any patient with Fabry disease in a population of 103 young stroke patients [22]. At least three ongoing studies examining the prevalence of Fabry disease in patients with stroke will shed more light on this controversial issue (SIFAP1, FIND, CFSSI, Table 8.3).

Table 8.2 Overview of 9 case finding studies among patients with heart disease

References	Study population	Country	AGAL	N (all)	% (all)	N (males)	% (males)	N (females)	% (females)
Nakao [47]	LVH, IVST > 13 mm, male	Japan	P			7/230	3		
Sachdev [10]	HCM, male, >40 years	UK	P			5/79	6.3		
	HCM, male, <40 years	UK	P			1/74	1.4		
Stöllberger [13]	LVHT, male	Austria	L			0/26			
Ommen [12]	SVSM	US	H	0/100		0/44		0/56	
Chimenenti [11]	HCM, female	Italy	P			0/44		4/43	12
Arad [14]	HCM	NA, SA, Europe	G	0/75		0/45		0/30	
Monserrat [15]	HCM	Spain	P	5/508		3/328	0.9	2/180	1.1
Gaspar, Abstract [16]	LVH, IVST ≥ 13 mm	Portugal	DBS	3/87		2/43		1/44	
Kleinert, Unpublished [19]	HTX, male	Austria	DBS			0/207			
Mundigler, VIEPAF, ongoing*	LVH, IVST > 12 mm	Austria	Urine Gb3	5,000	–	–	–	–	–

AGAL, alfa galactosidase A; P, plasma, L, leukocyte, H, histopathology; G, genetic analysis; DBS, dried blood spot; LVH, left ventricular hypertrophy; IVST, interventricular septum thickness; HCM, hypertrophic cardiomyopathy; LVHT, left ventricular hypertrabeculation/noncompaction; SVSM, subaortic ventricular septal myectomy for treatment of HCM; HTX, heart transplantation; NA, North America; SA, South America
*ClinicalTrials.gov identifier: NCT00871611

Table 8.3 Overview of five case finding studies among patients with stroke

References	Study population	Country	AGAL	N (all)	% (all)	N (males)	% (males)	N (females)	% (females)
Rolfs [21]	Cryptogenic stroke	Germany	L, G	28/721	3.883	21/432	4.9	7/289	2.4
Brouns [22]	Cryptogenic stroke	Belgium	DBS, G	0/103	–	0/64	–	0/39	–
Rolfs, SIFAP1, ongoing*	Cryptogenic stroke	Europe	L, G	5,000					
Moore, CFSSI, Abstract (2009), ongoing	Cryptogenic stroke	Canada	G	500					
Germain, FIND, ongoing**	Cryptogenic stroke, male	France	n.s.	889					

AGAL, alfa galactosidase A; L, leukocyte; G, genetic analysis; DBS, dried blood spot; n.s., not specified
*ClinicalTrials.gov identifier: NCT00414583
**ClinicalTrials.gov identifier: NCT00484549

8.5 Summary

After more than a decade of case finding studies among high risk patients that allowed for a proper diagnosis of Fabry disease in many cases and their families (Tables 8.1, 8.2, and 8.3), an expert group that met on the occasion of a satellite meeting of the World Congress of Nephrology in 2009 endorsed case finding studies within an organized frame among high risk populations such as male ESRD patients [23]. Others even suggest routine testing for Fabry disease among individuals with chronic kidney disease, stroke, or cardiac disease [24, 25]. In addition, case finding studies in populations presenting without life threatening complications of alfa-galactosidase A deficiency, such as ocular or skin manifestations, may also have the potential to facilitate an early diagnosis of Fabry disease [26, 27].

The methodology recommended for Fabry disease case finding strategies was recently summarized and includes testing for enzyme activity in dried blood spots or examination of urine specimen for increased excretion of globotriaosylceramide [24, 25, 28]. Other developments include testing for globotriaosyl-sphingosine [29] or urine proteomics [30].

Together with newborn screening [31, 32] the results of large case finding studies among patients with stroke, left ventricular hypertrophy, or chronic kidney disease stage 1–4 will allow a better approximation of the true prevalence of this hereditary disease and will probably result in an improvement of clinical care of affected individuals.

Financial Conflict of Interest Statement Gere Sunder-Plassmann: honoraria, research grants, travel grants from Shire HGT and Genzyme

Manuela Födinger: Research support from Genzyme.

References

1. Clarke JT (2007) Narrative review: Fabry disease. Ann Intern Med 146(6):425–433
2. Grimes DA, Schulz KF (2002) Uses and abuses of screening tests. Lancet 359(9309):881–884
3. Tsakiris D, Simpson HK, Jones EH, Briggs JD, Elinder CG, Mendel S et al (1996) Report on management of renale failure in Europe, XXVI, 1995. Rare diseases in renal replacement therapy in the ERA-EDTA Registry. Nephrol Dial Transplant 11(Suppl 7):S4–S20
4. Thadhani R, Wolf M, West ML, Tonelli M, Ruthazer R, Pastores GM et al (2002) Patients with Fabry disease on dialysis in the United States. Kidney Int 61(1):249–255
5. Kotanko P, Kramar R, Devrnja D, Paschke E, Voigtlander T, Auinger M et al (2004) Results of a nationwide screening for Anderson-Fabry disease among dialysis patients. J Am Soc Nephrol 15(5):1323–1329
6. Merta M, Reiterova J, Ledvinova J, Poupetova H, Dobrovolny R, Rysava R et al (2007) A nationwide blood spot screening study for Fabry disease in the Czech Republic haemodialysis patient population. Nephrol Dial Transplant 22(1):179–186
7. Shah T, Gill J, Malhotra N, Takemoto SK, Bunnapradist S (2009) Kidney transplant outcomes in patients with Fabry disease. Transplantation 87(2):280–285
8. Kleinert J, Kotanko P, Spada M, Pagliardini S, Paschke E, Paul K et al (2009) Anderson-Fabry disease: a case-finding study among male kidney transplant recipients in Austria. Transpl Int 22(3):287–292

9. Linhart A, Kampmann C, Zamorano JL, Sunder-Plassmann G, Beck M, Mehta A et al (2007) Cardiac manifestations of Anderson-Fabry disease: results from the international Fabry outcome survey. Eur Heart J 28(10):1228–1235

10. Sachdev B, Takenaka T, Teraguchi H, Tei C, Lee P, McKenna WJ et al (2002) Prevalence of Anderson-Fabry disease in male patients with late onset hypertrophic cardiomyopathy. Circulation 105(12):1407–1411

11. Chimenti C, Pieroni M, Morgante E, Antuzzi D, Russo A, Russo MA et al (2004) Prevalence of Fabry disease in female patients with late-onset hypertrophic cardiomyopathy. Circulation 110(9):1047–1053

12. Ommen SR, Nishimura RA, Edwards WD (2003) Fabry disease: a mimic for obstructive hypertrophic cardiomyopathy? Heart 89(8):929–930

13. Stöllberger C, Finsterer J, Voigtländer T, Slany J (2003) Is left ventricular hypertrabeculation/noncompaction a cardiac manifestation of Fabry's disease? Z Kardiol 92(11): 966–969

14. Arad M, Maron BJ, Gorham JM, Johnson WH Jr, Saul JP, Perez-Atayde AR et al (2005) Glycogen storage diseases presenting as hypertrophic cardiomyopathy. N Engl J Med 352(4):362–372

15. Monserrat L, Gimeno-Blanes JR, Marin F, Hermida-Prieto M, Garcia-Honrubia A, Perez I et al (2007) Prevalence of Fabry disease in a cohort of 508 unrelated patients with hypertrophic cardiomyopathy. J Am Coll Cardiol 50(25):2399–2403

16. Gaspar P, Azevado O, Rodrigues D, Providencia R, Gomes PL, Monteiro S et al (2009) Screening of Fabry disease in patients with left ventricular hypertrophy: preliminary results. Proceedings of the 9th international symposium on LSDs, Frankfurt, Shire HGT

17. Karras A, De Lentdecker P, Delahousse M, Debauchez M, Tricot L, Pastural M et al (2008) Combined heart and kidney transplantation in a patient with Fabry disease in the enzyme replacement therapy era. Am J Transplant 8(6):1345–1348

18. Cantor WJ, Daly P, Iwanochko M, Clarke JT, Cusimano RJ, Butany J (1998) Cardiac transplantation for Fabry's disease. Can J Cardiol 14(1):81–84

19. Kleinert J, Spada M, Pagliardini S, Kotanko P, Voigtländer T, Födinger M et al (Submitted) Lack of evidence for unrecognized cases with Fabry disease among male heart transplant recipients

20. Sims K, Politei J, Banikazemi M, Lee P (2009) Stroke in Fabry disease frequently occurs before diagnosis and in the absence of other clinical events: natural history data from the Fabry Registry. Stroke 40(3):788–794

21. Rolfs A, Böttcher T, Zschiesche M, Morris P, Winchester B, Bauer P et al (2005) Prevalence of Fabry disease in patients with cryptogenic stroke: a prospective study. Lancet 366(9499):1794–1796

22. Brouns R, Sheorajpanday R, Braxel E, Eyskens F, Baker R, Hughes D et al (2007) Middelheim Fabry Study (MiFaS): a retrospective Belgian study on the prevalence of Fabry disease in young patients with cryptogenic stroke. Clin Neurol Neurosurg 109(6): 479–484

23. Mignani R, Feriozzi S, Schaefer RM, Breunig F, Oliveira JP, Ruggenenti P et al (2010) Dialysis and transplantation in Fabry disease: indications for enzyme replacement therapy. Clin J Am Soc Nephrol 5(2):379–385

24. Öqvist B, Brenner BM, Oliveira JP, Ortiz A, Schaefer R, Svarstad E et al (2009) Nephropathy in Fabry disease: the importance of early diagnosis and testing in high-risk populations. Nephrol Dial Transplant 24(6):1736–1743

25. Auray-Blais C, Millington DS, Young SP, Clarke JT, Schiffmann R (2009) Proposed high-risk screening protocol for Fabry disease in patients with renal and vascular disease. J Inherit Metab Dis 32(2):303–308

26. Hauser AC, Lorenz M, Voigtlander T, Födinger M, Sunder-Plassmann G (2004) Results of an ophthalmologic screening programme for identification of cases with Anderson-Fabry disease. Ophthalmologica 218(3):207–209

27. Orteu CH, Jansen T, Lidove O, Jaussaud R, Hughes DA, Pintos-Morell G et al (2007) Fabry disease and the skin: data from FOS, the Fabry outcome survey. Br J Dermatol 157(2): 331–337
28. Schiffmann R, Waldek S, Benigni A, Auray-Blais C (2010) Biomarkers of Fabry disease nephropathy. Clin J Am Soc Nephrol 5(2):360–364
29. Aerts JM, Groener JE, Kuiper S, Donker-Koopman WE, Strijland A, Ottenhoff R et al (2008) Elevated globotriaosylsphingosine is a hallmark of Fabry disease. Proc Natl Acad Sci USA 105(8):2812–2817
30. Kistler AD, Wuthrich RP, Serra AL, Mischak H, Breunig F, Hughes DA et al (2009) Identification of biomarkers for Fabry disease by urine proteomics. Focus on Fabry nephropathy-biomarkers, progression and disease severity (Official Satellite of the World Congress of Nephrology). Fondazione Internazionale Menarini, Bergamo, 2009
31. Spada M, Pagliardini S, Yasuda M, Tukel T, Thiagarajan G, Sakuraba H et al (2006) High incidence of later-onset Fabry disease revealed by newborn screening. Am J Hum Genet 79(1):31–40
32. Bodamer OA (2008) Newborn screening in Fabry disease: what can be achieved with early diagnosis? Clin Ther 30(Suppl B):S41
33. Utsumi K, Kase R, Takata T, Sakuraba H, Matsui N, Saito H et al (2000) Fabry disease in patients receiving maintenance dialysis. Clin Exp Nephrol 4:49–51
34. Desnick RJ (2002) Fabry disease: unrecognized ESRD patients and effectiveness of enzyme replacement on renal pathology and function. J Inherit Metab Dis 25(Suppl 1):116
35. Spada M, Pagliardini S (2002) Screening for Fabry disease in end-stage nephropathies. J Inherit Metab Dis 25(Suppl 1):113
36. Linthorst GE, Hollak CE, Korevaar JC, Van Manen JG, Aerts JM, Boeschoten EW (2003) alpha-Galactosidase A deficiency in Dutch patients on dialysis: a critical appraisal of screening for Fabry disease. Nephrol Dial Transplant 18(8):1581–1584
37. Nakao S, Kodama C, Takenaka T, Tanaka A, Yasumoto Y, Yoshida A et al (2003) Fabry disease: detection of undiagnosed hemodialysis patients and identification of a "renal variant" phenotype. Kidney Int 64(3):801–807
38. Ichinose M, Nakayama M, Ohashi T, Utsunomiya Y, Kobayashi M, Eto Y (2005) Significance of screening for Fabry disease among male dialysis patients. Clin Exp Nephrol 9(3): 228–232
39. Bekri S, Enica A, Ghafari T, Plaza G, Champenois I, Choukroun G et al (2005) Fabry disease in patients with end-stage renal failure: the potential benefits of screening. Nephron Clin Pract 101(1):c33–c38
40. Tanaka M, Ohashi T, Kobayashi M, Eto Y, Miyamura N, Nishida K et al (2005) Identification of Fabry's disease by the screening of alfa-galctosidase A activity in male and female hemodialysis patients. Clin Nephrol 64(4):281–287
41. Maslauskiene R, Bumblyte IA, Sileikiene E, Grazulis S, Laurinavicius A, Pleckaitis M et al (2007) The prevalence of Fabry's disease among male patients on hemodialysis in Lithuania (a screening study). Medicina (Kaunas) 43(Suppl 1):77–80
42. Terryn W, Poppe B, Wuyts B, Claes K, Maes B, Verbeelen D et al (2008) Two-tier approach for the detection of alpha-galactosidase A deficiency in a predominantly female haemodialysis population. Nephrol Dial Transplant 23(1):294–300
43. Andrade J, Waters PJ, Singh RS, Levin A, Toh BC, Vallance HD et al (2008) Screening for Fabry disease in patients with chronic kidney disease: limitations of plasma alpha-galactosidase assay as a screening test. Clin J Am Soc Nephrol 3(1):139–145
44. Porsch DB, Nunes AC, Milani V, Rossato LB, Mattos CB, Tsao M et al (2008) Fabry disease in hemodialysis patients in southern Brazil: prevalence study and clinical report. Ren Fail 30(9):825–830
45. Rasaiah VI, Underwood JP, Oreopoulos DG, Medin JA (2008) Implementation of high-throughput screening for Fabry disease in Toronto dialysis patients. Nephrol Dial Transplant Plus 1(2):129–130

46. De Schoenmakere G, Poppe B, Wuyts B, Claes K, Cassiman D, Maes B et al (2008) Two-tier approach for the detection of alpha-galactosidase A deficiency in kidney transplant recipients. Nephrol Dial Transplant 23(12):4044–4048
47. Nakao S, Takenaka T, Maeda M, Kodama C, Tanaka A, Tahara M et al (1995) An atypical variant of Fabry's disease in men with left ventricular hypertrophy. N Engl J Med 333(5): 288–293

Chapter 9
Small Molecule Drug Discovery for Fabry Disease

Omid Motabar, Ehud Goldin, Wei Zheng, and Ellen Sidransky

Abstract Small molecule therapy has been widely used for the treatment of a variety of diseases. Small molecule drugs can be easily administered to patients, and are advantageous in that they can cross the blood-brain barrier, do not cause autoimmune responses, and have lower manufacturing costs. In this chapter, we focus on different strategies and methods for small molecule drug development as it applies to Fabry disease. The steps involved in developing an appropriate high throughput screen to identify activators and inhibitors of alpha galactosidase A are outlined. Assay development includes optimization of the assay pH, time course, enzyme and substrate concentration and the amount of sodium taurocholate used. The assay must then be validated and confirmed using additional screens. The optimized screens can be used to identify novel lead compounds that can serve as new starting points for drug development for Fabry disease.

Keywords Fabry disease · α-galactosidase · Drug discovery · High throughput screening · Small molecule chaperone therapy · Assay optimization

9.1 Introduction

Fabry disease is caused by mutations in the gene encoding for α-galactosidase A (GLA), which subsequently results in a mutant protein. To date, 431 mutations have been identified in the GLA gene (Human Gene Mutation Database, www.hgmd.cf.ac.uk). Of these, more than 57% are missense mutations. Studies of residual activity of mutant forms of the enzyme revealed that many of these mutants had kinetic properties similar to the wild-type enzyme, but were significantly less stable [1–3]. This finding suggests that the deficiency of enzymatic activity in

E. Sidransky (✉)
Medical Genetics Branch, National Human Genome Research Institute, National Institutes of Health, Bethesda, MD, USA
e-mail: sidranse@mail.nih.gov

D. Elstein et al. (eds.), *Fabry Disease*, DOI 10.1007/978-90-481-9033-1_9,

Fabry Disease is caused by misfolding, and/or the inability to traffic these mutant proteins to lysosomes. The mutant proteins are subsequently retained in the endoplasmic reticulum after synthesis and then degraded prematurely. The deficiency of GLA in Fabry patients causes the accumulation of the glycosphingolipid, globotriaosylceramide (Gb3), in many cells and organs, including endothelial cells and the smooth muscle cells of blood vessels [4]. Patients with Fabry disease present clinically with chronic neuronopathic pain, gastrointestinal disturbances, angiokeratomata, progressive renal impairment, cardiomyopathy, premature myocardial infarctions, and stroke. Both life expectancy and quality of life are severely compromised.

Enzyme replacement therapy (ERT) has been available since 2001 for the treatment of Fabry disease [5, 6]. ERT showed positive effects on the kidney and heart at an early phase of the disease, relieving pain and improving quality of life [6]. However, the long term clinical benefits of ERT for Fabry patients are still unclear, especially its ability to prevent premature strokes in patients [7, 8]. Some patients also develop immune responses to the infused enzyme [7]. In addition, the high cost of ERT is a burden to Fabry patients who require lifelong treatment.

Chemical chaperone therapy has recently emerged as a potential therapeutic alternative for Fabry disease. "Chemical chaperones" are small molecules that bind mutant proteins and assist in their correct folding, maturation, and trafficking to their functional site, such as the lysosome. It has been reported that some enzyme inhibitors and receptor antagonists can serve as chaperones for mutant enzymes and receptors [9, 10]. The effects of chemical chaperones have been explored in various lysosomal storage disorders, including Gaucher disease [11–14], Pompe disease [15, 16], Tay-Sachs/Sandhoff disease [17], GM1-gangliosidosis [18], as well as Fabry disease. One GLA inhibitor, 1-deoxygalactonojirimycin (DGJ, marketed as Amigal[TM] by Amicus Therapeutics, Inc.) is currently being studied under a phase 3 clinical trial as a chaperone therapeutic agent for Fabry disease [19]. However, the effect of DGJ is mutation-specific. Many mutant GLAs that have poor protein stability with nearly normal catalytic activity are not responsive to DGJ, such as ones with the R356W mutation [1, 20]. Therefore, the identification of novel lead compounds with broad chaperone activity that can serve as new starting points for drug development may prove beneficial.

9.2 Strategies for Drug Discovery and Drug Targets

Small molecule therapy has been widely used for the treatment of a variety of diseases, and accounts for approximately 80–90% of marketed drugs. Small molecule drugs can be easily administered to patients, have quick responses, and are effective. Compared to protein based drugs, such as ERT, small molecules are advantageous in that they can be administered orally, can cross the blood-brain barrier, do not cause autoimmune responses, and have lower manufacturing costs. This chapter focuses on the strategies and methods for small molecule drug development.

Enzyme activators enhancing GLA activity. Enzyme activators can stimulate enzyme activity above the normal level. Thus, small molecule activators may increase the residual activity of mutant GLA enzymes in the lysosomes of patients with Fabry disease, thereby correcting the lysosomal storage of substrate. However, the activators may not work if their efficacies are not high enough, or if there is not enough residual mutant enzyme remaining in the lysosomes. For the most part, it is difficult to discover enzyme activators in compound library screens.

Promoter activators increasing GLA expression. A small molecule promoter activator can increase the expression of target proteins. In this case, a small molecule would bind to the GLA promoter and increase the synthesis of proteins, including the mutant GLA. It has been reported that the enhancement of mutant enzyme expression can proportionally increase protein trafficking to the lysosome [21]. For mutations with significant residual enzyme activity, a small molecule promoter activator may correct the lysosomal storage by increasing the amount of the enzyme in lysosomes. While it is relatively simple to find specific GLA promoter activators, the hypothesis of a promoter activator being a drug for Fabry disease must be tested and validated with small molecule lead compounds. A cell line can be established by transfection with a cDNA plasmid containing the promoter region of the GLA gene linked with a reporter gene such as luciferase. The reporter gene based promoter activating assay can then be used for the screening of compound collections to identify potential lead compounds.

Chemical chaperones specifically targeting GLA. The chemical chaperones under consideration for the treatment of lysosomal storage disorders are all enzyme inhibitors. Several iminosugar inhibitors, the sugar analogs of enzyme reaction products, have shown promising chaperone activities in cell-based and animal disease models for Fabry disease, as well as for other lysosomal storage diseases [9, 13, 19]. However, iminosugar molecules may not be the best drug candidates due to issues with selectivity and compound stability. Thus, enzyme inhibitors with novel structures are needed for chaperone therapy drug development for Fabry disease. New GLA inhibitors can be identified in compound library screens using a fluorogenic enzyme assay.

The use of an inhibitor as a "chaperone" to enhance the activity of a mutant enzyme is not a perfect solution in vivo. Clearly, the chaperone action of an inhibitor may be functionally compromised due to its inhibition of enzyme activity. Therefore, the chaperone activity of these compounds must be balanced against the direct inhibition of the enzyme. In theory, an enzyme activator with chaperone activity would be a better choice for drug development. Both the chaperone and enzyme stimulatory actions of the activator would synergistically increase enzyme activity in the lysosomes. Currently, no such small molecule activators with chaperone activity are available.

Small molecule modulators regulating GLA homeostasis (proteostasis). In addition to the stabilization of the mutant protein by a chaperone mechanism, small molecule proteostasis regulators can increase the amount of folded protein in the ER by increasing the proteostasis network capacity [22]. This is achieved through the enhancement of signaling pathways and/or the transcription and translation of components in the proteostasis network. Increases and decreases in the proteostasis network capacity promote protein folding and degradation, respectively. Examples of small molecules increasing proteostasis network capacity are diltiazem and verapamil, known calcium channel blockers, which have been shown to partially restore glucocerebrosidase folding, trafficking, and function in patient fibroblasts [23]. If proteostasis regulators are combined with small molecule chaperones, their synergy could significantly increase the amount of folded protein trafficked to lysosomes.

9.3 The Process of Small Molecule Drug Discovery

The drug discovery process has evolved from disease model based screens with low throughput, to the mechanism/molecular target based screens with high throughput. Small molecule drug discovery includes target identification and validation, early lead discovery and optimization, preclinical safety development, and clinical trials, and requires an average of 10–15 years (Fig. 9.1). Modern target based drug discovery started in the late 1980s, when advancements in molecular biology and the Human Genome Project led to a wealth of new drug targets. Recombinant proteins/enzymes and target protein expressed cell lines became available as useful tools for the identification of small molecule activators and inhibitors. The demand for the rapid screening of molecular targets led to the development of new assay/detection technologies and drug screen robots in the 1990s. Synthetic chemical compounds for compound collections also became commercially available at reasonable costs. A screen using 1–3 million compounds to identify lead compounds for a single drug target has become a routine operation in the pharmaceutical industry over the last 10 years.

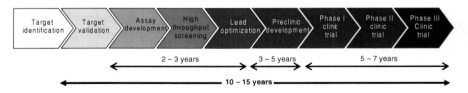

Fig. 9.1 Schematic representation of the drug discovery process

Drug screening methods have significantly improved in the last 20 years. They were initially done in test tubes (1–5 ml), then in 96-well plates (100–300 μl), and have recently advanced to high density 384-well (2,040 μl) and 1536-well (2–8 μl) plates. The increase in well density has greatly enhanced compound screening throughput, and has also reduced screening costs. Currently, most screening assays, including both biochemical/enzymatic and cell-based assays, can be performed in 1536-well plates with total assay volumes of 2–8 μl. The NIH Chemical Genomics Center has recently developed a quantitative high throughput screening (qHTS) method using 1536-well plates for the primary compound screen. Using this method, compounds are screened at a 1:5 titration, and concentration-response curves are obtained for the active compounds [24]. This method allows for the testing of a wide range of compound concentrations, with the highest concentrations reaching 50–80 μM. The use of multiple compound concentrations is particularly helpful for identifying potentially useful compounds that may be overlooked when using only one concentration.

Once active compounds are identified from the primary screen, they need to be confirmed in secondary and tertiary assays. The best lead compounds with drug-like chemical structures then would then undergo chemical optimization to improve potency and selectivity. Then, hundreds or thousands of newly synthesized analog compounds would be rescreened to determine structure-activity-relationships (SAR), and pharmacokinetic properties, such as drug absorption, distribution, metabolism and excretion properties. The optimized lead compounds with the highest potencies and selectivities, as well as the most drug-like pharmacokinetic properties, could then move to preclinical development to ensure safety and efficacy in animal models before entering clinical trials. It is clear that target selection and early lead discovery play key roles in the drug discovery and development process. Identification of high quality, drug-like lead compounds is vital for success in the later stages of drug development.

9.4 Assay Development and HTS to Identify New GLA Inhibitors/Activators

Once the drug development strategy is set and the drug target selected, assay development is the next step in lead discovery. Here, as an example, we describe the development, optimization and screen validation of a GLA enzyme assay.

The fluorogenic molecule, 4-methylumbelliferyl-α-D-galactopyranoside (4MU-α-Gala), is available as a substrate for GLA, where the enzyme reaction product (4MU) emits blue fluorescence at a peak of 440 nm upon excitement at 365 nm [25, 26]. However, due to its emission in the blue fluorescence wavelength, this assay is prone to interference from fluorescent compounds in the collection. A red fluorogenic substrate, resorufinyl α-D-galactopyranoside (res-α-Gala), which emits at 610 nm was developed for use in HTS and is less sensitive to fluorescence interference [27]. Chromogenic assays are also available that use p-nitrophenol-α-D-galactopyranoside [28, 29] or naphthyl-α-D-galactopyranoside [30] as substrates. But absorbance assays are usually less sensitive than fluorescence assays, and cannot be easily miniaturized into the 1536-well plate format for HTS.

GLA enzyme assay with a fluorogenic substrate. In order to perform a high throughput screen, the assay must be developed and optimized further. In the case of this GLA enzyme assay, a recombinant GLA enzyme (Fabrazyme) and the fluorogenic substrate, 4MU-α-Gala, are used. When the substrate is cleaved by GLA, galactose and fluorescent 4-methylumbelliferone (4MU) are produced, which emits in the blue spectrum at 440 nm (Fig. 9.2). This is a simple and homogenous assay. The enzyme is first incubated with the test compound for 5 min, followed by the addition of substrate and incubation at room temperature for 20 min. After

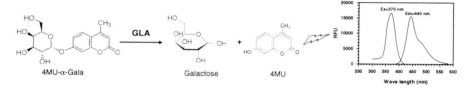

Fig. 9.2 Diagram of the assay principle for the fluorogenic GLA assay. The substrate, 4MU-α-Gala, is hydrolyzed to form galactose and the fluorescent product, 4MU. The *right panel* is a fluorescence spectrum of 4MU, which has an excitation peak at 370 nm and an emission peak at 440 nm

termination of the reaction, the resulting fluorescence in the assay plate is measured with a standard fluorescence plate reader. 1-deoxygalactonojirimycin (DGJ), a known GLA inhibitor, is used as the control compound in this assay. Because no GLA activator is currently available, the addition of a 2× concentration of GLA is used as a control for the activator effect. Thus, both activators and inhibitors can be identified in the same assay plate.

Typically, assay development is carried out in 384-well plates. Twenty microliters per well of enzyme solution is added followed by 10 μl/well of substrate solution in a citric acid buffer at pH 4.5. After an incubation of 20 min at room temperature, the reaction is terminated by the addition of 30 μl/well of stop solution (0.5 M NaOH, 0.5 M glycine, pH = 10). The plate is then read in a CCD-based imaging plate reader (ViewLux, PerkinElmer, Boston, MA) with an excitation at 365 nm and an emission at 440 nm. The fluorescence intensity results are converted to the amount of product formed using a 4MU standard curve.

In order to optimize this assay for HTS in 1536-well plates, various conditions need to be addressed, including the pH, bile salt concentration (sodium taurocholate), enzyme concentration, incubation time, substrate concentration, and DMSO concentration. The following is an example of the optimization of these conditions.

Effect of pH. GLA is a lysosomal enzyme whose activity is dependent upon the local environment in the lysosomes of cells. A series of assay buffers with pH values ranging from 4.0 to 7.4 was used to determine the optimal pH for enzyme activity. The enzyme activity reached a peak at pH 4.5 (Fig. 9.3a), consistent with the reported local acidic pH of 4–6 in the lysosomes. Therefore, an assay buffer at pH 4.5 was selected for this assay.

Effect of sodium taurocholate. Sodium taurocholate, a bile salt that may activate lysosomal enzymes in vitro, is generally included in the buffer for a GLA enzyme assay [20], but the optimal concentration has not been established. An experiment was performed to measure the effect of sodium taurocholate on GLA activity. It was found that GLA activity did not depend on this bile salt, and actually decreased with increasing concentrations of sodium taurocholate (Fig. 9.3b). This result contrasts with those obtained using other lysosomal hydrolases, including glucocerebrosidase, in which the enzyme activity in vitro depends on the presence of sodium

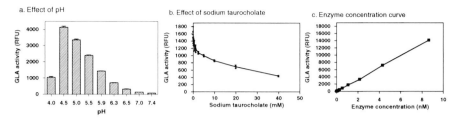

Fig. 9.3 (**a**) pH effect on GLA activity. (**b**) Effect of sodium taurocholate on GLA activity. (**c**) GLA enzyme concentration – response curve

taurocholate [14]. Therefore, sodium taurocholate was not included in the buffer for this GLA enzyme assay.

Enzyme concentration. To increase the assay sensitivity for compound screens, the enzyme concentration should be selected in the linear portion of the enzyme concentration-response curve, and a minimal concentration of GLA enzyme that produces enough signal should be chosen. Selection of a lower enzyme concentration does not only increase the assay sensitivity to compounds, but also reduces the amount of enzyme needed, lowering the cost of HTS. It was found that GLA enzyme activity increased linearly up to 9 nM (Fig. 9.3c). Based on this result, 1.1 nM (1:100 dilution of stock enzyme solution) was selected as the appropriate enzyme concentration for this assay, as it provided sufficient fluorescence intensity with less than 10% substrate consumption.

Time course. The time course for the GLA enzyme reaction is important for the determination of the proper incubation time. 1.1 nM enzyme and 600 μM substrate were incubated for various times at room temperature. The enzyme activity was found to be linear for up to a 40 min incubation time (Fig. 9.4a). With regards to assay sensitivity, the incubation time selected should be in the linear portion of the time course curve with sufficient signal. Thus, an incubation time of 20 min at room temperature was selected as an optimal assay condition.

Substrate concentration and kinetic assay. In balancing assay sensitivity with the proper assay signal, the concentration of the substrate for the enzyme assay is

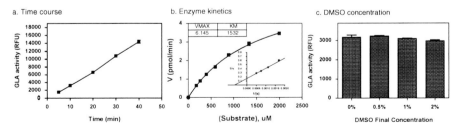

Fig. 9.4 (**a**) Time course of GLA activity. (**b**) Enzyme kinetics of GLA (Km = 1.53 mM). (**c**) DMSO effect on the GLA enzyme assay

usually selected around or below the K_m value. In a kinetic experiment, the substrate was titrated at seven concentrations up to 2 mM. A series of enzyme reactions was terminated by the addition of stop solution after incubation at 2, 4, 6, 8, 10 and 12 min, respectively. The rate of product formation was calculated with reference to a 4MU standard curve. The enzyme kinetics result was calculated using Prism software (GraphPad, San Diego, CA). The K_m value was found to be 1.5 mM (Fig. 9.4b). Based on this result, 600 μM of substrate was selected for the enzyme assay. The substrate consumption with 1.1 nM enzyme and a 20 min incubation time was approximately 3.6%.

DMSO concentration. The effect of DMSO on enzyme activity was also examined, as it is a solvent commonly used to dissolve compounds. It was determined that the effect of DMSO on GLA activity was negligible for up to a final concentration of 1.0% (Fig. 9.4c). In our HTS, the final concentration of DMSO with the addition of compound solution was 0.8%, which did not affect the performance of this enzyme assay.

IC$_{50}$ of a known inhibitor. Known inhibitors or activators are commonly used as the control compounds to assess the assay sensitivity for compound screens. DGJ, a known GLA inhibitor, was evaluated in this enzyme assay. The IC$_{50}$ value was determined to be 60 nM with 1.1 nM GLA enzyme and 600 μM 4MU-α-Gala (Fig. 9.5a), which is consistent with the value reported elsewhere [31]. This result indicates that this GLA assay is sensitive and suitable for compound screens.

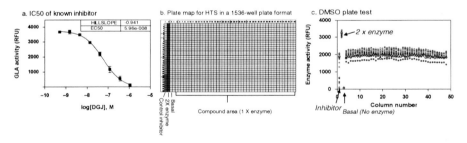

Fig. 9.5 (**a**) Concentration response of DGJ determined in the GLA assay. (**b**) Plate map of GLA enzyme HTS assay in a 1536-well plate. Column 1 is the concentration response of a control compound, DGJ; column 2 is the 2X concentration of enzyme (positive control for activators); column 3 is the basal without enzyme and column 4 is the 1X enzyme – same as columns 5–48 (compound area in HTS). (**c**) Scatter plot of a DMSO plate test in the GLA enzyme assay

Optimized GLA enzyme assay for HTS. Based on the above studies, the conditions selected for the GLA enzyme assay were 1.1 nM GLA enzyme, 600 μM substrate (4MU-α-Gala), and a 20 min incubation at room temperature. The assay buffer at pH 4.5 was composed of 50 mM citric acid and 0.01% tween-20, with the pH adjusted by the addition of ~100 ml of 1 M K_2HPO_4. The assay was then miniaturized into the 1536-well plate format for HTS. This was done by a 1:4 proportional reduction in reagent volume to adapt the 384-well plate format to the 1536-well plate format. The final assay protocol for the 1536-well plate format is shown in Table 9.1. Briefly, 2 μl/well of enzyme solution is added followed by 23 nl/well of compound

Table 9.1 GLA enzyme assay protocol in 1536-well plate format

Step	Parameter	Value	Description
1	Reagent – 1	2 ul	1.5X enzyme solution
2	Compound	23 nl	Control or compound solution
3	Incubation	5 min	Room temperature
4	Reagent – 2	1 ul	3X substrate
5	Incubation	20 min	Room temperature
6	Termination of reaction	3 ul	2X stop solution
7	Incubation	1 min	Room temperature
8	Detection	Ex = 365, Em = 440 nm	ViewLux plate reader (1 s)

in DMSO solution. After 5 min incubation at room temperature, the enzyme reaction is initiated by the addition of 1 μl/well of substrate. After 20 min incubation at room temperature, the reaction is terminated by the addition of 3 μl/well of stop solution and the assay plate is then measured in a fluorescence plate reader with an excitation at 365 ($\pm$20) nm and emission at 440 ($\pm$20) nm.

9.5 Assay Validation

To further validate the enzyme assay, a test screen with a DMSO plate was carried out. A plate using DMSO (a solvent) instead of compounds was first tested in this assay in 1536-well plate format (Fig. 9.5b). The signal-to-basal (S/B) ratio was found to be 32.6 fold, CV was 8.1% and the Z' factor was 0.76 in this experiment (Fig. 9.5c). The Z' factor is a commonly used parameter for judging the quality of a screening assay, with a value greater than 0.5 being acceptable for HTS. It can be calculated using the following equation: $Z' = 1 - (3^*s.d._{(1)} + 3^*s.d._{(2)})/(A-B)$, where $s.d._{(1)}$ is the standard deviation of enzyme activity, $s.d._{(2)}$ is the standard deviation of basal activity (without enzyme), A is the mean of enzyme activity and B is the mean of basal activity. The results above indicate that this assay in a 1536-well plate format is robust and suitable for HTS. The stability of reagents over the course of 24 h (enzyme and substrate) must be examined as well to make sure that the signal-to-basal ratio remains nearly constant throughout the continuous robotic screen.

9.5.1 Test Screen

Prior to the full-scale screen using a robot, a test screen with a smaller compound library was performed. The LOPAC (Library of Pharmacologically Active Compounds), which consists of 1,208 compounds (Sigma-Aldrich), is commonly used to validate assay performance [24]. A quantitative high throughput screen was performed, with each compound in the collection titrated 7 times at a 1:5 dilution ratio, with final concentrations ranging from 4.90 nM to 76.6 μM. A signal-to-basal ratio of 23.9 fold, CV of 3.0% and Z' factor of 0.90 were obtained from this LOPAC library screen. Four hits (all inhibitors), including DGJ, were identified from this screen, and the hit rate was 0.33%. These results confirmed that the GLA enzyme assay was robust and suitable for HTS.

9.6 Full-Scale Compound Screen (HTS)

Once the assay is validated using a DMSO plate and the LOPAC library, and the results indicate that the screening assay is of sufficient quality (S/B > 2 fold and Z' factor > 0.5), the full library screen using a robot can be planned and executed. HTS uses a significant amount of reagents, as several hundred to a few thousand plates are screened, depending on the size of the compound library. The robotic screen is usually run continuously, which requires the reagents to be stable at room temperature or 4°C for at least 24 h. The robotic screen for the full compound collection can take anywhere from a few days to 2 weeks.

After the screen is performed, the data is loaded into a database for analysis. Traditionally, the percent inhibition or activation is used to calculate the hit rate at the compound concentration selected for the screen. The hit rate is usually 0.1–1% of the compound collection. However, when evaluating qHTS results, active compounds are selected based on their potencies (EC_{50}/IC_{50}) and the quality of their concentration response curves. This increases the probability of identifying active compounds, including ones with biphasic or 'bell-shaped' concentration response curves.

Since concentration responses for all the compounds are available after the qHTS, the results can be further analyzed by structure clustering using the Leadscope® Hosted Client software (Leadscope Inc., Columbus, OH) to group the active compounds based on structural similarity. This analysis is particularly useful for screens that produce a large number of hits, as only two or three representative compounds from each structurally similar group can be selected for the confirmation test.

9.7 Confirmation and Secondary Screens

Confirmation. The active compounds selected from the primary screen, usually 30–100 compounds, are ordered for the confirmation test. These compounds are titrated at a 1:3 dilution for 12 concentrations, and tested in the same assay used in the primary screen.

Counterscreen. These compounds are also tested for selectivity using other lysosomal enzyme assays, such as the glucocerebrosidase, α-glucosidase, and β-N-acetylglucosaminidase assays. Similar to the GLA assay, these counter-screen assays are fluorogenic assays using 4MU as the fluorophore. Because the same fluorophore is used in these counterscreen assays, false positive compounds, including fluorescence quenchers and fluorescent compounds, can be eliminated. The ideal lead compound should have no effect, or should be at least 10 fold more potent in the GLA assay than in the other counterscreen enzyme assays.

Enzyme kinetic assay. The mode of inhibition of the confirmed inhibitors can be determined using the enzyme kinetic assay. A series of 5–6 substrate concentration response curves in the absence and presence of several concentrations of inhibitors are generated kinetically. The Lineweaver–Burk plot (double reciprocal plot) is commonly used for analysis of the kinetic results to determine the mode of inhibition (competitive, noncompetitive or uncompetitive) of these compounds. The K_i values can also be calculated from the plot. A rapid K_i assessment method has been developed, in which the K_i values of 6 compounds can be measured in one 1536-well plate using this type of fluorogenic enzyme assay [14].

9.8 Tertiary Screens

From the above secondary screens, false positives would be eliminated and the selectivity and mode of action of the remaining active compounds would be defined. Powder samples of a few lead compounds could then be purchased and tested in tertiary assays to further characterize their actions.

Native substrate assay. The compound activities were determined using a fluorogenic substrate for GLA. To assess the compounds in a more physiologically relevant environment, the natural substrate for GLA, globotriaosylceramide (Gb3), should be used. Several methods have been reported to measure Gb3, including gas chromatography/chemical ionization mass spectrometry (GC/CI-MS) after permethylation of glycolipids [32], HPLC with UV detection after perbenzoylation [33], and enzyme-linked immunosorbent assay [34]. Recently, a more sensitive and robust method has been developed which uses electrospray ionization mass spectrometry (ESI-MS) [35]. However, this method is still relatively low throughput, and would only be useful for confirming the activity of a small number of compounds.

Cell-based assays. Once active compounds from the HTS are confirmed, and the lead compounds selected, the most promising five to ten inhibitors and/or activators can be evaluated further. A cell-based assay using skin fibroblasts or lymphoblasts derived from patients could be used to test the effect of compounds on enzymatic activity in cells. Patient cells would be cultured with or without the compounds using standard cell culture conditions for 2–3 days, and intracellular GLA activity would be measured with a fluorogenic substrate, either 4MU-α-Gala or res-α-Gala. The substrate should be able to enter the cells after permeablization of cell membranes by treatment with 0.2 M sodium acetate buffer at pH 4.0 [14]. Compounds capable of enhancing GLA activity in patient cells would be considered potential chemical chaperones.

9.9 Western Blot and Immunofluorescence Analysis of GLA in Cells

Western Blot analysis of patient-derived cells can be compared with normal cells to evaluate GLA protein maturation after treatment with compounds. GLA is present in two main forms within cells, the immature ER form (51 kDa) and the mature lysosomal form (46 kDa) [20, 31, 36]. The intensity of each band on the Western Blot, and the relative ratio of the two bands, provides information about protein expression, processing and trafficking.

In fibroblasts derived from patients with Fabry disease, the accumulation of lysosomal Gb3 can be studied by confocal microscopy using double immunofluorescence staining of Gb3 and the lysosomal membrane protein 1 (LAMP1) [36, 37]. Active compounds should be able to reduce Gb3 storage in the lysosome, and thus, Gb3 staining in cells should become distinctively diminished after treatment with the active compounds.

9.10 Probe Identification and Optimization

Depending on the potency and selectivity of active compounds identified in the above processes, a probe can be defined if the potencies (IC_{50}/EC_{50}) of the identified agents are less than 1 μM, and if they selectively act on GLA and effectively reduce the Gb3 accumulation in patient cells. If the activity of the compounds is weak and/or the specificity is poor, probe optimization would be carried out by chemists. The bioavailability of the active compound(s) would also be optimized during this process.

9.11 Further Testing in Animal Models

Several mouse models have been reported for Fabry disease. A complete GLA knockout model was generated that shows some Gb3 accumulation in various organs and tissues [38]. This model has been used for experiments with ERT, substrate reduction, and gene therapy. However, this model is not useful for examining the effect of chemical chaperones because it has no mutant enzyme that can be enhanced by chaperones. However, a GLA knock-in mouse that contains the human mutation R301Q has been generated that may prove useful in answering this question [39]. Because the expression level of the human transgene is substantially higher than that of the endogenous gene, this mouse has no signs or symptoms of Fabry disease. However, it has been shown that the activity of the mutant GLA can be enhanced by DGJ in vivo [39]. Mouse models with mutations that still retain some enzyme activity will prove useful for testing the probes identified from HTS.

9.12 Conclusions

In summary, we have provided a brief overview of the small molecule drug discovery process from target selection to tests in animal models (Fig. 9.6). If the candidate drug shows promise, it could enter preclinical drug safety tests and clinical trials. This process usually takes 10–15 years and costs millions of dollars. With the rapid advancement of technologies in drug development, and a better understanding of the pathophysiology of rare genetic diseases, we hope that the cost of and time needed for drug development for these rare disorders may be significantly reduced in the future.

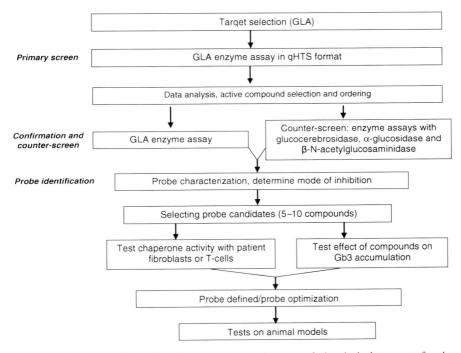

Fig. 9.6 Flowchart ↓ for the identification and development of chemical chaperones for the potential therapy of Fabry disease

References

1. Ishii S, Chang HH, Kawasaki K, Yasuda K, Wu HL, Garman SC et al (2007) Mutant alpha-galactosidase A enzymes identified in Fabry disease patients with residual enzyme activity: biochemical characterization and restoration of normal intracellular processing by 1-deoxygalactonojirimycin. Biochem J 406(2):285–295
2. Ishii S, Suzuki Y, Fan JQ (2000) Role of Ser-65 in the activity of alpha-galactosidase A: characterization of a point mutation (S65T) detected in a patient with Fabry disease. Arch Biochem Biophys 377(2):228–233

3. Ishii S, Kase R, Sakuraba H, Suzuki Y (1993) Characterization of a mutant alpha-galactosidase gene product for the late-onset cardiac form of Fabry disease. Biochem Biophys Res Commun 197(3):1585–1589
4. Desnick R, Ioannou Y, Eng C (2001) Alpha-galactosidase A deficiency: Fabry disease, 8th edn. McGraw-Hill Professional, New York
5. Brady RO (2006) Enzyme replacement for lysosomal diseases. Annu Rev Med 57:283–296
6. Lidove O, Joly D, Barbey F, Bekri S, Alexandra JF, Peigne V et al (2007) Clinical results of enzyme replacement therapy in Fabry disease: a comprehensive review of literature. Int J Clin Pract 61(2):293–302
7. Wilcox WR, Banikazemi M, Guffon N, Waldek S, Lee P, Linthorst GE et al (2004) Long-term safety and efficacy of enzyme replacement therapy for Fabry disease. Am J Hum Genet 75(1):65–74
8. Moore DF, Scott LT, Gladwin MT, Altarescu G, Kaneski C, Suzuki K et al (2001) Regional cerebral hyperperfusion and nitric oxide pathway dysregulation in Fabry disease: reversal by enzyme replacement therapy. Circulation 104(13):1506–1512
9. Bernier V, Lagace M, Bichet DG, Bouvier M (2004) Pharmacological chaperones: potential treatment for conformational diseases. Trends Endocrinol Metab 15(5):222–228
10. Ulloa-Aguirre A, Janovick JA, Brothers SP, Conn PM (2004) Pharmacologic rescue of conformationally-defective proteins: implications for the treatment of human disease. Traffic 5(11):821–837
11. Sawkar AR, Cheng WC, Beutler E, Wong CH, Balch WE, Kelly JW (2002) Chemical chaperones increase the cellular activity of N370S beta-glucosidase: a therapeutic strategy for Gaucher disease. Proc Natl Acad Sci USA 99(24):15428–15433
12. Sawkar AR, Adamski-Werner SL, Cheng WC, Wong CH, Beutler E, Zimmer KP et al (2005) Gaucher disease-associated glucocerebrosidases show mutation-dependent chemical chaperoning profiles. Chem Biol 12(11):1235–1244
13. Alfonso P, Pampin S, Estrada J, Rodriguez-Rey JC, Giraldo P, Sancho J et al (2005) Miglustat (NB-DNJ) works as a chaperone for mutated acid beta-glucosidase in cells transfected with several Gaucher disease mutations. Blood Cells Mol Dis 35(2):268–276
14. Zheng W, Padia J, Urban DJ, Jadhav A, Goker-Alpan O, Simeonov A et al (2007) Three classes of glucocerebrosidase inhibitors identified by quantitative high-throughput screening are chaperone leads for Gaucher disease. Proc Natl Acad Sci USA 104(32):13192–13197
15. Okumiya T, Kroos MA, Vliet LV, Takeuchi H, Van der Ploeg AT, Reuser AJ (2007) Chemical chaperones improve transport and enhance stability of mutant alpha-glucosidases in glycogen storage disease type II. Mol Genet Metab 90(1):49–57
16. Parenti G, Zuppaldi A, Gabriela Pittis M, Rosaria Tuzzi M, Annunziata I, Meroni G et al (2007) Pharmacological enhancement of mutated alpha-glucosidase activity in fibroblasts from patients with Pompe disease. Mol Ther 15(3):508–514
17. Tropak MB, Reid SP, Guiral M, Withers SG, Mahuran D (2004) Pharmacological enhancement of beta-hexosaminidase activity in fibroblasts from adult Tay-Sachs and Sandhoff Patients. J Biol Chem 279(14):13478–13487
18. Matsuda J, Suzuki O, Oshima A, Yamamoto Y, Noguchi A, Takimoto K et al (2003) Chemical chaperone therapy for brain pathology in G(M1)-gangliosidosis. Proc Natl Acad Sci USA 100(26):15912–15917
19. Fan JQ, Ishii S (2007) Active-site-specific chaperone therapy for Fabry disease. Yin and Yang of enzyme inhibitors. Febs J 274(19):4962–4971
20. Shin SH, Murray GJ, Kluepfel-Stahl S, Cooney AM, Quirk JM, Schiffmann R et al (2007) Screening for pharmacological chaperones in Fabry disease. Biochem Biophys Res Commun 359(1):168–173
21. Gelsthorpe ME, Baumann N, Millard E, Gale SE, Langmade SJ, Schaffer JE et al (2008) Niemann-Pick type C1 I1061T mutant encodes a functional protein that is selected for endoplasmic reticulum-associated degradation due to protein misfolding. J Biol Chem 283(13):8229–8236

22. Powers ET, Morimoto RI, Dillin A, Kelly JW, Balch WE (2009) Biological and chemical approaches to diseases of proteostasis deficiency. Annu Rev Biochem 78:959–991

23. Mu TW, Fowler DM, Kelly JW (2008) Partial restoration of mutant enzyme homeostasis in three distinct lysosomal storage disease cell lines by altering calcium homeostasis. PLoS Biol 6(2):e26

24. Inglese J, Auld DS, Jadhav A, Johnson RL, Simeonov A, Yasgar A et al (2006) Quantitative high-throughput screening: a titration-based approach that efficiently identifies biological activities in large chemical libraries. Proc Natl Acad Sci USA 103(31):11473–11478

25. Mapes CA, Sweeley CC (1973) Galactosyl (alpha 1–4)galactosylceramide: galactosyl hydrolase activity in normal and Fabry plasma. Biochem Biophys Res Commun 53(4):1317–1324

26. Hultberg B, Sjoblad S, Ockerman PA (1975) Glycosidases in human skin fibroblast cultures. Alpha-fucosidase, alpha-galactosidase, alpha-glucosidase, beta-mannosidase, and N-acetyl-alpha-glucosaminidase. Acta Paediatr Scand 64(1):123–131

27. Shi ZD, Motabar O, Goldin E, Liu K, Southall N, Sidransky E et al (2009) Synthesis and characterization of a new fluorogenic substrate for alpha-galactosidase. Anal Bioanal Chem 394(7):1903–1909

28. de Groot PG, Hamers MN, Westerveld A, Schram AW, Meera Khan P, Tager JM (1978) A new immunochemical method for the quantitative measurement of specific gene products in man-rodent somatic cell hybrids. Hum Genet 44(3):295–304

29. Yagi F, Eckhardt AE, Goldstein IJ (1990) Glycosidases of Ehrlich ascites tumor cells and ascitic fluid–purification and substrate specificity of alpha-N-acetylgalactosaminidase and alpha-galactosidase: comparison with coffee bean alpha-galactosidase. Arch Biochem Biophys 280(1):61–67

30. Tsou KC, Su HC (1964) A Study Of Yeast Alpha-Galactosidase With Naphthyl Alpha-D-Galactopyranosides As Chromogenic Substrates. Anal Biochem 8:415–423

31. Fan JQ, Ishii S, Asano N, Suzuki Y (1999) Accelerated transport and maturation of lysosomal alpha-galactosidase A in Fabry lymphoblasts by an enzyme inhibitor. Nat Med 5(1):112–115

32. Levery SB, Hakomori S (1987) Microscale methylation analysis of glycolipids using capillary gas chromatography-chemical ionization mass fragmentography with selected ion monitoring. Methods Enzymol 138:13–25

33. Oshima M, Asano K, Shibata S, Suzuki Y, Masuzawa M (1990) Urinary neutral glycosphingolipid analysis of patients with Fabry's disease; rapid isocratic elution from high-performance liquid chromatography as per-o-benzoyl derivatives. Biochim Biophys Acta 1043(2):157–160

34. Zeidner KM, Desnick RJ, Ioannou YA (1999) Quantitative determination of globotriaosylceramide by immunodetection of glycolipid-bound recombinant verotoxin B subunit. Anal Biochem 267(1):104–113

35. Fauler G, Rechberger GN, Devrnja D, Erwa W, Plecko B, Kotanko P et al (2005) Rapid determination of urinary globotriaosylceramide isoform profiles by electrospray ionization mass spectrometry using stearoyl-d35-globotriaosylceramide as internal standard. Rapid Commun Mass Spectrom 19(11):1499–1506

36. Yam GH, Bosshard N, Zuber C, Steinmann B, Roth J (2006) Pharmacological chaperone corrects lysosomal storage in Fabry disease caused by trafficking-incompetent variants. Am J Physiol Cell Physiol 290(4):C1076–C1082

37. Yam GH, Zuber C, Roth J (2005) A synthetic chaperone corrects the trafficking defect and disease phenotype in a protein misfolding disorder. Faseb J 19(1):12–18

38. Ohshima T, Murray GJ, Swaim WD, Longenecker G, Quirk JM, Cardarelli CO et al (1997) alpha-Galactosidase A deficient mice: a model of Fabry disease. Proc Natl Acad Sci USA 94(6):2540–2544

39. Ishii S, Yoshioka H, Mannen K, Kulkarni AB, Fan JQ (2004) Transgenic mouse expressing human mutant alpha-galactosidase A in an endogenous enzyme deficient background: a biochemical animal model for studying active-site specific chaperone therapy for Fabry disease. Biochim Biophys Acta 1690(3):250–257

Part II
Clinical

Chapter 10
Clinical Manifestations of Fabry Disease: An Overview

Atul Mehta

Abstract The last decade has seen an enormous expansion of interest in Fabry disease. The spectrum of clinical manifestations has been outlined in studies from single institutions and these observations have been confirmed and extended by publications from the registries which are associated with the two licensed forms of enzyme replacement therapy. It has become clear that Fabry disease, particularly atypical forms associated with residual enzyme activity, is much commoner that previously thought. Estimates range from 1:5,000 to 1:30,000. Fabry disease frequently presents as a stroke or isolated left ventricular hypertrophy. Skin manifestations appear to correlate well with overall disease severity. Some genotype/phenotype correlations have been demonstrated such that patients with miss- sense mutations generally have less severe clinical manifestations at a given age than patients with non-sense mutations. There is a very high prevalence of symptoms and clinical manifestations amongst females with Fabry disease. There is preliminary evidence that enzyme replacement therapy may be altering the natural history of the disease.

Keywords Fabry disease · Genotype/phenotype · Stroke · Enzyme replacement therapy · Left-ventricular hypertrophy · FOS · Fabry registry

10.1 Introduction

The enzyme alpha glactosidase A, in common with all other lysosomal enzymes, is expressed in all tissues to a greater or lesser extent. Cellular deficiency of this 'housekeeping' enzyme would be expected to result in a generalized metabolic disturbance and clinical manifestations in a range of organ systems [1]. It is encoded on

A. Mehta (✉)
Department of Haematology, Royal Free Hospital, University College London School of Medicine, London, UK
e-mail: atul.mehta@royalfree.nhs.uk

D. Elstein et al. (eds.), *Fabry Disease*, DOI 10.1007/978-90-481-9033-1_10,   181
© Springer Science+Business Media B.V. 2010

the X chromosome, therefore deficiency manifests more severely and at an earlier age in males than in females. The systemic nature of the condition was recognized even in its earliest descriptions [2, 3]. MacDermot and her colleagues gave a clear description of the clinical manifestations in males and females in the UK [4, 5]. Her group identified renal failure as a frequent cause of death, particularly in males; cardiac and cerebrovascular disease were the most frequent causes of death in females. Death occurs on average 15 years earlier in males than females and 20 years earlier in males compared with the general population. The advent of enzyme replacement therapy has led to a very substantial increase in interest in this disease [1]. The genetic mutations underlying the disease have been characterized [6]. Two formulations of enzyme replacement therapy are licensed in Europe, agalsidase, alpha (Replagal, Shire HGT, Basingstoke, UK) and agalsidase beta (Fabrazyme, Genzyme Corporation, Boston, USA). Concerted international attempts have also been made to improve diagnosis and management of rare diseases and to expand access to treatment [7].

10.2 Prevalence

Over the past decade, it has become clear that this disease is not as rare as was once believed. Thus whereas classic Fabry disease with a nonsense mutation of the *GLA* gene and undetectable levels of expressed enzyme may indeed occur only at a frequency of perhaps 1 in 100,000 X chromosomes [8, 9], attenuated forms of the condition characterized by a range of *GLA* mutations associated with residual enzyme activity may be much more common. Indeed one study of consecutive neo-natal dry blood test spot analysis indicated a prevalence of mutations in the *GLA* gene, a gene as high as 1 in 3,100 [10]. However of the twelve patients with mutations detected in this study, all mutations were misssense and only one had previously been associated with clinical disease. It remains possible that some of these patients with misssense mutations may develop atypical Fabry disease in later life. Such patients often have predominant involvement of a single organ system e.g. cardiac or renal.

Screening studies conducted in populations of patients who have suffered a clinical event associated with Fabry disease have also shown a surprisingly high prevalence. Thus amongst males with left ventricular hypertrophy, a number of studies have shown [11, 12] that 2–5% will have reduced alpha-galactosidase, A enzyme activity, usually associated with a relevant gene mutation. Importantly, some of the reported mutations [12] are considered in other studies to be polymorphisms [6]. An important study amongst stroke patients also reported a prevalence of Fabry disease of 2–5% amongst males aged less than 55 years presenting with cryptogenic stroke. A similar incidence was reported in females [13]. Screening studies have also confirmed that about 1% of males undergoing haemodialysis have Fabry disease [14].

10.3 Registry Studies

The advent of ERT has meant that the manufacturers have an obligation to report long term safety and efficacy data to regulators through the use of patient registries. A wealth of data has come from registry studies – Fabry outcome survey (FOS, Shire HGT, 15) and Fabry registry (Genzyme, 16). Publications from these studies have demonstrated the range of symptoms and organ systems that can be affected by Fabry disease. A major advantage of these registry studies is that they have been able to recruit much larger numbers of patients than were reported in the smaller series from individual centres. Reports from these registry studies have confirmed and extended observations on the natural history of Fabry disease.

Detailed studies of individual organ involvement among large populations of Fabry patients have been reported. A particular finding has been the prevalence of symptoms amongst females with Fabry disease. Data from FOS [15, 17], confirmed by data from the Fabry registry [18], show that not only do the majority of heterozygous females have symptoms but that organ disease is frequently as severe in females as in males. Thus heterozygous females should not merely be considered carriers of Fabry disease. Fabry disease frequently presents in childhood and manifestations in boys occur earlier than in girls [19, 20]. While the most common symptoms are pain, rash and abdominal pain, hearing loss, eye changes and early renal involvement (e.g. proteinuria) or even stroke have been reported. The Mainz group have made an excellent attempt at evaluating the overall severity of Fabry disease using the Mainz severity scoring index [21]. This has been adapted by FOS to give the FOS MSSI, which is also an integrated index of overall disease severity [17]. Interestingly, the dermatologic changes in Fabry disease and their extent correlate well with the overall disease severity [22]. Thus the skin, which was the original identified province of Fabry disease, is indeed an excellent mirror of the overall severity of this systemic condition. The spectrum of ocular and auditory changes in Fabry disease have been well illustrated with data from FOS [22, 23, 24]. A previously neglected aspect of the condition was gastro-intestinal symptomatology. This appears to be particularly prevalent amongst females, can easily be confused with irritable bowel syndrome and has as its cardinal features bloating, cramping abdominal pain, diarrhea and constipation [25]. The pathologic basis remains elusive but may relate predominately to neural mechanisms. It responds well to enzyme replacement therapy. Indeed, pain, temperature, sensitivity, sweating and hearing loss, all of which may have an important neural component, all respond well to enzyme replacement therapy [26]. Studies of the natural history of cardiac [27] and renal [28] manifestations in Fabry disease have substantially extended our understanding. Stroke has been confirmed to be an important presenting symptom of Fabry disease in publications from the Fabry registry [30]. Data from FOS have shown that patients with Fabry disease who suffer a stroke are far more likely to have cardiac and renal disease than patients with Fabry disease who have not suffered a stroke [31]. The prevalence of stroke and TIA amongst Fabry patients is reported to be approximately 10 and 15% respectively [31]. The strokes occur 10–15 years earlier than strokes in the standard population. These strokes are far more likely to affect the posterior cerebral circulation; and thrombosis and hemorrhage have both been reported [10, 14, 15].

These natural history data on stroke, cardiac and renal manifestations have set bench marks against which the effects of enzyme replacement therapy can be judged. It would not be ethical to conduct large scale double blind controlled clinical trials in rare diseases in which enzyme replacement therapy has already become available and is licensed. In the absence of such data, registry data showing the natural history of the disease alongside other registry data illustrating the impact of enzyme replacement therapy [29] may well be the best available 'real world' data.

10.4 Rarer Manifestations

The last decade has also seen an increasing appreciation of rarer manifestations of Fabry disease. Thus the facial appearance of Fabry disease has been better characterized and it is recognized that the changes respond to ERT [32]. Pulmonary involvement is common and smoking is particularly harmful [33, 34]. Hyperhidrosis is less common that hypohidrosis but is often an early sign [35]. Subclinical hypothyroidism [36], osteopenia [37], leukaemia [38] and azoospermia [39] all occur and have been reported in males and females [40]. Depression is common and frequently undiagnosed [41].

10.5 Is the Natural History Changing?

The natural history of Fabry disease in the pre ERT era is well described by MacDermot [4, 5] and Schiffmann [43]. A recent analysis from FOS reference sheds new light on the natural history of the condition [44]. The principal cause of death amongst 181 affected relatives of patients in FOS (the majority of whom had died before 2001) were renal failure in males (42%) and cerebrovascular disease in females (25%). In contrast amongst 42 patients enrolled in FOS whose deaths were reported between 2001 and 2007, cardiac disease had become the main cause of death in both males (34%) and females (57%). A recent publication from the Fabry registry [45] also reports cardiovascular disease to be the commonest cause of death in male and female Fabry patients. It may be that enzyme replacement therapy is altering the natural history of the condition. Certainly, a number of reports have demonstrated an impact of ERT on progression of renal impairment [29]. Encouragingly, ERT also has a favorable impact on most parameters of cardiac disease in Fabry patients [29]. Thus we look forward to an era where achievements in management of renal failure in Fabry patients are mirrored by similar achievements in managing cardiac disease amongst the Fabry population. Cerebrovascular disease remains a major challenge.

10.6 Genotype–Phenotype Correlations

Data on the underlying mutations amongst patients in the registries confirms that the full range of mutations (nonsense, a range of misssense mutations of variable severity, and mild misssense) are seen [6]. Registry data containing detailed information on the clinical spectrum of the disease amongst large numbers of patients are an ideal resource for studying genotype/phenotype correlations. Data from FOS (42 and Fig. 10.1) indicates that Fabry patients with the N215S mutation generally have less severe Fabry disease at a given age than the standard population. Extension of these data shows that patients with misssense mutations generally have milder disease manifestations than patients with nonsense mutations. Further studies are underway to confirm and extend these findings.

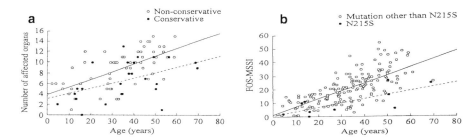

Fig. 10.1 (a) Correlation between the age at entry into FOS and the number of affected organs in male patients with *GLA* mutations that are predicted to result in conservative (*dotted line*; n = 25; r = 0.50; p = 0.011) or non-conservative (*solid line*; n = 61; r = 0.63; p <0.001) amino acid side chain changes in enzyme α-galactosidase A. Mutations affecting residues in the active site of the enzyme were excluded from the analysis. (b) Correlation between the age at entry into FOS and the FOS Severity Index (FOS-MSSI) in male patients with the mutation N215S (*dotted line*; n = 10; r = 0.73; p = 0.016) and in those carrying a different mutation (*solid line*; n = 160; r = 0.71; p = 0.001) in the gene encoding α-galactosidase A (reproduced from Schafer et al. [42])

It remains a matter of concern, however that this multisystem disorder, which is eminently treatable is often missed and the diagnosis is delayed [45, 46]. Awareness of the condition needs to be raised among all healthcare professionals.

References

1. Mehta A (2009) Anderson Fabry Disease: developments in diagnosis and treatment. Int J Clin Pharmacol Ther 47(Suppl 1):S66–S74
2. Anderson W (1898) A case of angiokeratoma. Br J Dermatol 18:113–117
3. Fabry J (1898) Ein Beitrag zur Kenntnis der Purpura haemorrhagica nodularis (Purpura papulosa haemorrhagica Hebrae). Arch Dermatol Syph 43:187–200
4. MacDermot KD, Holmes A, Miners AH (2001) Anderson Fabry disease clinical manifestations and impact of disease in a cohort of 98 hemizygous males. J Med Genet 38:750–760

5. MacDermot KD, Holmes A, Miners AH (2001) Anderson Fabry disease: clinical manifestations and impact of disease in a cohort of 60 obligate female carriers. J Med Genet 38:769–775
6. Garboczi DN, Garman SC (2004) The molecular defect leading to Fabry disease: structure of human alpha-galactosidase. J Mol Biol 337(2):319–335
7. Henter JI, Schieppatti A (2008) Why rare diseases are an important medical and social issue. Lancet 371:2039–2041
8. Meikle PJ, Hopwood JJ, Clague AE et al (1999) Prevalence of lysosomal storage disorders. JAMA 281(3):249–254
9. Poorthuis BJ, Wevers RA, Kleijer WJ et al (1999) The frequency of lysosomal storage diseases in The Netherlands. Hum Genet 105(1–2):151–156
10. Spada M, Pagliardini S, Yasuda M et al (2006) High incidence of later-onset Fabry disease revealed by newborn screening. Am J Hum Genet 79(1):31–40
11. Sachdev B, Takenaka T, Teraguchi H (2002) Prevalence of Anderson-Fabry disease in male patients with late onset hypertrophic cardiomyopathy. Circulation 105:1407–1411
12. Monserrat L, Gimeno-Blanes JR, Marin F et al (2007) Prevalence of Fabry disease in a cohort of 508 unrelated patients with hypertrophic cardiomyopathy. J Am Coll Cardiol 50(25): 2399–2403
13. Rolfs A, Bottcher T, Zschiesche M et al (2005) Prevalence of Fabry disease in patients with cryptogenic stroke: a prospective study. Lancet 366(9499):1794–1796
14. Kotanko P, Kramer R, Devrnja D et al (2004) Results of a nationwide screening for Anderson-Fabry disease among dialysis patients. J Am Soc Nephrol 15(5):1323–1329
15. Mehta A, Ricci R, Widmer U et al (2004) Fabry disease defined: baseline clinical manifestations of 366 patients in the Fabry Outcome Survey. Eur J Clin Invest 34:236–242
16. Eng CM, Fletcher J, Wilcox WR et al (2007) Fabry disease: baseline medical characteristics of a cohort of 1765 males and females in the Fabry Registry. J Inherit Metab Dis 30(2): 184–192
17. Deegan PB, Baehner AF, Hughes DA et al (2006) Natural history of Fabry disease in females in the Fabry Outcome Survey. J Med Genet 43(4):347–352
18. Wilcox WR, Oliveria JP, Hopkin RJ et al (2008) Females with Fabry disease frequently have major organ involvement: lessons from the Fabry Registry. Mol Genet Metab 93(2): 112–128
19. Ramaswami U, Whybra C, Parini R et al (2006) Clinical manifestations of Fabry disease in children: data from the Fabry Outcome Survey. Acta Paediatr 95(1):86–92
20. Hopkin RJ, Zarate AY (2008) Fabry disease. Lancet 372:1427–1435
21. Whybra C, Baehner F, Baron K (2006) Measurement of disease severity and progression in Fabry disease. In: Mehta A, Beck M, Sunder-Plassmann G (eds) Fabry disease: perspectives from 5 years of FOS. Oxford PharmaGenesis Ltd, Oxford, pp 315–322
22. Orteu C, Janssen T, Lidove O et al (2007) Fabry disease and the skin: data from the Fabry outcome Survey. Br J Dermatol 157:331–337
23. Sodi A, Ioannidis AS, Mehta A et al (2007) Ocular manifestations of Fabry disease: data from the Fabry Outcome Survey. Brit J Ophthal 91(2):210–214
24. Hegemann S, Hajioff D, Conti G et al (2006) Hearing loss in Fabry disease: data from the Fabry Outcome Survey (FOS). Europ J Clin Invest 36(9):654–662
25. Hoffman B, Schwarz M, Mehta A et al (2007) Gastrointestinal symptoms in 342 patients with Fabry disease: prevalence and response to enzyme replacement therapy. Clin Gastroenterol Hepatol 5(12):1447–1453
26. Mehta A, Beck M, Sunder-Plassmann G (eds) (2006) Fabry disease, perspectives from 5 years of FOS. Oxford Pharmagenesis, Oxford, p 427
27. Linhart A, Kampmann C, Zamorano JL et al (2007) Cardiac manifestations of Anderson Fabry Disease: results from the International Fabry Outcome Survey. Europ Heart J 28:228–235
28. Schwarting A, Dehout F, Feriozzi S et al (2006) Enzyme replacement therapy and renal function in 201 patients with Fabry disease. Clin Nephrol 66:77–84

29. Mehta A, Beck M, Elliott P et al (2009) Evidence of benefit of 5 years of enzyme replacement therapy with agalsidase alpha in patients with Fabry disease – A report from the Fabry outcome survey (FOS). Lancet 374:1986–1996

30. Sims K, Politei J, Basikazemi M, Lee P (2009) Stroke in Fabry disease frequently occurs before diagnosis and in the absence of other clinical events: natural history data from the Fabry Registry. Stroke 40(3):788–794

31. Mehta A, Ginsberg L, Investigators FOS (2005) Natural history of the cerebrovascular complications of Fabry disease. Acta Paediatr Suppl 94(447):24–27, discussion 9–10

32. Cox-Brinkman J, Vedder A, Hollak C et al (2007) Three dimensional face shape in Fabry disease. Europ J Human Genet 15(5):535–542

33. Brown LK, Miller A, Bhuptani A et al (1997) Pulmonary involvement in Fabry disease. Am J Respir Crit Care Med 155(3):1004–1010

34. Magage S, Lubanda JC, Susa Z et al (2007) Natural history of the respiratory involvement in Anderson – Fabry disease. J Inherit Metab Dis 30(5):790–799

35. Lidove O, Ramaswami U, Jaussaud R et al (2006) Hyperhidrosis: a new and often early symptom in Fabry disease. International experience and data from the Fabry Outcome Survey. Int J Clin Pract 60(9):1053–1059

36. Hauser AC, Gessl A, Lorenz M et al (2005) High prevalence of subclinical hypothyroidism in patients with Anderson-Fabry disease. J Inherit Metab Dis 28(5):715–722

37. Germain DP, Benistan K, Boutouyrie P et al (2005) Osteopenia and osteoporosis: previously unrecognized manifestations of Fabry disease. Clin Genet 68(1):93–95

38. Cybulla M, Kleber M, Walter KN et al (2006) Is Fabry disease associated with leukaemia? Br J Haematol 135(2):264–265

39. Papaxanthos-Roche A, Deminiere C, Bauduer F et al (2007) Azoospermia as a new feature of Fabry disease. Fertil Steril 88(1):212.e15–212.e18

40. Mehta A, Hughes DA Fabry disease. Gene reviews at GeneTests: medical genetics information resource [database online]. Copyright, University of Washington, Seattle (updated Feb 2008). Available at http://www.genetests.org

41. Cole AL, Lee PJ, Hughes DA et al (2007) Depression in adults with Fabry disease: a common and under-diagnosed problem. J Inherit Metab Dis 30(6):943–951

42. Schaefer E, Mehta A, Gal A (2005) Genotype and phenotype in Fabry Disease: analysis of the Fabry Outcome Survey. Acta Paediactrica 94(Suppl 447):87–92

43. Schiffmann R, Warnock DG, Banikazemi M et al (2009) Fabry disease: progression of nephropathy, and prevalence of cardiac and cerebrovascular events before enzyme replacement therapy. Nephrol Dial Transplant 24(7):2102–2111

44. Mehta A, Clarke J, Giugliani R et al (2009) Natural Course of Fabry disease: changing pattern of causes of death in FOS, the Fabry Outcome Survey. J. Med Genet 46(8):548–552

45. Waldek S, Patel MR, Banikazemi M, Lemay I, Lee P (2009) Life expectancy and cause of death in males and females with Fabry disease: findings from the Fabry Registry. Genet Med 11(11):1–7

46. Mehta A, Lewis S, Laverey C (2003) Treatment of lysosomal storage disorders (Editorial). Brit Med J 327:462–463

Chapter 11
The Heart in Fabry Disease – from Pathogenesis to Enzyme Replacement Therapy

Christoph Kampmann and Aleš Linhart

Abstract The cardiovascular involvement in Fabry disease is progressive, and accounts for one of the major reasons for abbreviated life expectancy and increased morbidity. The majority of patients develop signs and symptoms, related to heart failure and arrhythmias. Hypertrophic cardiomyopathy, in later stages combined with myocardial fibrosis, is one of the leading features. Both genders are affected, and females develop severe cardiac Fabry disease approximately 10–15 years later in life than male patients. Diastolic dysfunction and reduced longitudinal mid-wall related systolic function are the mechanical consequences of the myocardial and epithelial changes related to accumulation of the storage material in different cardiac components. The direct involvement of the conduction system and myocardial scar formation are the contributing factors for the development of complex arrhythmias, accompanied by disturbances in the autonomic control of the heart rate and its variability. Some of these changes are readily detectable in childhood and adolescence. Treatment of the cardiovascular involvement is crucial and consists of concomitant management of clinical symptoms and on enzyme replacement therapy. Different aspects of the cardiac disease and possible treatment options are discussed.

Keywords Fabry disease · Cardiomyopathy · Storage disease · Enzyme replacement therapy

11.1 Introduction

Together with cerebrovascular events and end-stage renal failure, the cardiovascular involvement accounts for the major cause of morbidity and mortality in Fabry disease [1, 2]. The un-degraded glycosphingolipid storage products are to be found in almost all cardiac tissues, including the cardiac myocytes, the cardiac nerves and the conduction system, and the endothelium of the coronary arteries. The

C. Kampmann (✉)
University Medicine, Johannes Gutenberg University Mainz, Mainz, Germany
e-mail: kampmann@uni-mainz.de

D. Elstein et al. (eds.), *Fabry Disease*, DOI 10.1007/978-90-481-9033-1_11,
© Springer Science+Business Media B.V. 2010

involvement of the different cardiac structures leads to a wide spectrum of progressive cardiac related features. The deposition of material within the myocytes is believed to be the major reason for development of the hypertrophic cardiomyopathy usually of all cardiac chambers, the involvement of the endocardium to valvular leaflet alterations, in terms of valvular thickening, as to be seen at the mitral and aortic valve; the involvement of the endothelium of the coronary arteries to an outstripping supply of the increased wall thicknesses; the involvement of the conduction system as one of the contributing factors for the development of arrhythmias; and the involvement of the autonomous nervous system to progressive disturbances in the regulation of the heart rate and its variability [3–10]. Clinically, these alterations result in a broad spectrum of cardiac signs and symptoms: patients may present with chest anginal pain, dyspnoea, fatigue, palpitations and syncope. And of note, there is a high coincidence between the clinical course of the disease and the degree of cardiac involvement [11, 12]. But, the main reason for cardiac death in this population seems not to be related to a high incidence of myocardial infarction, but presumably is more related to sudden cardiac death as a consequence of occult arrhythmias besides depressed cardiac function.

Although the inheritance of the disease is X-linked, large observational studies in heterozygous females could demonstrate, that even female patients do develop the classical signs and symptoms of cardiovascular involvement, but do so approximately 10 years later than male patients, but ultimately to the same degree [12–14].

But, because of the progressive nature of this inborn error of metabolism, the question must be raised, if any signs and symptoms of the disease are even to be seen in affected children. And indeed there are cardiovascular related alterations to be seen in childhood, which may contribute to a more advanced disease progression, as the reduced variability of the heart rate, to be seen in affected male children [15–18].

To understand the effects of enzyme substitution or enzyme activity enhancement therapy on the cardiovascular system, it is therefore of utmost importance to recognize and to understand the progressive nature of the disease and its life threatening nature.

11.2 Pathogenesis of the Cardiac Involvement

The glycosphingolipid storage, mainly globotriaosylceramid (Gb3 or GL3) is found in various cells and cell types of the heart, including the cardiomyocytes, conduction system cells, valvular fibroblasts, endothelial cells within all types of vessels, smooth muscle cells, and the cardiac nerves and the autonomic nervous system [5, 19]. In affected females, a mosaic pattern of storage is observed, most likely related to a random X-chromosome inactivation [8].

However, the storage of Gb3 by itself is unable to explain the observed level of cardiac hypertrophy, conduction abnormalities and other cardiac manifestations. Cardiac specimens of extremely hypertrophied hearts (>1,000 g) revealed a relatively limited amount of the stored material to the enormous increase in cardiac mass, and accounted for approximately around 2% of the wet heart weight [4]. It appears, that the storage of Gb_3 itself induces progressive lysosomal and other sub-cellular and cellular malfunction that, in turn, activates common signalling pathways leading to hypertrophy, apoptosis, autophagy, necrosis and fibrosis.

Energy depletion in sub-cellular components has been proposed to be the common denominator in a wide variety of metabolic and sarcomeric hypertrophic cardiomyopathies and might be a contributing factor in Fabry disease [20], as suggested by the impairment in energy handling seen in Fabry skin fibroblasts and the MRI spectrometry observation of a decreased ratio of adenosine – tri – phosphate (ATP) to inorganic ortho-phosphate, indicating mitochondrial energy depletion [21, 22]. Here, the unifying dysfunction is an increased energy demand owing to inefficient sarcomeric ATP utilization. This compromises the capacity of the myocytes to maintain energy levels in sub cellular compartments responsible for contraction resulting in hypertrophy [20].

Accepting the energy depletion hypothesis, which might be one of the major contributor to the cellular dysfunction, the involvement of the valvular tissues will result in a valve thickening (mainly mitral and aortic valve) with the development of a passager mitral valve prolapse (prolapse which is obvious at a certain age, but then vanishes when valve thickening occurs), with aortic root dilatation and usually mild regurgitation but moderate valvular stenosis (mainly aortic valve). The cellular dysfunction of the cardiomyocytes will activate hypertrophic signalling, autophagy and apoptosis, which ends up in fibre disarray, hypertrophy, autophagocytotic vacuoles and fibrosis, as has been shown in electron micrographs of myocardial cells. Furthermore, it is reported, that there is some degree of intravital desmin and troponin I degradation in Fabry cardiomyopathy, parallel to findings of myofibrillolysis. Both will contribute to a reduction in cardiomyocyte contractility explained by proteolysis. Here, the active tension of cardiomyocytes was four times lower in Fabry cardiomyocytes compared to normals, and this correlated well with the extent of myofibrillolysis. Furthermore, the resting tension was six times higher than in controls, indicating a reduced diastolic function, which was shown to correlate with tissue Doppler imaging data. These functional findings here, did not correlate with the extent of fibrosis or the degree of glycosphingolipid storage [23]. In addition to that, there are reports available, indicating the presence of circulating growth-promoting factors, which are able to induce in vitro a hypertrophic response of cardiomyocytes [24].

These alterations of the cardiac structure will result in impairment of systolic and diastolic function and this again is responsible for the clinical features as dyspnoea and heart failure. It has been shown, that the endothelial cells and the vascular smooth muscle cells are severely involved by deposition of storage material. As a result of that, it can be speculated, that this will result in a depressed coronary reserve, which in addition to diastolic dysfunction will contribute to ischemia leading to the clinical signs of chest anginal pain. Large coronary vessel disease, like in atherosclerosis is rarely reported in Fabry patients. The direct involvement and destruction of the conduction cells will be presented as an abbreviated PR interval in the ECG, as AV-conduction blocks and bradycardia, and in combination with the autonomic cardiac dysfunction, as a depressed heart rate variability finally end up in kinds of chronotropic incompetence. Clinically this can be related to fatigue and syncope. Furthermore, the conduction system involvement, the fibrosis, ischemia and the diastolic dysfunction, end up in complex arrhythmias which account for the high degree of palpitations and sudden death, which is reported in affected Fabry patients.

The natural history of Fabry disease is characterized by progressive hypertrophy of the cardiac muscle, with increasing interstitial and fibrotic changes [25] (Fig. 11.1). Almost all male patients once they have reached the age of 40 years and almost all females over 50 years of age present with a hypertrophic cardiomyopathy. This is consistent with the observations of relatively mild diastolic incompetence in early stages of the disease and with the late appearance of signs and symptoms that might be observed in patients with restrictive cardiomyopathy [26], enhanced and potentiated by absolute or relative ischemia, occurring even in the absence of significant epicardial coronary artery disease. This might be due to the increased oxygen demand of the hypertrophied muscle cells, the decreased capillary density, and increased diastolic filling pressures, that impair the blood flow throughout the subendocardial layers in diastole and to the infiltrative deposits of small arterioles and capillaries within endocardial cells and the vascular smooth muscle layers [19, 27, 28].

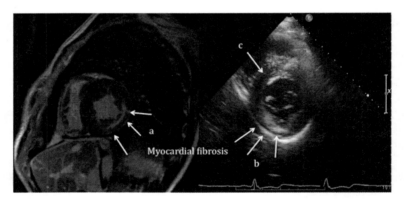

Fig. 11.1 MRI (*left*) and transthoracal ECHO (*right*) of the same 53 year old male patient with severe LV hypertrophy. Both in short axis view. Of note are the large areas of fibrosis. Gadolineum enhanced MRI (*left: arrows*; *a*) and the corresponding echocardiographic areas with increased echo-density (*right: arrows*; *b*). Additionally, the ECHO reveals a small area of endocardial increase in echodensity, with increase in echo-density, suspicious for endocardial fibro-elastosis (*right upper arrow*; *c*)

Interestingly, the Kaplan-Meier estimation of cumulative event freedom from severe hypertrophic cardiomyopathy fits exactly with the reported mean survival in male and female patients [1, 29, 30] (Fig. 11.2), and might be, as mentioned, one of the major contributors to the severely reduced life expectancy and high degree of morbidity in late stage Fabry disease.

Fig. 11.2 Progression of
Cardiomyopathy: Severe
Cardiomyopathy (50% above
upper limit of normal) was
detected in male patients at a
mean age of 42.3 ± 1.1
(SEM) (95% CI 40: 40–44.5
years) and in females at a
mean age of 53.5 ± 1.6
(SEM) (95% CI: 51.3–55.6
years) (P <0.00001)

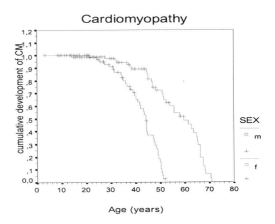

11.2.1 Cardiac Hypertrophy – Hypertrophic Cardiomyopathy

The cardiac hypertrophy is readily detectable by different techniques as echocardiography (ECHO) and magnetic resonance imaging (MRI) (Fig. 11.1) and electrocardiography (ECG) (Fig. 11.3). The hypertrophic cardiac changes are representable by increased wall thicknesses in ECHO and MRI and in the ECG by typical hypertrophy voltage signs [26, 31, 32]. Histological, this related hypertrophy is characterized

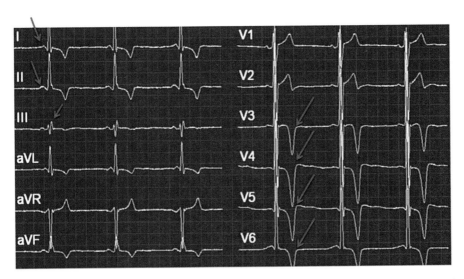

Fig. 11.3 ECG (25 mm/s; 10 mm/mV) of a 53 year old male patient. Of note are the abbreviated PR interval (133 ms; arrows in I and II), incomplete right bundle branch block (arrow in III), severe LV hypertrophy QRS complex widening (130 ms) with repolarisation disturbances, but without signs of ischemia (*arrows* in V3–V6)

by mild myofibril fibre disarray, lysosomal inclusions within myofibrils and vascular structures, large areas of autophagocytotic vacuoles and a variable degree of fibrosis depending on the stage of disease [4, 33]. Although the absolute amount of Gb_3 within the cardiac myocytes is low, the heart has the highest quantity of glycosphingolipid content compared to the kidney, liver or skin, and the heart has a much higher glycolipid turn over than other organs [4, 32].

The hypertrophic changes are progressive and occur earlier in males than in females [7, 11, 26], and are sometimes seen even in children and adolescents [15, 18]. Although females are heterozygous for this disease, it seems to be that there is an inability of cell expressing the wild type allele to cross-correct the metabolic defect [34, 35]. Several observational studies in female patients have indicated that cardiac involvement in females is common, slightly delayed relative to male patients and usually with a milder progression rate [11, 13, 36]. But, nevertheless, the severest cardiomyopathies with the highest left ventricular masses have been seen in female patients.

Early stages are predominantly characterized by a slight increase in myocardial mass, but without development of manifest hypertrophic changes as concentric remodelling. This feature is to be seen in approximately 50% of adolescents and children over the age of 10 years [15]. In later stages, the hypertrophic changes are symmetrical, as indicated by a concentric hypertrophy. Once there is a dramatic reduction in energy supplementation or increased energy depletion, eccentric changes can be seen, indicated by an increase in end-diastolic internal cavity dimensions. Asymmetric hypertrophic changes, as to be seen in asymmetrical septal hypertrophy as typically seen in sarcomeric cardiomyopathy is rarely seen in severe Fabry-related cardiomyopathy, but may account for approximately 5% of all cases with severe cardiac involvement [7, 26]. In case of severe left ventricular (LV) outflow obstruction, concomitant therapeutic approaches should be considered such as transcatheter alcohol ablation [37, 38].

Within the last few years, several MRI studies in small cohorts of affected patients have provided a deeper insight into the development of the Fabry-related cardiomyopathy. It could be demonstrated that in patients with LV hypertrophy a substantial number of patients show areas of late gadolinium enhancement, corresponding to myocardial fibrosis. This fibrosis occurs frequently within the mid-wall of the posterolateral basal segments, and the areas are interestingly not related to a specific coronary supply type [39, 40]. It appears, that these findings characterize the later stages of cardiac involvement and are associated with decreased regional functioning, as assessed by strain and strain-rate imaging studies [40].

Although LV hypertrophy is more severe in older than in younger patients with Fabry disease [12], longitudinal data describing the progression of left ventricular hypertrophy (LVH) in untreated patients are limited. Repeat serial echocardiograms of LV mass in 39 male and 39 female patients found, that the mean increase in LV mass in male patients is around 4.1 ± 1.0 g/m$^{2.7}$ and in females of around 2.3 ± 0.8 g/m$^{2.7}$. The rate of increase was greater when only patients with baseline LVH were analysed. Here, increase in LV mass was 6.6 ± 8.5 g/m$^{2.7}$ per year in males and 3.8 ± 7.7 g/m$^{2.7}$ in females, respectively [11].

The right ventricle also appears to be affected by storage and hypertrophy, and usually all cardiac biopsy–driven diagnoses and electron micrographs from vital patients are obtained from the right ventricular side, usually from the interventricular septum. However, there are only two reports available describing the functional impact of right ventricular infiltration, which is believed to be low, and isolated right ventricular failure rarely complicates the course of the disease [41].

11.2.2 Cardiac Systolic and Diastolic Function

Normally, the systolic function is estimated by traditional parameters such as ejection fraction (EF) or fractional shortening (FS). These parameters of systolic function are seldom decreased [26, 42], but once related to the mid-wall shortening (where usually the fibrosis is located) there is an age dependant progressive decline in mid-wall fractional shortening. This parameter reflects the contractility impairment that may be masked by geometrical structural changes and may be undetectable by the measurement of endocardial ejection fraction or endocardial fractional shortening. However, using more comprehensive and sophisticated techniques, such as tissue Doppler imaging and strain rate imaging, a substantial decrease in contractile performance, occurring earlier in the longitudinal than in the radial dimension, are to be seen, and this may contribute to the feature of systolic heart failure with 'preserved' radial endocardial fractional shortening [40, 43, 44].

Diastolic dysfunction is a common feature of Fabry disease, and can even be obvious in some cases with almost normal or only slightly increased left ventricular masses and is usually not related to mitral valve incompetence or stenosis. Unfortunately, there is no information available about the development of fibrosis and its influence on diastolic function in patients with almost normal LV mass or with mild cardiomyopathies. In contrast to genuine restrictive cardiomyopathies, restrictive filling patterns are found rarely, mostly in extremely advanced stages of cardiomyopathy with associated pronounced myocardial fibrosis [45]. But, end-stage cardiac involvement may present with restrictive pathophysiology [33, 46].

Together, reduced longitudinal function and impaired diastolic function account for the clinical features of dyspnoea and fatigue.

11.2.3 Ischemia, Coronary Artery Disease and Coronary Flow Reserve

Historically, the major course of cardiovascular related deaths in Fabry patients were believed being related to ischaemic events and myocardial infarction. However, large databases of Fabry patients (Fabry Outcome Survey and Fabry Registry) suggest a low incidence of proven myocardial infarctions. Nevertheless, the high incidence of reported chest anginal pain together with frequently disturbed ECG patterns, including ST–segment depressions and T–wave inversions, might be the cause for mis-diagnosis of either acute or sub-acute coronary artery disease and subsequently myocardial infarction [47]. Moreover, typical chest anginal pain and specific ECG changes are more frequently found in patients with severe LV hypertrophy, accompanied by a minor increase in myocardial destruction markers as troponin T or I in plasma. Large vessel coronary artery disease as of the epicardial coronary arteries, is rarely seen, and may be more correlated to classic causes of coronary artery disease, such as smoking and other precursors of atherosclerosis. In addition to the infiltrative changes within the endothelial and muscular layers of arteries, Fabry patients accumulate a large number of risk factors for (accelerated) atherosclerosis, including high levels of blood lipids, hypertension, renal insufficiency, and elevated levels of myeloperoxidase [48]. To what degree the prothrombotic state in some Fabry patients will contribute to vascular occlusive disorder remains unclear [19, 49]. It has been shown, that patients with Fabry cardiomyopathy do have a significantly reduced coronary flow reserve [50–53]. This could be related to the endothelial infiltration and dysfunction, potentiated by the increased oxygen demand of the hypertrophied hearts and further aggravated by elevated diastolic filling pressures, as to be seen in diastolic impairment and the enlargement of the left atrium. In some cases, vasospastic components of the small coronary arteries may contribute to the clinical sign of chest anginal pain, when neurohumoral stimuli cause inadequate vasodilatation of the coronary bed [54]. The ischaemic ECG changes are more likely to reflect left ventricular hypertrophy and the LV strain pattern, which is presumed to be related subendocardial ischemia and not infarction. But besides all that, it could be demonstrated, that Fabry patients with chest anginal pain, have myocardial perfusion defects, slow coronary blood flow, and luminal narrowing of intramural arteries, contributing to symptomatic limitation and progressive myocardial dysfunction.

Coronary artery interventions, such as coronary bypass surgery or trans-catheter performed revascularization therapy with angioplasty or stent placement in stenotic coronary artery lesions, are reported to have a prevalence of less than 1% in the Fabry patients' cohort. But nevertheless, there are case reports available where the risk of death due to coronary artery disease should not be underestimated [5].

11.2.4 Arrhythmias and Electrophysiological Abnormalities

Palpitations are the clinical symptom for underlying cardiac arrhythmias, and are common complains in patients with Fabry disease [12]. The most frequently encountered rhythm abnormalities include supraventricular tachycardias, atrial fibrillation and atrial flutter. Non-sustained ventricular tachycardias are more common than previously thought, and are reported in cases of fatal malignant arrhythmias resistant to implantable cardioverter defibrillator treatment [55, 56]. Complex and life threatening ventricular arrhythmias are usually related to intramural scar formation and the myocardial fibrosis, which are frequently found in Fabry cardiomyopathy, and these are a contributing factor [57]. Even the resting ECG patterns of Fabry patients are frequently altered. Common findings are high voltage signs, which reflect nicely the myocardial hypertrophy accompanied by repolarisation changes and prolongation of the QRS complex not only related to bundle branch blocks, but reflects the increase in cardiac muscle mass [31] (Fig. 11.3). A short PR–interval, one of the most frequent findings, is even to be seen in patients with no obvious increase in left ventricular mass and is due to an accelerated atrioventricular conduction [58]. Atrial arrhythmias and ECG changes due to the atria are frequently seen even in young children, and there is a need for close follow up in childhood.

As in other lysosomal and glycogen storage diseases, pre-excitation with accessory pathways may also be present in patients with Fabry disease [59, 60] and require in case of re-entry tachycardias transcatheter high frequency or cryoablation. With disease progression, conduction system dysfunction occurs, leading to bundle branch blocks and AV conduction blocks of varying degrees, sometimes requiring anti-bradycardiac pacemaker implantation. Some patients need pacemaker implantation for progressive sinus node dysfunction and chronotropic incompetence, which is relatively frequent in Fabry patients [61]. Of note here, is that in patients with isolated sinus node dysfunction, invasive electrophysiological testing of the AV node function should be performed to avoid choosing the wrong pacemaker. Therefore, a sequential atrio-ventricular pacing should be mandatory, once a patient fulfils the criteria for pacemaker implantation.

11.2.5 Autonomic Cardiac Control and Cardio Neuropathy

Information about the heart rate variability and the autonomic cardiac control can be easily derived from Holter ECGs. Heart rate variability can be measured using time-domain and or frequency-domain measurements and can therefore provide information about the cardiovascular control of the autonomic nervous system and allows a rough estimation of the influence of the parasympathetic and/or sympathetic activity. As for co-morbidities such as co-existing diabetes, a reduction in heart rate variability is associated with an increased risk of sudden cardiac death. It is worth to mention, that one of the first signs that affects the cardiovascular system, are depressed heart rate variability in boys with Fabry disease [15]. Observations regarding the heart rate variability patterns in adult Fabry patients have not been published so far.

11.2.6 Valvular Involvement in Fabry Disease

As in other lysosomal storage diseases, valvular involvement in Fabry disease is frequent observed. These changes are believed being caused by lipid storage and fibrosis of the valvular tissue. However, estimates of valvular involvement in Fabry disease differ significantly. Changes are almost exclusively found in the left heart valves, as the mitral and aortic valve, probably due to the higher hemodynamic stresses in the left side of the heart [7, 62]. Since the mid 1970s it is known, that mitral valve prolapse (MVP) is a common finding in Fabry patients [63], but compared to data from large cohorts of Fabry patients, the prevalence of mitral valve prolapse was overestimated. Subsequent reports confirmed the existence of MVP, but with a significantly lower prevalence [26]. Nevertheless, minor structural abnormalities on both mitral and aortic valves are frequent. Mitral valve alterations, leaflet thickening or prolapse are mostly seen in younger patients, while additional aortic abnormalities appear in the older patients. Most of the patients with mitral valve thickening have thickened papillary muscles, often accompanied by mild valvular regurgitation. In advanced stage of the disease with progression of cardiac involvement and left ventricular hypertrophy, there is a marked aortic root dilatation [42], which may contribute to mild aortic valve regurgitation. There are no differences in valvular changes between hemizygous or heterozygous patients; both genders are affected with more or less the same incidence. Severe alterations of the valves with the need of surgical valve repair are to date rare, but may increase in future.

11.2.7 Fabry Disease with the Main Manifestation in the Heart

Although Fabry disease is a complex disease affecting multiple organs, there are observations and reliable reports available, indicating that the manifestation of Fabry disease can be mainly limited to the heart in a small number of male hemizygotes [4, 32, 64–66]. Histopathologic studies revealed Gb$_3$ storage located almost exclusively in the heart and with less or almost no vascular endothelial involvement. Relatively high levels of residual alpha-galactosidase-A (AGALA) activity distinguished these cases, and with late onset disease [65, 66], these cases were described as cardiac variants.

It could be shown, that the cardiac variant type of Fabry disease seems to be more common than previously thought, and approximately 1–3% of all male patients with otherwise un-explained left ventricular hypertrophy suffer from this variant [36, 60, 67–69]. In all of these reported patients, the diagnosis was established by endomyocardial biopsies. Several studies have attempted to identify Fabry disease among patients with cardiac hypertrophy. Special attention should be paid to patients in whom unexplained LV hypertrophy is diagnosed after 40 years of age [70, 71]. At this age, most male patients with Fabry disease have at least LV hypertrophy, which is not necessarily obvious in younger patients. Screening studies in patients with asymmetrical septal hypertrophy and/or left ventricular outflow obstruction, revealed almost no patients to be found by this screening, because asymmetrical septal hypertrophy is per se a relatively rare finding in patients who manifest the complete picture of Fabry disease [68]. Regarding the prevalence of suspected cardiac variants among females, the published reports contrast dramatically, and finally this question cannot be answered to date [36, 60]. However, Fabry disease should be considered in the differential diagnosis of patients with otherwise unexplained LV hypertrophy, independent of gender, and cardiac biopsy should be performed in each of those suspected cases.

11.2.8 Cardiac Involvement in Children

Childhood and adolescence are usually characterized in Fabry children by severe attacks of neuropathic pain, and gastro-intestinal problems [16–18]. But, the increasing awareness, that Fabry disease is a congenital debilitating problem, has motivated investigators to examine the children of affected adult Fabry patients. Of interest are, that even strokes and white matter lesions are reported in the Fabry children cohort. Data analyses of both, Fabry Outcome Survey and Fabry Registry, indicate, that some of the cardiovascular features are even to be found in children around the age of 10–12 years [17, 18]. The most common cardiac abnormality was valvular dysfunction, which was found in approximately 22.6% of males and in approximately 13.9% of females [15]. Besides that, Holter ECG analyses of children revealed a substantial number of usually supraventricular arrhythmias, conduction abnormalities, and even left ventricular hypertrophy was documented. Affected children tend to have slightly higher left ventricular masses compared with age matched healthy children, and all have LV masses above the 75% for age. Besides that, there are children reported with concentric remodelling a precursor for concentric left ventricular hypertrophy and with eccentric left ventricular hypertrophy. Those children with abnormal left ventricular shape or mass had normal diastolic filling patterns [15]. But tissue Doppler imaging studies have not been published so far. Combinations with congenital cardiac malformations have been reported in single cases, with an AVSD and a Tetralogy of Fallot. On follow-up examinations in children, it is reported, that those children with a proteinuria above 200 mg/d, tend to have a larger increase in LV mass than those with no urinary protein excretion [15].

   In our center, none of the reported children had QRS duration times or PR intervals outside the limits of normal, or met age-appropriate electrocardiographic criteria for LV hypertrophy.

   Analyses of the heart rate variability in Fabry children revealed significantly depressed heart rate variability parameters such as pNN50% and r-MSSD but only in male children, and not in female children, compared to an age- matched normal gender-related control population [15, 72] (Fig. 11.4). HRV analyses may be used as a quantitative index of involvement of the parasympathetic and/or sympathetic nerves innervating the heart. The reduced parameters of pNN50% and r-MSSD are generally thought to measure parasympathetic influences on the heart rate and its variability. Additional analyses of frequency domain measures showed significantly lower power deviation and density in the parasympathetic HF spectrum. Therefore, it is suggested, that this findings would seem to show a withdrawal of parasympathetic rather than an increased sympathetic activity. It was speculated, that these findings were due to a disturbed acetylcholine metabolism [15]. Likewise, the findings described here were supported by previously reported data showing

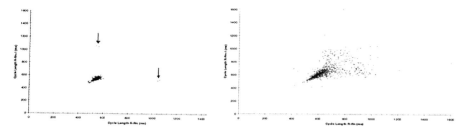

Fig. 11.4 Poincare plots where the RR distance (ms) is plotted against the RR distance of the previous beat. *Left side*: 10 year old male boy with Fabry disease, of note are the atrial arrhythmias (*arrows*); *right side*: plot of a healthy 10 year old boy

abnormal endothelial responses to intra-arterial acetylcholine administration in adult male Fabry patients.

If these findings of disturbed autonomic cardiac control in male children will contribute to a more advanced disease progression has to be elucidated with long-term follow up examinations in treated and untreated Fabry patients.

11.2.9 Clinical Signs and Symptoms

The major signs and symptoms of cardiac involvement are dyspnoea, chest anginal pain, palpitations, fatigue and syncope. In FOS, untreated male and female patients experienced a cumulative incidence of cardiac signs and symptoms of 10 and 6% respectively, by age 20 years; by age of 50 years, the cumulative incidence had increased to 45 and 25% in men and women, respectively. In most patients, these symptoms are related to LV hypertrophy, and there is a strong coincidence between the degree of cardiac involvement and the occurrence of symptoms. The presence and severity of LVH has been associated with significantly higher occurrences of heart failure, chest pain, arrhythmias, and valvular disease. Dyspnoea is mainly caused by diastolic dysfunction, and more rarely by systolic dysfunction. Valvular regurgitation is common, but usually mild and may only contribute in selected patients to this symptom. Chest anginal pain usually occurs even in the absence of stenotic coronary lesions and is mainly due to small vessel disease and an increase in oxygen consumption and a decreased coronary flow reserve. Palpitations are frequent complaints, and are almost always related to cardiac arrhythmias. In light of potential side effects of arrhythmias and potential benefits of either pharmacological treatment options or pacemaker and implantable cardioverter defibrillators, investigators should be encouraged to perform 24 h Holter monitoring in all patients. And even more than this, not everyone who has arrhythmias complains of palpitations. Syncope can be related to cardiac involvement, as it is known that a high degree of AV blocks or severe dynamic outflow obstruction or thrombembolic complications can cause overt neurological damage.

11.3 Treatment Options

11.3.1 Adjuvant Therapeutic Interventions

Treatment of the cardiovascular involvement is difficult, and because of the underlying mechanism of the disease being not only related to the enhancement of enzyme activity of the AGALA and should consider concomitant therapeutic options in all patients, and everything should be done to reduce the cardiovascular risk factors and to treat the classical cardiac signs and symptoms of the cardiovascular involvement. Adjuvant pharmacological treatment should therefore be included, such as in case of increased lipid levels the use of statins, and in case of borderline or manifest arterial hypertension, the use of antihypertensive treatment e.g. with ACE inhibitors and/or angiotensin receptor blocking agents (ARBs). Patients should be treated according to the signs and symptoms they experience. Anti-anginal treatment using nitroglycerine is needed in a substantial number of patients, but should be given with care. The use of beta-blockers might be crucial, because symptomatic bradycardia, the AV conduction impairment and the chronotropic incompetence of a large number of patients might be aggravated. Dihydropyridine calcium channel blockers are relatively effective and safe. Anti-aggregation and/or anti-coagulation should be considered and immediately started if patients experience ischaemic cerebrovascular accidents in light of occult cardiac arrhythmias, or have atrial flutter and other supraventricular arrhythmias known to be associated with a high incidence of thrombembolic complications. In patients with symptomatic bradycardia and/or AV conduction abnormalities, pacemaker implantation is frequently required, and will be helpful even in cases with chronotropic incompetence, in terms of inadequate or no physiological increase in heart rate under exercise. Patients with malignant ventricular arrhythmias will benefit from an implantable cardioverter defibrillator.

Treatment of heart failure should be given to all symptomatic patients, and ACE inhibitors or ARBs should be considered even more in asymptomatic patients but with any kind of obvious cardiac structural changes. Patients with advanced stages of congestive heart failure and severe and untreatable chest anginal pain may be candidates for heart transplantation, as the intrinsic enzyme production of the donor heart should prevent rapid deterioration. Biventricular pacing might, as it is used in other cases of hypertrophic cardiomyopathy, reduce the clinical signs of congestive heart failure and prolong the time to transplantation [46].

In patients with asymmetrical septal hypertrophy, septal alcohol ablation may be effective in reducing a significant LV outflow obstruction [37]. Other treatment options, like surgical myectomy or valve replacement should be individually considered, even in the light, that Fabry patients will have a higher complication rate and longer recovery times because of the multi-systemic nature and multi- organ involvement of the disease.

In general, once manifest organ destructions have occurred, in terms of fibrosis or myocardial necrosis, treatment benefits are limited. That does not mean, that treatment options should be deprived Fabry patients with severe cardiomyopathy, because recently published data of other cardiac diseases are suggestive of potential long term remodelling capacities of the myocardium after injuries have taken place.

11.3.2 Enhancement of Enzyme Activity and Enzyme Replacement Therapy

There are different terms available to describe the intravenous application of enzyme. The enhancement of enzyme activity means, that a patient must have at least some residual enzyme activity which can be enhanced by either supplementing bioactive molecules or substances, which are able to increase residual mutant enzyme activity by reversible competitive inhibition of AGALA (galactose) or by small molecule delivery which may stabilize the mutant mis-folded residual enzyme (chaperone). In general, in patients with residual enzyme activity or mutant activity, and patients with distinct mutations with some residual activity, treatment with chaperones or other options can be considered. The great advantage of chaperones is the route of administration: while enzyme replacement therapies and galactose are to be given intravenously, chaperones are (daily) orally taken.

One of the first reports on alternative treatment of a patient with cardiac variant of Fabry disease was published in 2001 [73]. This was a 55-year-old male patient with Fabry disease with the main manifestation of the heart who had some residual enzyme activity (2.4% of normal) as a result of a missense mutation. This patient was treated by galactose infusions every 2nd day for 2 years. Before and during this treatment, the patient was followed by serial heart biopsies, MRI, ECG and ECHO examinations, and blood samples. During this reported period, the patient dramatically improved from NYHA class IV to NYHA class I. Left ventricular masses decreased rapidly by 20% during the first 3 months, diastolic filling pressures declined, shortening and ejection fraction improved substantially to almost normal values. AGALA activity in lymphocytes and in endomyocardial tissue increased and the diameter of myocardial cells declined, while there was a substantial decrease in autophagocytotic vacuole areas.

In children and young adults, it is anticipated that enzyme substitution may be able to prevent development of the serious cardiac alterations described in adults. However, it may not be possible to demonstrate the benefits of ERT until there are data of patients available, who had undergone continuous enzyme replacement therapy over many years or even decades. However, there are reports of cases available that are receiving ERT for almost a decade, where ERT is suggestive for beneficial effects and for changing the natural course of the disease.

In a progressive disorder like Fabry cardiomyopathy, different aims of enzyme replacement therapy can be distinguished. Enzyme replacement can lead (1) to slowing down of the slope of progression, (2) to stop progression, (3) to a reduction in LV mass, (4) to normalization of LV mass, (5) to prevent disease-specific deterioration, and (6) to improve clinical signs and symptoms.

The development of enzyme replacement therapies for Fabry disease has raised the possibility of altering the natural history of the cardiac involvement by providing exogenous human AGALA. ERT for Fabry has been commercially available since 2001, and two distinct formulations are currently available. Agalsidase alfa (Replagal; Shire Human Genetic Therapies Inc, Cambridge Massachusetts, USA), is produced virus free in a continuous human cell line, and is administered every other week as a 0.2 mg/kg bodyweight intravenous infusion over 40 min. Agalsidase beta (Fabrazyme; Genzyme Corporation, Cambridge, Massachusetts, USA), produced in a Chinese hamster ovary cell line, is administered every other week as a 1.0 mg/kg body weight intravenous infusion over a periods ranging from 1.5 to over 4.5 h. There are dose recommendations for agalsidase beta starting at 0.3 mg/kg, but for others of these recommendations there are no evidence based data available. Therefore, for further discussion, the reported results of ERT with agalsidase beta will be solely related to the dose of 1.0 mg/kg EOW, as it has been used in different randomized controlled studies for approval.

Both formulations are reported to have clinical benefits besides the cardiovascular efficacy and are described elsewhere. Here, only the cardiovascular related efficacy will be elucidated.

11.3.2.1 Agalsidase Alfa

The first randomized controlled trial, which reported an effect of agalsidase alfa on the heart and cardiovascular system was published by Schiffmann et al., where there was a significant reduction in surface ECG derived QRS duration time compared to the placebo arm after 6 months of ERT (Evidence level T Ib) [74]. But, the cardiovascular efficacy was not the primary endpoint of the study, which was neuropathic pain. A small randomized controlled trial in 10 male patients with 6 months of ERT and thereafter a cross-over of all patients to treatment showed a significant change in wall thickness and an increase in long axis shortening, but was published as an abstract (Evidence level T Ib) [75]. The randomized controlled trial with cardiac primary endpoint of regression of LV mass, was published by Hughes et al. on 14 male patients with LVH assessed by MRI, where there was a statistically significant decrease in LV mass (−11.5 g) compared to placebo (+21.8 g) (Evidence level T Ib) [76]. Here, the investigators observed in 6 months of ERT a progression of LV mass in the placebo group, where in the treatment arm there was a decrease in LV mass. The amount of Gb3 storage, obtained by serial myocardial biopsies, decreased in the treatment arm and increased in the placebo group, but did not reach statistical significance. An open-label extension with treatment and further follow-up of 10 of the 14 patients by MRI, the LV mass did not decline further in these 10 patients, and remained stable over the 2 year follow-up; however, significant reduction in LV posterior wall thickness and septal thickness were observed, suggesting that cardiac remodelling occurred during treatment. Beck et al. reported that for 52 patients enrolled in FOS, 1 year of ERT was associated with a significant reduction in mean LV mass by 13 $g/m^{2.7}$ [77, 78]. A similar reduction was observed in 17 patients treated for 2 years for whom echocardiograms were available (Evidence level T III). In a 4 year prospective, open-label single-center trial, average LV mass in 25 female patients with baseline LVH was significantly reduced after 1 year of ERT, and the reduction was sustained through 4 years of treatment. Furthermore, there was a significant improvement in dyspnoea as demonstrated by a significant decrease in NYHA functional class (Evidence level T III) [79]. Kampmann et al. recently published a retrospective, blinded, pooled analysis of 4 industry-sponsored clinical studies conducted at the NIH, Bethesda, Maryland and the University of Mainz, Germany, that included assessments of the effects of ERT on echocardiographic variables [80]. The NIH study enrolled 26 adult male patients in a 6 month randomized, double-blind clinical trial assessing the safety profile and the efficacy of ERT, and continued as an open-label extension study for an additional 4 years [74, 81]. In another study of 80 patients, 10 adult male patients were included in a larger double-blind multicenter study that assessed the effects of ERT on neuropathic pain and renal function. From this latter trial, 15 adult male patients were enrolled in an open-label study assessing the safety profile. All available echocardiograms were pooled and blinded and analysed. Of 66 ptients enrolled in these studies, serial echocardiographic examinations obtained at baseline and after 12 and 36 months were available from 45 adult patients (34 men and 11 women). In summary, in those patients with baseline LV hypertrophy, the decline in LV mass was significant, 4 of those 22 male patients and none of the female patients with normal LV mass at baseline developed LV hypertrophy during follow up, indicating that the majority of patients with or without LV hypertrophy at baseline benefited from ERT with agalsidase alfa (Evidence level T IIb) [80].

The total number of reported single patients, in whom data on ERT and LV mass were published, comprised of 162 patients (excluded were those, who participated into different trials and overlap might occur). Treatment with agalsidase alfa seems consistently to decrease LV mass and to reduce the slope of progression in patients with Fabry disease and cardiac involvement. The treatment evidence levels were three times grade Ib, one grade IIb and twice grade III; therefore, the suggested level of recommendation of ERT with agalsidase alfa is grade A/B.

11.3.2.2 Agalsidase Beta

A search of PubMed database from January 1, 2001 to June 1, 2009, identified nine studies reporting the effects of 1.0 mg/kg body weight every other week agalsidase beta on LV mass. These studies were all non-controlled and included 125 patients, primarily male, who were treated for 12–36 months [51, 82–89]. Of those nine studies, three reported no change in LV mass [51, 85, 86], and the other six reported significant decrease in LV mass between 7% and around 22% in mean. It has been reported, that significant decrease in LV mass was only observed in patients without MRI confirmed myocardial fibrosis [88] and in patients, in whom estimated glomerular filtration rate >90 ml/min/1.73 m^2 [87]. Recently, it has been reported, that in 3 year follow-up under ERT, a significant reduction in LV mass was observed independent of no, mild or severe myocardial fibrosis, but interestingly an improvement in myocardial function was only observed in patients without MRI evidence of myocardial fibrosis [84]. The findings of these latter three studies suggest, that patients with LVH and advanced Fabry disease, as evidenced by myocardial fibrosis and/or kidney dysfunction, may have experienced irreversible changes in cardiac morphology and do not respond fully to enzyme replacement therapy with agalsidase beta.

One histopathological study on the pathophysiological mechanisms of chest anginal pain in Fabry patients has been published [52]. Here, the authors could show that chest anginal pain reflects a coronary small vessel disease in Fabry cardiomyopathy: 13 of those reported patients had serial histopathologic examinations, accompanied by Tissue Doppler Imaging and routine echocardiography. After at least 1 year of treatment, there was no evidence of decreased storage material, decreased LV mass or improvement in coronary blood flow and in chest anginal pain, compared to baseline under ERT with agalsidase beta [52]. Unfortunately, although cardiac biopsy specimens were obtained also during the randomized agalsidase beta trial, only endothelial, but not cardiomyocyte, storage changes were described [90]. Thus the available evidence suggests that at least in some patients agalsidase beta has limited access to non-vascular cardiac tissues.

The effects of treatment with agalsidase beta are inconsistent. Four of ten studies did not observe any change in LV mass. This inconsistency may be related to an incomparability between the patient populations reported in the studies; unfortunately, the age of the patients, one predictor for adverse outcome, is not given in every study, which makes a final conclusion difficult. But nevertheless, an observational finding, as LV mass which does not change over a certain treatment period, might be interpreted as a beneficial outcome in a progressive disease. The treatment evidence levels for beneficial effects in those six studies were all evidence level grade III; therefore, the suggested level of recommendation of ERT with agalsidase beta is grade B.

Nevertheless, the cardiovascular involvement in Fabry disease is a difficult target for treatment, and supposed to be more complex, than in most of the other organ systems. Once, the patient has reached a certain point of the disease, the influence of ERT on the heart might be reduced and the natural history, which was primary complicated by components like end-stage renal disease or stroke is shifting towards an untreatable cardiac condition, in terms of mortality [91]. But, using a composite end-point, including renal, cardiac and cerebrovascular events, ERT with agalsidase beta supposed to prolong the time to first clinical event. However, the difference in cardiac end-points alone, although showing a hazard ration of 0.42, did not reach significance [92].

References

1. MacDermot KD, Holmes A, Miners AH (2001) Anderson-Fabry disease: clinical manifestations and impact of disease in a cohort of 98 hemizygous males. J Med Genet 38(11):750–760
2. Mehta A, Ricci R, Widmer U, Dehout F, Garcia de Lorenzo A, Kampmann C et al (2004) Fabry disease defined: baseline clinical manifestations of 366 patients in the Fabry Outcome Survey. Eur J Clin Invest 34(3):236–242

3. Elleder M (2008) Cellular and tissue localization of globotriaosylceramide in Fabry disease. Virchows Arch 452(6):705, author reply 7–8
4. Elleder M, Bradova V, Smid F, Budesinsky M, Harzer K, Kustermann-Kuhn B et al (1990) Cardiocyte storage and hypertrophy as a sole manifestation of Fabry's disease. Report on a case simulating hypertrophic non-obstructive cardiomyopathy. Virchows Arch A Pathol Anat Histopathol 417(5):449–455
5. Schiffmann R, Rapkiewicz A, Abu-Asab M, Ries M, Askari H, Tsokos M et al (2006) Pathological findings in a patient with Fabry disease who died after 2.5 years of enzyme replacement. Virchows Arch 448(3):337–343
6. Kampmann C, Baehner F, Ries M, Beck M (2002) Cardiac involvement in Anderson-Fabry disease. J Am Soc Nephrol 13(Suppl 2):S147–S149
7. Linhart A, Lubanda JC, Palecek T, Bultas J, Karetova D, Ledvinova J et al (2001) Cardiac manifestations in Fabry disease. J Inherit Metab Dis 24(Suppl 2):75–83, discussion 65
8. Uchino M, Uyama E, Kawano H, Hokamaki J, Kugiyama K, Murakami Y et al (1995) A histochemical and electron microscopic study of skeletal and cardiac muscle from a Fabry disease patient and carrier. Acta Neuropathol 90(3):334–338
9. Hilz MJ (2002) Evaluation of peripheral and autonomic nerve function in Fabry disease. Acta Paediatr Suppl 91(439):38–42
10. Hilz MJ, Brys M, Marthol H, Stemper B, Dutsch M (2004) Enzyme replacement therapy improves function of C-, Adelta-, and Abeta-nerve fibers in Fabry neuropathy. Neurology 62(7):1066–1072
11. Kampmann C, Linhart A, Baehner F, Palecek T, Wiethoff CM, Miebach E et al (2008) Onset and progression of the Anderson-Fabry disease related cardiomyopathy. Int J Cardiol 130(3):367–373
12. Linhart A, Kampmann C, Zamorano JL, Sunder-Plassmann G, Beck M, Mehta A et al (2007) Cardiac manifestations of Anderson-Fabry disease: results from the international Fabry outcome survey. Eur Heart J 28(10):1228–1235
13. Kampmann C, Baehner F, Whybra C, Martin C, Wiethoff CM, Ries M et al (2002) Cardiac manifestations of Anderson-Fabry disease in heterozygous females. J Am Coll Cardiol 40(9):1668–1674
14. Whybra C, Kampmann C, Willers I, Davies J, Winchester B, Kriegsmann J et al (2001) Anderson-Fabry disease: clinical manifestations of disease in female heterozygotes. J Inherit Metab Dis 24(7):715–724
15. Kampmann C, Wiethoff CM, Whybra C, Baehner FA, Mengel E, Beck M (2008) Cardiac manifestations of Anderson-Fabry disease in children and adolescents. Acta Paediatr 97(4):463–469
16. Beck M, Whybra C, Wendrich K, Gal A, Ries M (2001) Anderson-Fabry disease in children and adolescents. Contrib Nephrol 136:251–255
17. Ramaswami U, Whybra C, Parini R, Pintos-Morell G, Mehta A, Sunder-Plassmann G et al (2006) Clinical manifestations of Fabry disease in children: data from the Fabry Outcome Survey. Acta Paediatr 95(1):86–92
18. Hopkin RJ, Bissler J, Banikazemi M, Clarke L, Eng CM, Germain DP et al (2008) Characterization of Fabry disease in 352 pediatric patients in the Fabry Registry. Pediatr Res 64(5):550–555
19. Hulkova H, Ledvinova J, Poupetova H, Bultas J, Zeman J, Elleder M (1999) Postmortem diagnosis of Fabry disease in a female heterozygote leading to the detection of undiagnosed manifest disease in the family. Cas Lek Cesk 138(21):660–664
20. Ashrafian H, Redwood C, Blair E, Watkins H (2003) Hypertrophic cardiomyopathy:a paradigm for myocardial energy depletion. Trends Genet 19(5):263–268
21. Lucke T, Hoppner W, Schmidt E, Illsinger S, Das AM (2004) Fabry disease: reduced activities of respiratory chain enzymes with decreased levels of energy-rich phosphates in fibroblasts. Mol Genet Metab 82(1):93–97

22. Jung WI, Sieverding L, Breuer J, Hoess T, Widmaier S, Schmidt O et al (1998) 31P NMR spectroscopy detects metabolic abnormalities in asymptomatic patients with hypertrophic cardiomyopathy. Circulation 97(25):2536–2542

23. Chimenti C, Hamdani N, Boontje NM, DeCobelli F, Esposito A, Bronzwaer JG et al (2008) Myofilament degradation and dysfunction of human cardiomyocytes in Fabry disease. Am J Pathol 172(6):1482–1490

24. Barbey F, Brakch N, Linhart A, Rosenblatt-Velin N, Jeanrenaud X, Qanadli S et al (2006) Cardiac and vascular hypertrophy in Fabry disease: evidence for a new mechanism independent of blood pressure and glycosphingolipid deposition. Arterioscler Thromb Vasc Biol 26(4):839–844

25. Funabashi N, Toyozaki T, Matsumoto Y, Yonezawa M, Yanagawa N, Yoshida K et al (2003) Images in cardiovascular medicine. Myocardial fibrosis in fabry disease demonstrated by multislice computed tomography: comparison with biopsy findings. Circulation 107(19):2519–2520

26. Linhart A, Palecek T, Bultas J, Ferguson JJ, Hrudova J, Karetova D et al (2000) New insights in cardiac structural changes in patients with Fabry's disease. Am Heart J 139(6):1101–1108

27. Olivotto I, Cecchi F, Camici PG (2004) Coronary microvascular dysfunction and ischemia in hypertrophic cardiomyopathy. Mechanisms and clinical consequences. Ital Heart J 5(8):572–580

28. Cecchi F, Olivotto I, Gistri R, Lorenzoni R, Chiriatti G, Camici PG (2003) Coronary microvascular dysfunction and prognosis in hypertrophic cardiomyopathy. N Engl J Med 349(11):1027–1035

29. MacDermot KD, Holmes A, Miners AH (2001) Anderson-Fabry disease: clinical manifestations and impact of disease in a cohort of 60 obligate carrier females. J Med Genet 38(11):769–775

30. MacDermot KD, Holmes A, Miners AH (2001) Natural history of Fabry disease in affected males and obligate carrier females. J Inherit Metab Dis 24(Suppl 2):13–14, discussion 1–2

31. Kampmann C, Wiethoff CM, Martin C, Wenzel A, Kampmann R, Whybra C et al (2002) Electrocardiographic signs of hypertrophy in fabry disease-associated hypertrophic cardiomyopathy. Acta Paediatr Suppl 91(439):21–27

32. von Scheidt W, Eng CM, Fitzmaurice TF, Erdmann E, Hubner G, Olsen EG et al (1991) An atypical variant of Fabry's disease with manifestations confined to the myocardium. N Engl J Med 324(6):395–399

33. Cantor WJ, Butany J, Iwanochko M, Liu P (1998) Restrictive cardiomyopathy secondary to Fabry's disease. Circulation 98(14):1457–1459

34. Morrone A, Cavicchi C, Bardelli T, Antuzzi D, Parini R, Di Rocco M et al (2003) Fabry disease: molecular studies in Italian patients and X inactivation analysis in manifesting carriers. J Med Genet 40(8):e103

35. Dobrovolny R, Dvorakova L, Ledvinova J, Magage S, Bultas J, Lubanda JC et al (2005) Relationship between X-inactivation and clinical involvement in Fabry heterozygotes. Eleven novel mutations in the alpha-galactosidase A gene in the Czech and Slovak population. J Mol Med 83(8):647–654

36. Chimenti C, Pieroni M, Morgante E, Antuzzi D, Russo A, Russo MA et al (2004) Prevalence of Fabry disease in female patients with late-onset hypertrophic cardiomyopathy. Circulation 110(9):1047–1053

37. Magage S, Linhart A, Bultas J, Vojacek J, Mates M, Palecek T et al (2005) Fabry disease: percutaneous transluminal septal myocardial ablation markedly improved symptomatic left ventricular hypertrophy and outflow tract obstruction in a classically affected male. Echocardiography 22(4):333–339

38. Burda CD, Winder PR (1967) Angiokeratoma corporis diffusum universale (Fabry's disease) in female subjects. Am J Med 42(2):293–301

39. Moon JC, Sachdev B, Elkington AG, McKenna WJ, Mehta A, Pennell DJ et al (2003) Gadolinium enhanced cardiovascular magnetic resonance in Anderson-Fabry disease. Evidence for a disease specific abnormality of the myocardial interstitium. Eur Heart J 24(23):2151–2155

40. Weidemann F, Breunig F, Beer M, Sandstede J, Stork S, Voelker W et al (2005) The variation of morphological and functional cardiac manifestation in Fabry disease: potential implications for the time course of the disease. Eur Heart J 26(12):1221–1227

41. Kampmann C, Baehner FA, Whybra C, Bajbouj M, Baron K, Knuf M et al (2005) The right ventricle in Fabry disease. Acta Paediatr Suppl 94(447):15–18, discussion 9–10

42. Goldman ME, Cantor R, Schwartz MF, Baker M, Desnick RJ (1986) Echocardiographic abnormalities and disease severity in Fabry's disease. J Am Coll Cardiol 7(5): 1157–1161

43. Pieroni M, Chimenti C, Russo A, Russo MA, Maseri A, Frustaci A (2004) Tissue Doppler imaging in Fabry disease. Curr Opin Cardiol 19(5):452–457

44. Pieroni M, Chimenti C, Ricci R, Sale P, Russo MA, Frustaci A (2003) Early detection of Fabry cardiomyopathy by tissue Doppler imaging. Circulation 107(15):1978–1984

45. Hasegawa H, Takano H, Shindo S, Takeda S, Funabashi N, Nakagawa K et al (2006) Images in cardiovascular medicine. Transition from left ventricular hypertrophy to massive fibrosis in the cardiac variant of Fabry disease. Circulation 113(16):e

46. Cantor WJ, Daly P, Iwanochko M, Clarke JT, Cusimano RJ, Butany J (1998) Cardiac transplantation for Fabry's disease. Can J Cardiol 14(1):81–84

47. Becker AE, Schoorl R, Balk AG, van der Heide RM (1975) Cardiac manifestations of Fabry's disease. Report of a case with mitral insufficiency and electrocardiographic evidence of myocardial infarction. Am J Cardiol 36(6):829–835

48. Kaneski CR, Moore DF, Ries M, Zirzow GC, Schiffmann R (2006) Myeloperoxidase predicts risk of vasculopathic events in hemizgygous males with Fabry disease. Neurology 67(11):2045–2047

49. DeGraba T, Azhar S, Dignat-George F, Brown E, Boutiere B, Altarescu G et al (2000) Profile of endothelial and leukocyte activation in Fabry patients. Ann Neurol 47(2):229–233

50. Kalliokoski RJ, Kalliokoski KK, Sundell J, Engblom E, Penttinen M, Kantola I et al (2005) Impaired myocardial perfusion reserve but preserved peripheral endothelial function in patients with Fabry disease. J Inherit Metab Dis 28(4):563–573

51. Elliott PM, Kindler H, Shah JS, Sachdev B, Rimoldi OE, Thaman R et al (2006) Coronary microvascular dysfunction in male patients with Anderson-Fabry disease and the effect of treatment with alpha galactosidase A. Heart 92(3):357–360

52. Chimenti C, Morgante E, Tanzilli G, Mangieri E, Critelli G, Gaudio C et al (2008) Angina in fabry disease reflects coronary small vessel disease. Circ Heart Fail 1(3):161–169

53. Dimitrow PP, Krzanowski M, Undas A (2005) Reduced coronary flow reserve in Anderson-Fabry disease measured by transthoracic Doppler echocardiography. Cardiovasc Ultrasound 3:11

54. Ogawa T, Kawai M, Matsui T, Seo A, Aizawa O, Hongo K et al (1996) Vasospastic angina in a patient with Fabry's disease who showed normal coronary angiographic findings. Jpn Circ J 60(5):315–318

55. Eckart RE, Kinney KG, Belnap CM, Le TD (2000) Ventricular fibrillation refractory to automatic internal cardiac defibrillator in Fabry's disease. Review of cardiovascular manifestations. Cardiology 94(3):208–212

56. Shah JS, Hughes DA, Sachdev B, Tome M, Ward D, Lee P et al (2005) Prevalence and clinical significance of cardiac arrhythmia in Anderson-Fabry disease. Am J Cardiol 96(6): 842–846

57. Igawa O, Miake J, Hisatome I (2005) Ventricular tachycardias and dilated cardiomyopathy caused by Fabry disease. Pacing Clin Electrophysiol 28(10):1142–1143

58. Pochis WT, Litzow JT, King BG, Kenny D (1994) Electrophysiologic findings in Fabry's disease with a short PR interval. Am J Cardiol 74(2):203–204

59. Murata R, Takatsu H, Noda T, Nishigaki K, Tsuchiya K, Takemura G et al (1999) Fifteen-year follow-up of a heterozygous Fabry's disease patient associated with pre-excitation syndrome. Intern Med 38(6):476–481

60. Arad M, Maron BJ, Gorham JM, Johnson WH Jr, Saul JP, Perez-Atayde AR et al (2005) Glycogen storage diseases presenting as hypertrophic cardiomyopathy. N Engl J Med 352(4):362–372

61. Ikari Y, Kuwako K, Yamaguchi T (1992) Fabry's disease with complete atrioventricular block: histological evidence of involvement of the conduction system. Br Heart J 68(3): 323–325

62. Matsui S, Murakami E, Takekoshi N, Hiramaru Y, Kin T (1977) Cardiac manifestations of Fabry's disease. Report of a case with pulmonary regurgitation diagnosed on the basis of endomyocardial biopsy findings. Jpn Circ J 41(9):1023–1036

63. Desnick RJ, Blieden LC, Sharp HL, Hofschire PJ, Moller JH (1976) Cardiac valvular anomalies in Fabry disease. Clinical, morphologic, and biochemical studies. Circulation 54(5):818–825

64. Ogawa K, Sugamata K, Funamoto N, Abe T, Sato T, Nagashima K et al (1990) Restricted accumulation of globotriaosylceramide in the hearts of atypical cases of Fabry's disease. Hum Pathol 21(10):1067–1073

65. Ishii S, Kase R, Sakuraba H, Suzuki Y (1993) Characterization of a mutant alpha-galactosidase gene product for the late-onset cardiac form of Fabry disease. Biochem Biophys Res Commun 197(3):1585–1589

66. Ishii S, Chang HH, Kawasaki K, Yasuda K, Wu HL, Garman SC et al (2007) Mutant alpha-galactosidase A enzymes identified in Fabry disease patients with residual enzyme activity: biochemical characterization and restoration of normal intracellular processing by 1-deoxygalactonojirimycin. Biochem J 406(2):285–295

67. Nakao S, Takenaka T, Maeda M, Kodama C, Tanaka A, Tahara M et al (1995) An atypical variant of Fabry's disease in men with left ventricular hypertrophy. N Engl J Med 333(5): 288–293

68. Ommen SR, Nishimura RA, Edwards WD (2003) Fabry disease: a mimic for obstructive hypertrophic cardiomyopathy? Heart 89(8):929–930

69. Monserrat L, Gimeno-Blanes JR, Marin F, Hermida-Prieto M, Garcia-Honrubia A, Perez I et al (2007) Prevalence of fabry disease in a cohort of 508 unrelated patients with hypertrophic cardiomyopathy. J Am Coll Cardiol 50(25):2399–2403

70. Sachdev B, Elliott PM (2002) Isolated cardiac manifestations in Fabry disease: the UK experience. Acta Paediatr Suppl 91(439):28–30

71. Sachdev B, Takenaka T, Teraguchi H, Tei C, Lee P, McKenna WJ et al (2002) Prevalence of Anderson-Fabry disease in male patients with late onset hypertrophic cardiomyopathy. Circulation 105(12):1407–1411

72. Ries M, Gupta S, Moore DF, Sachdev V, Quirk JM, Murray GJ et al (2005) Pediatric Fabry disease. Pediatrics 115(3):e344–e355

73. Frustaci A, Chimenti C, Ricci R, Natale L, Russo MA, Pieroni M et al (2001) Improvement in cardiac function in the cardiac variant of Fabry's disease with galactose-infusion therapy. N Engl J Med 345(1):25–32

74. Schiffmann R, Kopp JB, Austin HA III, Sabnis S, Moore DF, Weibel T et al (2001) Enzyme replacement therapy in Fabry disease: a randomized controlled trial. JAMA 285(21): 2743–2749

75. Kampmann C, Baehner F, Kim KS, Bajbouj M, Beck M (2002) Influence of Enzyme Replacement Therapy (ERT) on Anderson Fabry Disease associated Hypertrophic Infiltrative Cardiomyopathy (HIC). Eur J Pediatr 161(2):R5

76. Hughes DA, Elliott PM, Shah J, Zuckerman J, Coghlan G, Brookes J et al (2008) Effects of enzyme replacement therapy on the cardiomyopathy of Anderson-Fabry disease: a randomised, double-blind, placebo-controlled clinical trial of agalsidase alfa. Heart 94(2):153–158

77. Beck M (2009) Agalsidase alfa for the treatment of Fabry disease: new data on clinical efficacy and safety. Expert Opin Biol Ther 9(2):255–261
78. Beck M, Ricci R, Widmer U, Dehout F, de Lorenzo AG, Kampmann C et al (2004) Fabry disease: overall effects of agalsidase alfa treatment. Eur J Clin Invest 34(12):838–844
79. Whybra C, Miebach E, Mengel E, Gal A, Baron K, Beck M et al (2009) A 4-year study of the efficacy and tolerability of enzyme replacement therapy with agalsidase alfa in 36 women with Fabry disease. Genet Med 11(6):441–449
80. Kampmann C, Linhart A, Devereux RB, Schiffmann R (2009) Effect of agalsidase alfa replacement therapy on fabry disease-related hypertrophic cardiomyopathy: a 12- to 36-month, retrospective, blinded echocardiographic pooled analysis. Clin Ther 31(9):1966–1976
81. Schiffmann R, Ries M, Timmons M, Flaherty JT, Brady RO (2006) Long-term therapy with agalsidase alfa for Fabry disease: safety and effects on renal function in a home infusion setting. Nephrol Dial Transplant 21(2):345–354
82. Weidemann F, Breunig F, Beer M, Sandstede J, Turschner O, Voelker W et al (2003) Improvement of cardiac function during enzyme replacement therapy in patients with Fabry disease: a prospective strain rate imaging study. Circulation 108(11):1299–1301
83. Spinelli L, Pisani A, Sabbatini M, Petretta M, Andreucci MV, Procaccini D et al (2004) Enzyme replacement therapy with agalsidase beta improves cardiac involvement in Fabry's disease. Clin Genet 66(2):158–165
84. Weidemann F, Niemann M, Breunig F, Herrmann S, Beer M, Stork S et al (2009) Long-term effects of enzyme replacement therapy on fabry cardiomyopathy: evidence for a better outcome with early treatment. Circulation 119(4):524–529
85. Pisani A, Spinelli L, Sabbatini M, Andreucci MV, Procaccini D, Abbaterusso C et al (2005) Enzyme replacement therapy in Fabry disease patients undergoing dialysis: effects on quality of life and organ involvement. Am J Kidney Dis 46(1):120–127
86. Kalliokoski RJ, Kantola I, Kalliokoski KK, Engblom E, Sundell J, Hannukainen JC et al (2006) The effect of 12-month enzyme replacement therapy on myocardial perfusion in patients with Fabry disease. J Inherit Metab Dis 29(1):112–118
87. Breunig F, Weidemann F, Strotmann J, Knoll A, Wanner C (2006) Clinical benefit of enzyme replacement therapy in Fabry disease. Kidney Int 69(7):1216–1221
88. Beer M, Weidemann F, Breunig F, Knoll A, Koeppe S, Machann W et al (2006) Impact of enzyme replacement therapy on cardiac morphology and function and late enhancement in Fabry's cardiomyopathy. Am J Cardiol 97(10):1515–1518
89. Vedder AC, Breunig F, Donker-Koopman WE, Mills K, Young E, Winchester B et al (2008) Treatment of Fabry disease with different dosing regimens of agalsidase: effects on antibody formation and GL-3. Mol Genet Metab 94(3):319–325
90. Eng CM, Guffon N, Wilcox WR, Germain DP, Lee P, Waldek S et al (2001) Safety and efficacy of recombinant human alpha-galactosidase A–replacement therapy in Fabry's disease. N Engl J Med 345(1):9–16
91. Mehta A, Clarke JT, Giugliani R, Elliott P, Linhart A, Beck M et al (2009) Natural course of Fabry disease: changing pattern of causes of death in FOS – Fabry Outcome Survey. J Med Genet 46(8):548–552
92. Banikazemi M, Bultas J, Waldek S, Wilcox WR, Whitley CB, McDonald M et al (2007) Agalsidase-beta therapy for advanced Fabry disease: a randomized trial. Ann Intern Med 146(2):77–86

Chapter 12
Renal Manifestations of Fabry Disease

**David G. Warnock, Carmen Valbuena, Michael West,
and João Paulo Oliveira**

Abstract The majority of Fabry patients have kidney involvement (nephropathy), with significant proteinuria and progressive loss of kidney function leading to end-stage-renal-disease. Baseline assessment of the severity of Fabry nephropathy, institution of appropriate therapy, and close monitoring of the subsequent course is essential. Once present, target kidney damage is not reversed, so stopping further progression is the treatment goal. Fabry nephropathy is treatable, even in patients with fairly advanced disease. While the cornerstone of therapy remains enzyme replacement therapy with agalsidase preparations, this treatment alone does not reduce urine protein excretion. Treatment with angiotensin converting enzyme inhibitors or angiotensin receptor blockers must be added to enzyme replacement therapy to reduce urine protein excretion with the goal that this will stabilize kidney function. Kidney function, with estimated glomerular filtration rate based on serum creatinine, and measurements of urinary protein should be obtained at every clinic visit, and the rate of loss of function followed over time. Anti-proteinuric therapy can be dosed to a pre-specified urine protein target rather than a specific blood pressure goal, recognizing that successful therapy will usually lower the blood pressure below the goal of 130/80 mmHg used for other forms of kidney disease. The overall goal for treating Fabry nephropathy is to reduce the rate of loss of glomerular filtration rate to ≤ -1.0 ml/min/1.73 m^2/year, which is that seen in the normal adult population.

Keywords Chronic kidney disease · Focal glomerular sclerosis · Glomerular filtration rate · Proteinuria · Renal biopsy

Abbreviations

ACEI	Angiotensin converting enzyme inhibitor
ARB	Angiotensin receptor blocker
CKD	Chronic kidney disease

D.G. Warnock (✉)
Division of Nephrology, Department of Medicine, University of Alabama, Birmingham, AL, USA
e-mail: dwarnock@uab.edu

D. Elstein et al. (eds.), *Fabry Disease*, DOI 10.1007/978-90-481-9033-1_12,
© Springer Science+Business Media B.V. 2010

eGFR   Estimated GFR
EM   Electron microscopy
ESRD   End-stage renal disease
ERT   Enzyme replacement therapy
GFR   Glomerular filtration rate
GLA   The α-galactosidase A locus
GL-3   Globotriaosylceramide
mGFR   Measured GFR

12.1 Fabry Nephropathy

Chronic kidney disease (CKD), progressing to end-stage renal disease (ESRD), has been a major cause of morbidity and early mortality in adult male with the classical Fabry phenotype [1, 2]. As is typical for X-linked genetic diseases, heterozygous females with α-galactosidase A gene (*GLA*) mutations generally have a more variable, less severe and later-onset clinical course compared to males Fabry patients [1, 2]. However, a substantial proportion of heterozygous females ultimately develop significant clinical complications, including CKD and ESRD [3–9].

Although the patients originally described in 1898 by William Anderson and by Johannes Fabry had proteinuria, and despite subsequent reports of urinary abnormalities in typically affected patients, Fabry disease was long regarded as a dermatologic condition – '*Angiokeratoma Corporis Diffusum*'. It was not until the first autopsy studies [10, 11] that Fabry disease was recognized as a systemic lipoid storage disorder, with major involvement of the cardiovascular system and the kidneys [12]. Although the majority of classically affected patients were males [13–15], the kidney pathology was identical for males and females [16].

The main clinical features of Fabry nephropathy were described in the early 1960s [14, 17, 18]: proteinuria developing in childhood and adolescence, followed by continued decline of renal function in early adulthood, eventually reaching ESRD in the third to the fifth decade of life. It was later recognised that heterozygous females occasionally present with the classical phenotype of Fabry disease, including ESRD [19], and that patients who lacked the neuropathic, cutaneous and ocular manifestations of classical Fabry disease could still develop progressive CKD [20].

Not infrequently, patients without a family history of the Fabry disease are first diagnosed by nephrologists, in the investigation of proteinuric CKD, most often on renal biopsy [2]. Therefore, any physician involved in the diagnosis and treatment of Fabry patients should be aware of the renal manifestations of Fabry disease, just as nephrologists should be familiar with the most common extra-renal features.

12.2 Diagnosis of Fabry Nephropathy

In patients with the diagnosis of Fabry disease the finding of microalbuminuria, overt proteinuria and/or progressive CKD are presumptive evidence of Fabry nephropathy. Increased urinary excretion of globotriaosylceramide (GL-3) further supports the diagnosis of Fabry nephropathy in both genders, including children [21], although some females may have normal GL-3 excretion. Atypical clinical presentations for Fabry nephropathy, including acute nephritic syndrome, acute onset of the severe nephrotic syndrome, severe hypertension early in the course of progressive CKD, rapidly progressive loss of function, and macroscopic hematuria, are indications for diagnostic kidney biopsy [9, 22]. Minimal change nephropathy [23], IgA nephropathy [24–27], crescentic glomerulonephritis [28–30], granulomatous interstitial nephritis [30] and lupus nephritis [31, 32] have been described as coexisting renal disorders in patients with Fabry nephropathy, again requiring kidney biopsy for definitive diagnosis. The finding of multiple parapelvic renal cysts in the diagnostic workup of a patient with CKD also suggests consideration of Fabry disease in the differential diagnosis [33].

Electron microscopy intracellular lamellated inclusions similar to that seen in Fabry nephropathy have been reported in patients with silicosis [34, 35] or who have been exposed to certain drugs, including chloroquine [36–38]. Aminoglycoside antibiotics can cause lysosomal changes referred to as 'myelin bodies', but these are typically located in proximal tubules and not in the glomeruli [39]. The finding of typical glycosphingolipid deposits in a kidney biopsy specimen, especially when the glomerular epithelial cells are involved, is an important histologic clue for Fabry nephropathy, but the definitive diagnosis must be confirmed by identifying the causative *GLA* gene mutation, particularly in female patients [9, 40].

12.3 Clinical and Laboratory Manifestations of Fabry Nephropathy

The clinical and laboratory manifestations of Fabry nephropathy are expression of the accumulation of GL-3 and other neutral glycosphingolipids in the renal parenchyma and its consequences upon glomerular and tubular function, as reflected in the urine composition.

Even in early stages of Fabry nephropathy, red blood cells, white blood cells, and hyaline and granular casts can be found in the urine sediment [1, 41]. Birefringent lipid globules, with the characteristic 'Maltese cross' appearance, may also be noted with polarised light microscopy. These globules are present either free in the urine or within desquamated uroepithelial cells. Lipid-laden renal tubular cells account for about 75% of the exfoliated cells in the urine sediment of classically affected Fabry patients [42].

Studies of tubular reabsorption, and secretion were first described 50 years ago [16, 43, 44]. Defects of the proximal and distal tubules, out of proportion to the decrease of GFR, have also been demonstrated [44]. Signs of proximal tubular dysfunction included low tubular maximum reabsorption for glucose and low tubular maximum secretion for para-aminohippuric acid. Defective renal acidifying mechanisms, with reduced net acid excretion, particularly of urinary ammonium excretion, signify line distal tubule dysfunction. Hypokalemia has also been rarely observed as a very early manifestation of Fabry nephropathy [45], and can be accentuated when lymphedema is mistakenly treated with aggressive diuretic therapy [J-P Oliveira, personal observation]. It is possible that glycosphingolipid deposits in the principal and intercalated cells of the renal collecting ducts alter tubular potassium reabsorption, and enhance net potassium secretion [46]. The heterogeneity of the renal tubular disorders associated with the early stages of Fabry nephropathy may be related to the variable degrees of glycolipid accumulation in the tubule epithelial cells [44].

An inability to maximally concentrate the urine, and even isosthenuria, has been the most commonly reported tubular function abnormality in Fabry disease, and was demonstrated even in patients with normal glomerular filtration rate (GFR) [16, 43]. The urinary concentration defect may be the earliest functional manifestation of Fabry renal disease, leading to polyuria, nocturia, and polydipsia [2]. Vasopressin-resistant (nephrogenic) diabetes insipidus has been demonstrated in adult males with Fabry disease [16] as well as in children [45].

Most patients with classic Fabry disease develop proteinuria [1, 41], although the severity of the proteinuria is more marked in males than females [5, 8]. Before the age of 18 years, microalbuminuria or overt proteinuria are present in a minority of patients of both genders [47–49], even in children with residual α-galactosidase activity >1% normal [47]. By the age of 35 years, about 50% of the affected males are estimated to have proteinuria, and all patients who survive into the 6th decade of life eventually develop proteinuria [2]. In almost all cases, proteinuria is of glomerular origin, containing ≥50% albumin. Nephrotic range proteinuria develops in less than 20% of male Fabry patients with CKD [2, 5, 8]. However, the full clinical and laboratory presentation of nephrotic syndrome is not frequent [2]: hypoalbuminemia and hyperlipidemia were respectively seen in only 26 and 21% of patients with nephrotic-range proteinuria [50].

Progressive decline of renal function is a common complication of Fabry disease, particularly of the classically affected males [1, 2, 41]. Figure 12.1 shows the clinical course of a young male patient, who starting at age 14, rapidly progressed to ESRD. He had microalbuminuria, until age 18, with loss of nearly half of his GFR. He then developed hypertension and overt proteinuria, with continued inexorable decline in GFR at −11.5 ml/min/1.73 m^2/year [9]. Enzyme replacement therapy (ERT) was started very late in the course, but without control of his hypertension and proteinuria, he progressed to ESRD by the age of 23.4 years.

A minority of Fabry patients have decreased GFR before the age of 18 years [47, 49, 51], but cases of ESRD have been reported as early as in the second decade of life [52]. By 43 years of age, an estimated 50% of male Fabry patients have serum creatinine levels ≥1.5 mg/dl (estimated GFR (eGFR) <60 ml/min/1.73 m^2 by the CKD-EPI equation [53]), and an estimated 50% develop ESRD by the age of 53 years [2]. After serum creatinine reaches ≥1.5 mg/dl, the time of progression to ESRD is variable, ranging from ~1 year to >12 years [2]. The mean age of patients who have estimated GFR <30 ml/min/1.73 m^2 is not significantly different between genders and some of these patients reach the most advanced CKD stages only in

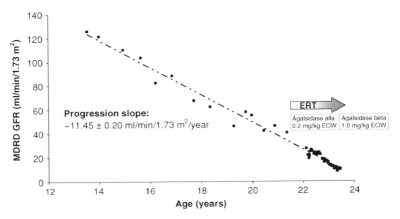

Fig. 12.1 Progressive, severe loss of glomerular filtration in a young male with Fabry disease. The urine albumin/creatinine ratio averaged 25 mg/mmol (221 mg/g) until age 18 and 188 mg/mmol (1,663 mg/g) thereafter (normal 3.8 mg/mmol; 33.6 mg/g). The systemic blood pressure averaged 114/76 until age 18, and 139/92 thereafter despite multiple antihypertensive agents. Agalsidase alfa was instituted at age 21.6 at 0.2 mg/kg every other week when the eGFR was 41 ml/min/ 1.72 m^2, and then switched to agalsidase beta at 1 mg/kg every week at age 23 when the eGFR was 15 ml/min/1.73 m^2. Kidney function steadily declined, attributable to late institution of enzyme replacement therapy, and inadequate control of the blood pressure and proteinuria. The rate of decline of kidney function was -11.45 ± 0.2 ml/min/1.73 m^2/year between the ages of 13.5 and 23.4 years (reprinted with permission from Oqvist et al. [9])

the eighth decade of life [5, 9]. The prevalence of anemia is higher among CKD patients with Fabry disease as compared to the general CKD population, at similar CKD stages [54, 55].

Regular assessment of eGFR and proteinuria is mandatory, with a frequency that should be related to the baseline severity. Changes in eGFR can be followed over time, recognizing the limitations of the estimating equations, especially when 'hyperfiltration' [56] >135 ml/min/1.73 m^2 is present [57]. Similar concerns have been expressed about estimates of GFR in children with Fabry disease. In a recent study from the Fabry Registry [49], the majority of children had estimated GFR values (using the Schwartz eGFR formula from 1976 [58]) that were higher than expected for healthy children and adolescents of the same age. The study by Tøndel et al. reported a significant increase in eGFR when compared to GFR measured as plasma iohexol clearance [59].

Plasma clearance techniques with clearance markers or radionuclide are currently viewed as the most accurate methods for measuring GFR, as indirect methods have previously overestimated GFR above 90 ml/min/1.73 m^2 [53]. It can be expected that the extended validation range of the CKD-EPI equation for eGFR [53] will reduce the prevalence of apparent hyperfiltration in patients with Fabry nephropathy. Figure 12.2 presents comparisons of estimated GFR versus measured GFR, comparing the Modification of Diet in Renal Disease eGFR equation [60] in Fig. 12.2a to the CKD-EPI equation for eGFR [53] in Fig. 12.2b; there is less variability around

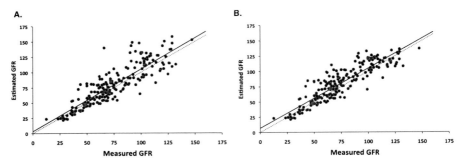

Fig. 12.2 Linear Regression Plots Comparing Measured Glomerular Filtration Rate to estimated GFR with 214 paired measurements. GFR was measured with [99]technetium DTPA clearance (data provided by M. West, personal communication). (**A**) Using the Modification of Diet in Renal Disease equation [60], the regression slope was 1.019 ± 0.038 (SE; 95% CI, 0.982–1.057, $P < 0.0001$; $r^2 = 0.772$), and the intercept was 3.229 ± 3.304 ml/min/1.73 m^2. (**B**) Using the CKD-EPI estimating equation [53], the regression slope was 0.980 ± 0.033 (SE; 95% CI, 0.948–1.013, $P < 0.0001$; $r^2 = 0.812$), and the intercept was 6.984 ± 2.587 ml/min/1.73 m^2

the regression with the CKD-EPI equation, and more importantly, there is a balanced distribution of data points above and below the solid regression line, especially for eGFR >90 ml/min/1.73 m^2.

The variability of eGFR compared to measured GFR is evaluated with Bland-Altman plots [61] in Fig. 12.3. The 2 Standard Deviation confidence band was narrower for the CKD-EPI estimating equation [53] compared to the Modification of Diet in Renal Disease equation [60]. The improved accuracy of the CKD-EPI estimating equation is not surprising because the Modification of Diet in Renal Disease equation had never been validated for GFR values >60 ml/min/1.73 m^2 [60]. Figure 12.3 shows that there were fewer outliers and a better distribution of values above and below the solid horizontal line, especially for GFR values >90 ml/min/1.73 m^2 for the CKD-EPI equation compared to the Modification of Diet in Renal Disease equation. It appears that much of the 'hyperfiltration' described in Fabry nephropathy can be explained by the limitations of the previous estimating equation, providing of course that these observations can be confirmed with other cohorts. For adult patients, the CKD-EPI equation [53] for eGFR should be used, and for children, the newly described Schwartz equation [62] appears to be the preferred approach for estimating GFR. Nonetheless, there remain a few adults with Fabry nephropathy and true hyperfiltration based on measured GFR [57]. Whether hyperfiltration presages a later fall in GFR in unknown; during ERT these patients had a rapid decline in GFR to the normal range consistent with disease progression or with treatment benefit. This normalization of GFR was also observed in children during ERT albeit with GFR calculated by the Counahan-Barratt formula [63] with the attendant overestimate of GFR [64].

For both genders, the proportion of patients with overt proteinuria, the magnitude of the proteinuria and the prevalence of nephrotic range proteinuria are higher with more advanced CKD stages [5, 8]. However, the role of proteinuria upon the rate

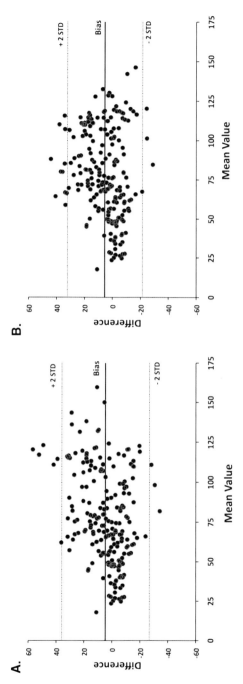

Fig. 12.3 Bland Altman Plots Comparing measured Glomerular Filtration Rate to estimated GFR with 214 paired measurements. GFR was measured ^{99}technetium DTPA clearance (data provided by M. West, personal communication). (**A**) Using the Modification of Diet in Renal Disease equation [60], the estimated GFR exceeded measured GFR by 4.36 ml/min/1.73 m^2 at the zero intercept (bias), and the ±2 standard deviation range was −26.6 to 36.0 ml/min/1.73 m^2. (**B**) Using the CKD-EPI estimating equation [53], the estimated GFR exceeded measured GFR by 5.11 ml/min/1.73 m^2 at the zero intercept (bias), and the ±2 standard deviation range was −21.4 to 32.3 ml/min/1.73 m^2

of CKD progression has been questioned [2, 4, 50]. Proteinuria develops in most patients with Fabry nephropathy, and there seems to be a general relation between the rate of loss of kidney function and the magnitude of the proteinuria, especially in male patients [8]. When adult males and females are stratified by baseline eGFR and proteinuria values, the rates of loss of kidney function are similar (Fig. 12.4). Among adult patients with an estimated GFR ≥ 60 ml/min/1.73 m^2, albuminuria can be demonstrated in 55% of the males and 35% of the females [5]. Nevertheless, about 10% of hemizygous males and 30% of heterozygous females reach stage 3 CKD without developing overt proteinuria [5], suggesting that other risk factors for progressive loss of GFR need to be considered, especially in females.

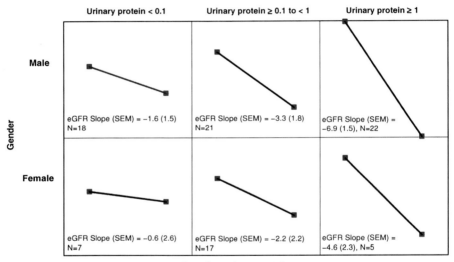

Fig. 12.4 Natural History of Fabry Nephropathy. eGFR progression slopes (ml/min/1.73 m^2/year) for male and female patients stratified by baseline 24-h urinary protein excretion (g/24 h). The y-axis represents eGFR (ml/min/1.73 m^2) and the x-axis in each panel represents a 12-month span. SEM = standard error of the mean (reproduced with permission from Schiffmann et al. [8])

Hypertension is less prevalent in CKD Fabry patients than in the general CKD population, at comparable levels of GFR [5]. More than 60% of the Fabry patients who developed hypertension did so concurrently with, or after serum creatinine reached ≥ 1.5 mg/dl (eGFR <60 ml/min/1.73 m^2) [2]. Proteinuria positively correlates with systolic blood pressure in adult males and females [5]. Kleinert et al. [65] observed systolic blood pressure ≥ 130 mmHg or diastolic blood pressure ≥ 80 mmHg in 57% of men and 47% of women among 391 patients with Fabry disease who were participating in the Fabry Outcome Survey. In both the Fabry Outcome Survey and the Fabry Registry, blood pressures were more elevated with more severe Fabry nephropathy as reflected in the eGFR [5, 65].

Among classically affected males and female carriers, renal ultrasonography and magnetic resonance imaging abnormalities, including renal atrophy, cortical and parapelvic cysts, decreased cortical thickness, increased echogenicity, and decreased corticomedullary differentiation, were detected in 64.5 and 60%, respectively [66], although this high prevalence has not been confirmed at other centers (D. Warnock, personal observation). No imaging abnormalities were present in males aged <12 years and females aged <20 years. In both genders, the occurrence and number of abnormalities increased with age in males and females. Cysts, particularly parapelvic cysts, were more common and appeared earlier than in the general population [66]. With magnetic resonance and computed tomography imaging, multiple renal sinus cysts were documented in 50% classically affected males with Fabry disease, aged 20–49 years [33]. An example of large non-communicating parapelvic cysts in a 42-year old male patient is shown in Fig. 12.5. The cause and significance of such cysts remain unknown.

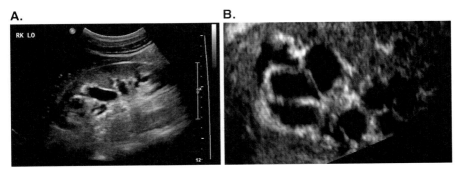

Fig. 12.5 Kidney ultrasonography of 42 year old male with Fabry disease (blood pressure 120/80; eGFR = 73 ml/min/1.73 m^2; urine protein/c.reatinine ratio = 0.10 g/g on 10 mg/day lisinopril). (**A**) Conventional gray-scale saggital image. (**B**) Coronal reformatted ultrasound false colored image generated from a volume acquisition showing multiple non-communicating parapelvic cysts embedded in the central echo complex of the right kidney (Images courtesy of Franklin Tessler, MD CM, Professor of Radiology, University of Alabama at Birmingham)

12.4 The Epidemiology of Fabry Disease and Nephropathy

Before the availability of kidney transplantation and dialysis for long-term renal replacement therapy, survival of classically affected males beyond the 5th decade of life was exceptional and most patients died in uremia [14, 67], at an average age of 41 years [68]. More recently, median [69] and mean [2] survival times of affected males were estimated as 50 years and death was attributed to a large variety of causes, other than ESRD. In patients undergoing long-term renal replacement therapy, the late cardiac and cerebrovascular complications of Fabry disease may become the major causes of morbidity and mortality [1, 70].

The prevalence of Fabry disease among patients on renal replacement therapy was 18.8/100,000 and 16.7/100,000, respectively in the European [71] and the United States ESRD registries [72]. These figures are about 10- to 45-fold higher than prevalence estimates in the general population [73, 74]. In both registries, approximately 12% of patients with the diagnosis of Fabry disease were women. The mean age of Fabry patients at the beginning of renal replacement therapy, was 38 years in Europe [71] and 42 years in the United States [72]. Overall, when renal replacement therapy was initiated, roughly 50% of the Fabry patients were aged between 35 and 44 years, slightly less than 10% were younger than 24 years and 10% were aged 55 or more years; these estimates that have not changed over the intervening 20 years [9].

In a large cohort of US patients who initiated dialysis between 1985 and 1993, the 3-year survival of Fabry patients was significantly lower (63% vs. 74%) and their median survival was roughly 2 years less as compared to matched non-diabetic hemodialysis controls [72]; diabetic and non-diabetic controls were matched with Fabry patients for age, gender, race, year of dialysis initiation and modality. The survival curves for Fabry patients and non-diabetic controls began to diverge after approximately 1.5 years. A comparable 3-year survival estimate of 60% was reported in Europe [71]: patient survival on dialysis was 41% at 5 years, compared to 68% in patients with non-diabetic ESRD. These studies need to be revisited now that the awareness of Fabry disease as a cause of ESRD is better recognized in the nephrology community [9].

Ten-year renal allograft and patient survival were similar in patients with Fabry disease and matched controls, in Europe [71] as well as in the United States [75]. In the American cohort, 1-, 5-, and 10-year graft survival (respectively 91, 76, and 56%) was statistically similar to the graft survival in control patients, reflecting the transplant experience in the late 1990s. Cumulative patient survival was estimated as 83% at 5 years and 67% at 10 years post-transplantation, also not significantly different from matched controls [75]. The analysis of a much larger cohort of Fabry patients who received a kidney transplant between 1997 and 2007 in the United States demonstrated 5-year graft and patient survival rates respectively of 74 and 81% [70]. Graft survival was similar, and dialysis-free patient survival was superior for patients with Fabry disease compared to a matched cohort of patients with other causes of ESRD, implying that Fabry disease did not recur in the allografts in any significant fashion [76]; the risk of returning to dialysis was 40% lower for the Fabry patients compared with the matched cohort, but their risk of death was roughly two-fold higher [70]. Overall, these data favour kidney transplantation as the renal replacement therapy of choice for appropriate patients with ESRD due to Fabry nephropathy, either pre-emptively or within a few years following the start of dialysis. In addition, the fact that Fabry patient survival was decreased despite equivalent graft survival and better dialysis-free survival could be used to argue for prospective studies of the efficacy of ERT for incident cardiovascular and cerebrovascular events in Fabry patients who have undergone renal transplantation.

12.5 Phenotype/Genotype Correlations and Residual Enzyme Activity

A broad correlation exists between the level of α-galactosidase A activity and the clinical manifestations of Fabry disease [1]. Residual α-galactosidase A activity is inversely related with the rate of deterioration of renal function in males with Fabry disease; patients with undetectable enzyme expression, or residual α-galactosidase activity in leukocytes below 1% normal, reached serum creatinine concentrations ≥1.5 mg/dl (eGFR <60 ml/min/1.73 m^2) at a younger age than patients with higher residual α-galactosidase activities [2]. In the former group, creatinine levels ≥1.5 mg/dl were already reached by patients <25 years of age, while none with residual α-galactosidase activities >1% normal reached that creatinine level before the age of 45 years. By the age of 55 years, none of the surviving patients with α-galactosidase activity <1% normal had serum creatinine <1.5 mg/dl, whereas a number of patients with higher residual enzyme activities had maintained their eGFR >60 ml/min/1.73 m^2 [2].

As expected from structural predictions [77, 78], the type of *GLA* mutation correlated with the level of α-galactosidase activity, thereby influencing the age of onset and progression of CKD, at least in male patients. Conservative missense mutations were associated with significantly higher mean residual α-galactosidase activity (6.8% of normal) as compared to non-conservative missense mutations (1.0% of normal) or with nonsense, deletion or insertion mutations (0.8% of normal) [2]. None of the male patients with missense conservative mutations had eGFR ≤60 ml/min/1.73 m^2, in contrast to male patients with the other types of mutations for whom eGFR ≤60 ml/min/1.73 m^2, could be observed as soon as the third decade of life. As mentioned before, there is a fairly large subset of female patients with Fabry nephropathy but minimal proteinuria [5]. With the exception of the distinctly unusual compound heterozygotes or homozygotes, female patients usually have some residual enzyme activity [79]. The association of measurable α-galactosidase activity, as well as other risk factors for progression (e.g., proteinuria, systolic hypertension, smoking, hyperlipidemia) needs to be carefully considered for female as well as male patients with Fabry nephropathy.

12.6 The Renal and Cardiac Variant Phenotypes

The residual α-galactosidase A activity threshold for progressive kidney disease appears to be lower than for heart disease, as patients with the 'renal phenotype' and progressive CKD also develop left ventricular hypertrophy, but patients with the 'cardiac phenotype' may have proteinuria but generally do not develop progressive CKD. Patients lacking the classic early presentation with neuropathic, cutaneous and ocular manifestations of Fabry disease, but who otherwise developed progressive CKD, have long been recognized [20]. More recently, screening of 514 Japanese adult males on maintenance hemodialysis led to the diagnosis of Fabry disease in six patients whose ESRD had been originally attributed to 'chronic glomerulonephritis' [80]. Their median age at the start of hemodialysis was 49 years, ranging from 25 to 56 years. Expressed as a percentage of the normal control mean, residual α-galactosidase A activity ranged from 2 to 28% (median: 4.5%) in lymphocytes and from 7 to 28% (median: 12%) in plasma. None of the patients had angiokeratomas or corneal dystrophy but five of six had left ventricular hypertrophy of moderate to severe degree. In one of the cases, a kidney biopsy was initially classified as 'glomerulosclerosis', but re-evaluation of the original biopsy specimen, with appropriate fixation for electron microscopy, demonstrated typical features of Fabry nephropathy; in retrospect, this patient appeared to have had classical Fabry disease and progressed to ESRD [80].

The 'renal variant' phenotype, especially in the absence of known family history of Fabry disease, may be particularly difficult to recognize. Even when a kidney biopsy is available, the diagnosis may be missed if the histological examination is limited to routine light microscopy [9]. In CKD or ESRD patients diagnosed with chronic glomerulonephritis, hypertension, or with an unknown cause for the ESRD, the presence of otherwise unexplained left ventricular hypertrophy of moderate to severe degree may be a clinical indication to specifically screen for Fabry disease [1].

In large scale, nationwide Fabry disease screening programs among patients with ESRD, either on chronic dialysis or transplanted, the frequency of undiagnosed cases of Fabry disease in males ranged from 0.07 to 0.15%, respectively in Austrian chronic dialysis [81] and transplant [82] cohorts, to 0.26% in Czech hemodialysis patients [83]. However, in both countries, the overall prevalence of Fabry disease among males on dialysis or transplanted, including the previously known cases as well as the newly discovered, was 263/100,000. These data are in agreement with results of a screening programme of 37,104 consecutive Italian male neonates [84], which demonstrated a 7- to 11-fold higher prevalence of *GLA* mutations associated with variant phenotypes of Fabry disease, as compared to mutations known to cause classic phenotype. In the combined analysis of several smaller case-finding studies among Japanese patients in maintenance hemodialysis [80, 85–87] the frequency of Fabry disease in males was as high as 0.72% (720/100,000), with an 80% rate of formerly unsuspected diagnoses. Other screening studies in Canada have failed to identify a single case of Fabry disease in over 1,300 patients [88] [M. West, personal communication]. Taken together, these data suggest that the prevalence of Fabry disease may vary widely in different populations and that many patients remain under-diagnosed, even in those with severe kidney involvement. It is also possible that *GLA* mutations associated with the 'renal variant' phenotype may have a non-homogeneous geographic distribution. While the prevalence, especially of 'late onset' variants reported by Spada et al. [84] was somewhat surprising, the concordance between the prevalence reported in that study, and the results from screening hemodialysis patients for Fabry disease has several important implications: the strategy of screening high risk cohorts for Fabry disease has merit [9]; the mutations associated with some residual activity that present with clinical findings later in life clearly have the potential of causing ESRD in some of the patients. The benefit of ascertaining index cases, even though they have already reached ESRD, is the opportunity to diagnose affected relatives at earlier stages of disease.

A 'cardiac variant' of Fabry disease, mainly presenting as left ventricular hypertrophy, has also been described [1, 89, 90]. Patients with hypertrophic cardiomyopathy represent an important population that merits systematic screening for Fabry disease [89, 90]. Patients with cardiac variant Fabry disease can develop proteinuria as early as the third decade, and usually have glycosphingolipid accumulation limited to podocytes. These patients do not usually have progressive CDK or reach ESRD. It has been postulated [1] that the development of progressive CKD in Fabry disease results from glycosphingolipid storage in the renal vascular endothelial cells and, to a lesser extent, in the interstitial and mesangial cells, and is not explained by glycosphingolipid inclusions limited to the podocytes. A mechanistic explanation is offered by the fact that patients with the cardiac variant phenotype are more likely to have residual α-galactosidase activities ranging from $\sim$1 to 10% of normal, with cases reported with up to 30% residual enzyme activity in plasma [91]. Altarescu and Elstein [92] posited that cardiac involvement is the sine qua non of Fabry disease, and hence will be seen in all male patients in an age-related association.

Males with the cardiac variant maintain renal function longer than classically affected males, and usually do not progress to ESRD. Their demise is attributable to severe left-sided heart failure and/or ventricular arrhythmias. Takenaka et al. [93] described severe left ventricular dysfunction and tachyarrhythmias in a group of 7 elderly males Fabry patients with the late-onset cardiac variant. From data in that report, it is possible to determine that their kidney function was well preserved in the terminal phases of their disease with an eGFR of 72.6 ml/min/ 1.73 m^2 (Table 12.1). On average, this group had 11.9 $\pm$ 1.8 (SEM) percent of residual enzyme activity, emphasizing that preservation of kidney function requires less residual α-galactosidase A enzyme activity than is required for protection against Fabry cardiomyopathy.

Table 12.1 Kidney function in males with end-stage cardiac variant Fabry disease*

Patient ID	Age (years)	Serum creatinine (mg/dl)	Plasma α-galactosidase A activity (% normal)	eGFR*
1	68	1.4	0.90	87.5
2	66	1.2	1.10	69.6
3	63	1.5	0.90	90.6
4	64	0.4	1.10	70.6
5	83	0.7	1.20	55.6
6	78	1.7	1.00	71.8
7	66	1.4	1.20	62.6
Mean $\pm$ SEM	69.7 $\pm$ 2.9	1.2 $\pm$ 1.8	1.10 $\pm$ 0.05	72.6 $\pm$ 4.8

*Data obtained from reference [93]. Estimated glomerular filtration rate (eGFR) estimated with the CKD-EPI equation [53]; expressed as ml/min/1.73 m^2

12.7 Glycosphingolipid Accumulation in Fabry Nephropathy

GL-3 and galabiosylceramide, the major neutral glycosphingolipids that accumulate in patients with Fabry disease, were first identified in extracts of kidney tissue obtained at the autopsy of a 28-year-old male with classic disease, who had died in renal failure [94]. The relative concentration of galabiosylceramide was one-third that of GL-3, which accumulates in all affected tissues of Fabry patients, while galabiosylceramide has more limited organ distribution [95]. The kidneys are major sites of glycosphingolipid deposition in Fabry disease and electron microscopy (EM) shows inclusions in all types of kidney cells, despite their normal appearance by conventional histology, even in patients with normal renal function and no proteinuria [96, 97]. The accumulation of glycosphingolipids in the kidneys starts in prenatal life and rudimentary deposits have been observed in podocytes of an aborted male foetus, at 19 weeks of gestational age [98]. Although the description of the pathology and most of the current concepts of Fabry nephropathy have been derived from autopsy and biopsy studies of affected males, it has since long been recognized that heterozygous females develop the same kidney lesions observed in males [96].

GL-3 is one of the most abundant glycolipids in the human kidney [99] and globoside, its metabolic precursor, is also a normal constituent of kidney tissue [100]. In all the neutral glycosphingolipid fractions isolated from the human kidney, C18-sphingosine constitute the predominant fraction and the fatty acid composition shows a characteristic common pattern with C22:0, C24:0, and C24:1 as the predominant isoforms [99]. GL-3 synthase is strongly expressed in the kidney [101] while the globoside synthase is expressed at a relatively low level [101]. Inhibitors of the first step in the biosynthetic pathway, glucosylceramide synthase, are currently being developed as small molecules for the treatment of lysosomal storage disease [102, 103].

GL-3 is a cell surface receptor for the B-subunit of Shiga-toxins (Verotoxins) [104]. It is expressed in the kidney [105], by many different cell types including podocytes, mesangial cells, endothelial cells, and proximal and distal tubular cells [106]. With standard immunohistochemistry of paraffin section, expression of GL3 can be observed in <1% of human tubular cortical cells [C. Valbuena, personal observation]. In human uroepithelial cells, GL-3 and globoside are iso-receptors for different molecular variants of the adhesin molecules of uropathogenic *Escherichia coli* [35]. In cultured human glomerular and tubular kidney epithelial cells, GL-3 expression at the cell membrane is inversely related to α-galactosidase expression [107].

Taken together, these data suggest that most of the neutral glycosphingolipids that accumulate in the kidneys of patients with Fabry disease is endogenously produced by normal metabolic and catabolic pathways. The fatty acid profiles of plasma GL-3 [108] and in the urine [109] are consistent with this assumption. Furthermore, the observations that Fabry nephropathy does not clinically recur in transplanted kidneys [76], and that the typical baseline kidney pathology of the transplanted kidney from an asymptomatic heterozygous donor to her non-affected daughter did not change over time [110], also supporting the foregoing hypothesis.

12.8 Pathology of Fabry Nephropathy

Glycosphingolipids consist of a hydrophilic carbohydrate moiety linked to a hydrophobic ceramide tail, which is composed of a sphingoid long-chain base in amide linkage to a fatty acid. Glycosphingolipids are important structural and functional components of cell membranes and their physiological breakdown occurs stepwise within lysososomes, by the action of acid hydrolases [108]. As ceramide tails are dissolved during the paraffin-embedding procedure, the most characteristic finding on routine light microscopy of kidney biopsies (Fig. 12.6) is vacuolation of podocytes, of parietal epithelial cells of Bowman's capsule, and of Henle's loop and distal tubular cells [96, 111–113]. Mesangial widening, focal segmental glomerular sclerosis and global sclerosis, tubular atrophy, interstitial fibrosis and other nonspecific lesions are additionally seen, even at the early stages of Fabry nephropathy [96]. In adolescents, these changes have been shown to be present in kidney biopsies even before any clinical signs of Fabry nephropathy are detected [59].

While in paraffin-embedded specimens the vacuoles look empty, and staining with lipid-soluble dyes is negative [96, 114, 115], the presence of GL-3 within vacuoles may still be demonstrated in formalin-fixed, paraffin-embedded kidney biopsy sections [116, 117] using immunostaining with a murine monoclonal antibody generated against the carbohydrate moiety of GL-3 [118]. On silver-stained ultra-thin sections of epoxy-embedded specimens, the stored glycosphingolipids appear as argyrophilic granules within the cytoplasmic vacuoles [96]. On light microscopy, the cellular distribution of glycosphingolipid deposits is best assessed in methylene blue or toluidine blue-stained semi-thin sections of epoxy-embedded tissue (Fig. 12.7) [27, 112, 119, 120]. In the glomeruli, the largest amounts of lipid material are seen in podocytes, followed by the parietal epithelial, mesangial, and glomerular endothelial cells [59, 96, 112, 119]. Progressive involvement of the parietal epithelial cells, of mesangial cells, of endothelial cells, and of the afferent and efferent glomerular arterioles, occurs as the disease worsens [46]. In heterozygous females, the parietal epithelium may be more extensively involved than the podocytes [27, 121].

On electron microscopy (Fig. 12.8), the largest inclusions are seen in podocytes and in cells of the proximal and distal tubules, and Henle's loop [96]. In these tubular segments, affected cells can be strikingly enlarged with giant inclusions measuring up 10 μm in diameter. The tubular involvement is not homogeneous and normal and affected cells may be found contiguously [96]. Proximal tubules and interstitial cells are frequently involved in Fabry nephropathy, and the presence of glycosphingolipid deposits in proximal tubular cells has been correlated with overt proteinuria in females with normal or only slightly decreased renal function [27]. Dense osmiophilic bodies have also been observed in the Bowman's space [96] and in the proximal tubular lumen [122].

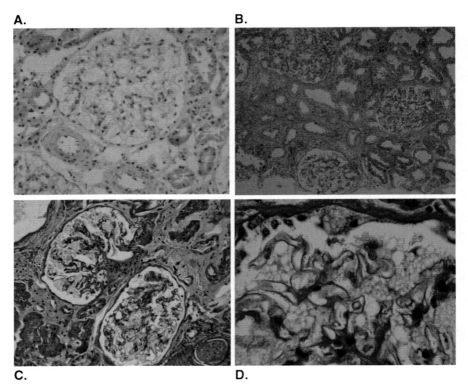

Fig. 12.6 Glomeruli showing extensive vacuolation of podocytes and GL-3 deposits in Fabry nephropathy. (**A**) Podocytes with extensive cytoplasmic vacuolation, and arteriolar vessel with hyaline droplets and reactive endothelial cells (*blue arrows*, 19 years old male patient. Hematoxylin and Eosin, magnification ×20 objective). (**B**) Focal and segmental glomerulosclerosis and localized tubular atrophy and interstitial fibrosis in a 45 years old heterozygous female patient (Special trichrome, magnification ×20 objective). (**C**) 41 year-old male patient; showing segmental sclerosis, vacuolation of visceral epithelial cells (podocytes) and parietal epithelial cells lining Bowman's capsule. There is also periglomerular and interstitial fibrosis (Periodic acid-Schiff stain. Magnification ×20 objective). (**D**) 41 year-old male patient; higher magnification of *panel* C, showing vacuolation of visceral epithelial cells (podocytes) and parietal epithelial cells lining Bowman's capsule (Periodic acid-Schiff stain. Magnification ×60 objective)

Most of the pathologic characterization of Fabry nephropathy has been derived from autopsy and biopsy studies of affected males [10, 16, 18, 43] but the heterozygous females develop the same type of kidney lesions described in males [16, 19, 96]. Descriptions of kidney pathology in heterozygous females are scarce and the largest published series describing kidney biopsy findings in affected females included only three [96] five [113] and four patients [27]. Valbuena et al. [27] recently reviewed the kidney biopsies of four affected females who had normal or only mildly impaired kidney function, two of them with overt proteinuria. Chronic

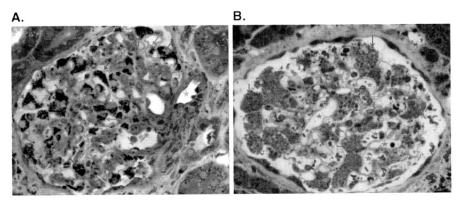

Fig. 12.7 Glomeruli showing extensive GL-3 deposits in Fabry nephropathy; plastic embedded tissue, semi-thin sections. (**A**) 7 year-old male patient; glomeruli show GL-3 osmiophilic inclusions in podocytes (*red arrows*), parietal epithelial cells along Bowman's capsule (*yellow arrows*), mesangial cells (*pink star*), and capillary endothelial cells (*green arrows*). (**B**) 19 year-old male patient; glomeruli show GL-3 osmiophilic inclusions in podocytes (*red arrows*), parietal epithelial cells along Bowman's capsule (*yellow arrows*), and capillary endothelial cells (*green arrows*), with glomerular capillary lumen marked by green star (Toluidine blue. Magnification ×60 objective)

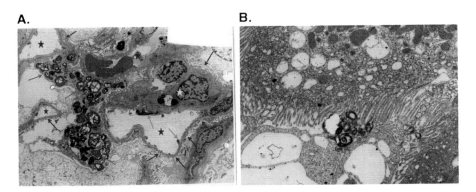

Fig. 12.8 Electron micrographs of glomerular and proximal tubule involvement in Fabry nephropathy. (**A**) Electron micrograph from a 42 years old female patient showing lamellar and amorphous osmiophilic inclusions in glomerular visceral epithelial cells (*red star*), endothelial (*green arrow*) and mesangial cells (*yellow star*). Glomerular capillary lumen are marked with a *blue star*, one of them is filled with two erythrocytes (*green star*). The podocyte foot processes remain intact (*blue arrows*. Magnification ×5,400). (**B**) Electron micrograph from a 19 years old male patient with nephrotic-range proteinuria showing lamellar osmiophilic inclusions in proximal tubular epithelial cells (*orange arrows*. Magnification ×15,900)

non-specific degenerative lesions and glycosphingolipid accumulation per cell type were semiquantitatively assessed by light and electron microscopy. Their data were combined with those of the previous series to identify significant clinico-pathologic correlations [27].

Non-specific degenerative lesions, including glomerular hyaline, increased mesangial matrix and widening of the mesangial stalks, focal segmental and global glomerular sclerosis, wrinkling of the capillary walls leading to capillary collapse, tubular atrophy and interstitial fibrosis are evident since the early stages of Fabry nephropathy [59, 96, 120]. Early signs of focal segmental glomerular sclerosis have been observed even in a female teenager with normal renal function and normal urinary albumin excretion [59]. Hyaline material or fibrinoid deposits in the media of arterioles and small and large renal arteries have been observed on routine light microscopy sections of kidney biopsies of teenagers of both genders, who had normal glomerular filtration rate and no overt proteinuria [96] or either normal or only a slightly increased urinary albumin excretion rate [59]. These fibrinoid deposits may result from necrosis of severely involved muscular cells. Valbuena et al. [27] found no histopathological evidence supporting a major role of vascular damage in the early pathogenesis of Fabry nephropathy in females. Females may develop similar degrees of arteriolar and arterial hyalinosis as males, although at an older age than males [27]. In older patients, intimal thickening can be superimposed on the vascular medial abnormalities [96]. In both genders, arterial sclerosis is generally more severe with more advanced CKD [120], but arterial and arteriolar lesions can even be observed in young males (Fig. 12.9).

The fine structure of the slit diaphragms of the foot processes may be spared despite the evidence of massive glycosphingolipid deposits in the cytoplasm of podocytes [46]. The ultrastructure of the glomerular basement membrane is usually

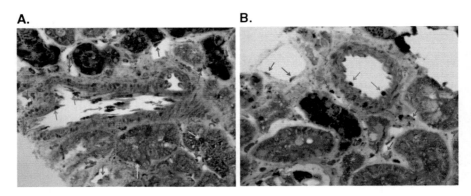

Fig. 12.9 Vascular lesions in a 7-year old male patient with Fabry nephropathy. (**A**) Artery showing osmiophilic inclusions in reactive endothelial cells (*orange arrows*) and smooth muscle cells (*orange star*). Inclusion bodies were also seen in peritubular capillary cells (*red arrows*), interstitial cells (*green arrows*) and proximal (*yellow arrows*) and distal tubular cells (Toluidine blue. Magnification ×40 objective). (**B**) Arteriolar vessel showing osmiophilic inclusions in endothelial cells (*orange arrows*) and smooth muscle cells (*green arrows*). Inclusion bodies were also seen in peritubular capillary cells (*red arrows*) and distal tubular cells (*pink star*). Part of a glomerulus with inclusions in podocytes and parietal epithelial cells is seen in botton left corner (*blue star*. Toluidine blue. Magnification ×60 objective)

normal, even alongside heavily affected podocytes. However, focal thickening and wrinkling of the glomerular basement membrane and extensive fusion of podocyte foot processes are associated with tortuosity, wrinkling and collapse of the capillary walls [96]. Furthermore, in both genders effacement of podocyte foot processes is correlated with the clinical presence of proteinuria or the nephrotic syndrome [27, 59, 113]. The basement membranes of atrophic tubules also appear thickened and wrinkled [96].

As in other chronic nephropathies, the progression of Fabry nephropathy is characterized by segmental and global glomerular sclerosis, tubular atrophy and interstitial fibrosis [46, 96, 97, 112, 113, 123]. In males, the presence of glomerular segmental or global sclerosis is the only significant pathologic association of proteinuria at early stages of Fabry nephropathy [2, 96, 120, 123]. Furthermore, negative correlations could be demonstrated between inulin clearance and histologic scores of either chronic glomerular pathology or tubulointerstitial pathology [2, 120]. In females, glomerular sclerosis and tubulointerstitial fibrosis were predictors of proteinuria and CKD stage [27].

The development of proteinuria and of late-onset CKD in some but not all patients with the cardiac variant, who have significant renal GL-3 deposits confined to podocytes [124], suggests that these cells may have a role in the pathogenesis of Fabry nephropathy. Lethal injury to GL-3-overloaded podocytes, through the formation of focal adhesions between the glomerular tuft and the Bowman's capsule [112, 125], loss of GL-3-laden podocytes in the urine, and increased hydraulic stress upon endothelial cells in the vicinity of damaged podocytes [46] are other possible mechanisms of glomerular sclerosis in Fabry nephropathy. By causing tubular injury, proteinuria can have a direct role in CKD progression and may provide a link between the aforementioned primarily glomerular pathologic processes and the development of tubulointerstitial disease [126, 127]. Mesangial cell necrosis [96], direct toxic injury to tubular cells [112] and diffuse involvement of interstitial cells [46] have also been suggested to play a role in the progression of Fabry nephropathy.

Quantitative approaches to assess the kidney pathology in biopsies of patients with Fabry disease [50, 119] have been developed as investigational tools to evaluate the short term [128, 129] and long term [130, 131] effects of agalsidase therapy in clinical trials. Thurberg et al. [119] developed a scoring system for changes in GL-3 deposits on semi-thin sections and electron micrographs in patients treated with agalsidase-beta. Figure 12.10 shows the characteristic GL-3 inclusions in vascular endothelial cells of peritubular capillaries. Clearance of these deposits, as well as form other cell types was fully achieved by 12 months of therapy [131], and maintained on follow-up biopsies after 5 years of ERT [130]. Most recently, Fogo et al. [120] systematically scored histologic lesions in kidney biopsies of a set of 35 males (mean age 36.4 years) and 24 females (43.9 years) who mostly had clinically mild Fabry nephropathy. Average serum creatinine was 1.3 mg/dl; eGFR was 82 ml/min/1.73 m^2, and urine protein to creatinine ratio was 1.08 g/g. A morphometric index of chronic damage was obtained for each biopsy. A validated scoring

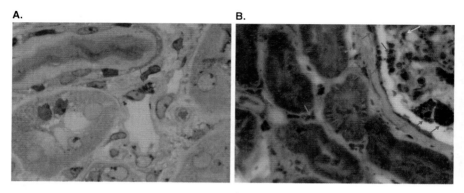

Fig. 12.10 Peritubular Capillary GL-3 Inclusions. (**A**) Plastic embedded tissue from a 32 years old female patient, showing osmiophilic inclusions in peritubular capillary cells (*Red arrow.* Methylene blue. Magnification ×40 objective). (**B**) Plastic embedded tissue from a 40 years old male patient. Tubulo-interstitial area and part of a glomerulus with round and spherical inclusion bodies in podocytes (*red arrows*), parietal epithelial cells (*green arrows*) and endothelial cells (*yellow arrow*). Inclusion bodies were also seen in peritubular capillary cells (*orange arrows*) and some interstitial cells (*pink arrow*) (Toluidine blue. Magnification ×60 objective)

system was developed, with the long-term goal to determine whether baseline histologic information can be related to the rate of progression and/or response to ERT in Fabry nephropathy. The development of a standardized scoring system of both disease-specific lesions, i.e., lipid deposition-related, and general lesions of progression, i.e., fibrosis and sclerosis, showed a spectrum of histologic appearances even in early clinical stage Fabry nephropathy. Males had greater podocyte vacuolization on light microscopy (mean score) and larger and more frequent glycosphingolipid inclusions on semi-thin sections than females. Males also had significantly more proximal tubule, peritubular capillary and vascular intimal inclusions. Arteriolar hyalinosis was similar, but females had significantly more arterial hyalinosis. Chronic kidney disease stage correlated with arterial and glomerular sclerosis scores. Significant changes, including segmental and global sclerosis, and interstitial fibrosis were seen even in patients with stage 1–2 chronic kidney disease with minimal proteinuria [120]. These findings support the role of kidney biopsy in the baseline evaluation of Fabry nephropathy, even with mild clinical disease. The validated scoring instrument developed by Fogo et al. [120] is shown in Fig. 12.11.

12.9 Dysfunction of the Microcirculation in Fabry Disease

The evidence supporting abnormal cerebral, coronary and renal blood flow, vessel architecture, endothelial function, and auto-regulation has been reviewed [44, 132–135]. The sub-cellular mechanisms linking glycosphingolipid accumulation to

• **INTERNATIONAL STUDY GROUP OF FABRY NEPHROPATHY SCORE SHEET** •

Case number: [   ]   **Scorer:** [   ]   **Date:** [   ]

• **LIGHT MICROSCOPY:** (Only score circled section indicated by a mark.)

1) PODOCYTE VACUOLIZATION		Total	Podocyte score (n affected x score)	Mean Podocyte Score (n affected x score) / total scorable counted
None	(score = 0)			
Mild	(score = 1; <25%)			
Moderate	(score = 2; 25-50%)			
Severe	(score = 3; >50%)			

Total scorable glomeruli [   ]

Not scoreable, indeterminate *(fragment or global GS)*

Total number of glomeruli *(sum scoreable + indeterminate)* [   ]

2) OTHER LESIONS	Total
Nonsclerotic glomerulus	
Segmental sclerosis, mild	
Segmental sclerosis, severe	
Global sclerosis	
Adhesion	
Ischemic/collapse	
Peri-glomerular fibrosis and/or Bowman's capsule reduplication	
Indeterminate *(fragment of glomerulus)*	

3) ARTERIES: Present ___ Absent ___

	Total
Average sclerosis (0-3)	
Most severe sclerosis(0-3)	

Hyalinosis:	Present	Absent
Arterioles: Medial		
Subendothelial		
Arteries: Medial		
Subendothelial		

4) TUBULOINTERSTITIUM Estimated — scored to nearest 10% (>0 and <5 scored as 5%)

Tubulointerstitial fibrosis	

Interstitial inflammation

Absent _____   Present _____

Scarred _____
Non-scarred _____

• **THICK SECTION:** (Only score circled section.)

0;   1 — rare, small;   2 — many, small;   3 — rare, large;   4 — ≥50% large

	Glomeruli available	Segmental sclerosis mild	severe	Global sclerosis
Number of:				

Inclusions	Glomerulus								
	1	2	3	4	5	6	7	8	Average
Podocyte (0-4+)									

	Present	Absent	Not Sampled
Parietal epithelial inclusions			
Proximal tubular inclusions			
Distal tubular inclusions			
Peritubular capillary inclusions			
Vascular intimal inclusions			
Vascular medial inclusions			

COMMENTS:

Revised 05/03/07

Fig. 12.11 Scoring sheet for Fabry nephropathy by light microscopy. Biopsy material was assessed on periodic acid-Schiff-stained slides. Of note, more than one lesion could be present on light microscopy in any one glomerulus, e.g. segmental sclerosis and ischemia/collapse could coexist in the same glomerulus, and both features were then scored as 'present' for that glomerulus. Optimal slides for scoring included >10 glomeruli for light microscopic assessment, and at least 3 glomeruli for semi-thin section scoring (reproduced with permission from Fogo et al. [120])

the clinical manifestations of Fabry disease are not clearly understood. The classical theory emphasized ischemic tissue damage resulting from microvascular endothelial disease and/or necrosis of vascular smooth muscle cells and/or pericyte injury [1, 136]. Recent studies provided evidence that GL-3 induces oxidative stress in vascular endothelial cells [137] and that circulating myeloperoxidase levels are significantly increased in males with Fabry disease, predicting the risk of subsequent vasculopathic events [138].

12.10 Progressive Loss of Glomerular Filtration in Fabry Nephropathy

An open-label extension study of the phase III study of agalsidase-beta has been published [130]. After 54 months of treatment, 8 patients had protocol kidney biopsies, which showed complete maintenance of GL-3 clearance of renal capillary endothelial cells. eGFR remained stable in 41 patients, but 6 patients with significant baseline proteinuria (>1.0 g/day) or segmental and global sclerosis in more than half of their glomeruli had rapid loss of GFR (Fig. 12.12).

The progression rates that have been reported for a number of prospective studies, trials and case reports have recently been reviewed [57, 139]. Very few of these studies have achieved slowing of progression to the optimal rate of –1.0 ml/min/

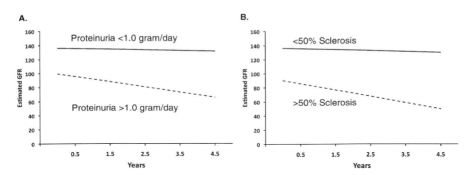

Fig. 12.12 Association between overt proteinuria, glomerular sclerosis and loss of glomerular filtration rate in Fabry nephropathy. (**A**) The 42 participants in the Phase III extension study with baseline estimated GFR of 136 ml/min/1.73 m² and less than 1.0 g of urine protein/day had a rate of loss of estimated GFR equal to –1.001 ml/min/1.73 m²/year, and the 10 participants who had baseline estimated GFR of 99.2 ml/min/1.73 m² and more than 1.0 g of urine protein/day had a rate of loss of estimated GFR equal to –7.40 ml/min/1.73 m²/year. The difference between these two slopes was 6.39, p-value = 0.004. (**B**) The 32 participants in the Phase III extension study with baseline estimated GFR of 136.4 ml/min/1.73 m² and focal or global sclerosis in less than 50% of their glomeruli had a rate of loss of estimated GFR equal to –1.40 ml/min/1.73 m²/year, and the 8 participants who had baseline estimated GFR of 90.2 ml/min/1.73 m² and focal or global sclerosis in more than 50% of their glomeruli had a rate of loss of estimated GFR equal to –8.96 ml/min/1.73 m²/year. The difference between these two slopes was 7.55, p-value = 0.003 (data re-plotted from Germain et al. [130])

1.73 m^2/year [57, 60]. Variability in the rates of change of GFR could reflect differences in baseline characteristics of the different patient populations, treatment duration, the prevalence of angiotensin converting enzyme inhibitor (ACEI) or angiotensin receptor blocker (ARB) use, achieved urine proteinuria reduction, as well as techniques of GFR measurement that complicate the comparison of different treatment groups.

12.11 Proteinuria, ERT and Progression of Fabry Nephropathy

Studies in CKD show that reno-protective treatments effectively limit the progressive decline in GFR to the extent that proteinuria is reduced [140, 141]. The rate of eGFR decline, especially for male patients largely depends on the level of proteinuria achieved during anti-proteinuric therapy [127]. With this approach, the goal is to achieve a rate of GFR decline equal to that observed in the general population [142]. It is not certain that proteinuria is as important in the progressive loss of GFR in females as it has been shown to be in male Fabry patients. Ortiz et al. [5] described a significant proportion of adult females with eGFR <60 ml/min/1.73 m^2 at baseline evaluation who did not have overt proteinuria, suggesting that other factors may be important determinants of loss of kidney function for females patients.

ERT does not reduce proteinuria, and pediatric patients have developed overt proteinuria despite ongoing ERT [59], emphasizing the need to monitor and treat proteinuria in patients already receiving ERT.

Treatment with ACEIs and/or ARBs was undertaken in an open-label study of 10 patients, most of whom had control of their proteinuria before initiation of ERT [143]. When urine protein excretion was controlled to ≤0.50 g/day in patients treated with agalsidase-beta at 1.0 mg/kg every 2 weeks, the rate of loss of eGFR was not significantly different from zero [143]. The response was much better than previously reported for patients with overt proteinuria and eGFR <60 ml/min/1.73 m^2 [144–147], but requires confirmation in an ongoing multi-center study [148]. There are patients described with progressive loss of kidney function and controlled urine protein excretion who showed greatly slowed rates of loss of function when ERT dosing was increased from 0.2 mg/kg of agalsidase-alfa given every other week to weekly dosing [146], or dosing with agalsidase-beta at 1 mg/kg given every 2 weeks [125].

Effective ACEI/ARB therapy is challenging for the physician and patient if the baseline blood pressure is relatively low. In addition, hyperkalemia and anemia, and other side effects, such as persistent cough with ACE inhibitors, can complicate the use of anti-proteinuric therapy in patients with CKD. Recent studies of Fabry disease reveal disappointing rates of use of renin-angiotensin-aldosterone system inhibitors under 50% despite multiple indications: hypertension, proteinuria, reduced GFR, hyperfiltration and others [14, 15, 17, 18]. This suggests that real barriers limit the use of ACEIs and ARBs in Fabry disease. As most physicians who care for patients with Fabry disease are not nephrologists and may not be familiar with use of these agents, education about the optimal use of these therapies is paramount. Referral of all Fabry disease patients with any of the above indications to a nephrologist is strongly recommended.

The response to ACEI/ARB therapy has to be optimized by adjusting the doses to achieve reduction of proteinuria to a pre-defined target level, but the optimal target has not been established for Fabry nephropathy. In addition, it is not known whether stabilization of kidney function can be achieved with control of proteinuria and ERT given at lower doses than used in the pilot study [143] or the FAACET trial [148].

Whether differences between 0.2 and 1.0 mg/kg, or between agalsidase-alfa (Replagal®, Shire Human Genetic Therapies, Cambridge, MA USA) versus agalsidase-beta (Fabrazyme®, Genzyme Therapeutics, Cambridge, MA USA) have an effect on renal outcomes is as of yet unknown. For example, in comparing the low risk groups of male patients with Fabry nephropathy and baseline proteinuria <1.0 g/day treated with agalsidase-alfa at 0.2 m/kg body weight every 2 weeks, West et al. [57] reported a progression rate of -2.1 ± 1.3 ml/min/1.73 m^2/year using a nucleide tracer technique. Germain et al. [130] used agalsidase-beta at 1.0 mg/kg every 2 weeks, and reported a progression rate of -1.01 ± 0.97 ml/min/1.73 m^2/year using the Modification of Diet in Renal Disease 4 variable equation to estimate GFR [149]. Statistically these rates are not different [57] by t-test. However, comparison is difficult due to non-randomized allocation of subjects to either treatment arm and different techniques for GFR determination.

The ongoing Canadian Fabry Disease Initiative study [150] is a randomized study that will evaluate the effects on progressive loss of GFR of agalsidase-alfa given at 0.2 mg/kg every 2 weeks compared to agalsidase-beta given at 1.0 mg/kg every 2 weeks. All patients will receive ACEI or ARB therapy at doses to achieve reduction of proteinuria to a similar degree. It is also important to demonstrated the progression rate in Fabry nephropathy be reduced to the 'normal' rate [60, 151] with optimal ACEI or ARB therapy and agalsidase-alfa given at 0.2 mg/kg every 2 weeks as has been demonstrated with agalsidase-beta given at 1.0 mg/kg every 2 weeks and control of urine protein excretion [130, 143].

The clinical significance of an absolute reduction of the progression rate by -1.0 ml/min/1.73 m^2/year could be questioned, but to put this change in perspective, this is exactly the magnitude of the reduction or the progression rate reported in the RENAAL [152] and IDNT [153] studies, which are generally accepted as important advances in the treatment of diabetic renal disease [154]. A similar effect was reported in the recent study of strict blood pressure control and progression of kidney disease in children [155]. In this study, there was not a significant difference between the eGFR slopes, but the intensively treated group of children had a significant delay in reaching the primary composite endpoint, which was defined as a 50% reduction in the eGFR or progression to ESRD. In all forms of chronic kidney disease, the beneficial effect of blood pressure control versus control of proteinuria has not been determined [156, 157]. The optimal goal for proteinuria reduction, and the effects of gender and age on setting and achieving these goals in Fabry nephropathy needs to be better defined [149].

12.12 Other Considerations for Treating Fabry Nephropathy

In addition to proteinuria, other potentially treatable factors in patients with CKD, including hypertension, smoking, and hyperlipidemia may contribute to progressive loss of GFR [126]. There is every reason to expect that this approach will apply to patients with Fabry nephropathy, so correction of these other risk factors should also be considered for interventions to slow CKD progression. Systemic blood pressure is generally lower in patients with Fabry disease [5, 158]. Beta-blockers and diuretics may cause hypotension and limit the use of anti-proteinuric therapy.

12.13 Treatment Goal for Fabry Nephropathy

The goal for treatment of Fabry nephropathy is reduction in the rate of loss of GFR to ≤ -1.0 ml/min/1.73 m^2/year [60, 151]. What can be done if this goal is not reached? Measuring proteinuria and urinary sodium excretion are important first steps. Control of dietary sodium is important to ensure ACEI/ARB effectiveness. Repeated measures of eGFR are needed; basing treatment decisions on only 2 measurements of serum creatinine is not recommended. If proteinuria is not controlled, then anti-proteinuric dosing increases are recommended, with the understanding that systemic blood pressure may further decrease. The doses can be split to minimize acute falls in blood pressure, and small dose increments are preferable. It may be necessary to reduce the dose of other anti-hypertensive agents (e.g., beta blockers, diuretics, calcium channel blockers) so that ACEI or ARB dosing can be increased. Aldosterone receptor blockers may lower proteinuria with modest effects on blood pressure [159]. Switch from one form of agalsidase to another, or increasing ERT dosing or frequency of administration has not been well studied, and would best done in the setting of a prospective clinical trial. The possibility of another form of kidney disease should be addressed with a kidney biopsy [160].

References

1. Desnick RJ, Ioannou YA, Eng CM (2001) Alpha-Galactosidase A deficiency: Fabry disease. In: Scriver C, Beaudet A, Sly W, Valle D (eds) The metabolic bases of inherited disease, 8th edn. McGraw-Hill, New York, pp 3733–3774
2. Branton MH, Schiffmann R, Sabnis SG, Murray GJ, Quirk JM, Altarescu G et al (2002) Natural history of Fabry renal disease: influence of alpha-galactosidase A activity and genetic mutations on clinical course. Medicine (Baltimore) 81(2):122–138
3. Mehta A, Ricci R, Widmer U, Dehout F, Garcia de Lorenzo A, Kampmann C et al (2004) Fabry disease defined: baseline clinical manifestations of 366 patients in the Fabry Outcome Survey. Eur J Clin Invest 34(3):236–242
4. Deegan PB, Baehner AF, Barba Romero MA, Hughes DA, Kampmann C, Beck M (2006) Natural history of Fabry disease in females in the Fabry Outcome Survey. J Med Genet 43(4):347–352

5. Ortiz A, Oliveira JP, Waldek S, Warnock DG, Cianciaruso B, Wanner C (2008) Nephropathy in males and females with Fabry disease: cross-sectional description of patients before treatment with enzyme replacement therapy. Nephrol Dial Transplant 9(23):1600–1607

6. Wilcox WR, Oliveira JP, Hopkin RJ, Ortiz A, Banikazemi M, Feldt-Rasmussen U et al (2008) Females with Fabry disease frequently have major organ involvement: Lessons from the Fabry Registry. Mol Genet Metab 93(2):112–128

7. Kobayashi M, Ohashi T, Sakuma M, Ida H, Eto Y (2008) Clinical manifestations and natural history of Japanese heterozygous females with Fabry disease. J Inherit Metab Dis online report #003 DOI 10.1007/s10545-007-0740-6

8. Schiffmann R, Warnock DG, Banikazemi M, Bultas J, Linthorst GE, Packman S et al (2009) Fabry disease: progression of nephropathy, and prevalence of cardiac and cerebrovascular events before enzyme replacement therapy. Nephrol Dial Transplant 24(7):2102–2111

9. Oqvist B, Brenner BM, Oliveira JP, Ortiz A, Schaefer R, Svarstad E et al (2009) Nephropathy in Fabry disease: the importance of early diagnosis and testing in high-risk populations. Nephrol Dial Transplant 24(6):1736–1743

10. Pompen AW, Ruiter M, Wyers HJ (1947) Angiokeratoma corporis diffusum (universale) Fabry, as a sign of an unknown internal disease; two autopsy reports. Acta Med Scand 128(3):234–255

11. Scriba K (1950) Zur Pathogenese des Angiokeratoma corporis diffusum Fabry mit cardio vasorenalem symptomenkomplex [Article in German]. Verhandlg Deutsch Path Gesellsch 34:221–226

12. Hornbostel H, Spier W, Koch H (1951) Angiokeratoma corporis diffusum universale (Fabry) with cardio-vaso-renal symptom complex as general disease (Article in German). Arztl Wochensch 6(3):49–55

13. Karr WJ Jr. (1959) Fabry's disease (angiokeratoma corporis diffusum universale). An unusual syndrome with multisystem involvement and unique skin manifestations. Am J Med 27:829–835

14. Wise D, Wallace HJ, Jellinek EH (1962) Angiokeratoma corporis diffusum. A clinical study of eight affected families. Q J Med 31:177–206

15. De Groot WP (1968) Angiokeratoma corporis diffusum Fabry. Dermatologica 136(5):432–433

16. Colley JR, Miller DL, Hutt MS, Wallace HJ, De Wardener HE (1958) The renal lesion in angiokeratoma corporis diffusum. Br Med J 1(5082):1266–1268

17. Rahman AN, Simeone FA, Hackel DB, Hall PW III, Hirsch EZ, Harris JW (1961) Angiokeratoma corporis diffusum universale (hereditary dystropic lipidosis). Trans Am Assoc Physicians 74:366–377

18. De Groot WP (1964) Angiokeratoma corporis diffusum Fabry. Dermatologica 128:321–349

19. Burda CD, Winder PR (1967) Angiokeratoma corporis diffusum universale (Fabry's disease) in female subjects. Am J Med 42(2):293–301

20. Clarke JT, Knaack J, Crawhall JC, Wolfe LS (1971) Ceramide trihexosidosis (Fabry's disease) without skin lesions. N Engl J Med 284(5):233–235

21. Kitagawa T, Suzuki K, Ishige N, Ohashi T, Kobayashi M, Eto Y et al (2008) Non-invasive high-risk screening for Fabry disease hemizygotes and heterozygotes. Pediatr Nephrol 23(9):1461–1471

22. Ortiz A, Oliveira JP, Wanner C, Brenner BM, Waldek S, Warnock DG (2008) Recommendations and guidelines for the diagnosis and treatment of Fabry nephropathy in adults. Nat Clin Pract Nephrol 4(6):327–336

23. Zarate YA, Patterson L, Yin H, Hopkin RJ (2009) A case of minimal change disease in a Fabry patient. Pediatr Nephrol 25(3):553–556

24. Kawamura O, Sakuraba H, Itoh K, Suzuki Y, Doi M, Kuwabara H et al (1997) Subclinical Fabry's disease occurring in the context of IgA nephropathy. Clin Nephrol 47(2):71–75

25. Pisani A, Sessa A, Sabbatini M, Andreucci MV, Fusco C, Balletta M et al (2005) Fabry nephropathy in a female with superposed IgA glomerulonephritis [in Italian]. G Ital Nefrol 22(4):385–389

26. Whybra C, Schwarting A, Kriegsmann J, Gal A, Mengel E, Kampmann C et al (2006) IgA nephropathy in two adolescent sisters heterozygous for Fabry disease. Pediatr Nephrol 21(9):1251–1256

27. Valbuena C, Carvalho E, Bustorff M, Ganhão M, Relvas S, Nogueira R et al (2008) Kidney biospy findings in heterozygous Fabry disease females with early nephropathy. Virchows Arch 453(4):329–338

28. Singh HK, Nickeleit V, Kriegsmann J, Harris AA, Jennette JC, Mihatsch MJ (2001) Coexistence of Fabry's disease and necrotizing and crescentic glomerulonephritis. Clin Nephrol 55(1):73–79

29. Shimazu K, Tomiyoshi Y, Aoki S, Sakemi T, Sugihara H (2002) Crescentic glomerulonephritis in a patient with heterozygous Fabry's disease. Nephron 92(2):456–458

30. Kriegsmann J, Otto M, Wandel E, Schwarting A, Faust J, Hansen T et al (2003) Fabry's disease, glomerulonephritis with crescentic and granulomatous interstitial nephritis. Case of one family [in German]. Pathologe 24(6):439–443

31. Rosenmann E, Kobrin I, Cohen T (1983) Kidney involvement in systemic lupus erythematosus and Fabry's disease. Nephron 34(3):180–184

32. Majima K, Ishizaki T, Inoue T, Hori Y, Egami J, Oohara A et al (1992) A case of Fabry's disease associated with lupus nephritis [in Japanese]. Nippon Jinzo Gakkai Shi 34(11): 1189–1194

33. Ries M, Bettis KE, Choyke P, Kopp JB, Austin HA III, Brady RO et al (2004) Parapelvic kidney cysts: a distinguishing feature with high prevalence in Fabry disease. Kidney Int 66(3):978–982

34. Banks DE, Milutinovic J, Desnick RJ, Grabowski GA, Lapp NL, Boehlecke BA (1983) Silicon nephropathy mimicking Fabry's disease. Am J Nephrol 3(5):279–284

35. Woywodt A, Hellweg S, Schwarz A, Schaefer RM, Mengel M (2007) A wild zebra chase. Nephrol Dial Transplant 22(10):3074–3077

36. Muller-Hocker J, Schmid H, Weiss M, Dendorfer U, Braun GS (2003) Chloroquine-induced phospholipidosis of the kidney mimicking Fabry's disease: case report and review of the literature. Hum Pathol 34(3):285–289

37. Albay D, Adler SG, Philipose J, Calescibetta CC, Romansky SG, Cohen AH (2005) Chloroquine-induced lipidosis mimicking Fabry disease. Mod Pathol 18(5):733–738

38. Bracamonte ER, Kowalewska J, Starr J, Gitomer J, Alpers CE (2006) Iatrogenic phospholipidosis mimicking Fabry disease. Am J Kidney Dis 48(5):844–850

39. Houghton DC, Campbell-Boswell MV, Bennett WM, Porter GA, Brooks RE (1978) Myeloid bodies in the renal tubules of humans: relationship to gentamicin therapy. Clin Nephrol 10(4):140–145

40. Ferreira S, Valbuena C, Carvalho F, Oliveira JP (2009) Novel human pathological mutations. Gene symbol: GLA. Disease: Fabry disease. Hum Genet 126(2):352

41. Desnick RJ, Banikazemi M, Wasserstein M (2002) Enzyme replacement therapy for Fabry disease, an inherited nephropathy. Clin Nephrol 57(1):1–8

42. Chatterjee S, Gupta P, Pyeritz RE, Kwiterovich PO Jr. (1984) Immunohistochemical localization of glycosphingolipid in urinary renal tubular cells in Fabry's disease. Am J Clin Pathol 82(1):24–28

43. Henry EW, Rally CR (1963) The renal lesion in angiokeratoma corporis diffusum (Fabry's disease). Can Med Assoc J 3(89):206–213

44. Pabico RC, Atancio BC, McKenna BA, Pamukcoglu T, Yodaiken R (1973) Renal pathologic lesions and functional alterations in a man with Fabry's disease. Am J Med 55(3): 415–425

45. Wornell P, Dyack S, Crocker J, Yu W, Accott P (2006) Fabry disease and nephrogenic diabetes insipidus. Pediatr Nephrol 21:1185–1188

46. Sessa A, Meroni M, Battini G, Righetti M, Maglio A, Tosoni A et al (2003) Renal involvement in Anderson-Fabry disease. J Nephrol 16(2):310–313

47. Ries M, Gupta S, Moore DF, Sachdev V, Quirk JM, Murray GJ et al (2005) Pediatric Fabry disease. Pediatrics 115(3):344–355

48. Ramaswami U, Whybra C, Parini R, Pintos-Morell G, Mehta A, Sunder-Plassmann G et al (2006) Clinical manifestations of Fabry disease in children: data from the Fabry Outcome Survey. Acta Paediatr 95(1):86–92

49. Hopkin RJ, Bissler J, Banikazemi M, Clarke L, Eng CM, Germain DP et al (2008) Characterization of Fabry disease in 352 pediatric patients in the Fabry Registry. Pediatr Res 64(5):550–555

50. Branton M, Schiffmann R, Kopp JB (2002) Natural history and treatment of renal involvement in Fabry disease. J Am Soc Nephrol 13(Suppl 2):S139–S143

51. Ries M, Ramaswami U, Parini R, Lindblad B, Whybra C, Willers I et al (2003) The early clinical phenotype of Fabry disease: a study on 35 European children and adolescents. Eur J Pediatr 162(11):767–772

52. Sheth KJ, Roth DA, Adams MB (1983) Early renal failure in Fabry's disease. Am J Kidney Dis 2(6):651–654

53. Levey AS, Stevens LA, Schmid CH, Zhang Y, Castro AF III, Feldman HI et al (2009) A new equation to estimate glomerular filtration rate. Ann Intern Med 150(9):604–612

54. Kleinert J, Dehout F, Schwarting A, de Lorenzo AG, Ricci R, Kampmann C et al (2005) Anemia is a new complication in Fabry disease: data from the Fabry Outcome Survey. Kidney Int 67(5):1955–1960

55. Oliveira JP, Valbuena C, Baldaia Moreira A, Fonseca E, Soares C, Leao Teles E et al (2008) Splenomegaly, hypersplenism and peripheral blood cytopaenias in patients with classical Anderson-Fabry disease. Virchows Arch 453(3):291–300

56. Rodriguez-Iturbe B, Herrera J, Garcia R (1985) Response to acute protein load in kidney donors and in apparently normal postacute glomerulonephritis patients: evidence for glomerular hyperfiltration. Lancet 2(8453):461–464

57. West M, Nicholls K, Mehta A, Clarke JT, Steiner R, Beck M et al (2009) Agalsidase alfa and kidney dysfunction in Fabry disease. J Am Soc Nephrol 20(5):1132–1139

58. Schwartz GJ, Haycock GB, Edelmann CM Jr., Spitzer A (1976) A simple estimate of glomerular filtration rate in children derived from body length and plasma creatinine. Pediatrics 58(2):259–263

59. Tondel C, Bostad L, Hirth A, Svarstad E (2008) Renal biopsy findings in children and adolescents with Fabry disease and minimal albuminuria. Am J Kidney Dis 51(5):767–776

60. Stevens LA, Coresh J, Greene T, Levey AS (2006) Assessing kidney function–measured and estimated glomerular filtration rate. N Engl J Med 354(23):2473–2483

61. Bland JM, Altman DG (1986) Statistical methods for assessing agreement between two methods of clinical measurement. Lancet 1(8476):307–310

62. Schwartz GJ, Munoz A, Schneider MF, Mak RH, Kaskel F, Warady BA et al (2009) New equations to estimate GFR in children with CKD. J Am Soc Nephrol 20(3):629–637

63. Counahan R, Chantler C, Ghazali S, Kirkwood B, Rose F, Barratt TM (1976) Estimation of glomerular filtration rate from plasma creatinine concentration in children. Arch Dis Child 51(11):875–878

64. Ries M, Clarke JT, Whybra C, Timmons M, Robinson C, Schlaggar BL et al (2006) Enzyme-replacement therapy with agalsidase alfa in children with Fabry disease. Pediatrics 118(3):924–932

65. Kleinert J, Dehout F, Schwarting A, de Lorenzo AG, Ricci R, Kampmann C et al (2006) Prevalence of uncontrolled hypertension in patients with Fabry disease. Am J Hypertens 19(8):782–787

66. Glass RB, Astrin KH, Norton KI, Parsons R, Eng CM, Banikazemi M et al (2004) Fabry disease: renal sonographic and magnetic resonance imaging findings in affected males and

carrier females with the classic and cardiac variant phenotypes. J Comput Assist Tomogr 28(2):158–168

67. Donati D, Novario R, Gastaldi L (1987) Natural history and treatment of uremia secondary to Fabry's disease: an European experience. Nephron 46(4):353–359

68. Colombi A, Kostyal A, Bracher R, Gloor F, Mazzi R, Tholen H (1967) Angiokeratoma corporis diffusum–Fabry's disease. Helv Med Acta 34(1):67–83

69. MacDermot KD, Holmes A, Miners AH (2001) Anderson-Fabry disease: clinical manifestations and impact of disease in a cohort of 98 hemizygous males. J Med Genet 38(11):750–760

70. Shah T, Gill J, Malhotra N, Takemoto SK, Bunnapradist S (2009) Kidney transplant outcomes in patients with Fabry disease. Transplantation 87(2):280–285

71. Tsakiris D, Simpson HK, Jones EH, Briggs JD, Elinder CG, Mendel S et al (1996) Report on management of renale failure in Europe, XXVI, 1995. Rare diseases in renal replacement therapy in the ERA-EDTA Registry. Nephrol Dial Transplant 11(Suppl 7):4–20

72. Thadhani R, Wolf M, West ML, Tonelli M, Ruthazer R, Pastores GM et al (2002) Patients with Fabry disease on dialysis in the United States. Kidney Int 61(1):249–255

73. Meikle PJ, Hopwood JJ, Clague AE, Carey WF (1999) Prevalence of lysosomal storage disorders. JAMA 281(3):249–254

74. Poorthuis BJ, Wevers RA, Kleijer WJ, Groener JE, de Jong JG, van Weely S et al (1999) The frequency of lysosomal storage diseases in The Netherlands. Hum Genet 105(1–2):151–156

75. Ojo A, Meier-Kriesche HU, Friedman G, Hanson J, Cibrik D, Leichtman A et al (2000) Excellent outcome of renal transplantation in patients with Fabry's disease. Transplantation 69(11):2337–2339

76. Sessa A, Meroni M, Battini G, Righetti M, Mignani R (2004) Chronic renal failure, dialysis, and renal transplantation in Anderson-Fabry disease. Semin Nephrol 24(5):532–536

77. Garman SC, Garboczi DN (2004) The molecular defect leading to Fabry disease: structure of human alpha-galactosidase. J Mol Biol 337(2):319–335

78. Matsuzawa F, Aikawa SI, Doi H, Okumiya T, Sakuraba H (2005) Fabry disease: correlation between structural changes in alpha-galactosidase, and clinical and biochemical phenotypes. Hum Genet 117(4):317–328

79. Desnick RJ, Allen KY, Desnick SJ, Raman MK, Bernlohr RW, Krivit W (1973) Fabry's disease: enzymatic diagnosis of hemizygotes and heterozygotes. Alpha-galactosidase activities in plasma, serum, urine, and leukocytes. J Lab Clin Med 81(2):157–171

80. Nakao S, Kodama C, Takenaka T, Tanaka A, Yasumoto Y, Yoshida A et al (2003) Fabry disease: Detection of undiagnosed hemodialysis patients and identification of a 'renal variant' phenotype. Kidney Int 64(3):801–807

81. Kotanko P, Kramar R, Devrnja D, Paschke E, Voigtlander T, Auinger M et al (2004) Results of a nationwide screening for Anderson-Fabry disease among dialysis patients. J Am Soc Nephrol 15(5):1323–1329

82. Kleinert J, Kotanko P, Spada M, Pagliardini S, Paschke E, Paul K et al (2009) Anderson-Fabry disease: a case-finding study among male kidney transplant recipients in Austria. Transpl Int 22(3):287–292

83. Merta M, Reiterova J, Ledvinova J, Poupetova H, Dobrovolny R, Rysava R et al (2007) A nationwide blood spot screening study for Fabry disease in the Czech Republic haemodialysis patient population. Nephrol Dial Transplant 22(1):179–186

84. Spada M, Pagliardini S, Yasuda M, Tukel T, Thiagarajan G, Sakuraba H et al (2006) High incidence of later-onset Fabry disease revealed by newborn screening. Am J Hum Genet 79(1):31–40

85. Utsumi K, Kase R, Takata T, Sakuraba H, Matsui N, Saito H et al (2000) Fabry disease in patients receiving maintenance dialysis. Clin Exp Nephrol 4(1):46–51

86. Ichinose M, Nakayama M, Ohashi T, Utsunomiya Y, Kobayashi M, Eto Y (2005) Significance of screening for Fabry disease among male dialysis patients. Clin Exp Nephrol 9(3):228–232

87. Tanaka M, Ohashi T, Kobayashi M, Eto Y, Miyamura N, Nishida K et al (2005) Identification of Fabry's disease by the screening of alpha-galactosidase A activity in male and female hemodialysis patients. Clin Nephrol 64(4):281–287

88. Andrade J, Waters PJ, Singh RS, Levin A, Toh BC, Vallance HD et al (2008) Screening for Fabry disease in patients with chronic kidney disease: limitations of plasma alpha-galactosidase assay as a screening test. Clin J Am Soc Nephrol 3(1):139–145

89. Nakao S, Takenaka T, Maeda M, Kodama C, Tanaka A, Tahara M et al (1995) An atypical variant of Fabry's disease in men with left ventricular hypertrophy. N Engl J Med 333(5):288–293

90. Sachdev B, Takenaka T, Teraguchi H, Tei C, Lee P, McKenna WJ et al (2002) Prevalence of Anderson-Fabry disease in male patients with late onset hypertrophic cardiomyopathy. Circulation 105(12):1407–1411

91. Yoshitama T, Nakao S, Takenaka T, Teraguchi H, Sasaki T, Kodama C et al (2001) Molecular genetic, biochemical, and clinical studies in three families with cardiac Fabry's disease. Am J Cardiol 87(1):71–75

92. Altarescu G, Elstein D (2005) Cardiac abnormalities in Fabry disease: natural history in hemizygote males suggests that cardiac pathology is universally present. Haema 8(1):103–108

93. Takenaka T, Teraguchi H, Yoshida A, Taguchi S, Ninomiya K, Umekita Y et al (2008) Terminal stage cardiac findings in patients with cardiac Fabry disease: An electrocardiographic, echocardiographic, and autopsy study. J Cardiol 51(1):50–59

94. Sweeley CC, Klionsky B (1963) Fabry's disease: classification as a sphingolipidosis and partial characterization of a novel glycolipid. J Biol Chem 238:3148–3150

95. Schibanoff JM, Kamoshita S, O'Brien JS (1969) Tissue distribution of glycosphingolipids in a case of Fabry's disease. J Lipid Res 10(5):515–520

96. Gubler MC, Lenoir G, Grunfeld JP, Ulmann A, Droz D, Habib R (1978) Early renal changes in hemizygous and heterozygous patients with Fabry's disease. Kidney Int 13(3):223–235

97. Sessa A, Toson A, Nebuloni M, Pallotti F, Giordano F, Battini G et al (2002) Renal ultrastructural findings in Anderson-Fabry disease. J Nephrol 15(2):109–112

98. Elleder M, Poupetova H, Kozich V (1998) Fetal pathology in Fabry's disease and mucopolysaccharidosis type I [in Czech]. Cesk Patol 34(1):7–12

99. Mårtensson E (1966) Neutral glycolipids of human kidney isolation, identification, and fatty acid composition. Biochim Biophys Acta 116(2):296–308

100. Makita A, Iwanaga M, Yamakawa T (1964) The chemical structure of human kidney globoside. J Biochem 55:202–204

101. Kojima Y, Fukumoto S, Furukawa K, Okajima T, Wiels J, Yokoyama K et al (2000) Molecular cloning of globotriaosylceramide/CD77 synthase, a glycosyltransferase that initiates the synthesis of globo series glycosphingolipids. J Biol Chem 275(20):15152–15156

102. Abe A, Gregory S, Lee L, Killen PD, Brady RO, Kulkarni A et al (2000) Reduction of globotriaosylceramide in Fabry disease mice by substrate deprivation. J Clin Invest 105(11):1563–1571

103. Cox T, Lachmann R, Hollak C, Aerts J, van Weely S, Hrebicek M et al (2000) Novel oral treatment of Gaucher's disease with N-butyldeoxynojirimycin (OGT 918) to decrease substrate biosynthesis. Lancet 355(9214):1481–1485

104. Cohen A, Hannigan GE, Williams BR, Lingwood CA (1987) Roles of globotriosyl- and galabiosylceramide in verotoxin binding and high affinity interferon receptor. J Biol Chem 262(35):17088–17091

105. Ergonul Z, Clayton F, Fogo AB, Kohan DE (2003) Shigatoxin-1 binding and receptor expression in human kidneys do not change with age. Pediatr Nephrol 18(3):246–253

106. Meyers KE, Kaplan BS (2000) Many cell types are Shiga toxin targets. Kidney Int 57(6):2650–2651

107. Thomaidis T, Relle M, Golbas M, Brochhausen C, Galle PR, Beck M et al (2009) Downregulation of alpha-galactosidase A upregulates CD77: functional impact for Fabry nephropathy. Kidney Int 75(4):399–407

108. Mills K, Johnson A, Winchester B (2002) Synthesis of novel internal standards for the quantitative determination of plasma ceramide trihexoside in Fabry disease by tandem mass spectrometry. FEBS Lett 515(1–3):171–176

109. Fuller M, Sharp PC, Rozaklis T, Whitfield PD, Blacklock D, Hopwood JJ et al (2005) Urinary lipid profiling for the identification of Fabry hemizygotes and heterozygotes. Clin Chem 51(4):688–694

110. Grunfeld JP, Le Porrier M, Droz D, Bensaude I, Hinglais N, Crosnier J (1975) La transplantation rénale chez les sujets atteints de maladie de Fabry. Transplantation du rein d'un sujet hétérozygote à un sujet sain [in French]. Nouv Presse Med 4(29):2081–2085

111. Sessa A, Meroni M, Battini G, Maglio A, Brambilla PL, Bertella M et al (2001) Renal pathological changes in Fabry disease. J Inherit Metab Dis 24(Suppl 2):66–70, discussion 65

112. Alroy J, Sabnis S, Kopp JB (2002) Renal pathology in Fabry disease. J Am Soc Nephrol 13(Suppl 2):S134–S138

113. Fischer EG, Moore MJ, Lager DJ (2006) Fabry disease: a morphologic study of 11 cases. Mod Pathol 19(10):1295–1301

114. Burkholder PM, Updike SJ, Ware RA, Reese OG (1980) Clinicopathologic, enzymatic, and genetic features in a case of Fabry's disease. Arch Pathol Lab Med 104(1):17–25

115. Faraggiana T, Churg J, Grishman E, Strauss L, Prado A, Bishop DF et al (1981) Light- and electron-microscopic histochemistry of Fabry's disease. Am J Pathol 103(2):247–262

116. Fukushima M, Tsuchiyama Y, Nakato T, Yokoi T, Ikeda H, Yoshida S et al (1995) A female heterozygous patient with Fabry's disease with renal accumulation of trihexosylceramide detected with a monoclonal antibody. Am J Kidney Dis 26(6):952–955

117. Askari H, Kaneski CR, Semino-Mora C, Desai P, Ang A, Kleiner DE et al (2007) Cellular and tissue localization of globotriaosylceramide in Fabry disease. Virchows Arch 451(4):823–834

118. Kotani M, Kawashima I, Ozawa H, Ogura K, Ariga T, Tai T (1994) Generation of one set of murine monoclonal antibodies specific for globo-series glycolipids: evidence for differential distribution of the glycolipids in rat small intestine. Arch Biochem Biophys 310(1):89–96

119. Thurberg BL, Rennke H, Colvin RB, Dikman S, Gordon RE, Collins AB et al (2002) Globotriaosylceramide accumulation in the Fabry kidney is cleared from multiple cell types after enzyme replacement therapy. Kidney Int 62(6):1933–1946

120. Fogo AB, Bostad L, Svarstad E, Cook WJ, Moll S, Barbey F et al (2010) Scoring system for renal pathology in Fabry disease: report of the International Study Group of Fabry Nephropathy (ISGFN). Nephrol Dial Transplant 25 (in press)

121. Tosoni A, Nebuloni M, Zerbi P, Vago L, Comotti C, Sessa A (2005) Ultrastructural study of renal involvement in two females with Anderson-Fabry disease. Ultrastruct Pathol 29(3–4):203–207

122. Faria V (1970) Fabry disease, a rare thesausrismosis [in Portugese]. Jornal do Médico. [Case report] 72(1423):5–11

123. Oliveira JP (2007) Staging of Fabry disease using renal biopsies. Clin Therap 29(Suppl A):S

124. Meehan SM, Junsanto T, Rydel JJ, Desnick RJ (2004) Fabry disease: renal involvement limited to podocyte pathology and proteinuria in a septuagenarian cardiac variant. Pathologic and therapeutic implications. Am J Kidney Dis 43(1):164–171

125. Warnock DG (2005) Fabry disease: diagnosis and management, with emphasis on the renal manifestations. Curr Opin Nephrol Hypertens 14(2):87–95

126. Remuzzi G, Benigni A, Remuzzi A (2006) Mechanisms of progression and regression of renal lesions of chronic nephropathies and diabetes. J Clin Invest 116(2):288–296

127. Ruggenenti P, Perna A, Remuzzi G (2003) Retarding progression of chronic renal disease: the neglected issue of residual proteinuria. Kidney Int 63(6):2254–2261

128. Eng CM, Guffon N, Wilcox WR, Germain DP, Lee P, Waldek S et al (2001) Safety and efficacy of recombinant human alpha-galactosidase A–replacement therapy in Fabry's disease. N Engl J Med 345(1):9–16

129. Schiffmann R, Kopp JB, Austin HA III, Sabnis S, Moore DF, Weibel T et al (2001) Enzyme replacement therapy in Fabry disease: a randomized controlled trial. JAMA 285(21): 2743–2749

130. Germain D, Waldek S, Banikazemi M, Bushinsky D, Charrow J, Lee P et al (2007) Sustained, long-term renal stabilization after 54 months of agalsidase beta therapy in patients with Fabry disease. J Am Soc Nephrol 18(5):1547–1557

131. Wilcox WR, Banikazemi M, Guffon N, Waldek S, Lee P, Linthorst GE et al (2004) Long-term safety and efficacy of enzyme replacement therapy for Fabry disease. Am J Hum Genet 75(1):65–74

132. Moore DF, Altarescu G, Ling GS, Jeffries N, Frei KP, Weibel T et al (2002) Elevated cerebral blood flow velocities in Fabry disease with reversal after enzyme replacement. Stroke 33(2):525–531

133. Hilz MJ, Kolodny EH, Brys M, Stemper B, Haendl T, Marthol H (2004) Reduced cerebral blood flow velocity and impaired cerebral autoregulation in patients with Fabry disease. J Neurol 251(5):564–570

134. Hughes DA, Mehta AB (2005) Vascular complications of Fabry disease: enzyme replacement and other therapies. Acta Paediatr Suppl 94(447):28–33, discussion 9–10

135. Elliott PM, Kindler H, Shah JS, Sachdev B, Rimoldi OE, Thaman R et al (2006) Coronary microvascular dysfunction in male patients with Anderson-Fabry disease and the effect of treatment with alpha galactosidase A. Heart 92(3):357–360

136. Desnick RJ, Brady R, Barranger J, Collins AJ, Germain DP, Goldman M et al (2003) Fabry disease, an under-recognized multisystemic disorder: expert recommendations for diagnosis, management, and enzyme replacement therapy. Ann Intern Med 138(4):338–346

137. Shen JS, Meng XL, Moore DF, Quirk JM, Shayman JA, Schiffmann R et al (2008) Globotriaosylceramide induces oxidative stress and up-regulates cell adhesion molecule expression in Fabry disease endothelial cells. Mol Genet Metab 95(3):163–168

138. Kaneski CR, Moore DF, Ries M, Zirzow GC, Schiffmann R (2006) Myeloperoxidase predicts risk of vasculopathic events in hemizygous males with Fabry disease. Neurology 67(11):2045–2047

139. Warnock DG, Daina E, Remuzzi G et al (2010) Enzyme replacement therapy and Fabry nephropathy. Clin J Am Soc Nephrol 5:371–378

140. Ruggenenti P, Schieppati A, Remuzzi G (2001) Progression, remission, regression of chronic renal diseases. Lancet 357(9268):1601–1608

141. Lea J, Greene T, Hebert L, Lipkowitz M, Massry S, Middleton J et al (2005) The relationship between magnitude of proteinuria reduction and risk of end-stage renal disease: results of the African American study of kidney disease and hypertension. Arch Intern Med 165(8): 947–953

142. Ruggenenti P, Perticucci E, Cravedi P, Gambara V, Costantini M, Sharma SK et al (2008) Role of remission clinics in the longitudinal treatment of CKD. J Am Soc Nephrol 19(6):1213–1224

143. Tahir H, Jackson LL, Warnock DG (2007) Antiproteinuric therapy and Fabry nephropathy: Sustained reduction in proteinuria in patients receiving enzyme replacement therapy with agalsidase-beta. J Am Soc Nephrol 18:2609–2617

144. Banikazemi M, Bultas J, Waldek S, Wilcox WR, Whitley CB, McDonald M et al (2007) Agalsidase-beta therapy for advanced Fabry disease: a randomized trial. Ann Intern Med 146(2):77–86

145. Breunig F, Weidemann F, Strotmann J, Knoll A, Wanner C (2006) Clinical benefit of enzyme replacement therapy in Fabry disease. Kidney Int 69(7):1216–1221

146. Schiffmann R, Askari H, Timmons M, Robinson C, Benko W, Brady R et al (2007) Weekly enzyme replacement therapy may slow decline of renal function in Fabry patients who are on long-term biweekly dosing. J Am Soc Nephrol 18(5):1576–1583

147. Schiffmann R, Ries M, Timmons M, Flaherty JT, Brady RO (2006) Long-term therapy with agalsidase alfa for Fabry disease: safety and effects on renal function in a home infusion setting. Nephrol Dial Transplant 21(2):345–354

148. Warnock DG (2007) The Fabrazyme® and Arbs and ACE Inhibitor Treatment (FAACET) Study (NCT00446862) 2007 [updated March 14, 2007; cited 2007 September 9]. Available from http://www.clinicaltrials.gov/ct/search;jsessionid=87169CD1104ADB522 E4B53168DEA01DD?term=NCT00446862&submit=Search

149. Warnock DG, Daina E, Remuzzi G, West M (2010) Enzyme replacement therapy and Fabry nephropathy. Clin J Am Soc Nephrol 5:371–378

150. Consortium CFR (2009) Canadian Fabry Disease Initiative (CFDI) Enzyme Replacement Therapy (ERT) Study (NCT00455104) 2009 [cited 2009 September 16]. Available from http://clinicaltrials.gov/ct2/show/NCT00455104?term=west+fabry&rank=1

151. Levey AS (2002) Clinical practice. Nondiabetic kidney disease. N Engl J Med 347(19):1505–1511

152. Brenner BM, Cooper ME, de Zeeuw D, Keane WF, Mitch WE, Parving HH et al (2001) Effects of losartan on renal and cardiovascular outcomes in patients with type 2 diabetes and nephropathy. N Engl J Med 345(12):861–869

153. Lewis EJ, Hunsicker LG, Clarke WR, Berl T, Pohl MA, Lewis JB et al (2001) Renoprotective effect of the angiotensin-receptor antagonist irbesartan in patients with nephropathy due to type 2 diabetes. N Engl J Med 345(12):851–860

154. Hofstetter TH (2001) Prevention of end-stage renal disease due to type 2 diabetes. N Engl J Med 345(12):910–912

155. The ESCAPE Trial Group (2009) Strict blood-pressure control and progression of renal failure in children. N Engl J Med 361(17):1639–1650

156. Kent DM, Jafar TH, Hayward RA, Tighiouart H, Landa M, de Jong P et al (2007) Progression risk, urinary protein excretion, and treatment effects of Angiotensin-converting enzyme inhibitors in nondiabetic kidney disease. J Am Soc Nephrol 18(6):1959–1965

157. de Zeeuw D (2007) Albuminuria: a target for treatment of type 2 diabetic nephropathy. Semin Nephrol 27(2):172–181

158. Eng CM, Germain DP, Banikazemi M, Warnock DG, Wanner C, Hopkin RJ et al (2006) Fabry disease: guidelines for the evaluation and management of multi-organ system involvement. Genet Med 8(9):539–548

159. Jain G, Campbell RC, Warnock DG (2009) Mineralocorticoid receptor blockers and chronic kidney disease. Clin J Am Soc Nephrol 4:1685–1691

160. Fervenza FC, Torra R, Warnock DG (2008) Safety and efficacy of enzyme replacement therapy in the nephropathy of Fabry disease. Biologics 2(4):1–22

Chapter 13
Neurological Manifestations in Fabry Disease

Arndt Rolfs, Ales Dudesek, Jan Lukas, and Tobias Böttcher

Abstract Neurological manifestations of Fabry disease occur in both the peripheral nervous system (PNS) and central nervous system (CNS), with globotriaosylceramide (Gb3) accumulation in neurons, Schwann cells and dorsal root ganglia. The abnormal Gb3 accumulation in neurons appears to have little clinical consequence on the natural history of Fabry disease. The vascular change in Fabry disease is considered to be responsible for increased regional cerebral blood flow (rCBF) documented in PET scans, especially in the posterior circulation. There is clear evidence for an increased number of lacunar infarctions, predominantly periventricular, as well as small cortical infarcts – in females as well as in males. However, the pathogenesis of Fabry vasculopathy remains mostly unclear, but is based on the combination of endothelial dysfunction and abnormal function control of the vessels. It is widely accepted that cerebral hyperperfusion, predominantly in the posterior cerebral circulation is an important cornerstone in the pathophysiology of stroke in Fabry disease. Additionally, inflammation seems to have an influence on the progress of the vasculopathy in Fabry disease. The majority of Fabry stroke patients both in the hemizygote and the heterozygote groups present symptoms and clinical signs of vertebrobasilar ischemia. Consequently, vertigo/dizziness, diplopia, dysarthria, nystagmus, ataxia are the most frequent symptoms in stroke patients with Fabry.

Keywords Cerebral hyperfusion · Stroke · Lacunar infarcts · Pulvinar sign · Enzyme replacement therapy · Cerebrovascular symptoms · Hearing loss · Pain

13.1 Fabry Disease and the Brain

In the central nervous system (CNS) of Fabry patients, diffuse storage occurs in the vascular endothelium, with more localized involvement of central neurons together

A. Rolfs (✉)
Medical Faculty, Albrecht-Kossel-Institute for Neuroregeneration, University of Rostock, Rostock, Germany
e-mail: arndt.rolfs@med.uni-rostock.de

D. Elstein et al. (eds.), *Fabry Disease*, DOI 10.1007/978-90-481-9033-1_13,
© Springer Science+Business Media B.V. 2010

with the dorsal root and autonomic ganglia in the peripheral nervous system. The pathophysiology of the cerebrovascular changes in Fabry disease remains unclear. PET investigations suggest a chronic alteration of the nitric oxide (NO) pathway in Fabry disease. On the other hand there is an increased endothelium-mediated vascular reactivity, where the increased vessel response to acetylcholine with and without N^G-monomethyl-L-arginine suggests altered functionality of non-NO endothelium-dependent vasodilatory pathways. Vessel wall alterations with narrowing of cerebral resistance vessels are likely to compromise cerebral blood flow velocity and contribute to the early and increased incidence of stroke. Increased cerebral blood flow in the posterior circulation, particularly in the thalamus, suggests that the dystrophic calcification is secondary to cerebral hyperperfusion and selective vulnerability of the pulvinar and adjacent thalamic structures.

The swollen vascular endothelial cells, often accompanied by endothelial cell proliferation, encroach upon the lumen of involved vessels and might lead to focal increase of intraluminal pressure, dilatation and angiectasis of small cerebral arteries. Grewal [1] described eight Fabry patients with cerebrovascular events (CVE) which in all cases involved the deep or penetrating arteries similar to those arteries which cause lacunar strokes. This is in accordance with the study from Rolfs and co-workers [2] as well as Schiffman and Ries [3] where nearly 50% of the Fabry patients with stroke demonstrate periventricular white-matter hyperintensities.

Several studies have reported an increased number of lacunar infarctions, predominantly periventricular, as well as small cortical infarcts [4]. As Fellgiebel and co-workers have demonstrated [5] Fabry patients more commonly exhibit radiological findings consistent with small-vessel disease, either as a cause of symptomatic stroke or as clinically silent lesions.

Beside the small vessels being involved in the pathogenesis, large vessels are also pathologically changed in Fabry disease. Dysfunction of cerebral circulation has been shown in different studies using cerebral blood flow velocity (CBFV [cm/s]), cerebrovascular reactivity as well as cerebral perfusion (CBF [ml/100 g of tissue/min]). Cerebral hyper-perfusion is also associated with calcifications in the cerebral white matter and in the pulvinar or posterior thalamic regions [6, 7]. In the study from Takanashi and co-workers [6] bilateral T1 shortening in the lateral pulvinar was recognized in at least seven out of 10 patients, all over the age of 30 years, who also had small areas of T2 prolongation in the white matter. CT and gradient echo images in one patient revealed no evidence of calcification or metallic deposits in the pulvinar. In the study from Moore and co-workers [7] overall, 22 patients (about 23%) demonstrated pulvinar hyperintensity on T1-weighted images (Fig. 13.1); the frequency increased with age to over 30% by age 50 years. Susceptibility-weighted T2* studies demonstrated a low-signal-intensity abnormality in the pulvinar in the more severe cases, whereas CT demonstrated the pulvinar to be mineralized. The group from Burlina and co-workers [8] has analysed 36 patients (16 males, 20 females) and was able to demonstrate the pulvinar sign only in 5 male patients. Seven patients had at least one stroke (territorial or lacunar). There was no correlation between stroke and the pulvinar sign. All patients with the pulvinar sign had hypertrophic cardiomyopathy. They conclude that the pulvinar sign is a highly

Fig. 13.1 MR finding in the posterior thalamus. T1-weighted image through the thalamus in a Fabry patient demonstrates moderate hyperintensity in the dorsolateral thalamus (Pulvinar)

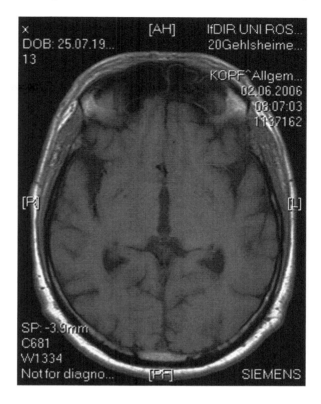

specific sign of Fabry disease, found in male patients with cardiac signs and severe kidney involvement.

Of the potential mechanisms of cerebral ischemia in patients with Fabry disease, the intracranial arterial dolichoectasia due to glycosphingolipid deposition in vascular smooth muscle, the progressive occlusion of small arteries or arterioles secondary to deposition of glycosphingolipid, endothelial and leukocyte activation, reduced cerebral blood flow velocity and impaired cerebral autoregulation, seem to be the most important aspects in the role of Fabry disease in stroke. Additional mechanisms, like cardiogenic embolism and impaired autonomic function, might play a less important role for cerebral ischemia, compared with the cerebrovascular changes induced by the enzymopathy.

There are also clear data of abnormalities of cerebrovascular autoregulation and vasoreactivity [9]. During the course of a randomized double-blind placebo-controlled 6-month ERT trial Moore and co-workers [10] investigated the functional blood flow response of the brain, the cerebral vasoactivity and PET in Fabry patients. They demonstrated that Fabry patients had a significantly greater increase in rCBF and that the time for recovery of the cerebral vasculature following acetazolamide was prolonged in Fabry patients. ERT was able to reverse the exaggerated cerebrovascular response. Similarly, Hilz and colleagues [9] speculate that both reduced rCBF and impaired cerebral autoregulation are likely to be involved in the increased risk of stroke in Fabry patients.

An increased endothelium-dependent vascular reactivity to acetylcholine in the forearm vascular bed has been described [11]. Interestingly, this seems to still be present after infusion of a competitive arginine inhibitor which indicates changing of function of the non-nitric oxide pathways [12]. Also based on the high incidence of vertebrobasilar dolichoectasia these data might argue that the vascular dysfunction in Fabry disease is due to increased release of reactive oxygen species, which induces increased oxidative stress and peroxynitrite formation potentially resulting in persistent vasodilatation [10].

13.1.1 Cerebrovascular Disease

The cerebrovascular manifestations consist of large-vessel ectasia, large vessel occlusive disease, and small vessel disease (Fig. 13.2). The vascular diathesis is

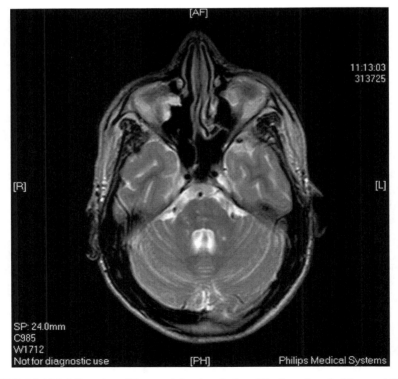

Fig. 13.2 Multiple bilateral small lacunar infarctions in the midbrain region of a 24-year old Fabry patient

reported to have a vertebrobasilar circulation distribution, although the reason for this is unclear.

The incidence of stroke together with vessel ectasia [13] is about 40% in hemizygous males, mainly seeming to affect younger subjects. The most frequent cerebrovascular symptoms in Fabry patients are hemiparesis, vertigo/dizziness, diplopia, nystagmus and ataxia of gait in the hemizygote group, and memory loss, dizziness, ataxia, hemiparesis, loss of consciousness and hemisensory symptoms in the heterozygote group [2].

Rolfs and co-workers [2] analysed 721 (432 male, 289 female) consecutive unrelated young patients (18–55 years of age) who had an apparently unexplained acute cerebrovascular event (CVE), a cryptogenic stroke. Mutations within the GLA gene were found in 28 patients (21 male, 7 female). The mean age of onset of symptomatic cerebrovascular disease was 38.4 ± 13.0 years in the male stroke patients and 40.3 ± 13.1 years in the female group, compared to the non-Fabry group with a mean age of 47.9 years. In a Belgian Fabry stroke study (BEFAS) Eyskens and co-workers [14] could show that over a period of 24 months four female patients (out of 1,000 patients with cryptogenic stroke) were diagnosed for heterozygosity of a known mutation. All patients had no signs of organ involvement besides stroke, transient ischemic attacks (TIA) and/or headache.

It is evident that acute stroke in young patients especially in Fabry disease is a multifactorial process. Fabry disease must be considered in all cases of unexplained stroke in young patients, particularly in cases with the combination of infarction in the vertebrobasilar artery system and proteinuria.

An important study from Sims and co-workers [15] analysed data from 2,446 patients in a Fabry Registry to identify clinical characteristics of patients experiencing stroke during the natural history period. A total of 138 patients (86 of 1,243 males [6.9%] and 52 of 1,203 females [4.3%]) had experienced strokes. Median age at first stroke was 39.0 years in males and 45.7 years in females. What is most important in this study is the fact that most patients (70.9% of males and 76.9% of females) had not experienced renal or cardiac events before their first stroke. Fifty percent of males and 38.3% of females experienced their first stroke before being diagnosed with Fabry disease.

13.1.2 Classification of Stroke in Fabry Disease

The cerebral vasculopathy of Fabry disease could be classified into large- and small-vessel disease pathology in addition to the cardioembolic sources of infarctions [5, 11, 16]. There is an increased likelihood of cerebral dolichoectasia (Fig. 13.3) or the elongation and dilation of the affected vessel. This most commonly involves the basilar artery [2] but the carotid artery may also be affected. Such arterial dilation may induce flow stagnation resulting in an increased risk of artery-to-artery embolization or thrombosis with consecutive cerebrovascular events. The majority of Fabry patients with stroke - both in the hemizygote and the heterozygote

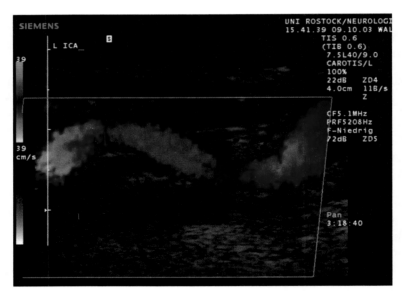

Fig. 13.3 Ectasia and elongation of the left carotid artery in a 28 year old female Fabry patient (duplex-sonography)

groups – presents with symptoms and clinical signs of vertebrobasilar ischemia, which argues from the clinical view for a general tendency for involvement of the posterior circulation arteries. These results support previous data, like the study from Mitsias and Levine [17] reporting vertigo/dizziness, diplopia, dysarthria, nystagmus, ataxia as the most frequent symptoms. The reason for the tendency for vertebrobasilar system involvement is not clear [2], as it seems reasonable to presume that the endothelial changes in the scope of Fabry disease should affect the cerebral arteries in a uniform manner. In their careful neuropathologic analysis of cerebrovascular complications in 12 hemizygotic and 3 heterozygotic Fabry patients Mitsias and Levine [17] reported a prevalence of thickened vessels (Fig. 13.4) of the circle of Willis with narrowing of the lumina in about one third of the cases, moderate atheroma of the major cerebral vessels or intracellular deposits in arteries and arterioles in about 15%. A massive dilatation of the basilar was seen in 1 case. There are a many reports of Fabry patients demonstrating the marked thickening of the medium- and small-sized arteries as well as the dolichoectasia in the posterior circulation [18–20]. In non-Fabry cases the incidence of dolichoectasia varies between 0.06 and 5.8% [21, 22]. Gavazzi and co-workers [19] have shown that men and women in Fabry disease showed a similar distribution of cerebral white matter changes, lacunar and cortical infarcts, small haemorrhages and vertebrobasilar dolichoectasia. Additionally, they found no significant differences between Fabry patients and control subjects for concentration of N-acetylaspartate, creatine and choline.

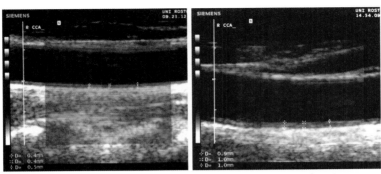

Normal control (0,5 mm)   Fabry disease (1,0 mm)

Fig. 13.4 Intima-media thickness (IM) in Fabry disease patient; artery IMT is increased to the same extent in male and female patients with Fabry disease (compared with that of the control population). In the Fabry group, IMT is not correlating with systolic blood pressure. Atherosclerotic plaques in the common carotid artery are rarely observed in Fabry patients

To determine the most promising imaging tool for the detection of CNS involvement in Fabry disease Fellgiebel and co-workers [23] were comparing the diagnostic utility of different MR imaging findings. With an accuracy of 87%, basilar artery diameters were superior to all other MR measures for separating patients with Fabry disease from controls.

However, besides abnormalities of the vessel wall, blood components, such as pro-coagulants and anticoagulants with additional abnormal hemodynamic also seem to play an important role [11] for the induction of vascular dysfunction in Fabry disease. The Schiffmann group [24] has shown in Fabry patients increased P-selectin, plasminogen activator inhibitor (PAI), soluble sICAM-1, sVCAM-1, and decreased thrombomodulin combined with increased integrin CD11b on monocytes (receptor for fibrinogen and factor X) expression. This data reveals measurable evidence for endothelium and leukocyte activation which argues for a prothrombotic state in Fabry patients.

13.1.3 Cerebrovascular Events in Women

Up to now no clear data exist about the frequency of Fabry disease in female stroke patients. From the Fabry Outcome Survey (FOS), a very recent databank from European clinics on the natural history of Fabry disease [25], it is now known that the most frequently reported signs and symptoms in proven cases of Fabry disease are neurological, and are reported for the majority of both male (84%) and female (79%) patients. The frequency of stroke, TIA and prolonged reversible ischemic neurological deficit is higher in women than in men, with 12% of male and 27% of female patients reporting these incidents. The mean age at onset of CVE is 28.8 years in males and 43.4 years in females. In addition, one female patient reported a TIA at the age of 25 years, and other CVE were reported for five further females aged less than 30 years. This is somewhat in contrast to the results of Rolfs and co-workers [2] who reported a mean age at onset of symptomatic cerebrovascular disease in the male stroke group of 39.6 ± 13.4 years.

The mean age of onset in the female stroke group described by Rolfs and co-workers [2] is 42.7 ± 14.2 years, thereby identical to the FOS databank; there was no significant difference between the age of onset of CVE between males and females in that study. In general, there are no clear data demonstrating an earlier manifestation of CVE in the Fabry group compared to the non-Fabry group [2, 13]. According to the recent evaluation of the FOS the principal causes of death among 181 affected relatives of patients in FOS (most of whom had died before 2001) were renal failure in males (42%) and cerebrovascular disease in females (25%) [26]. Interestingly, the Italian group from Padua [8], analysing 36 patients (16 males, 20 females) was able to demonstrate the pulvinar sign only in 5 male patients, and not at all in female patients.

13.1.4 Cerebrovascular Pathology in Fabry Disease and Enzyme Replacement Treatment

Little is known regarding the influence of enzyme replacement treatment (ERT), either with agalsidase alpha or beta, on cerebrovascular pathologies in Fabry disease. Leech and Johnson [27] reported a case of a 32-year-old man with large pontine and small basal ganglia infarct who was treated with 1 mg/kg biweekly of agalsidase beta. After 26 months of treatment he developed a pseudobulbar palsy and worsening weakness and spasticity, and repeated CT confirmed new areas of cerebral infarction in bilateral internal capsule. This is a hint that progression of cerebrovascular complications of Fabry disease can occur while on enzyme replacement therapy. On the other hand, patients have been reported with serious neurological problems due to CVE, who have responded well during the enzyme replacement therapy with agalsidase beta [28].

In a recent report Yamadera and co-workers [29] describe a 27-year-old man with Fabry disease who had widespread white-matter lesions (WMLs) despite the absence of renal or cardiac manifestations. After 12 months of enzyme replacement therapy, most of the WMLs had disappeared. Cell counts and protein levels in the cerebrospinal fluid also decreased. Until effective therapy becomes a reality, primary and secondary prevention of strokes is critical in Fabry disease. Besides antiplatelet agents other treatable risk factors should be appropriately addressed with statins, angiotensin-converting-enzyme inhibitors, or angiotensin receptor blockers.

There is a European study (www.sifap.eu) running which is controlled by a non-treated-group. This study is analysing the efficiency of ERT in recurrent stroke in Fabry patients in a trial extending for up to 45 months. First data will be available in 2012.

13.1.5 Fabry Disease Mimicking Multiple Sclerosis

As regions of massive periventricular signal intensities are seen in some Fabry patients, this constellation might be misinterpreted not only as multiple sclerosis, but also as demyelinating disease, neuropathies, and stroke. Although there have been some recent studies [30], Fabry disease mimicking multiple sclerosis has not been evaluated extensively. In a case reported by Saip and co-workers [31] the age of onset, repeated occurrence of cerebrovascular events and similar MRI findings of both diseases has lead an initial diagnosis of multiple sclerosis, but oligoclonal band was negative and there was no demyelinating process in brain biopsy specimens obtained from the lesions found in cerebral MRI. However, there are also some cases in the literature where oligoclonal bands have been reported in those patients [32]. Therefore, it remains open whether this is a co-incidence of two diseases or whether Fabry disease can also resemble such a clinical picture.

13.1.6 Fabry Disease and Hearing

Hearing loss and tinnitus are common symptoms in Fabry disease and increase in prevalence with age. Pure-tone audiograms from 101 children (53 girls, 48 boys) have been analysed [33]. When assessed by age-appropriate audiometry, 19 of 101 patients (19%) had a persistent hearing loss in at least one frequency range. Of these, 14 had a high-frequency hearing loss, 4 a pan-frequency hearing loss, and 1 a pattern typical of noise-induced loss. Of the 101 children with audiometry, 44 complained of tinnitus. Only 2 children reported sudden hearing loss, which was not verified by audiometry. Palla et al. [34] analysed the progressive hearing and vestibular loss in Fabry disease. Pure tone audiometry (PTA) was done at baseline in 47 patients (25 male, 18–60 years; 22 female, 17–74 years).

Of the 47 patients, 38 (24 males) were tested both before and during ERT (follow-up ≤60 months). ERT consisted of agalsidase alfa infusions. At baseline, progressive hearing loss was present in 88% of males and 86% of females. Over all tested frequencies (range: 0.5–6 kHz), progressive hearing loss (pHL) was significantly greater at higher ages and in males, with largest deficits at high frequencies. The authors speculate that progressive hearing and progressive vestibular loss emerge from lesions within the vestibulocochlear labyrinth, because no specific patterns of vestibulo-cochlear deficits were observed, which would be expected if lesions were more proximal along the inferior or superior branch of the vestibulo-cochlear nerve or labyrinthine artery. ERT stabilizes auditory and even improves vestibular function.

Ries and co-workers [35] conducted a retrospective cross sectional analysis of hearing loss in 109 male and female Fabry patients (85 males aged 6–58 years; 24 females aged 22–72 years). HL (95), defined as a hearing threshold above the 95th percentile for age and gender matched normal controls, was present in 56%

of the males. Prevalence of HL (95) was lower in the group of patients with residual GLA enzyme activity compared with those without detectable activity (33% vs. 63%). Male patients with HL (95) had a higher microvascular cerebral white matter lesion load and more pronounced cold perception deficit. Of the females, 38% had HL (95). According to this study hearing loss in Fabry disease is involving all frequency regions significantly contributes to morbidity in patients with Fabry disease.

ERT with agalsidase alfa appears to reverse the hearing deterioration in these patients. This improvement, however, is gradual, suggesting the need for long-term ERT [36].

13.2 Peripheral Nervous System in Fabry Disease

Pain and somatosensory disturbances are prominent manifestations of this disease [37]. In an animal model, the Fabry mice, sensorimotor assessment revealed diminished locomotor activity and warm hypoalgesia, as assessed with the hot-plate test [38]. Moreover Fabry mice displayed alterations both in balance and co-ordination. By histological analysis, the cytoarchitecture of Fabry mice sciatic nerves showed an increase in mean cross-sectional area accompanied by a decrease in the density of non-myelinated fibers as well as a trend for a decreased number of small myelinated fibers, a well established feature of Fabry disease. A relative preservation of large myelinated fibers and nerve conduction velocity was observed. These findings demonstrate that Fabry knockout mice have Gb3 accumulation in the peripheral nervous system, alterations in sensorimotor function, hypoalgesia and no impairment of motor nerve conduction.

To explore the frequency of symptoms and the functional and structural involvement of the nervous system in female patients Torvin-Moller and co-workers [37] examined the presence of pain, manifestations of peripheral neuropathy and nerve density in skin biopsies in 19 female patients with Fabry disease and 19 sex- and age-matched controls. Diaries, quantitative sensory testing, neurophysiologic tests and skin biopsies were performed. Daily pain was present in 63% of patients. Tactile detection threshold and pressure pain threshold were lower and cold detection thresholds increased in patients. Sensory nerve action potential amplitude and maximal sensory conduction velocity were not different, whereas there was a highly significant reduction in intraepidermal nerve fiber density. These data demonstrate that careful evaluation of symptoms in female Fabry patients is important as small fiber disease manifestations are present.

Maag et al. [39] used a quantitative sensory testing to determine the detailed somatosensory profile of male Fabry patients and compare this profile with somatosensory profiles of other painful sensory neuropathies. The profile revealed a small-fiber sensory neuropathy selectively affecting C- and A-delta fibers. The comparison with different somatosensory profiles of painful sensory neuropathies, including painful small-fiber sensory neuropathies of other etiologies, showed that the Fabry disease profile differs significantly and is characterized by a severe impairment of thermal discrimination and preserved vibratory and mechanical discrimination.

In a study where neurography, vibratory and thermal quantitative sensory testing (QST), skin biopsy for measuring intraepidermal nerve fiber density, heart rate variability and sympathetic skin response tests for detecting autonomic dysfunction, pain-, depression- and somatic symptom questionnaires and clinical examination were used [40], only two women had no persistent symptoms or signs of polyneuropathy; 10 had symptoms of small fiber neuropathy. Neurological examination was normal in most patients. In QST, A-delta-fiber function for innocuous cold was more often impaired than C-fiber function. Conventional nerve conduction studies were mostly normal.

In a retrospective analysis of the data of 752 patients with Fabry disease (393 females, 353 males) enrolled in the Fabry Outcome Survey, the prevalence of pain in male patients was 81.4% (females 65.3%) [41]. Mean age at onset of pain was 14.8+/−1.0 year in males (females 19.8+/−1.4 year). Pain was most frequently reported in the hands (males 76%, females 60%) and feet (males 73%, females 52%), but often affected the whole body. Interference of pain with daily life was higher in females than in males, and was observed predominantly for general activities, mood, and normal work. After 36 months, 'average pain' and 'pain now' were significantly reduced with ERT.

Summarizing, pain is one of the most prevalent symptoms in Fabry disease with onset early in childhood. ERT seems of benefit in this debilitating disorder.

References

1. Grewal RP (1994) Stroke in Fabry's disease. J Neurol 241:153–156
2. Rolfs A, Böttcher T, Zschiesche M et al (2005) High prevalence of Fabry disease in young stroke patients. Lancet 366:1794–1796
3. Schiffman R, Ries M (2005) Fabry's disease—an important risk factor for stroke. Lancet 366:1754–1756
4. Crutchfield KE, Patronas NJ, Dambrosia JM et al (1998) Quantitative analysis of cerebral vasculopathy in patients with Fabry disease. Neurology 50:1746–1749
5. Fellgiebel A, Albrecht J, Dellani PR et al (2007) Quantification of brain tissue alterations in Fabry disease using diffusion tensor imaging. Acta Paediatr Suppl 96:33–36
6. Takanashi J, Barkovich AJ, Dillon WP et al (2003) T1 hyperintensity in the pulvinar: key imaging feature for diagnosis of Fabry disease. AJNR Am J Neuroradiol 24:916–921
7. Moore DF, Ye F, Schiffmann R, Butman JA (2003) Increased signal intensity in the pulvinar on T1-weighted images: a pathognomonic MR imaging sign of Fabry disease. Am J Neuroradiol 24:1096–1101
8. Burlina AP, Manara R, Caillaud C et al (2008) The pulvinar sign: frequency and clinical correlations in Fabry disease. J Neurol 255:738–744
9. Hilz MJ, Kolodny EH, Brys M et al (2004) Reduced cerebral blood flow velocity and impaired cerebral autoregulation in patients with Fabry disease. J Neurol 251:564–570
10. Moore DF, Scott LTC, Gladwin MT et al (2001) Regional cerebral hyperperfusion and nitric oxide pathway dysregulation in Fabry disease. Reversal by enzyme replacement therapy. Circulation 104:1506–1512

11. Moore D, Kaneski CR, Askari H et al (2007) The cerebral vasculopathy of Fabry disease. J Neurol Sci 257:258–263
12. Altarescu G, Moore DF, Pursley R et al (2001) Enhanced endothelium-dependent vasodilation in Fabry disease. Stroke 32:1559–1562
13. Fellgiebel A, Muller MJ, Ginsberg L (2006) CNS manifestations of Fabry's disease. Lancet Neurol 5:791–795
14. Eyskens FJ, De Deyn PP (2009) Belgian Fabry stroke study (BEFAS): a national, multicentre, prospective study on the prevalence of Fabry disease in young stroke patients with stroke. Mol Genet Metabol 98:1–2
15. Sims K, Politei J, Banikazemi M et al (2009) Stroke in Fabry disease frequently occurs before diagnosis and in the absence of other clinical events: natural history data from the Fabry Registry. Stroke 40(3):788–794
16. Moore DF, Herscovitch P, Schiffmann R (2001) Selective arterial distribution of cerebral hyper-perfusion in Fabry disease. J Neuroimaging 11:303–307
17. Mitsias P, Levine SR (1996) Cerebrovascular complications of Fabry's disease. Ann Neurol 40:8–17
18. Taglianini F, Pietrini V, Gemignani F, Lechi A, Pallini R, Federico A (1982) Anderson-Fabry's disease: neuropathological and neurochemical investigation. Acta Neuropathol (Berl) 56: 93–98
19. Kaye EM, Kolodny EH, Logigian EL et al (1988) Nervous system involvement in Fabry's disease: clinicopathological and biochemical correlation. Ann Neurol 23:505–509
20. Gavazzi C, Borsini W, Guerrini L et al (2006) Subcortical damage and cortical functional changes in men and women with Fabry disease: a multifaceted MR study. Radiology 241: 492–500
21. Resta M, Gentile A, Cuonzo FD (1984) Clinical-angiographic correlations in 132 patients with megadolichovertebrobasilar anomaly. Neuroradiology 26:213–216
22. Yu Y, Mosely IF, Pullicino P et al (1982) The clinical picture of ectasia of the intracerebral arteries. J Neurol Neurosurg Psychiatry 45:29–36
23. Fellgiebel A, Keller I, Marin D et al (2009) Diagnostic utility of different MRI and MR angiography measures in Fabry disease. Neurology 72(1):63–68
24. DeGraba T, Azhar S, Dignat-George F et al (2000) Profile of endothelial and leukocyte activation in Fabry patients. Ann Neurol 47:229–233
25. Mehta A, Ricci R, Widmer U et al (2004) Fabry disease defined: baseline clinical manifestations of 366 patients in the Fabry Outcome Survey. Europ J Clin Invest 34: 236–242
26. Mehta A, Clarke JT, Giugliani R et al (2009) Natural course of Fabry disease: changing pattern of causes of death in FOS – Fabry Outcome Survey. J Med Genet 46(8):548–552
27. Leech N, Johnson K (2003) Enzyme replacement treatment in "cerebrovascular" Fabry disease – when is it too late? The 4th European round table on Fabry disease. Expectations of enzyme replacement therapy, Oct 17–18, 2003, Munich, Germany
28. Suresh S, Thompson L, Kenny M et al (2003) The effect of enzyme replacement therapy on the neurological complications of Anderson Fabry disease. The 4th European round table on Fabry disease. Expectations of enzyme replacement therapy, Oct 17–18, 2003, Munich, Germany
29. Yamadera M, Yokoe M, Beck G et al (2009) Amelioration of white-matter lesions in a patient with Fabry disease. J Neurol Sci 279(1–2):118–120
30. Callegaro D, Kaimen-Maciel DR (2006) Fabry disease as a differential diagnosis of MS. Int MS J 13(1):27–30
31. Saip S, Uluduz D, Erkol G (2007) Fabry disease mimicking multiple sclerosis. Clin Neurol Neurosurg 109(4):361–363
32. Invernizzi P, Bonometti MA, Turri E et al (2008) A case of Fabry disease with central nervous system (CNS) demyelinating lesions: a double trouble? Mult Scler 14(7): 1003–1006

33. Keilmann A, Hajioff D, Ramaswami U, on behalf of the FOS Investigators (2009) Ear symptoms in children with Fabry disease: data from the Fabry Outcome Survey. J Inherit Metab Dis 32(6):739–744
34. Palla A, Hegemann S, Widmer U et al (2007) Vestibular and auditory deficits in Fabry disease and their response to enzyme replacement therapy. J Neurol 254(10):1433–1442
35. Ries M, Kim HJ, Zalewski CK et al (2007) Neuropathic and cerebrovascular correlates of hearing loss in Fabry disease. Brain 130(Pt 1):143–150
36. Hajioff D, Enever Y, Quiney R et al (2003) Hearing loss in Fabry disease: the effect of agalsidase alfa replacement therapy. J Inherit Metab Dis 26(8):787–794
37. Torvin Møller A, Winther Bach F, Feldt-Rasmussen U et al (2009) Functional and structural nerve fiber findings in heterozygote patients with Fabry disease. Pain 145(1–2):237–245
38. Rodrigues LG, Ferraz MJ, Rodrigues D et al (2009) Neurophysiological, behavioral and morphological abnormalities in the Fabry knockout mice. Neurobiol Dis 33(1):48–56
39. Maag R, Binder A, Maier C et al (2008) Detection of a characteristic painful neuropathy in Fabry disease: a pilot study. Pain Med 9(8):1217–1223
40. Laaksonen SM, Röyttä M, Jääskeläinen SK, Kantola I, Penttinen M, Falck B (2008) Neuropathic symptoms and findings in women with Fabry disease. Clin Neurophysiol 119(6):1365–1372
41. Hoffmann B, Beck M, Sunder-Plassmann G et al (2007) Nature and prevalence of pain in Fabry disease and its response to enzyme replacement therapy–a retrospective analysis from the Fabry Outcome Survey. Clin J Pain 23(6):535–542

Chapter 14
Dermatological Manifestations of Fabry Disease

Catherine H. Orteu

Abstract The term 'angiokeratoma corporis diffusum' (ACD) has been used synonymously with Anderson-Fabry disease since its original description. Since the availability of effective therapy, the drive to identify patients has increased. As a result, we are becoming more aware of a broader spectrum in the cutaneous and systemic phenotype of the condition. Not all patients have widespread angiokeratomas. Macular (flat) angiomas without any overlying hyperkeratosis and papular- 'cherry' angiomas are also seen. Telangiectases may occur at sun exposed sites including the face and 'V' of the neck, more rarely they are present in unusual sites, such as flanks and elbow flexures. In addition to these cutaneous vascular lesions, skin signs include characteristic facial features, oedema and lymphoedema of the lower limbs, abnormalities of sweating and Raynaud's phenomenon. Skin signs are an obvious, outward manifestation of disease and as such are important signs for diagnosis. They represent a significant source of morbidity, have a recognised impact on self-esteem and quality of life, and should be treated appropriately. Of particular interest, is whether the cutaneous phenotype may be helpful not only in making the diagnosis of Fabry disease, but also in assessing or predicting overall disease severity.

Keywords Angiokeratoma · Cherry angioma · Cutaneous vascular lesions · Fabry facial features · Lymphoedema · Hyperhidrosis · Hypohidrosis · Raynaud's phenomenon

Abbreviations

ACD	Angiokeratoma corporis diffusum
AK	Angiokeratoma
CVL	Cutaneous vascular lesions
ERT	Enzyme replacement therapy
FD	Fabry disease

C.H. Orteu (✉)
Department of Dermatology, Royal Free Hospital, London, UK
e-mails: cate.orteu@royalfree.nhs.uk; kateorteu@hotmail.com

D. Elstein et al. (eds.), *Fabry Disease*, DOI 10.1007/978-90-481-9033-1_14,
© Springer Science+Business Media B.V. 2010

FOS   Fabry outcome survey
LSD   Lysosomal storage disorders
MSSI   Mainz severity scoring index
SD   Standard deviation
TIA   Transient ischaemic attack
VEGF   Vascular endothelial growth factor
VEGFR   Vascular endothelial growth factor receptor

14.1 Cutaneous Vascular Lesions

14.1.1 Angiokeratoma

Angiokeratomas are the cutaneous hallmark of Fabry disease [1–3]. Current epidemiological data suggests that they are present in 70% of males and 39% of females [4, 5]. Angiokeratoma are dark red to blue-black, macular (flat) and papular (raised) lesions, which do not blanch on pressure (Fig. 14.1). If overlying hyperkeratosis is present, they feel rough to the touch. They may be widespread or grouped. Their size range is from pin-point to 4 mm in diameter. They are produced by vascular abnormalities predominantly involving the dermal papillae. Ultrastructurally the dilated vessels resemble the small collecting veins, which are normally found at the

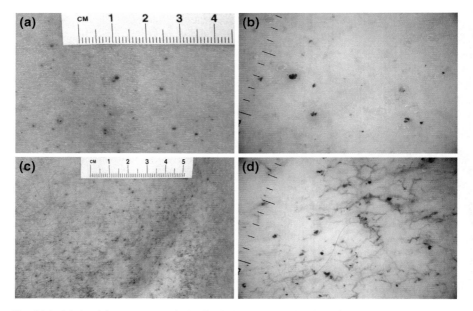

Fig. 14.1 (a) Angiokeratomas on the back. (b) Dermatoscopic view of (a). (c) Angiokeratomas and telangiectatic vessels on the flank in a patient with Angiokeratoma corporis diffusum. (d) Dermatoscopic view showing angiokeratomas and upper dermal vessel tortuosity

dermal-subcutaneous interface [6]. Histology typically shows dilated, ectatic capillaries in the papillary dermis, epidermal acanthosis, most prominent at the edges of the lesion, and variable degrees of focal compact orthohyperkeratosis. Lamellated intracytoplasmic vacuolar inclusions are typically seen on electron microscopy [7]. Histopathology and electronmicroscopic findings are described in detail elsewhere.

Angiokeratomas tend to appear between the ages of 5 and 15 years in males and 3–10 years later in females [8–10]. Numbers of lesions increase gradually thereafter. The distribution of angiokeratomas is illustrated in Fig. 14.2. In males lesions are typically within the 'bathing trunk' area, which includes the penis, scrotum, buttocks, inner thighs and sacral area. Classical angiokeratomas with overlying hyperkeratosis tend to be found mainly in these areas and in and around the umbilicus. Lesions at other sites, may be macular, with minimal or no hyperkeratosis [4, 11]. Angiokeratomas are also seen on the proximal limbs, particularly their medial aspects, the elbows and knees, the palms and soles, and around the proximal nail folds of the digits. Lesions may occur on the lips, particularly along the vermillion border, and occasionally on the mucosal surfaces. The commonest sites for lesions in females are the trunk and proximal limbs [4]. Genital lesions are relatively infrequent. Lesions are often quite sparse, and may occasionally occur in a dermatomal distribution [4, 10]

Widespread angiokeratomas are not specific to Fabry disease. Other lysosomal storage disorders should be considered in the differential diagnosis, most notably fucosidosis, where more than 50% of patients have the changes, alpha-N-galactosaminidase deficiency and galactosialidosis [12–15] (Table 14.1). Chloroquine therapy may result in storage of biochemically and ultrastructurally similar inclusions in many of the same cells as Fabry disease and may result in similar clinical manifestations, including the development of angiokeratoma [16]. Solitary and localised forms of angiokeratoma are also described, and occur in the absence of underlying systemic disease [17] (Table 14.1).

14.1.2 Other Cutaneous Vascular Lesions

Not all patients with Fabry disease (FD) have angiokeratomas [9–11]. At our centre we systematically examine the skin and can confirm that a proportion of patients have no cutaneous vascular lesions. Some patients exhibit macular, bright red, angiomatous lesions. These are indistinguishable from lesions seen frequently in the general population, particularly in females in the 4th–6th decades. It is not clear whether these lesions represent early angiokeratomas or macular haemangiomas. We have also identified patients with widespread papular angiomas [18]. These are clinically and histologically in keeping with cherry angiomas and distinct from angiokeratomas (Fig. 14.3). They are larger than angiokeratomas, dome shaped, smooth, bright red to blue-ish papules. They do not blanch on pressure. Ultrastructurally they are produced by spherical and tubular dilatations of capillary

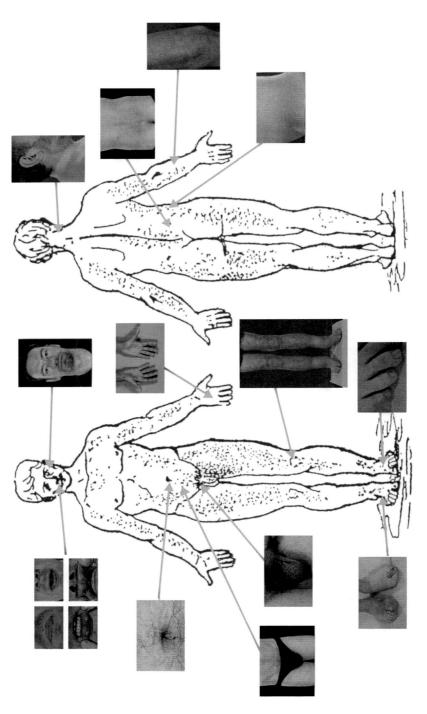

Fig. 14.2 Distribution of angiokeratomas and other dermatological signs in Fabry disease. Background diagram from Anderson [1]

Table 14.1 Other causes of angiokeratoma

Localised forms of angiokeratoma (AK)	Other lysosomal storage diseases associated with Angiokeratoma Corporis Diffusum
AK of Fordyce: commonest form, 1–4 mm, scrotal lesions, increased incidence with age. Degenerative disorder due to local venous hypertension AK of the vulva: analogous to AK of Fordyce occur on labia majora in older women Solitary papular AK: both sexes, age of onset 10–40 years, 2–10 mm, any site, often bleed/thrombose AK of Mibelli: mainly in females, familial predisposition, onset typically age 10–15 years, association with chilblains and acrocyanosis, grouped lesions on extremities AK circumscriptum naeviformis: rare, both sexes, unilateral plaque of keratotic vascular papules, may be dermatomal, early onset, may be present from birth	Fucosidosis (α-L-fucosidase) Kanzaki disease (α-N-acetylgalactosaminidase) Aspartylglycosaminuria (aspartylglycosaminidase) Galactosialidosis (β-galactosidase& α-neuraminidase) Sialidosis (α-neuraminidase) β-Mannosidosis (β-mannosidase) GM1- gangliosidosis (β-galactosidase)

loops in dermal papillae with tortuous cross-connections between individual loops [6]. The prevalence of such lesions in the general population may be as high as 50% [19] and their significance in patients with Fabry disease is as yet unknown. They may occur alone or in combination with macular angiomas, and/or classical angiokeratomas. It is possible that different types of cutaneous vascular lesion correlate with different Fabry disease phenotypes. For example, in one study, patients with a predominantly cardiac phenotype rarely had classical angiokeratoma. Interestingly, a third of males in this group had widespread (>100) cherry angiomas [18].

Telangiectases are thought to be due to dilatation of postcapillary venules in the upper horizontal plexus, and are not specific to Fabry disease (Fig. 14.4). In common telangiectases, vessel wall thickening due to peripheral deposition of basement membrane-like material admixed with reticulin fibers is seen ultrastructurally [6].

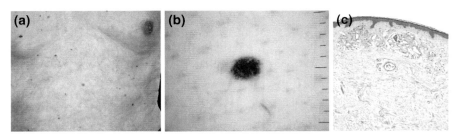

Fig. 14.3 (**a**) Cherry angiomas on the abdomen, (**b**) dermatoscopic view of a single lesion, (**c**) histopathologic section of cherry angioma haematoxylin and eosin stain

Fig. 14.4 Telangiectatic
vessels on the upper chest

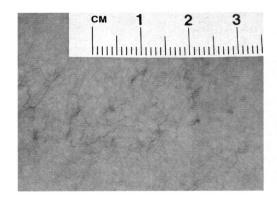

It is not known whether these changes occur in the telangiectases associated with Fabry disease. Clinically they may be distinguished from angiokeratomas and cherry angiomas by the presence of blanching on diascopic pressure. Fabry outcome survey (FOS) data shows that they are commoner in males (23%) than females (9%) [4, 5]. Although based on patient recall, data suggests that they appear later than angiokeratomas, with a mean age at onset of 26 years in males (SD 17, range 3–70) and 42 years in females (SD 22, range 5–73) [4]. In a majority of cases, telangiectases occur at sun exposed sites such as the face and V of the neck, often in patients with skin type I or II. Occasionally, telangiectases may be seen at unusual sites such as the flanks, groins, elbow & knee flexures. This tends to be in patients with ACD and a classical severe disease phenotype.

14.1.3 Therapy

Several studies have shown clearance of Gb3 from the skin following enzyme replacement therapy (ERT) [20, 21] this, unfortunately does not translate to clearance of angiokeratomas. In some patients on ERT individual lesions resolve and new lesions appear. Fortunately, quasi-continuous wave and pulsed lasers, and intense pulsed light systems can effectively treat the variety of vascular lesions seen in Fabry disease [22, 23]. Their benefits include non-invasiveness, ease of use, and short recovery time. The 585-nm flashlamp-pumped pulsed-dye laser follows the theory of selective photothermolysis, is safe for infants and children, and has a low incidence of side effects. It is successful in treating telangiectasias, spider and cherry angiomas, and angiokeratomas. Nd:Yag laser treatment although more painful, may be more effective in larger lesions. Newer lasers, which combine a high-powered pulse-dye laser and a 1,064-nm long – pulse Nd:YAG laser penetrate deeper and seem to work particularly well for the larger genital angiokeratomas [24–26].

14.1.4 Relationship to Disease Severity

Published data from FOS has shown that in both sexes, the presence of cutaneous vascular lesions (CVL), namely telangiectases and/or angiokeratoma is associated with higher disease severity scores [4, 5]. The FOS database categorises patients according to the overall severity of their disease using the Mainz severity scoring index (MSSI and FOS-MSSI). Figure 14.5 shows the mean MSSI for males and females at different age ranges (<20, 20–39, 40–59 and >60 years) that have or do not have cutaneous vascular lesions (angiokeratomas and telangiectases). The severity scores, as expected, increase with advancing age. Patients (males and females) with CVL have a higher MSSI score at each of the age ranges. Each comparison (non-parametric rank sum test) within sex and age group if significant ($p < 0.01$) except for men aged over 60 years, where patient numbers were small ($p = 0.088$) [4].

More recent data confirms this finding and shows that patients with CVL are significantly more likely to have major organ involvement [5]. Thus, cerebrovascular involvement (stroke & TIA) was present in 38% females & 32% males with CVL, but only 12% females and 9% males without. Cardiac involvement occurred in 80% females and 73% males with CVL vs. 38% females and 49% males without; renal involvement in 62% females and 72% males with CVL vs. 29%females and 42% males without. Similar differences are observed for hypertension, eye, ear, gastrointestinal and other neurological involvement. These findings demonstrate the importance of dermatological assessment and its possible predictive value in terms of systemic morbidity.

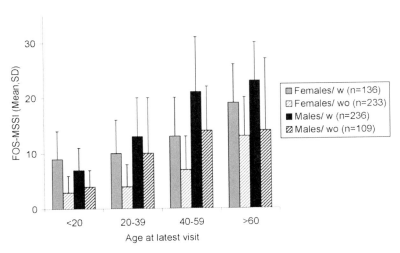

Fig. 14.5 Patients with (w) cutaneous vascular lesions have higher disease severity scores than patients without (wo) CVL. FOS data, adapted from Orteu [4]

14.2 Facial Features

A characteristic 'pseudo-acromegalic' facial appearance has been described in males with Fabry disease. Adult photographs of Fabry's original patient show that he had them to a mild degree. They are clearly demonstrated in the male in Fig. 14.6. The changes vary in severity from one family to another. Within individual families they tend to be of a similar degree, and it is usually possible to identify affected males in family groups. Features in females are much more subtle, and more easily missed.

There have been two larger studies of facial features published to date. The first was a cross-sectional, single centre, independent dysmorphology assessment by a panel of three clinical geneticists, based on standardized medical photography [27]. Thirty-eight patients were examined and the features identified were, in order of decreasing frequency: periorbital fullness, prominent ear lobes, bushy eyebrows, recessed forehead, pronounced nasal angle, generous nose/bulbous nasal tip, prominent supraorbital ridges, shallow midface, full lips, prominent nasal bridge, broad alar base, coarse features, posteriorly rotated ears, and prognathism. The second was a cross-sectional study using a 3D photogrammetric camera, in which facial dysmorphism was objectively assessed by three dimensional (3D) dense surface modelling and anthropometric analysis [28]. Facial features in 20 males and 22 females with Fabry disease were compared to controls. The mean male Fabry face had periorbital fullness, more prominent supraorbital ridges, a larger bitemporal width, bushier eyebrows, ptosis of the eyelids, a more acute nasal angle, a broader nasal base, a slightly shorter and more bulbous nose, fuller lips, some additional fullness to the cheeks and a slightly larger chin. There was also a suggestion of very localised, minor, midfacial hypoplasia. Minor face shape differences were also seen in females. The mean

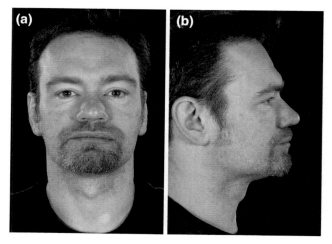

Fig. 14.6 Typical facial features: prominent supraorbital ridges, periorbital fullness, large bitemporal width, bushy eyebrows, broad nasal base, full lips, and prominent chin

female Fabry face had a more prominent forehead, was wider at the temples, and had a shorter nose with a wider alar base. The accuracy rates for detection of face shape differences were 85% for males and 67% for females, confirming that diagnostic screening based on facial features alone would be inappropriate. Nevertheless, the presence of the above facial features should prompt appropriate investigations for Fabry disease.

Experience at our centre suggests that the Fabry face occurs in patients with classical disease at the more severe end of the spectrum. Moderate or marked facial changes were present in 26/41 males (63%) with a classical disease phenotype; 16/26 (61%) of these males also had the classical cutaneous phenotype of angiokeratoma corporis diffusum. In contrast, facial features were present to a very mild degree (periorbital puffiness only) in 2/19 males (10.5%), with a predominantly cardiac phenotype of disease [18]. The mechanism underlying the development of these changes is not yet clear, but they do not reflect oedema. Similar periorbital puffiness is seen in patients with autoimmune thyroid and parathyroid disease, the other changes are sometimes indistinguishable from acromegaly. This suggests a possible underlying endocrine abnormality, although none has been found to date. Coarse facies are also described in fucosidosis, suggesting that abnormal lipid storage in the skin may be causally involved [12]. Facial changes with more widespread skin thickening and ivory white nodules or 'pebbly lesions' on the upper back are seen in the mucopolysaccharidoses, particularly MPS I and II. In this group increased tissue mucin and fragmented, hyalinised dermal collagen may be seen [29]. Further investigation of the histological and electron microscopic appearances of facial skin and soft tissues in Fabry patients is awaited.

Interestingly, the skin was noted to become finer and softer in a 3 year old boy with Hunter syndrome following idursulfase replacement therapy [30]. Likewise, serial photography in a small number of Fabry patients suggests that facial appearances do appear to change gradually, 6–12 months after starting enzyme replacement therapy [31].

14.3 Raynaud's Phenomenon

The term Raynaud's phenomenon describes an abnormal vasospastic response to cold or emotional stress. It is a common condition with a prevalence of 3–10% of the population [32, 33]. An attack of Raynaud's phenomenon is classically manifested as triphasic colour changes [34]. The white phase is due to excessive vasoconstriction and cessation of regional blood flow. This phase is followed by a cyanotic phase, as the residual blood in the finger desaturates. The red phase is due to hyperaemia as the attack subsides and blood flow is restored. There is frequently associated pain and/or paraesthesia due to sensory nerve ischaemia. Raynaud's phenomenon can be subdivided into primary, or idiopathic, and secondary forms. In the latter, associated diseases or causes can be identified. Thirty percent of first degree relatives of patients with primary Raynaud's phenomenon have the condition [35]. Pathologic changes have been observed primarily in vascular smooth muscle cells, endothelial cells and perineuronal microvasculature. Postulated mechanisms include increased activation of the sympathetic nerves, and an alteration in vascular function, possibly related to increased sensitivity to cold of the adrenergic receptors on the digital artery vascular smooth muscle. In some cases, locally released or systemically circulating vasoconstrictors or increased oxidative stress may be involved [34].

'Cold intolerance' and the development of pain in the extremities in cold environments is a common complaint amongst Fabry patients. In FOS, Raynaud's was documented in 8% of 710 females and 11% of 644 males (unpublished data). This may be an underestimate. In a subset of 98 patients at our centre (58 females and 40 males), 34% of females and 25% of males described cold, blue, painful fingers in summer as well as winter. In half of these cases, bi- or triphasic colour changes with pain on rewarming were described (unpublished observation). A representative thermography study in a male Fabry patient, confirming slow fingertip rewarming (under 18% temperature recovery) 10 min after cold challenge, and the diagnosis of Raynaud's phenomenon is shown in Fig. 14.7. Raynaud's phenomenon is usually commoner in women. The high prevalence in males in our cohort, and the fact that the sex ratio is reversed in FOS, suggest that this is not just isolated primary Raynaud's phenomenon, but that it is causally linked to the underlying Fabry disease.

In patients with primary Raynaud's, capillaroscopy is usually normal. In Fabry patients our experience to date has been intermediate, in that capillary density is usually normal, but with some capillary dilatation. A recent fluoroscopic nailfold capillaroscopy study [36] examined 25 Fabry patients (17 males) and showed significantly more bushy capillaries and clusters in cases (72%) than controls (10%). Enhanced natrium-fluorescein diffusion into the pericapillary area was observed in three patients. The authors conclude that morphological and functional abnormalities of nailfold capillaries were present. This abnormal vasoreactivity of digital vessels could in part be caused by Fabry related autonomic dysfunction. Abnormalities of nitric oxide synthetase and increased oxidative stress in vascular endothelium and smooth muscle might also be important triggers.

Current therapeutic strategies include supportive treatments, topical therapeutic approaches and systemic medication [37]. Standard measures such as stopping smoking, avoiding vasoconstricting medications such as beta-blockers and maintaining warm hands and feet with suitable clothing during winter months are generally recommended. Suggested non-medical therapies include increasing intake of anti-oxidant vitamins, and ginkgo biloba. Drug therapies with proven efficacy in other patient groups include Angiotensin II receptor antagonists such as Losartan 25 mg daily, calcium channel blockers such as longer acting formulations of nifedipine e.g. 10–20 mg or diltiazem 60 mg daily, and Sildenafil [37]. Possible cardiac and renal contraindications should be taken into account before prescribing these drugs in Fabry patients. The selective serotonin re-uptake inhibitor Fluoxetine at a dose of 20 mg daily has recently been shown to be of benefit in patients with primary Raynaud's [38]. Deposition of sphingolipid in vascular endothelium activates platelets, thus a drug such as fluoxetine which reduces 5HT release from platelets may also prove to be helpful in Fabry patients.

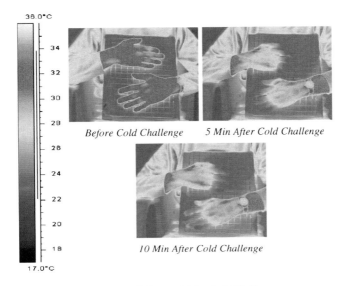

Fingertip Temperature Before and After Cold Challenge

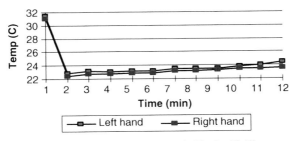

Left fingertips percentage temperature recovery in 10 min: 17.4%
Right fingertips percentage temperature recovery in 10 min: 12.8%

Fig. 14.7 Thermography study in a male Fabry patient with symptoms of Raynaud's phenomenon. *Bottom Chart* shows average fingertip temperatures (before cold challenge and during recovery) calculated from all four fingers of the left and right hands. Thumbs not included in analysis (courtesy of Mr K Howell, Dept Rheumatology, Royal Free Hospital, London UK)

14.4 Lower Limb Oedema and Lymphoedema

The lymphatic network functions to return fluid, cells and macromolecules to the circulation. Lymphoedema is defined as the abnormal accumulation of protein-rich fluid in soft tissues. It results from an imbalance between lymph formation and its absorption into the initial lymphatics [39]. Primary lymphoedema is largely due to anatomical abnormalities, such as hypoplasia or aplasia of lymphatics. Secondary lymphoedema commonly develops when lymphatic function is impaired due to lymphatic damage. Associated complications include reduced mobility due to 'heavy limbs', increased susceptibility to bacterial skin infections such as cellulitis and skin ulceration. In a recent UK community survey, the prevalence of lymphoedema was 1.33/1,000, increasing to 5.4/1,000 in those aged over 65 years. It was commoner in women (2.5 vs. 0.41/1,000) [40]. Although it is not a specific feature, the suggestion that the development of oedema and lymphoedema in Fabry patients is pathogenically linked to the underlying disease is supported by a number of observations.

Lymphoedema was cited in the original description of FD and is recognised in other LSDs such as alpha-N-acetylgalactosaminidase deficiency [41]. Case reports document it as an unusual presenting feature of the condition [42] and some suggest that familial lymphoedema and Fabry disease might be linked [43]. Available FOS data confirms that reversible peripheral oedema of the lower limbs was present in 87/345 males (25%) and 61/369 females (17%). The mean age at onset was 32 years (SD13) and 42 years (SD16) respectively. Lymphoedema was present in 55/345 males (16%) and 23/369 females (7%). The male: female ratio was reversed in Fabry patients compared to the community. The mean age of onset was 37 years (range 13–70) and 47 years (range 11–72) respectively [4]. The presence of oedema and lymphoedema does not appear to correlate with underlying renal or cardiac involvement, although it may be aggravated by either of these complications.

The mechanism underlying the changes is still unclear. Recurrent episodes of reversible lower limb oedema may gradually cause or increase lymphatic damage. The presence of glycosphingolipids within the lymphatic vessels may also contribute [44]. It is not clear, at present, whether glycosphingolipid accumulation affects lymphatic function. Two studies suggest a primary abnormality of the lymphatics, at least in a proportion of patients with Fabry disease [45, 46]. Using the technique of fluorescence microlymphography and measurement of lymph capillary pressure, Amann-Vesti et al. demonstrated fragmentation of the microlymphatic network in 5/5 hemizygous males and 5/5 heterozygous females but in none of 12 healthy controls. Microvessel diameter was increased, and in patients with lymphoedema, microlymphatic hypertension was present. Severe structural and functional changes in the initial lymphatics of the skin were present, even when lymphoedema was not manifest.

The recent identification of mediators of lymphangiogenesis has improved our understanding of lymphatic biology [47]. Reduced vascular endothelial growth factor receptor 3 (VEGFR-3) tyrosine kinase activity and subsequent failure in transducing sufficient physiological VEGF-C/-D signals may inhibit lymphangiogenesis. Recently an endogenous selective inhibitor of lymphatic vessel growth soluble VEGFR-2 has been identified. VEGFR-2 inhibits developmental and reparative lymphangiogenesis by blocking VEGF-C function [48]. The possibility that abnormalities in expression or function of these mediators may be involved in the development of lymphoedema in Fabry disease remains to be investigated. Some of these mediators represent good therapeutic candidates for stimulating lymphangiogenesis and it is hoped that in future, they may be used to facilitate the controlled regrowth of damaged, dysfunctional, or obliterated lymphatics [49]. In the meatime, regular application of moisturisers can help to avoid fissures. Prophylactic therapy with grade II graduated below knee compression hosiery can prevent the development of lymphoedema in patients whose oedema is still fully reversible. Once lymphoedema is established, control can be maintained in up to 80% of patients by regular skin care, exercise, manual lymphatic draining &/or self massage, and the use of appropriate specialist bandaging and hosiery for lymphoedema [40].

14.5 Abnormalities of Sweating

Reduced sweating is a classical feature of Fabry disease. In a series reported by Larralde et al., all six hemizygotes and none of the 5 heterozygotes had hypohidrosis [50]. Reduced production of tears and saliva is also associated with hypohidrosis in AFD and is thought to be the consequence of an autonomic neuropathy [51]. Although the data are subjective and self reported by patients, an analysis of FOS has confirmed that abnormalities are common. Hypohidrosis was seen in 53% of males, 28% of females, with earlier onset in males (23 vs. 26 years). Anhidrosis was seen in 25% of males, but only 4% females [4]. Heat intolerance is a common and frequently disabling symptom. Patients may be unable to tolerate exercise and may suffer nausea, dyspnoea, light-headedness and headache, or complete collapse with loss of consciousness [52]. It is widely held that the hypohidrosis of Fabry disease results principally from an autonomic peripheral neuropathy, though substrate accumulation within sweat glands may play a role. Previous studies [53, 54] have demonstrated an improvement in sweating in Fabry patients undergoing ERT. Interestingly, in some patients, hyperhidrosis occurs. This manifestation was commoner in females than males, present in 11.9% of 369 females vs. 6.4% of 345 males [55]. This is higher than the estimated prevalence of 1–2.8% of the general population in the US [56]. In a majority of Fabry patients it affects palms and soles and is not generalised [55]. Hyperhidrosis has a significant negative impact on daily activities and quality of life. Treatment options include the use of topical agents such aluminium chloride hexahydrate, regular tap water iontopheresis and local botulinum toxin injections repeated 6–12 monthly [57, 58]. Oral glycopyrrolate sodium up to 2 mg tds, is a well tolerated anticholinergic with minimal side effects, provided there are no cardiac contraindications. Endoscopic transthoracic sympathectomy may be used as a last resort, but may be complicated by gustatory and compensatory hyperhidrosis [58].

14.6 Summary

Like the systemic phenotype in Fabry disease, the cutaneous phenotype in this condition is highly variable. At one end of the spectrum there are patients with classical angiokeratoma corporis diffusum and facial features, who will typically have more severe systemic manifestations of disease. At the other, there are patients with no cutaneous vascular lesions or with cherry angiomata, and lower overall disease severity scores. Available data suggests that cutaneous vascular lesions and facial features may not only have a significant psychosocial impact, they may also be important predictors of overall disease severity.

In terms of cutaneous morbidity, the lower limb lymphoedema, Raynaud's phenomenon, hypo~ and hyperhidrosis can prove very debilitating in a proportion of patients. It is not yet known whether these cutaneous manifestations bear any relationship to disease severity.

Although it is likely that small fibre neuropathy and vascular smooth muscle and endothelial cell dysfunction contribute, the mechanisms underlying the skin complications in Fabry disease remain to be elucidated.

Acknowledgments I would like to thank the patients for participating and allowing us to use their clinical photographs and Dr P Elliott for his helpful comments during the preparation of this manuscript.

References

1. Anderson W (1898) A case of angiokeratoma. Br J Dermatol 18:113–117
2. Fabry J (1898) Ein Beitrag zur Kenntnis der Purpura haemorrhagica nodularis (Purpura papulosa haemorrhagica Hebrae). Arch Dermatol Syph 43:187–200
3. Desnick RJ, Ioannou YA, Eng CM (2001) α-Galactosidase A deficiency: Fabry disease. In: Scriver CR, Beaudet Al, Sly WS, Valk D (eds) The Metabolic and molecular basis of inherited disease, vol 3, 8th edn. McGraw Hill, New York, 3733–3774
4. Orteu CH, Jansen T, Lidove O et al (2007) Fabry disease and the skin: data from FOS the Fabry outcome survey. Br J Dermatol 157(2):331–337
5. Dhoat S, Orteu CH, Navarro C, Lidove O, Jansen T, Clarke J (2009) Patients with Fabry disease with cutaneous vascular lesions have higher disease severity scores and more multi-system involvement: data from 1354 patients registered on FOS, the Fabry outcome survey. Br J Dermatol 161(Suppl 1):45
6. Braverman IM (1989) Ultrastructure and organization of the cutaneous microvasculature in normal and pathologic states. J Invest Dermatol 93(2 Suppl):2S–9S
7. Navarro C, Teijeira S, Dominguez C et al (2006) Fabry disease: an ultrastructural comparative study of skin in hemizygous and heterozygous patients. Acta Neuropathol (Berl) 7:1–8
8. Ramaswami U, Whybra C, Parini R et al (2006) Clinical manifestations of Fabry disease in children: data from FOS – the Fabry Outcome Survey. Acta Paediatrica 95:86–92
9. MacDermott KD, Holmes A, Miners AH (2001) Anderson-Fabry disease: clinical manifestations and impact of disease in a cohort of 98 hemizygous males. J Med Genet 38:750–760
10. MacDermott KD, Holmes A, Miners AH (2001) Anderson-Fabry disease: clinical manifestations and impact of disease in a cohort of 60 obligate carrier females. J Med Genet 38:769–775
11. Weidemann F, Strotmann JM, Breunig F et al (2008) Misleading terms in Anderson-Fabry disease. Eur J Clin Invest 38(3):191–196
12. Fleming C, Rennie A, Fallowfield M, McHenry PM (1997) Cutaneous manifestations of fucosidosis. Br J Dermatol 136(4):594–597
13. Kanzaki T, Yokota M, Irie F et al (1993) Aniokeratoma corporis diffusum with glycopeptiduria due to deficient lysosomal alpha-N-acetylgalactosaminidase activity. Clincal, morphologic and biochemical studies. Arch Dermatol 129:460–465
14. Rodriguez-Serna M, Botella-Estrada R, Chabas A et al (1996) Angiokeratoma corporis diffusum associated with beta-mannosidase deficiency. Arch Dermatol 132(10): 1219–1222

15. Paller SA (1987) Metabolic disorders characterized by angiokeratomas and neurologic dysfunction. Neurol clin 5(3):441–446
16. Albay D, Adler SG, Philipose J, Calescibetta CC, Romansky SG, Cohen AH (2005) Chloroquine-induced lipidosis mimicking Fabry disease. Mod Pathol 18(5):733–738
17. Schiller PI, Itin PH (1996) Angiokeratomas: an update. Dermatology 193(4):275–282
18. Orteu CH, Mehta AB, Dhoat S, Hughes DA (2009) Fabry disease and angiokeratoma corporis diffusum are not synonymous: cutaneous vascular lesions and facial features in 100 patients with Fabry disease. Br J Dermatol 161(Suppl 1):46
19. Plunkett A, Merlin K, Gill D, Zuo Y, Jolley D, Marks R (1999) The frequency of common nonmalignant skin conditions in adults in central Victoria, Australia. Int J Dermatol 38(12):901–908
20. Eng CM, Banikazemi M, Gordon RE et al (2001) A phase 1/2 clinical trial of enzyme replacement in fabry disease: pharmacokinetic, substrate clearance, and safety studies. Am J Hum Genet 68(3):711–722
21. Thurberg BL, Randolph Byers H, Granter SR, Phelps RG, Gordon RE, O'Callaghan M (2004) Monitoring the 3-year efficacy of enzyme replacement therapy in fabry disease by repeated skin biopsies. J Invest Dermatol 122(4):900–908
22. Ross BS, Levine VJ, Ashinoff R (1997) Laser treatment of acquired vascular lesions. Dermatol Clin 15(3):385–396
23. Morais P, Santos AL, Baudrier T, Mota AV, Oliveira JP, Azevedo F (2008) Angiokeratomas of Fabry successfully treated with intense pulsed light. J Cosmet Laser Ther 10(4): 218–222
24. Pfirrmann G, Raulin C, Karsai S (2009) Angiokeratoma of the lower extremities: successful treatment with a dual-wavelength laser system (595 and 1064 nm). J Eur Acad Dermatol Venereol 23(2):186–187
25. Ozdemir M, Baysal I, Engin B, Ozdemir S (2009) Treatment of angiokeratoma of Fordyce with long-pulse neodymium-doped yttrium aluminium garnet laser. Dermatol Surg 35(1): 92–97
26. Bechara FG, Jansen T, Wilmert M, Altmeyer P, Hoffmann K (2004) Angiokeratoma Fordyce of the glans penis: combined treatment with erbium: YAG and 532 nm KTP (frequency doubled neodynium: YAG) laser. J Dermatol 31(11):943–945
27. Ries M, Moore DF, Robinson CJ et al (2006) Quantitative dysmorphology assessment in Fabry disease. Genet Med 8(2):96–101
28. Cox-Brinkman J, Vedder A, Hollak C et al (2007) Three-dimensional face shape in Fabry disease. Eur J Hum Genet 15(5):535–542
29. Freeman RG (1977) A pathologic basis for the cutaneous papules of mucopolysaccharidosisII (The Hunter syndrome). J Cutan Pathol 4:318–328
30. Galan-Gomez E, Guerrero-Rico A, Caceres-Marzal C et al (2008) Early response to idursulfase treatment in a 3 year-old boy affected of Hunter syndrome. Eur J Med Genet 51(3):268–271
31. Richfield L, Orteu CH, Fox N et al (2005) Fabry disease, changes in typical facial features in response to enzyme replacement therapy with agalsidase alpha. Acta Paediatr Suppl 447:122
32. Suter LG, Murabito JM, Felson DT, Fraenkel L (2005) The incidence and natural history of Raynaud's phenomenon in the community. Arthritis Rheum 52(4):1259–1263
33. Brand FN, Larson MG, Kannel WB, McGuirk JM (1997) The occurrence of Raynaud's phenomenon in a general population: the Framingham Study. Vasc Med 2(4):296–301
34. Cooke JP, Marshall JM (2005) Mechanisms of Raynaud's disease. Vasc Med 10(4):293–307
35. Cherkas LF, Williams FM, Carter L et al (2007) Heritability of Raynaud's phenomenon and vascular responsiveness to cold: a study of adult females twins. Arthritis Rheum 57(3): 524–528
36. Wasik JS, Simon RW, Meier T, Steinmann B, Amann-Vesti BR (2009) Nailfold capillaroscopy: specific features in Fabry disease. Clin Hemorheol Microcirc 42(2):99–106
37. Pope JE (2007) The diagnosis and treatment of Raynaud's phenomenon. Drugs 67(4):517–525

38. Coleiro B, Marshall SE, Denton CP et al (2001) Treatment of Raynaud's phenomenon with the selective serotonin reuptake inhibitor fluoxetine. Rheumatology (Oxford) 40(9):1038–1043
39. Rockson SG (2008) Diagnosis and management of lymphatic vascular disease. J Am Coll Cardiol 52(10):799–806
40. Moffatt CJ, Franks PJ, Doherty DC et al (2003) Lymphoedema: an underestimated health problem. QJM 96(10):731–738
41. Chabas A, Coll MJ, Aparicio M, Rodriguez Diaz E (1994) Mild phenotypic expression of alpha-N-acetylgalactosaminidase deficiency in two adult siblings. J Inhert Metab Dis 17(6):724–731
42. Lozano F, Garcia-Talavera R, Gomez-Alonso A (1988) An unusual cause of lymphoedema–confirmed by isotopic lymphangiography. Eur J Vasc Surg 2(2):129–131
43. Gemignani F, Pietrini V, Tagliavini F et al (1979) Fabry's disease with familial lymphedema of the lower limbs. Case report and family study. Eur Neurol 18(2):84–90
44. Jansen T, Bechara FG, Orteu CH, Altmeyer P, Mehta A, Beck M (2005) The significance of lymphoedema in Fabry Disease. Acta Paediatr Suppl 447:117
45. Amann-Vesti BR, Gitzelmann G, Widmer U, Bosshard NU, Steinmann B, Koppensteiner R (2003) Severe Lymphatic micrangiopathy in Fabry disease. Lymphat Res Biol 1(3):185–189
46. Gitzelmann G, Widmer U, Bosshard NU, Steinmann B, Koppensteiner R, Amann-Vesti BR (2006) Lymphoedema in Fabry disease: pathology and therapeutic perspectives. Acta Pardiatr Suppl 451:122
47. Lohela M, Bry M, Tammela T, Alitalo K (2009) VEGFs and receptors involved in angiogenesis versus lymphangiogenesis. Curr Opin Cell Biol 21(2):154–165
48. Albuquerque RJ, Hayashi T, Cho WG et al (2009 Sep) Alternatively spliced vascular endothelial growth factor receptor-2 is an essential endogenous inhibitor of lymphatic vessel growth. Nat Med 15(9):1023–1030
49. Jin da P, An A, Liu J, Nakamura K, Rockson SG (2009) Therapeutic responses to exogenous VEGF-C administration in experimental lymphedema: immunohistochemical and molecular characterization. Lymphat Res Biol 7(1):47–57
50. Larralde M, Boggio P, Amartino H, Chamoles N (2004) Fabry disease: a study of 6 hemizygous men and 5 heterozygous women with emphasis on dermatologic manifestations. Arch Dermatol 140(12):1440–1446
51. Cable WJ, Kolodny EH, Adams RD (1982) Fabry disease, impaired autonomic function. Neurology 32:498–502
52. Shelley ED, Shelley WB, Kurczynski TW (1995) Painful fingers, heat intolerance, telangiectases of the ear: easily ignored childhood signs of Fabry disease. Pediatr Dermatol 12:215–219
53. Hilz MJ, Brys M, Marthol H, Stemper B, Dutsch M (2004) Enzyme replacement therapy improves function of C-adelta-, and Abeta-nerve fibers in Fabry neuropathy. Neurology 62(7):1066–1072
54. Schiffmann R, Floeter MLK, Dambrosia JM et al (2003) Enzyme replacement therapy improves peripheral nerve and sweat function in Fabry disease. Muscle Nerve 28(6):703–710
55. Lidove O, Ramaswami U, Jaussaud R et al (2006) Hyperhidrosis: a new and often early symptom in Fabry disease. International experience and data from the Fabry Outcome Survey. Int J Clin Pract 60(9):1053–1059
56. Strutton DR, Kowalski JW, Glaser DA, Stang PE (2004) US prevalence of hyperhidrosis and impact on individuals with axillary hyperhidrosis: results from a national survey. J Am Acad Dermatol 51(2):241–248
57. Ram R, Lowe NJ, Yamauchi PS (2007) Current and emerging therapeutic modalities for hyperhidrosis, part 1: conservative and non-invasive treatments. Cutis 79(3):211–217
58. Ram R, Lowe NJ, Yamauchi PS (2007) Current and emerging therapeutic modalities for hyperhidrosis, part 2: moderately invasive and invasive procedures. Cutis 79(4):281–288

Chapter 15
Histopathology of Skin in Fabry Disease

Carmen Navarro, Susana Teijeira, Saida Ortolano, Jose M. Fernandez,
Beatriz San Millan, Carmen Fachal, Francisco Allegue, and Soraya Barrera

Abstract Fabry disease (FD) is a lysosomal storage disorder (LSD) with multi-system manifestations among which skin lesions are common and well-recognized. They may appear early in childhood in both hemizygous males and heterozygous females, their frequency increasing with age. In addition to dermatological lesions, normal-looking skin, as occurs with other tissues, accumulates unmetabolized products in multiple cells of different embryonic origin with variable distribution, biochemical and staining properties and morphological features, according to the type of stored material and the physiopathology of the disease. Globotryaosil-ceramide (Gb3), the most abundant glycosphyngolipid accumulated in FD, can be specifically documented with immunocytochemical methods using a particular monoclonal antibody. On the other hand, ultrastructural characteristics of Gb3 and its distribution in dermal cells are well-defined. Furthermore, the study of unmyelinated and small myelinated fibers in epidermal nerve endings is a reflection of the impaired sensory innervation and the characteristic painful neuropathy present in FD. Therefore, a combination of different technologies in tissues obtained with non-invasive techniques, such as skin biopsy, is advisable and should be considered in order to obtain better insights into FD. This is essential in the case of heterozygous women in whom biochemical diagnosis is often controversial.

Keywords Angiokeratoma · Dermal nerve endings · Electron microscopy · Immunocytochemistry · Lysosomal storage

15.1 Introduction

Skin lesions are one of the commonest manifestations of Fabry disease (FD), both in hemizygous men and heterozygous women and can be present at an early age. As previously reported, angiokeratoma (AK) are the most characteristic

C. Navarro (✉)
Department of Pathology and Neuropathology, University Hospital of Vigo, Vigo, Spain
e-mail: cnavfer@sergas.es; c.navarro.fb@gmail.com

D. Elstein et al. (eds.), *Fabry Disease*, DOI 10.1007/978-90-481-9033-1_15,
© Springer Science+Business Media B.V. 2010

dermatologic lesions, followed by telangiectases [1–7] or other vascular lesions preceding or related to AK. Angiokeratoma is also a feature in other lysosomal storage disorders (LSD) especially oligosaccharidoses, such as fucosidosis [8, 9], ß-mannosidosis [10, 11] or galactosialidosis [12], and can appear in asymptomatic persons with no known LSD [13].

Electron microscopic (EM) studies demonstrate that the lysosomal storage found within vessels and dermal cells in these lesions is different in cases of FD and in oligosaccharidoses and therefore ultrastructure is essential for diagnosis. In FD, electron-dense deposits characteristic of ceramide-amino acid compounds are present in lysosomes whereas in oligosaccharidoses electron-lucent deposits, typical of sugar-amino acid compounds, are observed [14, 15].

In addition to skin lesions, dermal cells of clinically unaffected skin of FD patients accumulate glycosphyngolipids, the most abundant of which is globotryaosil-ceramide or Gb3 [16–18]. Intralysosomal storage of unmetabolized products also occur in the dermis of patients with other LSD [14, 15, 19, 20]. This is the reason why, skin, an easily accessible tissue, has been the target for specific histopathological and ultrastructural studies included in the diagnostic methodology of most LSD and some neurodegenerative disorders [21–26].

More recently, detection of Gb3 by immunocytochemistry (IHC) in fresh tissues has turned out to be an attractive and reliable method for complementary diagnosis of FD.

Focusing on clinical practice, Gb3 detection is of great value in the cases where enzymatic assays are not conclusive, since to date, a more suitable biological marker for this purpose has not been identified. Although the levels of Gb3 (or lyso-Gb3) in body fluids do not really correlate with the severity of the pathology, the presence of an abnormal concentration of these glycosphyngolipids can be considered as an appropriate indicator for the disease and facilitate the identification of patients with difficult diagnosis, such as heterozygous females. In fact, Gb3 can be easily detected by immunofluorescence in all cells and structures identifiable in skin biopsy, and therefore Gb3 IHC constitutes a reliable screening method to be considered before the performance of other time-consuming studies such as EM [27]. Moreover, the examination of unaffected skin allows one to perform a careful study of sensory nerve epidermal endings and into the deep dermis, as well as the innervation of eccrine sweat glands. These analyses provide interesting information regarding the pathology of pain and hypohidrosis, two of the main clinical features of FD.

15.2 Methodology

15.2.1 Biopsy Procedure

For these purposes, clinically normal skin samples can be obtained using a power-driven 2–5 mm punch, under local anesthesia. The forearm is the selected site by some authors [15], although we prefer the subscapular or the flank areas, which are well vascularized and are not easily visible in the rare case of unpleasant scars. Other authors prefer the axillary region due to the presence of apocrine sweat glands. Apocrine sweat gland cells and eccrine ducts accumulate Lafora bodies in Lafora disease, a neurodegenerative disorder, but their examination is not relevant in most LSD since findings do not differ from those observed in eccrine glands [21–23, 28].

15.2.2 Electron Microscopy

Specimens should be immediately sent to a specialized laboratory without fixatives or other laboratory solutions. We divide each specimen into two portions perpendicularly to the dermis, so that both parts contain epidermis and dermis. We immerse one half in liquid nitrogen-chilled isopentane and keep it at $-80°C$ for further procedures. The second half is trimmed into tiny rectangular blocks, fixed in 2.5% glutaraldehyde for several hours, washed in buffer solution, progressively dehydrated in ascending concentrations of acetone, and routinely embedded in Epon. Epon blocks are sectioned using a conventional ultramicrotome with both glass and diamond knives. One micron thick sections are stained with toluidine blue for examination by light microscopy. Ultra-thin sections are mounted in copper grids, double-stained with uranyl acetate and lead citrate, and examined with a transmission electron microscope.

15.2.3 Gb3 Immunocytochemistry

Gb3 IHC is performed in 7 μm cryostat sections obtained from the stored frozen specimen. Sections are fixed with paraformaldehyde 4% w/v, permeabilized with triton 0.1% v/v and incubated overnight at 4°C with a monoclonal antibody against Gb3 receptor (CD77, BD Pharmingen, reference 551352). The specificity of this antibody in the immunoreaction has been extensively characterized and proved in previous works [29–31]. Following incubation with a fluorescent secondary antibody, sections are observed with a 60× oil immersion objective on an up-right fluorescence microscope.

15.2.4 Epidermal Nerve Endings

To assess nerve endings along dermo-epidermal junction skin samples are fixed according to the method described by Kennedy et al. [32] in Zamboni buffer (at 4°C overnight) and placed in 20% sucrose with PBS. After washing, the tissue is instantly frozen. Cryostat sections of about 50 μm are additionally treated with 0.5% Triton X-100 in PBS containing 5% donkey serum for deactivation of endogenous peroxidases. Sections are then incubated with rabbit polyclonal antibody against human PGP 9.5 (protein gene product 9.5, UltraClone Ltd., UK) at a dilution of 1:1,000 (at 4°C, overnight) and appropriate Cy 2-labeled secondary antibody (Jackson ImmunoResearch Laboratories, Inc.) is then applied. Sections are viewed under a confocal laser scanning microscope.

An alternative method to study epidermal nerve endings is using the avidin–biotin complex (ABC) technique [33, 34]. Skin biopsies are fixed in paraformaldehyde lysine periodate (PLP) overnight, rinsed in 0.1 M Sorenson phosphate buffer, transferred to a cryoprotectant solution (20% glycerol in 0.1 M Sorenson's buffer) and stored at 4°C. Fifty micron frozen sections are cut, soaked in 0.25% potassium permanganate for 15 min and washed in 5% oxalic acid for 2 min. The sections are blocked with normal goat serum in TBS, incubated at 4°C overnight with polyclonal antibody to human PGP 9.5 and incubated in secondary antibody for 1 h at room temperature. The Avidin-Biotin Complex routine technique is used.

15.3 Results

15.3.1 Histopathology of Clinically Normal Skin in Fabry Disease

In all the suspected or known cases of FD, males or females, it is advisable to study a sufficient number of sections as to examine all types of cells and appendages present in the skin, i.e. fibroblasts, endothelial and perithelial cells (pericytes) from capillaries, smooth muscle from small- and medium-sized vessels and from *arrector pili*, fascicles of myelinated and unmyelinated nerve endings, and eccrine sweat glands.

Fibroblasts. Fibroblasts are the most common cells of the dermal connective tissue. As other cells of the dermis, they are derived from primitive mesenchyme. They are morphologically heterogeneous with a branched cytoplasm surrounding an elliptical speckled nucleus with one or two nucleoli, and a variably active rough endoplasmic reticulum [35]. Skin fibroblasts of FD patients are among the cell types where storage products are mainly accumulated. Detection of Gb3 in these cells, performed by immunofluorescence with the monoclonal antibody CD 77, reveals that the glycosphyngolipid is mostly confined to cytosolic and membrane compartments and appears to be excluded from the nucleus (Fig. 15.1). The dotted pattern showed by the fluorescent tag is compatible with the localization of glycosphingolipids in the lysosome, though their presence in Golgi or ER compartments cannot be excluded.

On EM examination, lysosomes appear spherical of a size ranging from 0.2 to 2.5 μm in diameter, and are multiple, as many as 20–50 per cell, somehow deforming the usual elongated shape of the fibroblast to a rounded or globulous appearance (Fig. 15.2). At high magnification the intralysosomal inclusions are of different morphology. Most of them are composed of irregularly placed lamellae with alternating dark and light bands of a periodicity of 40–60 Å which correspond to the well-known typical Fabry inclusions, denominated 'zebra bodies' (Fig. 15.3). Other storage material consists of concentric alternating bands of different electronic

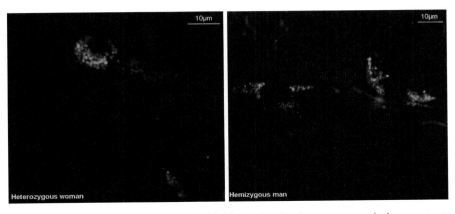

Fig. 15.1 Immunohistochemistry for Gb3 of the dermis in a hemizygous man and a heterozygous woman with FD. Gb3 is markedly fluorescent tracing the round shadows of stored lysosomes. Note the globulous cytoplasm and the negative shape of the nuclei

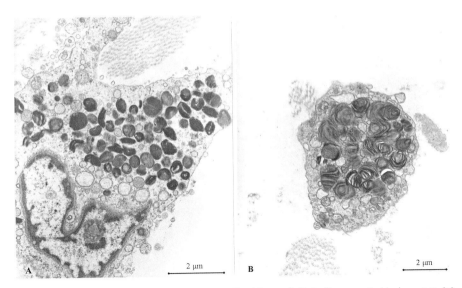

Fig. 15.2 Electron micrographs of two dermal fibroblasts of clinically normal skin in a man (**a**) and a woman (**b**) with FD. There are numerous lysosomal inclusions which deform the usual cytoplasmic shape. Lysosomes measure from 0.2 to 1 μm in diameter, and are composed of multilaminar and 'zebra-like' bodies

density and a periodicity of 150–200 Å, often close or at the periphery of electron-dense cores [36]. There are no obvious modifications of other organelles such as mitochondria or endoplasmic reticulum. Ultrastructural morphology is somehow homogeneous in fibroblasts, but displays a number of variable complex inclusions in other cell types.

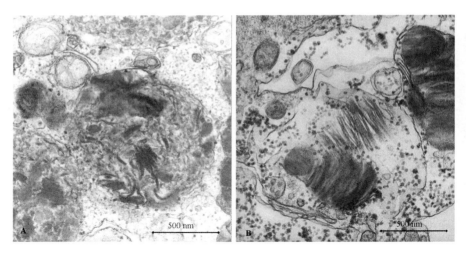

Fig. 15.3 High magnification of several lysosomes. Membrane bound inclusions are formed by alternating dark and clear bands with a periodicity of 40–60 Å

Vessels. The large vessels that supply the skin are located in the deep subcutaneous tissue, not present in regular punch biopsies. Smaller arteries, venules and capillaries constitute the main vasculature seen in the dermis. Zebra and laminated bodies are observed in endothelial and perithelial cells of capillaries (Fig. 15.4), as

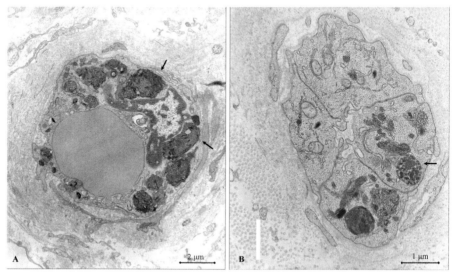

Fig. 15.4 Electron micrographs of two dermal capillaries in two different cases of FD. In **a**, a red blood cell occupies the lumen. Endothelial cells in both cases are filled with complex inclusions with undulating profiles and darker bodies, described as 'sunburst-like' inclusions (*arrows*)

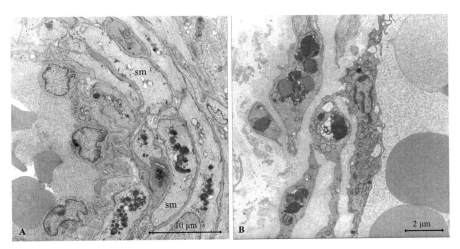

Fig. 15.5 Electron micrographs of two arterioles showing electron-dense inclusions in endothelial cells as well as in smooth muscle fibers (sm) from their wall

well as in smooth muscle cells of larger vessels (Fig. 15.5). Other complex storage inclusions have been described, such as undulating and fingerprint profiles, mixed inclusions combining zebra bodies and neutral lipid inclusions, or radiating periodic bands, all of which are surrounded by a single membrane, thus demonstrating their lysosomal origin [37]. Large inclusions with a 'sunburst-like' configuration have been reported in endothelial cells of dermal capillaries [38, 39], and observed in some of our cases (Fig. 15.4). Swollen endothelial cells can invade and narrow the vascular lumen and detach from the vascular inner layer (Fig. 15.6), which may contribute to the formation of small thrombi at the terminal part of small vessels producing microinfarcts.

Nerve endings. Small nerve fascicles and bundles with both myelinated and unmyelinated axons are present throughout the skin reaching the papillary dermis. Fascicles are surrounded by perineural cells or epithelioid myofibroblasts forming a protective sheath altogether with collagen fibers. Glycosphyngolipid lysosomal storage is invariably present in perineural cells (Fig. 15.7). Most reports indicate that Schwann cell itself is normal, with no lysosomal accumulation [38, 40]. We have carefully examined Schwann cells in serial sections and found no abnormalities. At the most, complex lipid inclusions of small diameter are occasionally seen and we interpret them as physiologic Schwann cell inclusions known as 'Pi granules' due to their similarity with the Greek letter Π. Endoneural fibroblasts can be similarly affected as those within the dermis. It is interesting to note that Schwann cell pathology is not expected in FD, since neurophysiological and histological studies (vide infra) indicate the selective involvement of unmyelinated and small myelinated fibers. On the contrary, Schwann cells are the target of lysosomal storage in LSD with central white matter and peripheral nerve demyelination, especially metachromatic and globoid cell leucodystrophies [25, 26]. In unmyelinated axons, axonal

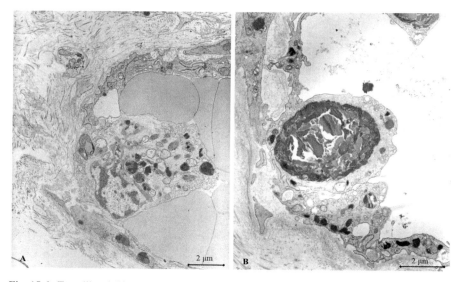

Fig. 15.6 Two dilated thin-walled capillaries with prominent endothelial cells protruding into the lumen. In **b**, the lysosomal inclusion has a diameter of 5 μm and has a complex electron-dense appearance

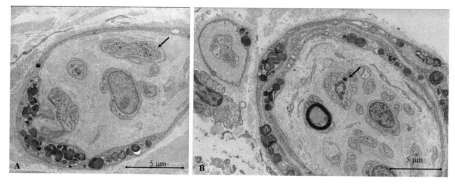

Fig. 15.7 Electron micrographs of three bundles of unmyelinated and myelinated nerve fibers. In the three bundles, perineural cells are filled with 'zebra-like', multilaminar and dense inclusions. Note the presence of small dense bodies in several unmyelinated axons (*arrows*)

damage is suspected by axonal swelling, occasional dense amorphous inclusions and loss of organelles (Fig. 15.7).

Eccrine sweat glands. Eccrine sweat glands develop from the fetal epidermis. Ducts and the secretory portion are lined by two cell layers, the tall columnar secretory cells and a basal layer that undergoes differentiation into secretory cells and myoepithelial cells. In addition to their secretory and excretory properties, the eccrine sweat glands are responsible for thermoregulation, their most important function. Myoepithelial cells are contractile spindle cells that surround the

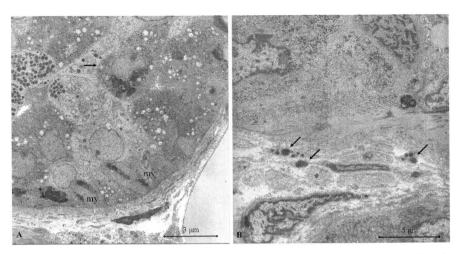

Fig. 15.8 Sections of eccrine sweat glands. In **a**, note the presence of lysosomal inclusions in basal myoepithelial cells (my) and in one 'dark' epithelial cell (*arrow*). Round droplets at the *left upper corner* represent secretion products. In **b**, note unmyelinated axonal dense bodies (*arrows*) at the periphery of the gland wall, which probably represent axonal degeneration

secretory coil and contract in response to cholinergic stimuli, therefore providing a mechanical support against a high hydrostatic pressure [35].

In eccrine glands, intralysosomal inclusions are seen in the three described cellular types. The most commonly affected are the myoepithelial cells (Fig. 15.8) although lysosomal storage can also be observed in the other two cellular components, i.e. clear and dark epithelial cells [15, 35]. Other inclusions seen in the basal cells consist of 'mulberry-like' cytoplasmic inclusions [41]. These lysosomes are composed of a number of rounded structures of about 0.3–2 μm in diameter surrounded by concentric dark and clear lines of a periodicity of 40–60 Å. Glycosphyngolipid storage in myoepithelial cells is supposed to be one of the factors that influences and limits the contractile capacity of the sweat gland thus giving rise to sweating abnormalities, common in FD. While examining eccrine sweat glands it is advisable to carefully study unmyelinated axon clusters twining around the gland. Axons appear morphologically normal, although some laminated bodies and fingerprint inclusions have been reported and could be interpreted as axonal degenerative changes [41]. Among the factors that could cause hypo- or anhidrosis in FD, peripheral or autonomic dysfunction has been strongly considered, since there is evidence of impaired autonomic function and Gb3 has been demonstrated to accumulate in peripheral autonomic ganglia as well as in sensitive posterior ganglia [38, 40, 42, 43].

Smooth muscle. Smooth muscle cells from vessels or from *arrector pili* are a good target to focus the study in suspected cases of FD, especially in women. Zebra bodies and other types of lysosomal inclusions are generally present in most muscle fibers and are diagnostic of FD. Inclusions are often placed in the center of the fiber,

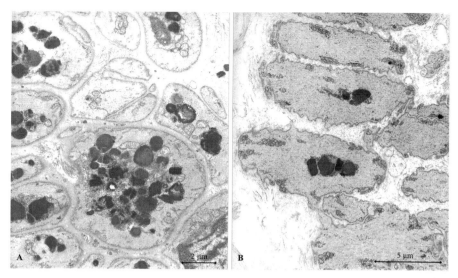

Fig. 15.9 Several smooth muscle cells from *arrector pili* in a male (**a**) and a woman (**b**) with FD. Dense irregular inclusions are present in most fibers, occupying an important part of the cytoplasm

where they can occupy an important part of the cytoplasm, as much as 30% of it (Fig. 15.9).

Smooth muscle involvement is intriguing and could account, in part, for some of the gastrointestinal symptoms that are common in FD.

15.3.2 Histopathology of Skin Lesions in Fabry Disease

Skin lesions in FD are described in detail in the previous chapter, and consist mainly in telangiectases, angiokeratoma, capillary angioma, cherry-like angioma and lymphangioma. Each of these lesions can appear in normal individuals, therefore fine histological studies including immunohistochemistry and electron microscopy are crucial for the diagnosis of a FD-associated dermatologic lesion [5, 44, 45].

Telangiectases are dilated, thin-walled vascular spaces that occur in the papillary dermis, with no major epidermal changes (Fig. 15.10). They are probably one of the earliest dermatological manifestations of FD and may lead to diagnosis in childhood [46]. Although angiectases may not be readily apparent in some patients, careful examination of the skin, especially the scrotum and umbilicus, may reveal isolated lesions.

Angiokeratoma are true blood vessel ectasias of the superficial dermis. They consist of numerous, dilated, thin-walled, congested capillaries located in the papillary dermis. The underlying epidermis shows variable degrees of acanthosis with elongation of the rete ridges and hyperkeratosis (Fig. 15.10). Partial or virtually complete

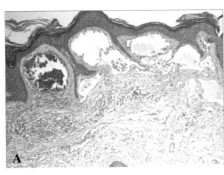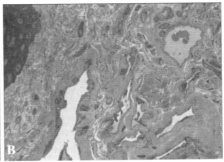

Fig. 15.10 (**a**) Light microscopy of an angiokeratoma showing typical superficial vascular dilatations bordered by epithelium. (**b**) semi-thin section of cutaneous telangiectases in a case of FD. Note swollen endothelial cells, some of which disclose dense bodies, as indicators of lysosomal Gb3 storage

occlusion of these dilated vessels by intravascular fibrin thrombi, at various degrees of organization, is common.

FD-associated angiokeratoma and telangiectases may show subtle vacuolization of the endothelium, *arrector pili* muscles, fibroblasts and pericytes, observed by regular histochemical techniques and light microscopy (Fig. 15.10). These vacuoles are better seen using lipid stains such as Sudan Black B, Oil red O in frozen sections or with periodic acid-schiff (PAS) which stains in dark pink the glycolipidic part of the inclusion contents. The lipid fraction is doubly refractile and can be visualized in frozen tissue sections examined with polarized light. Electron microscopy shows characteristic FD intralysosomal inclusions as previously described in endothelial and perithelial cells, smooth muscle and fibroblasts.

Capillary angioma or hemangioma is composed of numerous newly formed capillaries with narrow lumina and prominent endothelial cells arranged in a lobular way in the subpapillary region. Depending on the age of the lesion, the capillaries may become dilated.

Cherry-like angioma is also known as senile angioma or Campbell de Morgan spot. It is a variant of the capillary hemangioma. It is a very common lesion, often present in large numbers, which may appear in early adulthood, with the number of lesions increasing with age. Cherry angiomas are composed of fairly well-defined lobules of thin-walled dilated vascular channels, largely confined to the papillary dermis with a thin epidermal collarette. Intercapillary stroma shows edema and homogenization of the surrounding collagen fibers. Vascular channels that form this abnormal proliferation are mainly composed of venules. Several immmnunocytochemical markers for endothelial cells are useful to better typify these vascular lesions. These are factor VIII-related antigen, *Ulex europaeus,* CD31 and CD34. The latter is a rather poor specific marker and CD31 also stains macrophages. Fli-1 protein antibody, recently commercialized, is probably the best choice for endothelial cells.

Lymphangioma. Classic lymphangioma circunscriptum, acquired lymphedema and lymphangiectases are histologically indistinguishable [47]. They are composed of numerous dilated lymphatic vessels in the dermis. Within their lumina, a clear fluid or, less frequently, red blood cells, are present. The overlying epidermis is normal or acanthotic.

Endothelial cells in lymphangiomas are mostly negative for factor VIII-related antigen as opposed to hemangioma endothelial cells which are immunostained with this antibody, and show a negative or weakly positive reaction with *Ulex Europaeus*. A number of presumed specific markers of lymphatic endotelium have been described including LYVE-1, podoplanin, D2-40 and Prox-1.

15.3.3 Epidermal Nerve Endings in Fabry Disease

The axons within the epidermis arise entirely within the dorsal root ganglia and are presumed to represent the terminals of C and Aδ nociceptors [32, 48, 49], therefore they are affected in diseases with painful sensory neuropathy such as FD. The study and quantification of epidermal nerve fiber (ENF) density constitutes an ideal method for the evaluation of the degree of neuropathic involvement. In addition to FD [50, 51] ENF density is impaired in other diseases with neuropathic pain [33, 52], namely diabetic neuropathy [34, 53, 54], familiar dysautonomia or Riley-Day syndrome [55], HIV-associated sensitive neuropathy [56], and less commonly in chronic inflammatory demyelinating polyneuropathy or some connective tissue disorders [57].

Acroparesthesias and pain attacks are among the most frequent and characteristic symptoms in FD, usually beginning in early childhood [40]. Pain occurs in the distal part of the hands and feet, spreading proximally and may have exacerbations with lancinating attacks of different duration, from minutes to days. Pain can be triggered by pyrexia or extreme temperatures, either warm or cold [40, 58]. Painful neuropathy, in general, has been an enigma to clinicians due to the discordance between severe pain and little neurological and neurophysiological findings. In fact, sural nerve biopsy examination has been repeatedly reported as normal, although some authors have reported a loss of unmyelinated fibers [59]. In general, evaluation of small myelinated and unmyelinated fibers on sural nerve biopsy requires laborious ultrastructural and quantitative methods [59, 60] and may fail to reflect the degree of distal nerve degeneration [59, 61]. An explanation for this apparent contradiction is that nerve fibers at the level of the sural nerve undergo considerable branching before entering their sensory territory in the epidermis.

Post mortem examination of several cases of FD has demonstrated severe pathological changes in the dorsal root ganglion cells, with widely distributed deposits of Gb3 in interstitial cells and macrophages, decrease number of ganglion cells, proliferation of satellite cells and formation of residual 'Nageotte nodules' that follows neuronal death. Lysosomal storage has not been described in neurons, which present signs of neurodegeneration such as central chromatolysis (pale cytoplasm devoid of rough endoplasmic reticulum) and axonal degeneration in the form of axonal swellings or 'retraction balls' [40, 50, 62, 63]. Pathological changes in sensitive dorsal ganglia are in accordance with and account for degeneration and diminished density of ENFs.

We have studied the density and quantified the ENFs in several cases of hemizygous and heterozygous FD patients, and found decreased numbers of ENFs in all cases. We have followed the method of IHC and ABC technique [33, 64] described in 'Methodology', and immunostained nerve endings with the monoclonal antibody CD77 against Protein Gene Product 9.5. We have counted the number of axons that cross the basement membrane at the dermo-epidermal junction in several 1 mm lengths for each case. In normal subjects, ENFs that originate in the smaller neurons of the dorsal root ganglia, reach the skin and form a horizontal plexus, the subepidermal nerve plexus. Single ENFs separate from the bundles and penetrate the dermis, piercing the dermo-epidermal basement membrane, to innervate the epidermis (Fig. 15.11). In FD, there are a reduced number of axons crossing the basement lamina and epidermal branching is scarce (Fig. 15.12).

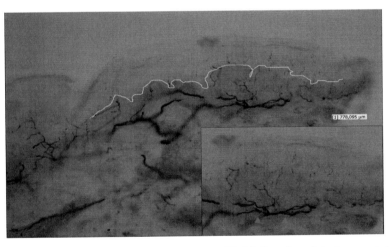

Fig. 15.11 Punch skin biopsy immunostained with PGP 9.5. Drawing of the basement dermo-epidermal basement membrane to quantify axons crossing the line to innervate the epidermis (*arrows* in insert). *Arrowheads*: subepidermal nervous plexus

Normal ENF density has been estimated at 25 ± 0.53 per lineal millimetre [32, 59, 64], with different degrees of severity according to the diminution in the number of epidermal axons. In all our cases, loss of ENF was severe, less than 8 ENF per mm (Fig. 15.12). Other pathologic findings such as ENF periodic swellings have been reported in patients with diabetic neuropathy [53] or in capsaicin-treated skin [65]. Although axonal swelling may represent ENF degeneration, they are difficult to quantify and can be occasionally seen in normal subjects.

Eccrine sweat gland innervation can also be observed by this IHC method. Eccrine glands are located at the superficial and deep dermis and their pathological

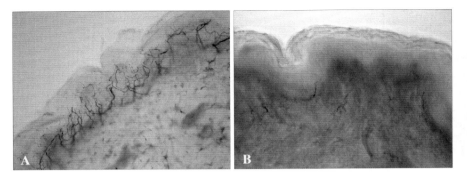

Fig. 15.12 IHC for PGP 9.5 in control skin and in a patient with FD. In the control, epidermal nerve endings arise from the subepidermal plexus and cross the basement membrane. In a FD patient some fibers seem to approach the dermo-epidermal junction but do not cross the basement membrane

features regarding lysosomal storage have been described in previous paragraphs. Eccrine glands innervation in FD appeared to be scarce and disorganized as compared to control subjects (Fig. 15.13). Further studies are necessary to objectively assess the degree of defective sweat gland innervation in FD.

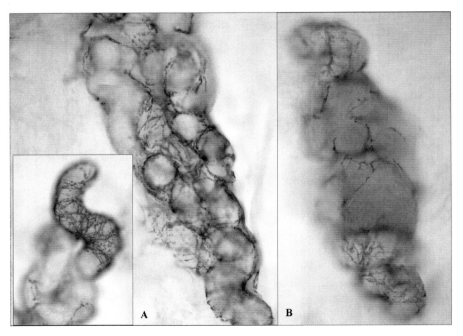

Fig. 15.13 Two views of eccrine sweat gland innervation immunostained with PGP 9.5. Note decreased nerve endings in a patient with FD (**b**) as compared to a control (**a**)

15.4 Summary

In summary, skin biopsy provides an enormous amount of information, crucial for the diagnosis of FD, especially in heterozygous women in whom clinical and biochemical analyses lead to a debatable diagnosis. Accumulation of Gb3 occurs in most dermal cells and appendages of clinically normal skin. In our experience, immunocytochemical evidence of Gb3 accumulation and ultrastructural changes occur both in hemizygous men and in heterozygous women. We believe that extensive and careful studies have to be performed by an expert in order to avoid erroneous interpretations or premature negative results. Examination of multiple types of dermal cells is necessary before a negative diagnosis is made. Under the electron microscope, intralysosomal inclusions are complex structures of different kinds, the commonest but not exclusive being the so-called zebra bodies, and clearly differ from other lysosomal accumulation in other storage disorders.

AK and telangiectases display similar clinical and histological features in FD to those in other LSD or in patients not known to have any metabolic disorder, thus Gb3 immunolabeling and electron microscopy studies are necessary as complementary investigations.

Finally, dermo-epidermal nerve endings that represent the terminals of C and Aδ nociceptors can be evaluated and quantified in clinically normal skin biopsy by IHC methods, which is essential to evaluate the degree of neuropathic pain present in FD patients, and eventually to assess the response to treatment.

Acknowledgements To all patients and their families for their generous and disinterested cooperation. To James Stilwell-Stronge for his help with the English version of this work and to Tania Vázquez for editorial assistance. This work was supported in part by grants from *Fondo de Investigacion Sanitaria* (PI07/1257 and PI07/90043) and *Xunta de Galicia* (PGIDIT06PXIB905328PR, INCITE07PXI905221ES and PS08/38).

References

1. Desnick RJ, Ioannou YA, Eng CM (2001) Alpha-galactosidase A deficiency: Fabry disease. In: Scriver C, Beaudet A, Sly W, Valle D, Kinzler DE, Volgestein B (eds) The metabolic and molecular basis of inherited disease, 8th edn. McGraw-Hill Inc, New York, pp 3733–3774
2. Orteu CH, Jansen T, Lidove O et al (2007) Fabry disease and the skin: data from FOS, the Fabry outcome survey. Br J Dermatol 157:331–337
3. Ries M, Ramaswami U, Parini R et al (2003) The early clinical phenotype of Fabry disease: a study on 35 European children and adolescents. Eur J Pediatr 162:767–772
4. Larralde M, Boggio P, Amartino H, Chamoles N (2004) Fabry disease: a study of 6 hemizygous men and 5 heterozygous women with emphasis on dermatologic manifestations. Arch Dermatol 140:1440–1446
5. Mohrenschlager M, Braun-Falco M, Ring J, Abeck D (2003) Fabry disease: recognition and management of cutaneous manifestations. Am J Clin Dermatol 4:189–196
6. Barba Romero MA, Garcia de Lorenzo y Mateos A, Groupo Espanol de Estudio de FOS (2004) Fabry's disease in Spain. Study of 24 cases. Med Clin (Barc) 123:57–60
7. Jansen T, Graue N, Dissemond J, Hillen U, Hentschke M, Grabbe S (2006) Telangiectasias on the neck as a presenting cutaneous sign of Fabry disease. J Dermatol 33:652–654

8. Fleming C, Rennie A, Fallowfield M, McHenry PM (1997) Cutaneous manifestations of fucosidosis. Br J Dermatol 136:594–597

9. Kanitakis J, Allombert C, Doebelin B et al (2005) Fucosidosis with angiokeratoma. Immunohistochemical & electronmicroscopic study of a new case and literature review. J Cutan Pathol 32:506–511

10. Rodriguez-Serna M, Botella-Estrada R, Chabas A et al (1996) Angiokeratoma corporis diffusum associated with beta-mannosidase deficiency. Arch Dermatol 132: 1219–1222

11. Molho-Pessach V, Bargal R, Abramowitz Y et al (2007) Angiokeratoma corporis diffusum in human beta-mannosidosis: report of a new case and a novel mutation. J Am Acad Dermatol 57:407–412

12. Kawachi Y, Matsu-ura K, Sakuraba H, Otsuka F (1998) Angiokeratoma corporis diffusum associated with galactosialidosis. Dermatology 197:52–54

13. Kelly B, Kelly E (2006) Angiokeratoma corporis diffusum in a patient with no recognizable enzyme abnormalities. Arch Dermatol 142:615–618

14. Navarro C (1995) Estudio ultraestructural de la piel. Su contribución al diagnóstico de las enfermedades metabólicas que afectan al Sistema Nervioso Central. University of Barcelona, Barcelona

15. de Groote CM (1998) Het Electronmicroscopisch Onderzoek van Huidbiopten als Metabole Aandoeningen van het. Zenuwestel. Born-Bunge Stichting, University of Antwerpen, Antwerpen

16. Brady RO, Gal AE, Bradley RM et al (1967) Enzymatic defect in Fabry's disease. Ceramidetrihexosidase deficiency. N Engl J Med 276:1163–1167

17. Khine AA, Firtel M, Lingwood CA (1998) CD77-dependent retrograde transport of CD19 to the nuclear membrane: functional relationship between CD77 and CD19 during germinal center B-cell apoptosis. J Cell Physiol 176:281–292

18. Tetaud C, Falguieres T, Carlier K et al (2003) Two distinct Gb3/CD77 signaling pathways leading to apoptosis are triggered by anti-Gb3/CD77 mAb and verotoxin-1. J Biol Chem 278:45200–45208

19. Ceuterick C, Martin JJ (1984) Diagnostic role of skin or conjunctival biopsies in neurological disorders. An update. J Neurol Sci 65:179–191

20. Hashimoto K, Gross BG, Lever WF (1965) Angiokeratoma Corporis Diffusum (Fabry). Histochemical and Electron Microscopic Studies of the Skin. J Invest Dermatol 44:119–128

21. Carpenter S (1987) Skin biopsy for diagnosis of hereditary neurologic metabolic disease. Arch Dermatol 123:1618–1621

22. Goebel HH (1999) Extracerebral biopsies in neurodegenerative diseases of childhood. Brain Dev 21:435–443

23. Abramovich CM, Prayson RA, McMahon JT, Cohen BH (2001) Ultrastructural examination of the axillary skin biopsy in the diagnosis of metabolic diseases. Hum Pathol 32: 649–655

24. Newton GA, Sanchez RL, Swedo J, Smith EB (1987) Lafora's disease. The role of skin biopsy. Arch Dermatol 123:1667–1669

25. Ceuterick-de Groote C, Martin JJ (1998) Extracerebral biopsy in lysosomal and peroxisomal disorders. Ultrastructural findings. Brain Pathol 8:121–132

26. Alroy J, Ucci AA (2006) Skin biopsy: a useful tool in the diagnosis of lysosomal storage diseases. Ultrastruct Pathol 30:489–503

27. Askari H, Kaneski CR, Semino-Mora C et al (2007) Cellular and tissue localization of globotriaosylceramide in Fabry disease. Virchows Arch 451:823–834

28. Malur PR, Davanageri RS, Bannur HB, Suranagi VV (2008) Lafora's disease diagnosed on axillary skin biopsy in 3 patients. Indian J Dermatol Venereol Leprol 74:672–673

29. Kotani M, Hosoya H, Kubo H et al (1994) Evidence for direct binding of intracellularly distributed ganglioside GM2 to isolated vimentin intermediate filaments in normal and Tay-Sachs disease human fibroblasts. Cell Struct Funct 19:81–87

30. Kanekura T, Fukushige T, Kanda A et al (2005) Immunoelectron-microscopic detection of globotriaosylceramide accumulated in the skin of patients with Fabry disease. Br J Dermatol 153:544–548

31. Rozenfeld PA, Croxatto O, Ebner R, Fossati CA (2006) Immunofluorescence detection of globotriaosylceramide deposits in conjunctival biopsies of Fabry disease patients. Clin Exp Ophthalmol 34:689–694

32. Kennedy WR, Wendelschafer-Crabb G (1993) The innervation of human epidermis. J Neurol Sci 115:184–190

33. McCarthy BG, Hsieh ST, Stocks A et al (1995) Cutaneous innervation in sensory neuropathies: evaluation by skin biopsy. Neurology 45:1848–1855

34. Lauria G, McArthur JC, Hauer PE, Griffin JW, Cornblath DR (1998) Neuropathological alterations in diabetic truncal neuropathy: evaluation by skin biopsy. J. Neurol. Neurosurg. Psychiatry 65:762–766

35. Urmacher CD (1997) Normal skin. In: Sternberg SS (ed) Histology for pathologists, 2nd edn. Lippincott-Raven, Philadelphia, pp 25–45

36. Sagebiel RW, Parker F (1968) Cutaneous lesions of Fabry's disease: glycolipid lipidosis; light and electron microscopic findings. J Invest Dermatol 50:208–213

37. Navarro C, Teijeira S, Dominguez C et al (2006) Fabry disease: an ultrastructural comparative study of skin in hemizygous and heterozygous patients. Acta Neuropathol 111: 178–185

38. Cable WJ, Dvorak AM, Osage JE, Kolodny EH (1982) Fabry disease: significance of ultrastructural localization of lipid inclusions in dermal nerves. Neurology 32:347–353

39. Dvorak AM, Cable WJL, Osage JE, Kolodny EH (1981) Diagnostic electron microscopy: II. Fabry's disease: use of biopsies from uninvolved skin: acute and chronic changes involving the microvasculature and small unmyelinated nerves. In: Summers SC, Rosen PP (eds) Pathology annual. Appleton-Century-Crofts, New York, pp 139–158

40. Kahn P (1973) Anderson-Fabry disease: a histopathological study of three cases with observations on the mechanism of production of pain. J Neurol Neurosurg Psychiatry 36:1053–1062

41. Lao LM, Kumakiri M, Mima H et al (1998) The ultrastructural characteristics of eccrine sweat glands in a Fabry disease patient with hypohidrosis. J Dermatol Sci 18:109–117

42. Kolodny EH, Cable WJ (1982) Inborn errors of metabolism. Ann Neurol 11:221–232

43. Tabira T, Goto I, Kuroiwa Y, Kikuchi M (1974) Neuropathological and biochemical studies in Fabry's disease. Acta Neuropathol 30:345–354

44. Mohrenschlager M, Ring J, Abeck D (2001) Skin manifestations of Fabry disease. JAMA 286:1315

45. Fischer EG, Moore MJ, Lager DJ (2006) Fabry disease: a morphologic study of 11 cases. Mod Pathol 19:1295–1301

46. Eggert AO, Wossner R, Knoll A, Hamm H, Wanner C, Breunig FB (2006) Umbilical angiectases as the sole clinical sign of Fabry disease in a 9-year-old boy. Eur J Pediatr 165:205–206

47. Amann-Vesti BR, Gitzelmann G, Widmer U, Bosshard NU, Steinmann B, Koppensteiner R (2003) Severe lymphatic microangiopathy in Fabry disease. Lymphat Res Biol 1: 185–189

48. Navarro X, Verdu E, Wendelschafer-Crabb G, Kennedy WR (1997) Immunohistochemical study of skin reinnervation by regenerative axons. J Comp Neurol 380:164–174

49. Kennedy WR (2004) Opportunities afforded by the study of unmyelinated nerves in skin and other organs. Muscle Nerve 29:756–767

50. Onishi A, Dyck PJ (1974) Loss of small peripheral sensory neurons in Fabry disease. Histologic and morphometric evaluation of cutaneous nerves, spinal ganglia, and posterior columns. Arch Neurol 31:120–127

51. Scott LJ, Griffin JW, Luciano C et al (1999) Quantitative analysis of epidermal innervation in Fabry disease. Neurology 52:1249–1254

52. Holland NR, Crawford TO, Hauer P, Cornblath DR, Griffin JW, McArthur JC (1998) Small-fiber sensory neuropathies: clinical course and neuropathology of idiopathic cases. Ann Neurol 44:47–59

53. Kennedy WR, Wendelschafer-Crabb G, Johnson T (1996) Quantitation of epidermal nerves in diabetic neuropathy. Neurology 47:1042–1048

54. Kennedy WR, Wendelschafer-Crabb G (1996) Utility of skin biopsy in diabetic neuropathy. Semin. Neurol 16:163–171

55. Hilz MJ, Axelrod FB, Bickel A et al (2004) Assessing function and pathology in familial dysautonomia: assessment of temperature perception, sweating and cutaneous innervation. Brain 127:2090–2098

56. Polydefkis M, Yiannoutsos CT, Cohen BA et al (2002) Reduced intraepidermal nerve fiber density in HIV-associated sensory neuropathy. Neurology 58:115–119

57. Chiang MC, Lin YH, Pan CL, Tseng TJ, Lin WM, Hsieh ST (2002) Cutaneous innervation in chronic inflammatory demyelinating polyneuropathy. Neurology 8(59):1094–1098

58. Hilz MJ, Stemper B, Kolodny EH (2000) Lower limb cold exposure induces pain and prolonged small fiber dysfunction in Fabry patients. Pain 84:361–365

59. Herrmann DN, Griffin JW, Hauer P, Cornblath DR, McArthur JC (1999) Epidermal nerve fiber density and sural nerve morphometry in peripheral neuropathies. Neurology 53:1634–1640

60. Llewelyn JG, Gilbey SG, Thomas PK, King RH, Muddle JR, Watkins PJ (1991) Sural nerve morphometry in diabetic autonomic and painful sensory neuropathy. A clinicopathological study. Brain 114:867–892

61. Periquet MI, Novak V, Collins MP et al (1999) Painful sensory neuropathy: prospective evaluation using skin biopsy. Neurology 53:1641–1647

62. Rahman AN, Lindenberg R (1963) The Neuropathology of Hereditary Dystopic Lipidosis. Arch Neurol 9:373–385

63. Steward VW, Hitchcock C (1968) Fabry's disease (angiokeratoma corporis diffusum). A report of 5 cases with pain in the extremities as the chief symptom. Pathol Eur 3:377–388

64. McArthur JC, Stocks EA, Hauer P, Cornblath DR, Griffin JW (1998) Epidermal nerve fiber density: normative reference range and diagnostic efficiency. Arch Neurol 55:1513–1520

65. Nolano M, Simone DA, Wendelschafer-Crabb G, Johnson T, Hazen E, Kennedy WR (1999) Topical capsaicin in humans: parallel loss of epidermal nerve fibers and pain sensation. Pain 81:135–145

Chapter 16
Bone and Muscle Involvement in Fabry Disease

Dominique P. Germain

Abstract Descriptive, cross-sectional studies investigating bone mineral density (BMD) using dual energy X-ray absorptiometry scan (DEXA) have shown that patients with Fabry disease have significantly reduced bone mineral density at both the lumbar spine and femoral neck. Osteopenia was present in approximately 50% of patients with untreated FD. Here, we further confirm these findings and report for the first time on a case of severe osteoporosis with spontaneous vertebral fractures in a 72-year-old male. With the emerging enzyme replacement therapy and the hope for increased life expectancy, the assessment of BMD should be recommended in patients with FD. Whether BMD and bone metabolism will improve after enzyme replacement therapy warrants further studies. Meanwhile, prophylactic therapy of osteoporotic fractures should be considered in patients with significantly decreased BMD

Keywords Fabry disease · Bone mineral density · DEXA · Osteopenia · Osteoporosis

16.1 Introduction

Fabry disease (FD, OMIM 301500) is a progressive X-linked inherited disorder of glycosphingolipid metabolism. Absent or deficient activity of the lysosomal exoglycohydrolase α-galactosidase A (α-D-galactoside galactohydrolase, EC 3.2.1.22; α-Gal A) results in progressive accumulation of globotriaosylceramide (Gb_3) and related glycosphingolipids (galabiosylceramide) within lysosomes in a variety of cell types, including capillary endothelial cells, renal (podocytes, tubular cells, glomerular endothelial, mesangial and intersticial cells), cardiac (cardiomyocytes

D.P. Germain (✉)
Medical Genetics, Centre de référence de la maladie de Fabry et des maladies héréditaires du tissu conjonctif, U.F. de Génétique Médicale, Hôpital Raymond Poincaré (AP-HP), Garches, France;
University of Versailles – St Quentin en Yvelines (UVSQ), Versailles, France
e-mail: dominique.germain@rpc.aphp.fr

D. Elstein et al. (eds.), *Fabry Disease*, DOI 10.1007/978-90-481-9033-1_16,
© Springer Science+Business Media B.V. 2010

and fibroblasts) and nerve cells [1]. With age, progressive damage to vital organ systems develops in both genders [2] leading to organ failure, but while the classic form of Fabry disease is known to be a multi-system disorder with protean clinical manifestations [1], few data are available regarding the skeletal involvement. However, the successful introduction of enzyme replacement therapy (ERT) for Fabry disease and the potential improvement in the clinical course of the disease warrants increased knowledge and awareness of co-morbidities such as osteoporosis, as more patients may live to have disease-related complications.

16.2 Skeletal Involvement in Fabry Disease

In a seminal study, osteopenia was demonstrated as a common feature of Fabry disease [3]. Bone mineral density of the lumbar spine and the femoral neck was assessed by dual-energy X-ray absorptiometry (DEXA) in 23 hemizygous male patients with a mean age of 31 years (range: 16–60 years) affected with classic FD. Using the World Health Organization classification of bone mineral density (BMD) abnormalities: [normal: T score >-1 SD; osteopenia: -2.5 SD$\leq$ T score <-1SD; osteoporosis: T score <-2.5 SD; and severe osteoporosis: T score <-2.5 SD with spontaneous fracture [4], 20 of the 23 male patients (88%) had either osteopenia ($n = 11$) or osteoporosis ($n = 9$) [3, 5].

Skeletal involvement was subsequently confirmed in a larger cohort of 53 untreated Fabry patients (21 males, 32 females), aged 15–63 years (mean = 40), in which osteopenia was present in approximately 50% of cases [6].

Following our first description of a high prevalence of osteopenia and osteoporosis in Fabry disease, additional patients were enrolled in the original cross-sectional, descriptive study of patients with FD. Bone mineral density (lumbar spine and femoral neck T scores) was assessed in a total of 49 male patients (aged 18–72, mean = 37). In addition, forearm T score was obtained for 45% of the patients ($n = 22$). Bone densitometry revealed a statistically significant decrease in BMD at both femoral neck and lumbar spine (L1–L4) (Fig. 16.1) with 33 hemizygotes (67%) found to have either osteopenia ($n = 18$) or osteoporosis ($n = 15$). Results are shown in Table 16.1. Demographics, anthropometry, kidney function and individual T scores are shown in Table 16.2 for all 33 patients who presented with osteopenia or osteoporosis. Of note, the oldest patient of the study population, a 72-year-old male who was 67 at the time of DEXA assessment and has been on recombinant enzyme therapy since then, complained of acute lower back pain during his last visit to the hospital. While X-rays failed to identify any lesion, lumbar MRI revealed a pathological fracture of L5 pedicula together with previous vertebral body fractures, illustrating the possible occurrence of severe osteoporosis in Fabry patient with prolonged life expectancy (Fig. 16.2).

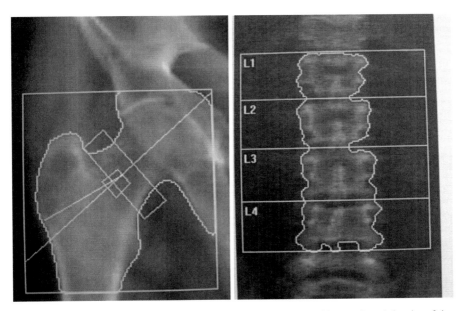

Fig. 16.1 Dual-energy X-ray absorptiometry (DEXA) assessment of bone mineral density of the femoral neck and the lumbar spine in a 53-year-old male patient affected with Fabry disease. T scores of –4.2 and –4.3 were found at the hip and L1–L4, respectively

Table 16.1 Prevalence of osteopenia and osteoporosis in 49 hemizygous males (age 18–68 years, mean = 37) affected with Fabry disease

Sites	Osteopenia (–2.5 SD ≤ T score <–1 SD) n (%)	Osteoporosis (T score <–2.5 SD) n (%)
Lumbar spine *T* score	14/47 (29.79%)	11/47 (23.40%)
Femoral neck *T* score	13/45 (28.89%)	4/45 (8.89%)
Forearm *T* score	9/22 (40.91%)	1/22 (4.55%)
At least one site	18/49 (36.73%)	15/49 (30.61%)

16.3 Muscular Involvement

The accumulation of storage material in muscle fibers has been reported only rarely in Fabry disease [7–9]. Inclusions have been found mostly in the intermyofibrillar and subsarcolemmal [8]. By light microscopy, muscle biopsy specimens obtained from a 26-year-old male patient appeared normal, except for biopsies stained with periodic acid – Schiff (PAS) stain, which showed small granular deposits in the endothelium of endomysial capillaries, beneath the sarcolemma

Table 16.2 Demographics, anthropometry, renal function, and lumbar spine, femoral neck and forearm T scores for the 33 male patients with osteopenia or osteoporosis

Patient ID	Age (years)	BMI (g/m^2)	eGFR (ml/min/1.73 m^2)	Lumbar spine (L1–L4) T score (DEXA)	Femoral neck T score (DEXA)	Forearm T score (DEXA)
1	49	20	99	−3.2	−1.6	−2.2
2	32	19	109.5	−1.9	−1.6	−2
3	33	27	89.8	0	−2.9	ND
4	31	18	64.4	−1.4	−0.8	−0.5
5	27	19	96.3	−2.2	−0.7	ND
6	36	24	75.1	−2.3	−1.7	−1.8
7	41	23	75.6	−1.4	−0.6	−0.1
8	39	17	89.4	−2.6	−2.3	ND
9	36	19	95.1	−2.1	−0.6	ND
10	18	19	149.3	−3	−2.2	ND
11	27	21	125.3	−2.5	−1	ND
12	47	23	122.6	−2.4	−1.9	ND
13	41	23	92.2	−3.2	−2	−2
14	22	17	148.3	−2.4	−2.4	ND
15	31	20	112.0	−0.8	−1	−2.8
16	28	19	118.2	−0.9	−0.6	−2.1
17	32	25	152.9	−3.1	−1.8	−2.4
18	29	19	130.8	−2.2	−1.6	ND
19	34	25	77.6	−1.9	−1.4	−1.3
20	36	19	87.1	−2	−1.9	−2.1
21	50	21	88.5	−2.1	−2.2	−1.8
22	36	20	62.3	−0.4	ND	−1.9
23	22	25	118.1	−2.4	ND	−0.7
24	69	28	26.3	−1.3	−1.4	ND
25	52	22	27.9	−1.4	−1.3	−0.3
26	40	28	112.0	−1.6	−1.1	0.1
27	38	19	104.0	−1.9	−2.7	−1.4
28	44	22	71.3	−2.5	−0.5	ND
29	57	22	91.8	−2.9	−1.2	ND
30	51	17	42.4	−4.3	−4.2	ND
31	50	18	62.9	−2.6	−3.5	ND
32	60	30	79.8	−1.9	−0.9	ND
33	58	19	87.5	−4.9	−2.4	ND

BMI: Body Mass Index; eGFR: estimated Glomegular Filtration Rate (MDRD formula); ND: Not done (Tran TC et al., unpublished data).

and in the intermyofibrillar network of some fibers [9]. By electron microscopy, pleiomorphic inclusions were found in the subsarcolemmal and intermyofibrillar spaces of muscles fibers and in the capillary endothelium. Muscle fiber components remained normal. Some satellite cells contained inclusions. Fibroblasts also enclosed dense and membranous structures. In the vessel walls, inclusions were found in the endothelial and perithelial cells [9].

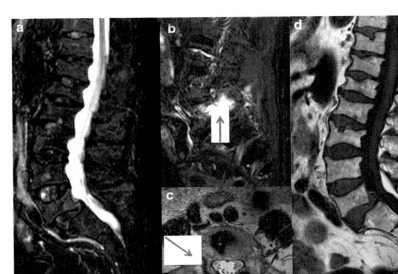

Fig. 16.2 MRI illustrating bone fragility with bone insufficiency of L5 (isthm), ancient fractures of the vertebral bodies and a recent fracture of L5 right pedicula, in a 72-year-old patient with severe osteoporosis. *Panel* **a** (STIR, sagittal view) and *Panel* **d** (T1, sagital median): several vertebral bodies fractures are seen, without signal anomaly in T1 or T2, in favour of ancient fractures. A mild spondylolisthésis of L5 on S1 can be observed. *Panel* **b** (STIR, sagital right lateral view): hypersignal corresponding to a bone oedema of the right pedicula of L5 (*arrow*). *Panel* **c** (T2, axial): fracture of the right pedicula of L5

16.4 Pathological Hypotheses

Fabry disease is frequently complicated by osteopenia or osteoporosis of the lumbar spine and femoral neck [3, 6]. Normal bone development with achievement of peak bone mass is influenced by several factors: genetics, nutritional status, hormones, exercise, and other physical factors. Among the causes of secondary osteoporosis which can be discussed in Fabry disease, malnutrition due to the gastrointestinal manifestations of FD including diarrhoea and vitamin D malabsorption are likely to lower BMI and thereby BMD. In our study, BMD of the lumbar spine and femoral neck were lower in patients with impaired renal function compared with those with preserved renal function. Secondary hyperparathyroidism is an important factor in the osteopenia of end stage renal disease, causing osteoclastic bone resorption and progression of renal impairment may further reduce bone mineralization and contribute to the development of osteoporosis in patients with Fabry disease. It is known that physical exercise with resistance exercise and mechanical loading favors increased bone mass. Patients with FD are prone to avoiding exercise because of depression, hypohidrosis and heat intolerance which may further add to the secondary osteoporosis. Finally, glycosphingolipids accumulation may also affect the bones and account for part of the bone manifestations [10, 3].

16.5 Conclusions

With the emerging enzyme replacement therapy and the hope for increased life expectancy, the assessment of bone mineral density should be recommended in patients with Fabry disease. Whether bone mineral density will improve after enzyme replacement therapy remains to be established. Meanwhile, prophylactic therapy of osteoporotic fractures with adjunctive therapies should be considered in patients with significantly decreased bone mineral density.

Acknowledgments The author is grateful to Karelle BENISTAN, MD, Robert CARLIER, MD, Caroline LEBRETON, MD and Thi-Chien TRAN, MSc for their help in preparing the manuscript.

References

1. Germain DP (2010) Fabry disease. Orphanet J Rare Dis (in press)
2. Wilcox WR, Oliveira JP, Hopkin RJ et al (2008) Females with Fabry disease frequently have major organ involvement: lessons from the Fabry Registry. Mol Genet Metab 93(2):112–128
3. Germain DP, Benistan K, Boutouyrie P, Mutschler C (2005) Osteopenia and osteoporosis: previously unrecognized symptoms of Fabry disease. Clin Genet 68:93–95
4. Kanis JA (1994) Assessment of fracture risk and its application to screening for post-menopausal osteoporosis: synopsis of a WHO report. WHO Study Group. Osteoporos Int 4:368–381
5. Germain DP, Benistan K, Khatchikian L, Mutschler C (2005) Bone involvement in Fabry disease. Med Sci (Paris) 21(11 Suppl):43–44
6. Mersebach H, Johansson JO, Rasmussen AK et al (2007) Osteopenia: a common aspect of Fabry disease. Predictors of bone mineral density. Genet Med 9(12):812–818
7. Sima AA, Robertson DM (1978) Involvement of peripheral nerve and muscle in Fabry's disease. Histologic, ultrastructural, and morphometric studies. Arch Neurol 35(5):291–301
8. Tome FM, Fardeau M, Lenoir G (1977) Ultrastructure of muscle and sensory nerve in Fabry's disease. Acta Neuropathol (Berl) 38(3):187–194
9. Pellissier JF, Van Hoof F, Bourdet-Bonerandi D, Monier-Faugere MC, Toga M (1981) Morphological and biochemical changes in muscle and peripheral nerve in Fabry's disease. Muscle Nerve 4(5):381–387
10. Horiuchi H, Saito N, Kobayashi S, Ota H, Taketomi T, Takaoka K (2002) Avascular necrosis of the femoral head in a patient with Fabry's disease: identification of ceramide trihexoside in the bone by delayed-extraction matrix-assisted laser desorption ionization-time-of-flight mass spectrometry. Arthritis Rheum 46(7):1922–1925

Chapter 17
The Eye in Fabry Disease

Andrea Sodi

Abstract The more specific ocular manifestations of Fabry Disease (FD) are represented by corneal opacities (cornea verticillata), cataract, and conjunctival and retinal vascular abnormalities. Cornea verticillata is the most common ocular finding and consists of bilateral whorl-like opacities, located in the superficial corneal layers. These corneal opacities have been described in the large majority of the patients and so, at present, cornea verticillata is usually considered the most reliable ophthalmological marker of FD. Recently corneal deposits have been investigated by confocal microscopy, a diagnostic technology able to study the corneal structure layer by layer; this technique may provide more detailed information about the physiopathology of cornea verticillata and its changes with time. FD patients may also show a typical posterior subcapsular cataract with a 'spoke-like' appearance: this is a rare finding and cannot be routinely used for diagnosis and monitoring the disease. Conjunctival and retinal vessels tortuosity is very common but it is not specific of FD, as it can be observed in other vascular disorders. Moreover the evaluation of vessels tortuosity is very subjective and it can be difficult to quantify. Our group is presently developing a specific software for computer-assisted analysis of vessels tortuosity in digital fundus pictures.

Keywords Cornea verticillata · Vessels tortuosity · Posterior subcapsular cataract

17.1 Ocular Manifestations in Fabry Disease (FD)

17.1.1 Specific Ocular Abnormalities

The most common ocular signs associated with Fabry Disease (FD) are conjunctival vessels abnormalities, corneal opacities, lens opacities and retinal vessels tortuosity [1, 2].

A. Sodi (✉)
Eye Clinic, University of Florence, Florence, Italy
e-mail: andrea.sodi@unifi.it

D. Elstein et al. (eds.), *Fabry Disease*, DOI 10.1007/978-90-481-9033-1_17,
© Springer Science+Business Media B.V. 2010

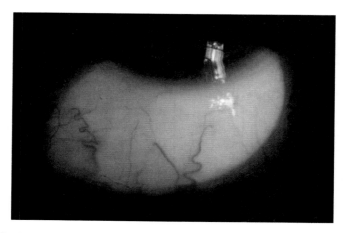

Fig. 17.1 Conjunctival vessels tortuosity in an FD patient

Conjunctival vessels abnormalities consist of increased tortuosity sometimes associated with aneurysmatic dilations and blood sludging (Fig. 17.1); they are determined by the deposition of glycosphingolipids within the vessel walls which become less resistant to bloodstream pressure [3].

The anomalous course of the conjunctival vessels is not absolutely specific of FD; in fact it may be associated with other vascular systemic disorders (like diabetes, carotid-cavernous fistula, multiple mieloma, sickle cell anemia, Sturge-Weber syndrome, and some others).

Corneal opacities are represented by deposits in the corneal superficial layers, with a typical whorl-like pattern (Fig. 17.2) in most cases with a clockwise disposition, which is the cause of the name 'cornea verticillata' [1–5] commonly used

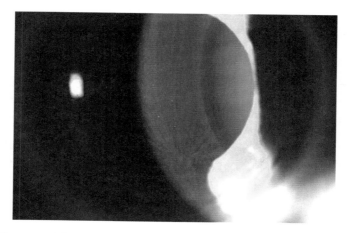

Fig. 17.2 Cornea verticillata

to indicate this corneal appearance. They are usually bilateral and symmetrical and are often more evident in the inferior part of the cornea. The mechanisms determining the vortex pattern are still unknown; possible explanations include the effect of blinking and the influence of periocular electromagnetic fields [6]. Cornea verticillata can be observed in almost all hemizygous male patients but also in most of heterozygous females. A diffuse subepithelial corneal haze has sometimes been reported in FD [5], but it is unclear if it represents an independent entity or a stage of evolution of cornea verticillata; it is usually not considered a typical ocular manifestation of FD.

Imaging of cornea verticillata is very difficult because corneal deposits are usually very thin and pale and are located within a transparent structure. A standardized procedure for cornea verticillata imaging is advisable. In our experience better quality pictures of the corneal deposits with the vortex pattern can be obtained by means of a slit-lamp camera with tangential illumination, high basic illumination, low intensity or absent flash light and anterior defocusing (accurate focus on the corneal surface with iris out of focus).

With very few exceptions, other than FD, cornea verticillata can be caused by long-term therapy with a number of drugs (especially amiodarone and cloroquine) [7]; so this ocular sign has a high specificity for FD.

Corneal alterations with a vortex disposition can also be seen in the so-called 'hurricane keratopathy', a whorl-like pattern reported in patients where the corneal epithelial cells turnover is abnormally increased; but this is a clinical picture significantly different from cornea verticillata. In fact hurricane keratopathy doesn't depend on the deposition of any substance, it is usually seen in corneal graft patients and corneal lens wearer, often after steroid treatment; it is often associated with mild ocular symptoms (like ocular irritation, foreign body sensation, lacrimation, photophobia) and it often shows spontaneous resolution. Moreover, the pattern is highlighted by fluorescein staining [8].

Some studies investigated the pathology of cornea verticillata showing that it corresponds to duplication of corneal epithelium basement membrane, subepithelial deposits of amorphous material and intraepithelial lipid deposits [9–12]

Two kinds of *lens opacities* [1–5] have been described in FD. The first one is an anterior capsular and subcapsular cataract with a wedge shape and a radial disposition (the base near the equator of the lens and the apex towards the center). In our experience this sign is rather uncommon and when present, it is not really specific of the disease. The second type of cataract consists of linear whitish opacities located in the posterior part of the lens, near the capsule, with a spoke-like appearance. This pattern is more typical of FD and this kind of cataract is often reported as 'Fabry cataract '.

Retinal vessels abnormalities [1–5] are represented by increased vessels tortuosity (Fig. 17.3) often associated with segmental dilation and narrowing of the vessels. Both arteriolar and venular retinal circulations are usually involved. Retinal vessels tortuosity in FD is caused by pathologic deposits in some structures of the vessels walls (smooth muscles, endocytes, pericytes) [13]. Again retinal vessels abnormalities are not specific of FD; they can be found in some ocular vascular disorders (like

Fig. 17.3 Retinal vessels
tortuosity in an FD patient

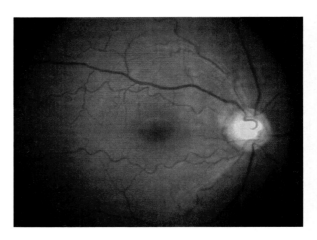

hypertensive retinopathy and retinal vein occlusion), in some patients affected by systemic cardiovascular diseases (like leukaemia, sickle cells anemia, polycythemia, and others), and even in a few number normal subjects, as a variant of the normal vascular course.

There are several studies reporting the prevalence of the various eye signs in different series of FD patients, including both hemizygous males and heterozygous females [4, 5, 14–16]. The data of some of them are summarized in Table 17.1.

Table 17.1 Prevalence of eye abnormalities in Fabry disease (M = hemizygous males, F = heterozygous females)

	Spaeth [4]		Sher [5]		Orssaud [15]	Nguyen [16]	
	6 M	3F	37 M	25 F	32 M	34 M	32 F
Conjunctival vessels abnormalities (%)	41.6		78	46	68.7	97.1	78.1
Cornea verticillata (%)	91.6		94.5	88	43.7	94.1	71.9
Posterior subcapsular cataract (%)	50		37	14	37.5	11.8	none
Retinal vessels abnormalities (%)	25		70	25	56.2	76.5	18.8

Fabry Outcome Survey (FOS) is a centralized database for all FD patients who are receiving or are candidates for enzyme replacement therapy (ERT) with agalsidase alfa [17]. FOS ophthalmological data have been reviewed in 2007 considering 173 patients; at present this is the largest study reporting the prevalence of the ocular manifestations in FD patients [18]. In the FOS study, the prevalence of cornea verticillata was 73.1% in males and 76.9% in females; the prevalence of vessels tortuosity (conjunctival and/or retinal) was 48.7% in males and 21.9% in females; while Fabry cataract was reported in 23.1% of males and 9.8% of females.

There are significant differences in the prevalence of ocular abnormalities in the various studies; they are probably related to the size of the samples, their demographic features (mainly age and sex), the systemic involvement, the underlying genotype, the influence of ERT in subgroups of patients, the technologies used for eye investigation.

In FD patients ocular manifestations can be detected even in young children [2] (Fig. 17.4); in FOS, the youngest patient with ophthalmological abnormalities was 3 years old. An early presence of cornea verticillata has been previously reported even in a 6-month-old child [4] and in a fetus [19].

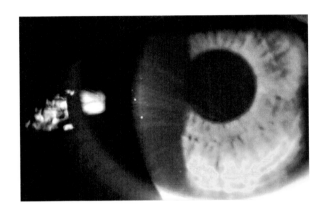

Fig. 17.4 Cornea verticillata in an 8 year old girl. She is still clinically asymptomatic; her father died because of a stroke at 35 years of age

The possible association between ocular manifestations and the systemic clinical picture is still uncertain. The absence of a clear relationship between ocular abnormalities and cardiac and renal manifestations has been reported in a small group of FD patients [20]. Conversely in FOS [18], increased vessels tortuosity seemed to be associated with a more rapid worsening of indices of cardiac and renal function and more progressive increase in the FOS-MSSI (a scoring system developed to measure FD severity) [21]. These data suggest a possible predictive value of eye investigation for the systemic involvement in FD; in any case, they are absolutely preliminary and need further investigation.

17.1.2 Uncommom Ocular Findings

Some other ocular disorders have been described in a few isolated patients of FD but in most of the cases a physiopathological link with FD is merely hypothetical. They include retinal vascular occlusive disorders [22, 23], ischemic optic neuropathy [24], myelinated nerve fibers [5], retinal pigment epithelium abnormalities [25], and uveitis [26]. We have reported the case of a FD patient with early-onset choroidal neovascularization in the macula without any traditional risk factor; we speculated that the vascular complications of FD may facilitate the neovascular process [27].

In FD some rare ocular abnormalities may also affect the eye anterior segment, like lid oedema [5] and conjunctival chemosis [28].

17.2 Clinical Interest of Ocular Abnormalities in FD

The clinical interest of the FD ophthalmological abnormalities may involve the diagnosis and the screening of FD, the monitoring of the natural course of the disease and its response to treatments.

The ophthalmologic contribution to FD *diagnosis* is essentially based on the detection of cornea verticillata, which can be considered an 'ophthalmological marker' for FD. In fact cornea verticillata represents a sign with high sensitivity and specificity: it is present in almost all FD patients and it is rarely found in non-FD subjects. Moreover, its detection is not expensive and time-consuming. Fabry cataract can be found only in a minority of patients while vessels tortuosity is not specific and its evaluation is subjective.

On the other hand, cornea verticillata doesn't determine visual symptoms stimulating the patients to see an ophthalmologist and – unfortunately – it is usually not easily recognized by basic ophthalmologists. So the efficacy of ophthalmologic *screening* programs of FD is still questionable [29]. However among the patients included in the Fabry Registry, another observational database for FD, ophthalmological signs were reported as the presenting symptoms in 11% of males and 12%of females [30].

Finally, the technical obstacles in imaging cornea verticillata prevent its use for *monitoring* disease evolution; without reproducible and reliable documentation it is very difficult to detect accurately subtle changes in corneal opacities related to the natural progression of the disease or to the effect of treatments. So, at present, there are only very limited data about the influence of ERT on ocular signs in FD.

17.3 Technological Developments for the Study of Ocular Signs in FD

Recently, eye abnormalities in FD have been investigated by means of sophisticated technologies with the goal to obtain reliable and quantitative measurements to be used both for scientific research and clinical practice.

Corneal deposits have been investigated by confocal microscopy (CM), a diagnostic technology able to study the corneal structure layer by layer. In three hemizygous male patients CM showed the presence of hyper-reflective roundish intracellular inclusion in the basal epithelial cells while in three heterozygous female patients a diffuse accumulation of reflective substances in the basal epithelial layers could be appreciated [31]. Another group reported with the same technique the presence of hyper-reflective intra-cellular deposits in the basal epithelial cells layers;

more interestingly they noted in one patient a reduction in inclusions 15 months after the start of ERT [32].

A dedicated software for the evaluation of retina vessels tortuosity was recently developed by our group; after semi-automatic extraction of the vessels profile, the vessel segment under consideration was automatically analysed, and then some parameters describing vessels tortuosity were calculated.

Finally, other investigators have reported mild visual field abnormalities in FD patients, suggesting a possible subclinical optic neuropathy in FD and the interest of perimetric test in the ophthalmic evaluation of FD [33, 34].

17.4 Summary

The study of ophthalmological manifestations in FD may represent a useful tool to refine the diagnosis of the disease. Further technological developments are required to use eye abnormalities for monitoring the natural history of FD and patients' response to enzyme replacement therapy.

References

1. Sodi A, Ioannidis A, Pitz S (2006) Ophthalmological manifestations of Fabry disease. In: Metha A, Beck M, Sunder-Plassman G (eds) Fabry disease. Perspective from 5 years of FOS. Oxford Pharmagenesis, Oxford, pp 249–261
2. Samiy N (2008) Ocular features of Fabry disease: diagnosis of a treatable life-threatening disorder. Surv Ophthalmol 53(4):416–423
3. Dufier JL, Gubler MC, Dhermy P, Lenoir G, Paupe J, Haye C (1980) La maladie de Fabry et ses manifestations ophthalmologiques. J Fr Ophthalmol 3:625–630
4. Spaeth GL, Frost P (1965) Fabry's disease. Its ocular manifestations. Arch Ophthalmol 74:760–769
5. Sher NA, Letson RD, Desnick RJ (1979) The ocular manifestations in Fabry's disease. Arch Ophtahlmol 97:671–676
6. Dua HS, Singh A, Gomes JA, Laibson PR, Donoso LA, Tyagi S (1996) Vortex or whorl formation of cultured human corneal epithelial cells induced by magnetic fields. Eye 10: 447–450
7. Mantyjarvi M, Tuppurainen K, Ikaheimo K (1998) Ocular side effects of Amiodarone. Surv Ophthalmol 42:360–366
8. Dua HS, Gomes JA (2000) Clinical course of hurricane keratopathy. Br J Ophthalmol 84: 285–288
9. Weingeist TA, Blodi FC (1971) Fabry's disease: ocular findings in a female carrier. A light and electron microscopy study. Arch Ophtahlmol 85:169–176
10. François J, Hanssens M, Teuchy H (1978) Corneal ultrastructural changes in Fabry's disease. Ophthalmologica 176(6):313–330
11. Macrae WG, Ghosh M, McCulloch C (1985) Corneal changes in Fabry's disease: a clinico-pathological case report of a heterozygote. Ophthalmic Pediatr Genet 5(3):185–190
12. Hirano K, Murata K, Miyagawa A et al (2001) Histopathologic findings of cornea verticillata in woman heterozygous for Fabry's disease. Cornea 20(2):233–236
13. Riegel EM, Pokorny KS, Friedman AH et al (1982) Ocular pathology of Fabry's disease in a Hemizygous male following renal transplantation. Surv Ophthalmol 26(5):247–252

14. Galanos J, Nicholls K, Grigg L, Kiers L, Crawford A, Becker G (2002) Clinical features of Fabry's disease in Australian patients. Intern Med J 32:575–584
15. Orssaud C, Dufier JL, Germain DP (2003) Ocular manifestations in Fabry disease: a survey of 32 hemizygous male patients. Ophthalm Genet 24(3):129–139
16. Nguyen TT, Gin T, Nicholls K, Low M, Galanos J, Crawford A (2005) Ophthalmological manifestations of Fabry disease: a survey of patients at the Royal Melbourne Fabry disease treatment centre. Clin Exp Ophthalmol 33:164–168
17. Mehta A, Ricci R, Widmer U et al (2004) Fabry disease defined: baseline clinical manifestations of 366 patients in the Fabry outcome survey. Eur J Clin Invest 34(3):236–242
18. Sodi A, Ioannidis A, Metha A, Davey C, Beck M, Pitz S (2007) Ocular manifestations of Fabry disease: data from the Fabry outcome survey. Br J Ophthalmol 91:210–214
19. Tsutsumi A, Uchida Y, Kanai T et al (1984) Corneal findings in a Foetus with Fabry's disease. Acta Ophthalmologica 62:923–931
20. Fumex-Boizard L, Cochat P, Fouilhoux A, Guffon N, Debips P (2005) Relation entre les manifestations ophtalmologiques et les atteintes générales chez dix patients atteints de la maladie de Fabry. J Fr Ophtalmol 28:45–50
21. Whybra C, Kampmann C, Krummenauer F, Ries M, Mengel E, Miebach E, Baehner F, Kim K, Bajbouj M, Schwarting A, Gal A, Beck M (2004) The Mainz severity score index: a new instrument for quantifying the Anderson-Fabry disease phenotype, and the response of patients to enzyme replacement therapy. Clin Genet 65(4):299–307
22. Andersen MVN, Dahl H, Fledelius H, Nielsen NV (1992) Central retinal artery occlusion in a patient with Fabry's disease documented by scanning laser ophthalmoscopy. Acta Ophthalmologica 72:635–638
23. Dantas MA, Fonseca RA, Kaga T, Yannuzzi RA, Spaide RF (2001) Retinal and choroidal vascular changes in heterozygous Fabry disease. Retina 21(1):87–89
24. Abe H, Sakai T, Sawaguchi S et al (1992) Ischemic optic Neuropathy in a female carrier with Fabry's disease. Ophthalmologica 205:83–88
25. Jourdel D, Deefort-Dhelemmes S, Labalette P, Ryckewaert M, Hache JC (1998) Retinal pigment anomalies associated with Fabry's disease. J Fr Ophtalmol 21:755–760
26. Shen YD, Yang CM, Huang JS (2007) Fabry disease manifesting as chronic uveitis-treated with enzyme replacemnt therapy. Eye 21:431–432
27. Sodi A, Bini A, Mignani R, Minuti B, Menchini U (2009) Subfoveal choroidal neovascularization in a patient with Fabry's disease. Int Ophthalmol 29:435–437
28. Edwards JD, Bower KS, Brooks DB, Walter A (2009) Fabry disease and chemosis. Cornea 28(2):224–227
29. Hauser A, Lorenz M, Voigtlander T, Fodinger M, Sunder-Plassmann G (2004) Results of an ophthalmological screening programme for identification of cases with Anderson-Fabry disease. Ophthalmologica 218:207–209
30. Eng CM, Fletcher J, Wilcox WR et al (2007) Fabry disease: baseline medical characteristics of a cohort of 1765 males and females in the Fabry registry. J Inherit Metab Dis 30:184–192
31. Mastropasqua L, Nubile M, Lanzini M, Carpineto P, Toto L, Ciancaglini M (2006) Corneal and conjunctival manifestations in Fabry disease: in vivo confocal microscopy study. Am J Ophthalmol 141:709–718
32. Falke K, Buttner A, Schittkowski M, Stachs O, Kraak R, Zhivov A, Rolfs A, Guthoff R (2009) The microstructure of cornea verticillata in Fabry disease and amiodarone-induced keratopathy: a confocal laser-scanning microscopy study. Graefes Arch Clin Exp Ophthalmol 247:523–534
33. Orssaud C, Dufier JL, Germain DP (2003) Ocular manifesattions in Fabry disease: a survey of 32 hemizygous male patients. Opthalm Genet 24(3):29–139
34. Pitz S, Grube-Einwald K, Renieri A, Reinke J (2009) Subclinical optic neuropathy in Fabry disease. Ophthalm Genet 30:165–171

Chapter 18
Pulmonary, Ear and Less Commonly Appreciated Manifestations

Julian A.J. Raiman and Joe T.R. Clarke

Abstract The widespread organ involvement associated with the deficiency of alpha galactosidase in Fabry disease (FD) [OMIM 301500] is well recognized in the renal, cardiac, neurological and cutaneous manifestations of the disorder. However, beyond these major sites of disease burden the accumulation of glycosphingolipids has been found in other areas. Apart from sporadic case reports, descriptions of primary pulmonary, visual, auditory and other less prominent systems involvement have not been prominent in the Fabry literature until recent times. The emergence of novel therapies, such as enzyme replacement, has led to the need for greater information about the natural history and extent of this disease. The impact of this combined morbidity, often beginning in childhood, and in particular the effect on quality of life is beginning to be recognized. In a time of improving techniques for clinical surveillance, monitoring of such systems will allow for a better understanding of timing of treatment as well as offering diagnostic leads when the more common features may yet have occurred. The purpose of this chapter is to provide a review of FD and these organ systems, a summary of the clinical, epidemio-logical data and results of therapy which are currently available to those who look after Fabry patients.

Keywords Fabry · Hearing · Lung · Pulmonary

18.1 Fabry Disease and the Lung

18.1.1 Background

While not as prominent as the other systemic manifestations associated with the disease, pulmonary manifestations, including dyspnea, asthma, emphysema and hemoptysis, have all been reported periodically in the Fabry literature in case reports and increasingly recognized in more recent series.

J.A.J. Raiman (✉)
Division of Clinical and Metabolic Genetics, Hospital for Sick Children, Toronto, ON, Canada
e-mail: julian.raiman@sickkids.ca

D. Elstein et al. (eds.), *Fabry Disease*, DOI 10.1007/978-90-481-9033-1_18,
© Springer Science+Business Media B.V. 2010

Macdermot's study of 98 male patients from the United Kingdom described three patients from the cohort treated with bronchodilators and one having extensive emphysema with recurrent pneumothorax [1]. Eng at al noted 3% of male (total 713) and 2% of female (total 430) patients included respiratory manifestations in their initial symptoms of the disease [2] while Mehta and colleagues reported dyspnea amongst the cluster of cardiac symptoms, in 69% (total 201) of male and 65% (total 165) of female patients [3].

Indeed in the first clinical description by Johannes Fabry [4], the patient was described as suffering from asthma and frequent infections. Pulmonary disease was stated as a possible cause of death [5]. Subsequent review of that original case disclosed that the patient had 'frequent colds and influenza,' 'productive sputum' on occasion, and 'asthmatic troubles' with no cause of death mentioned [6]. Likewise case reports since then, reporting lung involvement, were unable to clearly separate the impact of the primary disease process compared to secondary factors including smoking and cardiac disease [6, 7].

18.1.2 Aetiology

With the application of more systematic pulmonary evaluation, other groups have reported more discernable differences. In a series of 25 patients, consisting of 18 non-smokers, three ex and four current smokers, Brown found symptoms were similar in the smokers and non-smokers. Thirty-six percent complained of dyspnea, and 24% had cough and/or wheezing. Nine (36%) had airway obstruction (FEV1:FVC, ratio of forced expiratory volume in 1 s to forced vital capacity, < 0.7) on spirometry; this finding correlated with age ≥ 26 year ($p < 0.05$) and dyspnea or wheezing ($p < 0.005$), but only weakly with smoking (p = 0.062) [8].

Other results from this study showed a significant increase in FEV1 following bronchodilator administration in 5/8 (63%) of the 'airway obstruction group'. However none of the patients tested showed a positive response (decline of FEV1 > 20%) to methacholine challenge (an indicator of bronchial hyper-reactivity, such as asthma, cystic fibrosis or chronic bronchitis) [9]. Although two patients had a history of spontaneous pneumothorax, a finding reported elsewhere [1, 7, 10], there was no radiological evidence of bullous change. This was contrary to those previous reports, in which smoking may have been a major factor. It was concluded the finding of airway obstruction and normal diffusing capacity suggested that airway obstruction was the cause of the pneumothorax in FD [8].

In the study by Magage and colleagues [11] static spirometry was performed on 50 Fabry patients (27 females, 23 males, mean age 40+ 14 years) and 50 matched controls. In hemizygous men a significant decrease in all predicted spirometric variables with increasing age was noted, when compared to controls. In the women there was a significant decrease in %FVC with increasing age in Fabry patients compared with the control group.

The same group also had the opportunity to undertake longitudinal follow up in all the men and 16 of the women for a median of 24 months. There was a greater deterioration in the older subgroup in %FVC and %FEV1, while the decrease in 25–75% forced expiratory flow (%FEF25–75), was similar in both the older and younger subgroups, consistent with the idea of progressive bronchial disease affecting the small airways first.

18.1.3 Pathophysiology

Inconsistent findings from studies of airway reactivity and anatomical change within the lungs suggest neither is the primary mechanism of the airway obstruction. Glycosphingolipid accumulation has been noted in airway epithelial cells collected at alveolar lavage, brush biopsy and from induced sputum [10, 12]. Electron micrographs demonstrating the electron dense, concentric parallel arrangements of lamellar bodies are reminiscent of histological findings in other organs of Fabry patients (Fig. 18.1). Similar findings have been recorded at autopsy in endothelial cells from the pulmonary vasculature [13] and suggest that local globotriacylceramide accumulation maybe the responsible mechanism.

18.1.4 Treatment

In light of these findings, the avoidance of smoking and other risk factors is deemed to be imperative. Rosenberg postulated that tobacco induced lung disease appeared more aggressive in the Fabry population when compared to non Fabry smokers [10]. A trial of $\beta2$ agonist/anti cholinergic bronchodilators should also be offered to assess response. In a study of the impact of enzyme replacement therapy (ERT) reported by Bierer [14], 15 patients underwent baseline cardiopulmonary assessment. Six were randomized (2:1) to receive either ERT (agalsidase beta; Fabrazyme, Genzyme, Cambridge, MA, USA) or placebo. Improvements were observed in the VO_{2max} (maximum oxygen uptake measured at peak exercise), VO_2/HR (mean oxygen pulse) and stroke volume compared to placebo, though not reaching statistical significance. Kim et al. reported a 38-year-old female with FD presenting with dyspnea and requiring constant supplemental oxygen [15]. After 21 months of treatment with agalsidase beta, she showed marked improvement in her pulmonary symptoms, pulmonary function tests and chest CT examination, and she eventually no longer needed supplemental oxygen and returned to an active lifestyle. Of the 44 patients (27 men, 17 women) reported by Babery et al., 15 patients underwent spirometry and imaging after 15+9 months of ERT (biweekly agalsidase alpha; Replagal, Shire HGT, Cambridge, MA, USA) which had no demonstrable impact on pulmonary function [16].

18.2 Fabry Disease and the Ear

Both sudden-onset and slowly progressive hearing loss has been frequently reported in FD. It may be sensorineural or conductive. Other manifestations include tinnitus and vertigo, and all have presented from childhood throughout life as the disease progresses.

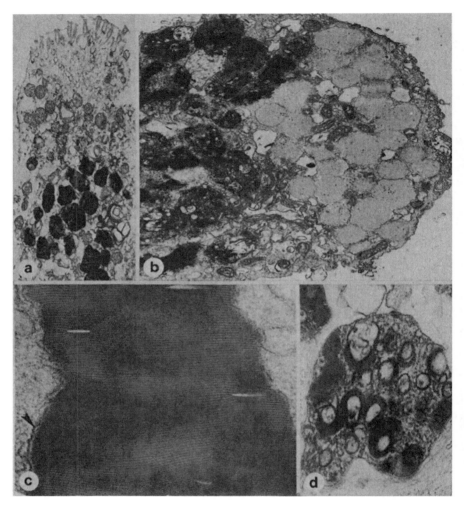

Fig. 18.1 Electron micrographs of cells brushed from the airway epithelium of Fabry patient (Rosenberg et al. [10])

18.2.1 Epidemiology

From the cohort of 98 UK male patients, MacDermot noted 41% reported hearing loss at a mean age of onset of 29 years. Audiograms showed mild to severe high frequency bilateral or unilateral sensorineural hearing loss in the 2–3 kHz range. Three patients without a family history of deafness had confirmed severe sensorineural and conductive hearing loss diagnosed before the age of 10 years [1]. From the corresponding cohort of 60 female patients, hearing loss was self reported in 23% [17].

In the baseline survey of 366 patients by Mehta and colleagues, auditory symptoms, such as tinnitus and hearing loss, were reported in 57%[115/201] of male and 47%[76/165] of female patients [3].

18.2.2 Audiological Spectrum

Germain et al. reported on 22 hemizygous males [18]. A total of 12 patients (54.5%) with classic FD were found to have abnormal audiograms. Five patients had progressive hearing loss and seven (32%) experienced sudden deafness. Interestingly, a high frequency hearing loss was found in seven out of the ten remaining patients without clinical impairment. Tinnitus was also found in six patients (27%). They concluded the origin and the mechanisms of deafness probably involve the inner ear, as no patient had conductive hearing loss, all tympanograms were consistent with normal middle ear mobility and pressure, and brainstem audiometry suggested cochlear rather than retrocochlear pathology.

Conti [19] reported further baseline data on the auditory and vestibular findings in 14 patients (ten males, four females) aged 14–57 years. Fifty percent complained of hearing symptoms (hearing loss, tinnitus, ear fullness). Subjective hearing loss was present in six, and it was the first reported symptom of FD in three. In 6/7 cases the onset and/or progression of hearing symptoms were sudden. Vertigo or dizziness was reported by four patients and associated with hearing symptoms in two cases. Audiological evaluation showed sensorineural hearing loss in eight patients (five males, three females). In the majority, the hearing loss was unilateral (six cases) and bilateral in the remaining two cases. The lesion was always cochlear. Vestibular examination showed abnormalities in four patients, which were not related to either the audiological results or the history of vertigo/dizziness.

Hajioff et al. reported on 25 patients, 15 of whom received ERT or placebo in a double blind/randomized trial and ten who joined on extension open label therapy [20]. At baseline, nine patients (36%) had bilateral and ten (40%) had unilateral high-frequency sensorineural hearing loss (SNHL). Three (12%) had unilateral middle ear effusions with conductive losses persisting beyond 6 months. Only five patients (20%) had normal hearing.

In a follow up report of the multi centre cohort originally reported by Mehta [3], Hegemann et al. reported on 566 Fabry patients, of who 316 reported ear-related symptoms [21]. Overall data from this study suggested a lesser degree of clinical impairment and rate of sudden hearing loss when compared to the earlier reports.

Patients were asked whether they had experienced subjective hearing loss, sudden hearing loss, vertigo or tinnitus. Pure-tone audiograms were performed in 86 and compared to an age and sex-matched population (International Organization for Standardization, ISO 7029). 74% of patients had a threshold elevated above the 95th centile in at least one tested frequency. However, only 14(16%) were clinically affected by hearing impairment according to the age-independent World Health Organization (WHO) classification. Hearing loss was sensorineural in 63 patients (73%) of whom seven patients (8%) also had a conductive component. Hearing seemed to be affected at all frequencies, especially in the low-frequency range. One patient had a purely conductive hearing loss. Episodes of sudden hearing loss seemed to occur more frequently than in the general population. Thirty two cases (5·6%) were found in the 566 patients with a complete symptom checklist. Men were affected earlier and more severely than women [21].

18.2.3 Hearing Loss in Children

In a further study from this dataset, the baseline demographic and clinical characteristics of the 82 patients (40 boys, 42 girls) below the age of 18, hearing loss and tinnitus was reported in 55% of the girls and 39% of the boys [22]. In a recent follow up, questionnaires were completed for 543 children with FD [23]. Thirty three percent of the children ($n = 179$) reported subjective hearing impairment. However, when assessed by audiometry, only 19 of 101 (19%) patients tested (53 girls, 48 boys) had a persistent hearing loss. Fourteen had high-frequency hearing loss, four had hearing loss at all frequencies, and one had a pattern typical of noise-induced loss. Forty-four of the children undergoing audiometry complained of tinnitus. Two reported sudden hearing loss, though this was not confirmed by testing. Vertigo was reported by 16 girls (30%) and ten boys (21%). This was not differentiated further from nonspecific dizziness. The authors suggested that the inconsistencies between the reported subjective hearing impairment and the results of formal audiometry may have been due to middle-ear effusions in many cases. This was consistent with previous reports on inner-ear function in children showing that most pediatric patients with FD hear normally [24]. It also confirmed tinnitus as a well-recognized symptom in FD which may present in childhood [23].

18.2.4 Pathogenesis and Disease Association

There are few reports in the literature of the histopathological findings of the auditory system in FD. The most extensive by Schachern et al. are the clinical, audiometric and autopsy findings of two male patients affected by sensorineural hearing loss [25]. Findings included bilateral hyperplastic mucosa of the middle ear and seropurulent effusions, evidence of glycosphingolipid accumulation in vascular endothelial cells of the middle and inner ear, as well as in various ganglion cells.

Strial/spiral ligament atrophy and outer hair cell loss in the cochlea were also common findings. The combination of these with evidence of new bone formation and fibrous tissue in the superior semicircular canal may have been due to vascular obstruction. The authors concluded the findings to be due to both a local direct effect and the indirect effect of glycosphingolipid accumulation in the temporal cortex, kidney, endothelial and smooth muscle cells.

With regard to an association of auditory disease and other system involvement, Germain and colleagues found the incidence of hearing loss appeared significantly increased in patients with kidney failure or cerebrovascular lesions, whereas there was no correlation with left ventricular hypertrophy [18]. Reis et al. [26], also reported that male patients with hearing loss had a higher load of microvascular cerebral white matter lesions, more pronounced deficit of cold perception and lower kidney function compared to those without. They also noted the prevalence of hearing loss was lower in the group of patients with residual enzyme activity compared with those without detectable activity (33% vs. 63%).

18.2.5 Response to Treatment

A number of recent reports has now assessed changes in hearing after starting ERT. In the study by Hajioff et al. [20], the high frequency sensorineural hearing loss noted at baseline deteriorated over the first 6 months in both placebo and active treatment groups by a median 6.3 dB ($p < 0.0001$). This subsequently improved on ERT above baseline by 1.5 dB at 18 months ($p = 0.07$), by 5.0 dB at 30 months ($p = 0.006$) and by 4.0 dB at 42 months ($p = 0.01$). In a follow up report by the same author [27], after a median of 12 months of treatment in 26 patients, results did not change significantly in ears with normal hearing or those with severe hearing loss at baseline. In ears with a mild or moderate hearing loss at baseline, hearing thresholds improved significantly by 4–7 dB at most frequencies. The authors concluded that agalsidase alpha stabilizes, and possibly improves, hearing in Fabry patients who have not already progressed to severe hearing loss. Further follow-up of these patients will determine the longer-term effects of ERT.

18.3 Less Commonly Appreciated Manifestations

18.3.1 Less Common Manifestations: Cognition

An association between FD and an increased risk of cerebrovascular events is well documented. Dementia can appear in middle or later life, secondary to diffuse leukomalacia, multiple strokes or possibly to lipid storage in hippocampal and frontal lobe neurons [28–30]. Likewise, the secondary burden of the multisystem involvement puts both male and female patients at risk of psychiatric disease [31].

There are few formal reports of the cognitive status of patients with the condition. In the report by MacDermot et al. [1], dementia was present in 18% and was associated in all cases with recurrent CVAs or TIAs. Two males had mild learning difficulty of unknown cause. Overall, the educational status of the male cohort compared favourably to the UK male population. However, 17% stated that they had never had a job because of the diagnosis of Fabry. Only 56.8% were currently employed. It would appear that other system involvement was the main factor here rather than overt neurocognitive deficits. A total of 70.2% of patients stated that pain interfered with their job and necessitated taking time off work. Other manifestations including, diarrhea and fatigue, were reported as interfering with the ability to work. Depression is a common feature, but is often under recognised and likely under treated [32]. A recent report showed specific psychological scores in Fabry that were worse than those of patients with Gaucher disease, chronic heart disease, and were comparable to those of other chronic pain populations [33].

18.3.2 Less Common Manifestations: Dysmorphic Features

Dysmorphic features of the face, trunk and extremities have been noted. They were reported present on careful inspection in about half of the patients evaluated by MacDermot [1] In a single centre study of 38 patients, the following core features were noted in descending frequency: periorbital fullness, prominent lobules of the ears, bushy eyebrows, recessed forehead, pronounced nasal angle, generous nose/bulbous nasal tip, prominent supraorbital ridges, shallow midface, full lips, prominent nasal bridge, broad alar base, coarse features, posteriorly rotated ears, and prognathism. Abnormalities in the hands included broad fingertips, short fingers, prominent superficial vessels of hands, 5 digit brachydactyly, and 5 digit clinodactyly [34]. The knowledge and recognition of these features may facilitate the identification and diagnosis of patients and their affected family members leading to earlier diagnosis and treatment.

18.3.3 Less Common Manifestations: Gastrointestinal Disease

Gastrointestinal [GI] symptoms are a very common, but underappreciated manifestation of FD. They were rated the second and third most frequently reported presenting feature in the cohort of 809 females and 956 males respectively, reported by Eng et al. [35]. Similar figures ranging from 40 to 69% were reported by the other large series [1, 3, 17].

Symptoms consist of recurrent bouts of colicky, burning pain, located in the mid and lower abdomen. Typically the episodes are post-prandial and are accompanied by bloating followed by multiple bowel movements and diarrhea. Other gastrointestinal symptoms include nausea, vomiting, and early satiety [36]. Such effects result in a reluctance to eat, individuals becoming housebound, compounding the social isolation and overall poor quality of life patients' experience. FD patients have undergone numerous gastrointestinal investigations, including contrast imaging and upper/lower GI endoscopy which are invariably normal. Diverticular disease has also occurred and led to bowel perforation on occasion [1, 37].

Children report gut involvement as an early feature of the disease, often in the first decade [22]. The lack of positive findings on investigation, adding to diagnostic confusion in younger FD patients.

When present in adults, morphological changes have included smoothing or lack of colonic haustrae in the descending and sigmoid colon segments and indeed throughout the colon. Additional radiographic studies have demonstrated thickened, edematous colonic folds, mild dilatation of the small bowel, and granular-appearing ileum [36].

Examination of intestinal biopsies typically demonstrate a normal villous pattern but may show 'foamy' cell deposits, more so in males, with enlargement and vacuolation of the ganglion cells in Meissner's plexus [38]. As reported in other tissues, electron microscopic examination has shown the characteristic electron dense, intralysosomal 'zebra-like' bodies within ganglion cells of the submucosal plexus, within smooth muscle cells of the muscularis mucosae, endothelial cells lining arterioles, venules, and capillaries, as well as in the cytoplasm of small unmyelinated neurons, and perineurial cells [39].

From a pathophysiological basis, delayed gastric emptying has been reported and assumed to be a cause of the satiety [40]. This has been correlated to abnormal autonomic function on testing [41]. Microvascular ischemia, due to glycosphingolipid accumulation of the splanchnic and mesenteric vessels has been implicated in the basis of the abdominal pain [39].

Dietary restrictions, the use of antispasmodics, dysmotility and prokinetic agents such as metaclopramide and tetracycline have all been tried with incomplete success [40]. Following the advent of ERT, however results suggest a positive impact on GI manifestations following treatment.

Dehout and colleagues reported a survey of 11 patients assessing abdominal pain and diarrhea prior to, 6 and 12 months following commencement of ERT [42]. Pain was reported in 10/11 patients and diarrhea in 6/11 patients at baseline. Following 6 months of treatment with agalsidase alpha, there was a significant decrease in both the severity and frequency score of abdominal pain ($p < 0.02$) in seven patients. The diarrhea had also improved after ERT in 5/6 patients who reported it at baseline. Both these findings were maintained in those who completed 12 months ERT. Similar findings were reported by Banikazemi, in four male patients using agalsidase beta, up to 3 years in follow up. All patients had stopped their other GI medications and experienced a weight gain of 3–9 kg [36].

The largest series reporting GI response to ERT, from Hoffmann et al., came from 342 patients, in whom information on GI symptoms was available prior to starting therapy [43]. Overall incidence was 52%, though this was higher in females than males and children more than adults. Results after ERT were available for 62 patients at 12 months and for 58 at 24 months respectively.

Overall, pain decreased from 49 to 39% in adults and from 64 to 36% ($p < 0.05$) in children at 12 months. At 24 months the overall change for pain from baseline was 43–29% ($p < 0.05$). Diarrhea was reported by 27% at baseline, which reduced by 8% at 12 months improvement was more pronounced among male than female patients (10% vs. 5%). The prevalence in children was significantly reduced from 36 to 7% after 12 months of ERT ($p < 0.05$). The results at 24 months were smaller for diarrhea than pain. Data was available for 57 patients completing 24 months of ERT. At baseline, the prevalence was 28%, and after 24 months of ERT this was reduced to 26%. In the subgroup of male patients, 41% of patients reported diarrhea at baseline and 34% after 24 months. In contrast to this, the prevalence of diarrhea in female patients (12% vs. 16%) and adults (24% vs. 26%) was higher after 2 years of ERT compared with baseline. However, in children, the prevalence was markedly reduced from 45 to 27%. In conclusion, the authors recommended that prospective studies be performed to assess whether these functional improvements can be correlated with changes in the morphology and function of enteric nerves and the microvasculature.

18.3.4 Less Common Manifestations: Psychosexual Disturbance

Psychosexual disturbance, sexual dysfunction and infertility have also all been noted and appear to be seriously under-reported.

In the UK male cohort ($n = 46$) a total of 73.8% reported a rash on their genitals, 64.4% were embarrassed by it. A small group (16%) reported genital pain. This has affected enjoyment of sex for over half the sample (55%) and reportedly affected both libido (48.7%) and self esteem (68.3%). Almost two-thirds (61.5%) of patients noted that these manifestations of FD resulted in a fear of initiating sexual relationships, particularly in the teenage years. Only 42% of the group was married and two of these were separated or divorced [1]. One of us (JTRC) has encountered serious priapism in two patients with FD (unpublished).

18.3.5 Less Common Manifestations: Spermatic Dysfunction

Further to this are reports of spermatic dysfunction. A case report of two males with Fabry identified azoospermia as a risk factor of the condition. Testicular biopsies from both cases showed hypospermatogenesis with a scarcity of spermatids and spermatozoa [44].

Histologic analysis revealed thickened tubule basement membranes; and vitreous tables of the interstitial blood vessels were thickened with diminishing of the vascular lumen. In both testes, the number of Leydig cells was in the normal range, some of them were increased in size. Their cytoplasm contained microvacuoles, giving the appearance of stored lipid. The Leydig cells had a distorted nucleus. The cytoplasm was full of numerous inclusions that had a lamellar appearance. Other inclusions had the appearance of an onion bulb, with concentric lamellae of irregular thickness such as myelin-like bodies, similar to those in the Fabry kidney. In noting that most men with FD are fertile, and the possible risk of azoospermia is probably higher after 30–40 years of age, the authors' reccommended a routine sperm analysis in the follow-up of young patients with FD.

Both the reported cases had also been on ERT without an improvement in sperm production leading to the recommendation that sperm cryopreservation should also be advised in these patients, to circumvent developing azoospermia in the future.

Faggiano et al., also found asthenozoospermia, oligozoospermia, or both in 5/5 men tested, in their investigation of endocrine dysfunction of 18 Fabry patients (nine females and nine males). Ten of the 18 patients were receiving ERT during the study [45].

18.3.6 Less Common Manifestations: Endocrine Dysfunction

As part of the above study, thyroid, gonadal, adrenal, and GH/IGF-I axes were all evaluated. The Fabry patients had higher baseline TSH levels than controls ($p < 0.01$) and three subjects were diagnosed with an early stage of sub clinical primary hypothyroidism associated with negative antithyroid antibodies.

A history of menses abnormalities, miscarriage, or assisted delivery was found in eight of the nine women (89%). Abnormalities were consistent with oligomenorrhea in four and polymenorrhea in two women. There was a significant difference in adrenal function compared to controls. Fabry patients had higher circulating ACTH and lower cortisol levels than controls ($p < 0.05$). ACTH stimulation tests performed in patients on ERT revealed a suboptimal cortisol response in one patient, with normal gland morphology, GFR and negative autoantibodies. The GH/IGF-I axis was normal in all patients.

The authors suggested the wide spectrum of latent endocrine dysfunctions that may occur in patients and the susceptibility of endocrine glands to globotriaosylceramide accumulation because of their high vascularization and low cellular proliferation rate, provides the rationale to investigate the endocrine function in patients with Fabry.

18.3.7 Less Common Manifestations: Bone Mineral Density

Bone mineral density [BMD] has also been shown to be affected in FD. In a prospective study of 23 consecutive hemizygous male patients, Germain et al. found a statistically significant decrease in BMD [46].

Twenty patients (87%) were found to have either osteopenia [11] or osteoporosis [9] Beyond kidney failure or hypoparathyroidism, that was present in four, suggested secondary causes of osteoporosis/osteopenia in Fabry, included malabsorption, an association with depression, reduced physical activities and the secondary effect of carbamazepine, used for the relief of neuropathic pain, on calcium and bone metabolism. The authors concluded that bone density is assessed in all patients with FD and prophylactic therapy of osteoporosis be considered.

18.4 Conclusions

The systems described in this chapter, though not typically associated with mortality in FD, can be a major source of morbidity to the individual and often at an early stage of the disease. Enhanced awareness of the associated problems is required along with serial follow up when considering the diagnosis, the introduction of treatment and its response.

References

1. MacDermot KD, Holmes A, Miners AH (2001) Anderson-Fabry disease: clinical manifestations and impact of disease in a cohort of 98 hemizygous males. J Med Genet 38(11):750–760

2. Eng CM, Fletcher J, Wilcox WR, Waldek S, Scott CR, Sillence DO et al (2007) Fabry disease: baseline medical characteristics of a cohort of 1765 males and females in the Fabry Registry. J Inherit Metab Dis 30(2):184–192

3. Mehta A, Ricci R, Widmer U, Dehout F, Garcia de Lorenzo A, Kampmann C et al (2004) Fabry disease defined: baseline clinical manifestations of 366 patients in the Fabry Outcome Survey. Eur J Clin Invest 34(3):236–242

4. Fabry J (1898) Ein Beitrag zur Kenntniss der purpura hemorrhagica nodularis (purpura papula hemorrhagica Hebrae). Arch Derm u Syph 43:187–201

5. Ferrans VJ, Hibbs RG, Burda CD (1969) The heart in Fabry's disease. A histochemical and electron microscopic study. Am J Cardiol 24(1):95–110

6. Bartimmo EE Jr, Guisan M, Moser KM (1972) Pulmonary involvement in Fabry's disease: a reappraisal follow-up of a San Diego kindred and review of literature. Am J Med 53(6): 755–764

7. Kariman K, Singletary WV Jr, Sieker HO (1978) Pulmonary involvement in Fabry's disease. Am J Med 64(5):911–912

8. Brown LK, Miller A, Bhuptani A, Sloane MF, Zimmerman MI, Schilero G et al (1997) Pulmonary involvement in Fabry disease. Am J Respir Crit Care Med 155(3):1004–1010

9. Crapo RO, Casaburi R, Coates AL, Enright PL, Hankinson JL, Irvin CG et al (2000) Guidelines for methacholine and exercise challenge testing-1999. This official statement of the American Thoracic Society was adopted by the ATS Board of Directors, July 1999. Am J Respir Crit Care Med 161(1):309–329

10. Rosenberg DM, Ferrans VJ, Fulmer JD, Line BR, Barranger JA, Brady RO et al (1980) Chronic airflow obstruction in Fabry's disease. Am J Med 68(6):898–905

11. Magage S, Lubanda JC, Susa Z, Bultas J, Karetova D, Dobrovolny R et al (2007) Natural history of the respiratory involvement in Anderson-Fabry disease. J Inherit Metab Dis 30(5):790–799

12. Kelly MM, Leigh R, McKenzie R, Kamada D, Ramsdale EH, Hargreave FE (2000) Induced sputum examination: diagnosis of pulmonary involvement in Fabry's disease. Thorax 55(8):720–721

13. Smith P, Heath D, Rodgers B, Helliwell T (1991) Pulmonary vasculature in Fabry's disease. Histopathology 19(6):567–569

14. Bierer G, Balfe D, Wilcox WR, Mosenifar Z (2006) Improvement in serial cardiopulmonary exercise testing following enzyme replacement therapy in Fabry disease. J Inherit Metab Dis 29(4):572–579

15. Kim W, Pyeritz RE, Bernhardt BA, Casey M, Litt HI (2007) Pulmonary manifestations of Fabry disease and positive response to enzyme replacement therapy. Am J Med Genet A 143(4):377–381

16. Barbey FWU, Brack T, Vogt B, Aubert J (2005) Spirometric abnormalities in patients with Fabry disease and effect of enzyme replacement therapy. Acta Paediatr Suppl:447

17. MacDermot KD, Holmes A, Miners AH (2001) Anderson-Fabry disease: clinical manifestations and impact of disease in a cohort of 60 obligate carrier females. J Med Genet 38(11):769–775

18. Germain DP, Avan P, Chassaing A, Bonfils P (2002) Patients affected with Fabry disease have an increased incidence of progressive hearing loss and sudden deafness: an investigation of twenty-two hemizygous male patients. BMC Med Genet 11(3):10

19. Conti G, Sergi B (2003) Auditory and vestibular findings in Fabry disease: a study of hemizygous males and heterozygous females. Acta Paediatr Suppl 92(443):33–37, discussion 27

20. Hajioff D, Goodwin S, Quiney R, Zuckerman J, MacDermot KD, Mehta A (2003) Hearing improvement in patients with Fabry disease treated with agalsidase alfa. Acta Paediatr Suppl 92(443):28–30, discussion 27

21. Hegemann S, Hajioff D, Conti G, Beck M, Sunder-Plassmann G, Widmer U et al (2006) Hearing loss in Fabry disease: data from the Fabry Outcome Survey. Eur J Clin Invest 36(9):654–662

22. Ramaswami U, Whybra C, Parini R, Pintos-Morell G, Mehta A, Sunder-Plassmann G et al (2006) Clinical manifestations of Fabry disease in children: data from the Fabry Outcome Survey. Acta Paediatrica (Oslo, Norway: 1992) 95(1):86–92

23. Keilmann A, Hajioff D, Ramaswami U (2009) Ear symptoms in children with Fabry disease: data from the Fabry Outcome Survey. J Inherit Metab Dis:27

24. Keilmann A (2003) Inner ear function in children with Fabry disease. Acta Paediatr Suppl 92(443):31–32, discussion 27

25. Schachern PA, Shea DA, Paparella MM, Yoon TH (1989) Otologic histopathology of Fabry's disease. Ann Otol Rhinol Laryngol 98(5 Pt 1):359–363

26. Ries M, Kim HJ, Zalewski CK, Mastroianni MA, Moore DF, Brady RO et al (2007) Neuropathic and cerebrovascular correlates of hearing loss in Fabry disease. Brain 130(Pt 1):143–150

27. Hajioff D, Hegemann S, Conti G, Beck M, Sunder-Plassmann G, Widmer U et al (2006) Agalsidase alpha and hearing in Fabry disease: data from the Fabry Outcome Survey. Eur J Clin Invest 36(9):663–667

28. Kolodny EH, Pastores GM (2002) Anderson-Fabry disease: extrarenal, neurologic manifestations. J Am Soc Nephrol 13(Suppl 2):S150–S153

29. Okeda R, Nisihara M (2008) An autopsy case of Fabry disease with neuropathological investigation of the pathogenesis of associated dementia. Neuropathology 28(5):532–540

30. Mendez MF, Stanley TM, Medel NM, Li Z, Tedesco DT (1997) The vascular dementia of Fabry's disease. Dement Geriatr Cogn Disord 8(4):252–257

31. Grewal RP (1993) Psychiatric disorders in patients with Fabry's disease. Int J Psychiatry Med 23(3):307–312

32. Cole AL, Lee PJ, Hughes DA, Deegan PB, Waldek S, Lachmann RH (2007) Depression in adults with Fabry disease: a common and under-diagnosed problem. J Inherit Metab Dis 30(6):943–951

33. Crosbie TW, Packman W, Packman S (2009) Psychological aspects of patients with Fabry disease. J Inherit Metab Dis:31

34. Ries M, Moore DF, Robinson CJ, Tifft CJ, Rosenbaum KN, Brady RO et al (2006) Quantitative dysmorphology assessment in Fabry disease. Genet Med 8(2):96–101

35. Eng CM, Fletcher J, Wilcox WR, Waldek S, Scott CR, Sillence DO et al (2007) Fabry disease: baseline medical characteristics of a cohort of 1765 males and females in the Fabry Registry. J Inherit Metab Dis 30(2):184–192

36. Banikazemi M, Ullman T, Desnick RJ (2005) Gastrointestinal manifestations of Fabry disease: clinical response to enzyme replacement therapy. Mol Genet Metab 85(4):255–259

37. Friedman LS, Kirkham SE, Thistlethwaite JR, Platika D, Kolodny EH, Schuffler MD (1984) Jejunal diverticulosis with perforation as a complication of Fabry's disease. Gastroenterology 86(3):558–563

38. Sheth KJ, Werlin SL, Freeman ME, Hodach AE (1981) Gastrointestinal structure and function in Fabry's disease. Am J Gastroenterol 76(3):246–251

39. O'Brien BD, Shnitka TK, McDougall R, Walker K, Costopoulos L, Lentle B et al (1982) Pathophysiologic and ultrastructural basis for intestinal symptoms in Fabry's disease. Gastroenterology 82(5 Pt 1):957–962

40. Argoff CE, Barton NW, Brady RO, Ziessman HA (1998) Gastrointestinal symptoms and delayed gastric emptying in Fabry's disease: response to metoclopramide. Nucl Med Commun 19(9):887–891

41. Cable WJ, Kolodny EH, Adams RD (1982) Fabry disease: impaired autonomic function. Neurology 32(5):498–502
42. Dehout F, Roland D, Treille de Granseigne S, Guillaume B, Van Maldergem L (2004) Relief of gastrointestinal symptoms under enzyme replacement therapy [corrected] in patients with Fabry disease. J Inherit Metab Dis 27(4):499–505
43. Hoffmann B, Schwarz M, Mehta A, Keshav S (2007) Gastrointestinal symptoms in 342 patients with Fabry disease: prevalence and response to enzyme replacement therapy. Clin Gastroenterol Hepatol 5(12):1447–1453
44. Papaxanthos-Roche A, Deminiere C, Bauduer F, Hocke C, Mayer G, Lacombe D (2007) Azoospermia as a new feature of Fabry disease. Fertil Steril 88(1):212.e15–212.e18
45. Faggiano A, Pisani A, Milone F, Gaccione M, Filippella M, Santoro A et al (2006) Endocrine dysfunction in patients with Fabry disease. J Clin Endocrinol Metab 91(11):4319–4325
46. Germain DP, Benistan K, Boutouyrie P, Mutschler C (2005) Osteopenia and osteoporosis: previously unrecognized manifestations of Fabry disease. Clin Genet 68(1):93–95

Chapter 19
Neuropsychiatric Manifestations of AFD

Perri Segal and Annick Raas-Rothschild

Abstract There is growing evidence that both male and female AFD patients are at risk for developing neuropsychiatric symptoms. An expanding number of studies have demonstrated that these patients suffer from psychiatric disorders, especially from depression. Results of studies of the patients' cognitive function are variable, ranging from severe impairment to normal functioning. Living with a chronic and painful disease, might be related to the difficult psychosocial adjustment of AFD patients. More attention should be given to the psychiatric and cognitive needs of the patients. We recommend that neuropsychiatric evaluation, and treatment should be included in the multidisciplinary care of AFD patients.

Keywords Anderson-Fabry disease · Psychiatric · Cognitive · Psychosocial

19.1 Introduction

In recent years there is growing awareness that the clinical manifestations of Anderson-Fabry Disease (AFD) may have profound psychosocial effects. Many aspects of the patients' quality of life (QoL), namely physical function, body pain, general health, vitality, social functioning and mental health have been found to be reduced in AFD patients [1, 2]. Other indexes of psychosocial adjustment such as marriage rates and employment are also reduced [3].

Female patients are not asymptomatic carriers as once thought. Indeed, they present with symptoms of variable severity, at a later age of onset than their male counterparts [1, 4, 5].

Both male and female AFD patients are at risk for developing neuropsychiatric symptoms, including psychiatric [6–8], and neuropsychological symptoms [9–11].

P. Segal (✉)
Department of Human Genetics and Metabolic Diseases, Hadassah Hebrew University Medical Center, Ein Kerem, Jerusalem, Israel
e-mail: perri.segal@mail.huji.ac.il

D. Elstein et al. (eds.), *Fabry Disease*, DOI 10.1007/978-90-481-9033-1_19,
© Springer Science+Business Media B.V. 2010

19.2 Neuro-Psychiatric Manifestations

Psychiatric manifestations in AFD patients were first documented in 1962 [12]; the most common reported psychiatric finding is depression [3, 7, 13, 14]. Cole et al. reported that up to 46% and 28% of the cohort studied met the criteria for depression, and for severe depression respectively [7]. In addition, AFD patients suffer from additional psychiatric manifestations besides depression, such as suicide ideation, suicide attempts [3, 13, 15, 16], psychosis and paranoid ideation [17, 18], confusional states [6, 10].

Recently, Crosbie et al. [9] assessed the psychological functioning of a cohort of AFD patients, using the MMPI-2 test (Minnesota Multiphase Personality Inventory) and compared the results to a population of patients affected with Gaucher disease, chronic heart disease and chronic pain. The authors found that most of the scales were elevated, including the scales associated with personality disorders, such as Psychopathic Deviate (Pd) and Schizophrenia (SC).

Substantial cerebral ischemia is commonly reported in AFD patients [15, 19, 20]. Significant cognitive impairment following such incidents has been noted in a few single case studies [6, 9, 10]. Muller [11] refers to an unpublished study, in which he found no evidence for reduced intelligence scores in a cohort of 36 AFD patients. Low et al. [21] using the MMSE (Mini Mental State Examination) [22] found no significant differences between AFD patients and controls in 5 cognitive domains as well (attention, memory, visuo-construction, executive functioning and language).

19.3 Brain Imaging Studies

AFD patients commonly suffer from cerebral microangiopathy, with the most common finding in brain imaging studies being white matter lesions (WML), usually localized in the periventricular white matter [23–25]. Interestingly, studies including healthy elderly patients, elderly patients with pre-existing vascular disease, diabetes patients and post stroke patients have found a correlation between periventricular WML and a decline in information processing speed and executive functions [26, 22]. This suggest that AFD patients could be also affected. Interestingly, a possible connection between WML and depression has been found [27].

19.4 Summary

In summary, the neuropsychiatric deficits of AFD patients might reflect the consequences of living with a chronic and painful disease, which has significant effects on psychological well being [9]. There is evidence that the L-arginine-nitric oxide (NO) pathway is impaired in both AFD [28, 29] and depressive patients [30], raising the possibility that NO pathway abnormalities could be related to the neuro-psychiatric findings in Fabry patients.

As Muller points out, there is most probably an interaction between both the pathophysiological and psychosocial aspects of AFD, which remains to be explained in future studies [11].

We recommend that special attention should be given to the psychiatric and cognitive phenotype of AFD patients and that psychiatric and cognitive evaluation, follow up and appropriate treatment should be included in the multidisciplinary care of AFD patients.

References

1. Wilcox WR, Oliveira JP, Hopkin RJ et al (2008) Females with Fabry disease frequently have major organ involvement: lessons from the Fabry registry. Mol Genet Metab 93(2): 112–128
2. Hoffmann B, Garcia de Lorenzo A, Mehta A, Beck M, Widmer U, Ricci R (2005) Effects of enzyme replacement therapy on pain and health related quality of life in patients with Fabry disease: data from FOS (Fabry Outcome Survey). J Med Genet 42(3):247–252
3. MacDermot KD, Holmes A, Miners AH (2001) Anderson-Fabry disease: clinical manifestations and impact of disease in a cohort of 98 hemizygous males. J Med Genet 38(11):750–760
4. Mehta A, Clarke JT, Giugliani R et al (2009) Natural course of Fabry disease: changing pattern of causes of death in FOS – Fabry outcome survey. J Med Genet 46(8):548–552
5. Mehta A, Ricci R, Widmer U et al (2004) Fabry disease defined: baseline clinical manifestations of 366 patients in the Fabry outcome survey. Eur J Clin Invest 34(3):236–242
6. Grewal RP (1993) Psychiatric disorders in patients with Fabry's disease. Int J Psychiatry Med 23(3):307–312
7. Cole AL, Lee PJ, Hughes DA, Deegan PB, Waldek S, Lachmann RH (2007) Depression in adults with Fabry disease: a common and under-diagnosed problem. J Inherit Metab Dis 30(6):943–951
8. Crosbie TW, Packman W, Packman S (2009) Psychological aspects of patients with Fabry disease. J Inherit Metab Dis 32(6):745–753
9. Mendez MF, Stanley TM, Medel NM, Li Z, Tedesco DT (1997) The vascular dementia of Fabry's disease. Dement Geriatr Cogn Disord 8(4):252–257
10. Mohanraj R, Leach JP, Broome JC, Smith DF (2002) Neurological presentation of Fabry's disease in a 52 year old man. J Neurol Neurosurg Psychiatry 73(3):340–342
11. Muller MJ (2006) Neuropsychiatric and psychosocial aspects of Fabry disease. In: Mehta A, Beck M, Sunder-Plassmann G (eds) Fabry disease: perspectives from 5 years of FOS. Oxford PharmaGenesis Ltd, Oxford
12. Wise D, Wallace HJ, Jellinek EH (1962) Angiokeratoma corporis diffusum. A clinical study of eight affected families. Q J Med 31:177–206
13. Grewal RP (1993) Psychiatric disorders in patients with Fabry's disease. Int J Psychiatry Med 23(3):307–312
14. Sadek J, Shellhaas R, Camfield CS, Camfield PR, Burley J (2004) Psychiatric findings in four female carriers of Fabry disease. Psychiatr Genet 14(4):199–201
15. MacDermot KD, Holmes A, Miners AH (2001) Anderson-Fabry disease: clinical manifestations and impact of disease in a cohort of 60 obligate carrier females. J Med Genet 38(11):769–775
16. Sadek J, Shellhaas R, Camfield CS, Camfield PR, Burley J (2004) Psychiatric findings in four female carriers of Fabry disease. Psychiatr Genet 14(4):199–201

17. Liston EH, Levine MD, Philippart M (1973) Psychosis in Fabry disease and treatment with phenoxybenzamine. Arch Gen Psychiatry 29(3):402–403

18. Shen YC, Haw-Ming L, Lin CC, Chen CH (2007) Psychosis in a patient with Fabry's disease and treatment with aripiprazole. Prog Neuropsychopharmacol Biol Psychiatry 31(3):779–780

19. MacDermot KD, Holmes A, Miners AH (2001) Natural history of Fabry disease in affected males and obligate carrier females. J Inherit Metab Dis 24(Suppl 2):13–14, discussion 1–2

20. Moore DF, Kaneski CR, Askari H, Schiffmann R (2007) The cerebral vasculopathy of Fabry disease. J Neurol Sci 257(1–2):258–263

21. Low M, Nicholls K, Tubridy N et al (2007) Neurology of Fabry disease. Intern Med J 37(7):436–447

23. Albrecht J, Dellani PR, Muller MJ et al (2007) Voxel based analyses of diffusion tensor imaging in Fabry disease. J Neurol Neurosurg Psychiatry 78(9):964–969

24. Jardim L, Vedolin L, Schwartz IV et al (2004) CNS involvement in Fabry disease: clinical and imaging studies before and after 12 months of enzyme replacement therapy. J Inherit Metab Dis 27(2):229–240

25. Moore DF, Altarescu G, Barker WC, Patronas NJ, Herscovitch P, Schiffmann R (2003) White matter lesions in Fabry disease occur in 'prior' selectively hypometabolic and hyperperfused brain regions. Brain Res Bull 62(3):231–240

26. Jokinen H, Kalska H, Mantyla R et al (2005) White matter hyperintensities as a predictor of neuropsychological deficits post-stroke. J Neurol Neurosurg Psychiatry 76(9):1229–1233

22. Tiehuis AM, Vincken KL, Mali WP et al (2008) Automated and visual scoring methods of cerebral white matter hyperintensities: relation with age and cognitive function. Cerebrovasc Dis 25(1–2):59–66

27. Herrmann LL, Le Masurier M, Ebmeier KP (2008) White matter hyperintensities in late life depression: a systematic review. J Neurol Neurosurg Psychiatry 79(6):619–624

28. Moore DF, Scott LT, Gladwin MT et al (2001) Regional cerebral hyperperfusion and nitric oxide pathway dysregulation in Fabry disease: reversal by enzyme replacement therapy. Circulation 104(13):1506–1512

29. Shu L, Park JL, Byun J, Pennathur S, Kollmeyer J, Shayman JA (2009) Decreased nitric oxide bioavailability in a mouse model of Fabry disease. J Am Soc Nephrol 20(9):1975–1985

30. Pinto VL, Brunini TM, Ferraz MR, Okinga A, Mendes-Ribeiro AC (2008) Depression and cardiovascular disease: role of nitric oxide. Cardiovasc Hemat Agents Med Chem 6(2): 142–149

Chapter 20
Genetic Counseling and Psychosocial Issues for Individuals and Their Families with Fabry Disease

Robin L. Bennett

Abstract Fabry disease is an X-linked disorder with severe and chronic disease manifestations beginning in childhood. Genetic counseling is important as part of the multidisciplinary care of individuals and their families with Fabry disease. This chapter reviews the key aspects of genetic counseling for persons and their families with Fabry disease and many of the psychological issues. Genetic counseling may occur over multiple visits during various times (such as when establishing a diagnosis, when identifying relatives at risk for Fabry disease, and when making reproductive decisions).

Keywords Genetic counseling · Family history · Fabry disease · Psychosocial issues

20.1 Introduction

Fabry disease can affect many areas of a person's psychological, medical, financial and social life. The diagnosis of Fabry disease in a person or a relative may change the individual's perception of self and his or her world views. A plethora of emotions and questions can surround the diagnosis [1]: 'What is my prognosis? Will I develop all the manifestation of Fabry disease? Is there treatment? Will I need treatment for the rest of my life? When and how should I share this information with my family? When and how do I share this information with a person I am dating? Will my siblings develop Fabry disease? Why me? Will Fabry disease affect my ability to have children? Is it my fault that my children have this disease? Is there anything I can do to prevent this from happening to my children or my siblings? Will I or my family face discrimination in social situations or in seeking insurance coverage, or in employment?' The process of genetic counseling not only can identify individuals

R.L. Bennett (✉)
Division of Medical Genetics, Department of Medicine, UWMC Medical Genetics Clinic, University of Washington Medical Center, Seattle, WA, USA
e-mail: robinb@u.washington.edu

D. Elstein et al. (eds.), *Fabry Disease*, DOI 10.1007/978-90-481-9033-1_20,
© Springer Science+Business Media B.V. 2010

and their at-risk relatives with Fabry disease, but also provide such persons with education about Fabry disease and psychosocial support to help the individual and family with healthy adjustment to living with Fabry disease and facilitate making informed decisions.

20.1.1 Definition of Genetic Counseling

The field of genetic counseling developed from the need to educate, manage and counsel individuals and families diagnosed with, or at risk for genetic disorders. Genetic counseling encompasses more than reproductive counseling or advising as to the risks and benefits of genetic tests.

The definition of genetic counseling as adopted by the National Society of Genetic Counselor is as follows [2]: 'Genetic counseling is the process of helping people understand and adapt to the medical, psychological and familial implications of genetic contributions to disease. This process integrates:

- Interpretation of family and medical histories to assess the changes of disease occurrence or recurrence;
- Education about inheritance, testing, management, prevention, resources and research;
- Counseling to promote informed choices and adaptation to the risk of the condition.'

Genetic counseling is designed to reduce the client's anxiety, enhance the client's control and mastery over life circumstances, increase the client's understanding of the genetic disorder and options for testing and disease management, and provide the individual and family with the tools required to adjust to potential outcomes [1]. Genetic counseling can help individuals understand their options and make decisions that are appropriate in view of their perceptions of risk, religion, life beliefs, and family goals [3]. Table 20.1 summarizes the process of genetic counseling for persons with Fabry disease.

20.1.2 A Multidisciplinary Approach is Best

Fabry disease can affect virtually any organ system. A multidisciplinary team approach is optimal for care of an individual with Fabry disease [4]. Professionals on the team may include experts in genetics, hematology, cardiology, pulmonology, gastroenterology, nephrology, organ transplantation, neurology, otolaryngology, urology, dermatology, ophthalmology, pain management, psychology, psychiatry, occupational and physical therapy, obstetrics and gynecology, and social work. These experts should work with the patient's primary care practitioner (e.g., pediatrician, general internal medicine physician, etc.) for coordination of this complex care.

Physician medical geneticists often take the lead in managing the coordination of care of the person with Fabry disease including management of enzyme

Table 20.1 Summary of the process of genetic counseling for persons with Fabry disease

- Contracting: what are the client's needs and what are the mutual goals of the session?
- Develop rapport; explore client's beliefs and concerns about Fabry disease
- Obtaining and assessing family history (3–4 generation pedigree)
- Determine tobacco use
- Assessing issues with substance abuse (alcohol, street drugs, possible self medication)
- Psychosocial assessment
- Interpretation of medical and family history
- Obtain medical records to confirm diagnosis in consultand and relatives
- Diagnostic confirmation with enzyme analysis and DNA testing
- Discussion regarding DNA testing (including estimate of costs, specificity and sensitivity, chance of identifying gene variant of uncertain significance) and options if not tested
- Education about pattern of inheritance
- Discussion of possible emotional consequences of genetic diagnosis and/or testing
- Review of management options and prevention, and refer to specialists as appropriate
- Discussion of reproductive options
- Discussion of key ethical issues
- Plans for test result disclosure
- Plans for sharing information with relatives and others; discussion of resources for genetic counseling and/or additional tests/evaluations for relatives, as needed
- Education about resources (such as Fabry disease advocacy groups)
- Refer for psychological support and social work services, as needed
- Referral to research as appropriate
- Supporting a patient's decisions in the context of individual values, beliefs and goals
- Counseling to promote informed choices and adaptation to the condition

Source: References [3, 6, 12, 20, 21].

replacement therapy. Genetic counselors who are usually Masters degree trained individuals with specialty training certification by groups such as the American Board of Genetic Counseling (www.abgc.net), the Canadian Board of Genetic Counselors, and similar professional programs around the world (International Genetic Counseling Education: http://igce/med/sc.edu). Nurse genetic professionals are also often a leading member of the care team for a person with Fabry disease. Genetic counselors, medical geneticists, and advanced practice nurse genetics professionals can be located through the GeneTests Clinic Directory (http://www.genetests.org).

20.2 X-Linked Inheritance Pattern

Women have two X chromosomes in every cell and men have an X and a Y chromosome. Because Fabry disease is inherited in an X-linked pattern, a woman who carries a mutation for Fabry disease has a 50:50 chance to pass the gene mutation on to each son or daughter. Females often have manifestation of Fabry disease although they may be detected at a later age than is typical for males. Men with Fabry disease have a 100% chance to pass the mutation to each daughter but will have no affected sons.

Women with a Fabry disease mutation have more clinical manifestations than was first appreciated; for a family with an established diagnosis of Fabry disease of many years, it is important to review inheritance patterns and address any misconceptions regarding inheritance. A woman in a family with Fabry disease may have been advised that she would not develop symptoms of Fabry disease and advised that her problems were psychosomatic [5].

Because both men and women have manifestations of Fabry disease, it is best to simply refer to it as an X-linked disorder rather than describing it as an X-linked dominant or recessive disorder [6]. Women who are homozygous or compound heterozygotes have been reported [7]; this is a possible outcome for a daughter of a man with Fabry disease and his partner who is heterozygous for a *GLA* mutation.

20.3 Family Health History

Recording a family health history in the form of a pedigree is an important component of genetic counseling and diagnostic evaluation of Fabry disease. A pedigree is a multi-generational diagram that references biological relationship, demographic information and health history. The pedigree is not only a valuable tool for diagnosis and for identifying at-risk relatives, it also can be used as a means of identifying potential psychosocial issues that may be of concern to the client and his or her family. The pedigree should be available in the medical record for reference to in future clinical visits.

Table 20.2 lists the key health and demographic information and a sample of targeted queries to guide the clinician recording a family health history for diagnostic and genetic evaluation of a person with Fabry disease or possible Fabry disease, or for a person with a family history of Fabry disease. Individuals with de novo mutations have been identified (though this is uncommon), and therefore some persons with Fabry disease will not have a family history suggestive of Fabry disease.

The pedigree can identify relatives at risk to have inherited Fabry disease. Because of the availability of enzyme replacement therapy and the importance of medical management of the many medical complications of Fabry disease, it is important to be aggressive in helping the client with Fabry disease contact at risk relatives to assure appropriate genetic counseling and diagnostic evaluation. This approach can help to alleviate the traditional extreme diagnostic lag-time that has been observed to-date between the manifestations of symptoms of Fabry disease and the confirmation of a diagnosis.

20.3.1 A Pedigree Has Multiple Functions

The pedigree can serve as an education tool such as to demonstrate variable expression in the family (e.g., varying ages at diagnosis in relatives, reduced penetrance of

Table 20.2 Key information to include on a pedigree and targeted queries for diagnostic assessment and genetic counseling for Fabry disease

- Record biological relationships and basic demographic information, including: Two generations of ascendants and two generations of descendants from the proband or consultand (e.g., siblings and half-siblings, children, parents, aunts and uncles, grandparents, and often first cousins and grandchildren); Age or year of birth; Age at death (year if known) (obtain any available autopsy reports); Distinguish full- from half-sibs
- Record relevant health information on consultand and close biological relatives, including:

 1. *Cardiovascular disease* (obtain any records of echocardiograms, cardiac MRI, angiograms, and EKGs): Is there a history of heart disease? Specifically, has anyone been told they have heart murmurs or problems with their heart valve(s)? Does anyone have a history of chest pain (angina)? Has anyone died of heart disease such as an enlarged heart (cardiomyopathy)? Does anyone have a history of irregular heart rhythm? A pacemaker? Has anyone received a heart transplant?
 2. *Respiratory disease*: Is there a history of bronchitis, wheezing or shortness of breath (dyspnea)? Is there a current or past history of tobacco use?
 3. *Cerebrovascular disease*: Is there a history of strokes, seizures, or aneurysms? (Obtain brain MRI, interventional radiology reports, autopsy reports)? Is there history of dementia? Any history of thromboses?
 4. *Renal disease*: Is there a history of kidney problems (hypertension, protein in the urine, chronic renal disease)? Has anyone needed dialysis or a kidney transplant?
 5. *Auditory problems*: Is there a history of hearing loss? If so, at what age did it begin and is it both ears? Is there a history of 'ringing in the ears' (tinnitus)
 6. *Ophthalmologic evaluation*: Check for presence of the typical cataracts and corneal anomalies, and retinal vascular changes associated with hypertension and uremia including retinal artery thrombosis
 7. *Dermatological*: Does anyone have unusual rashes or birthmarks (angiokeratomas)? Note distribution; Has there been any treatment to remove these (e.g., laser therapy)?
 8. *Gastrointestinal*: Is there a history of abdominal pain, cramping, vomiting, and diarrhea?
 9. *Endocrine*: Does anyone have problems with sweating (anhidrosis–not sweating enough)?
 10. *Pain (acroparesthesias)*: Describe where the pain occurs and how often? Is there anything that triggers the pain (particularly heat or rapid temperature changes, fatigue, or stress); What have been effective strategies to reduce pain?
 11. *Psychological*: Is there a history of depression? Is there any history of suicide? (assess history of treatment both with medications and with counseling; it is appropriate to ask if there are guns in the home)

- Record information on who recorded the pedigree and when: Include name and title of recorder of information; Note name of the historian and relationship if not the consultant/proband (e.g. spouse, mother); Note date taken or updated

Source: References [3, 6].

the disease, and pattern of transmission). The process of obtaining a pedigree is a way of developing client rapport and engendering patient trust. Also, it is a simple way to identify possible fears and concerns of the patient. For example, if a patient's sibling had a renal transplant at age 40, the patient is likely to have concerns about also needing a renal transplant. If relatives in the family have had few manifestations of Fabry disease or have had success with treatment, then the patient may have a different attitude about Fabry disease then if many relatives have died from Fabry disease at a young age.

20.3.2 *Standard Pedigree Symbols*

The standard system for symbolizing a pedigree was developed through a consensus process of the Standardized Pedigree Task Force of the National Society of Genetic Counselors and published in 1995 [8], and has since been adopted as the international standard [9].

Common pedigree symbols and conventions for recording a genetic family history are shown in Figs. 20.1 and 20.2. For more details on some of the less common pedigree symbols (such as for pregnancies conceived by donor gametes, refer to the standard pedigree nomenclature of the National Society of Genetic Counselors [9]). For a more complete summary of how to take and record a genetic family health history refer to Bennett [3], A Practical Guide to the Genetic Family History.

20.4 Psychosocial Issues

There is a need for further study of the unique psychosocial issues in relation to Fabry disease. Overall the psychosocial issues in relation to a diagnosis of Fabry disease are similar to those associated with a diagnosis of other chronic genetic disorders [10–12]. A person diagnosed with Fabry disease may have feelings of anxiety, anger, grief, denial, blame, and hopelessness. A diagnosis may influence self-esteem and self-identity. There can be changed relationships with the family of origin.

Because the manifestations of Fabry disease begin in childhood, the requirements of lifelong management of this condition can cause stress on relationships, and there does seem to be higher rates of depression, unemployment, and suicide.

Providing accommodations in school and employment settings to anticipate and avoid settings that may exacerbate the symptoms of Fabry disease (such as rapid changes in the environmental temperatures, humidity, and extreme physical exertion) can help an individual with Fabry disease reach full potential in their educational and employment environments [6].

It is important to address issues of substance abuse. Because pain can be one of the most debilitating features of Fabry disease, there can be problems with substance abuse as a form of self-medication [6].

20.5 Sexuality

Both men and women with Fabry disease may have concerns about body image, intimacy, and sexuality in relation to Fabry disease. The angiokeratomas may be a significant source of embarrassment and psychological stress. MacDermot et al. [13]. found a substantial proportion of individuals with angiokeratomas feared

Instructions:
— Key should contain all information relevant to interpretation of pedigree (e.g., define fill/shading)
— For clinical (non-published) pedigrees include:
  a) name of proband/consultand
  b) family names/initials of relatives for identification, as appropriate
  c) name and title of person recording pedigree
  d) historian (person relaying family history information)
  e) date of intake/update
  f) reason for taking pedigree (e.g., abnormal ultrasound, familial cancer, developmental delay, etc.)
  g) ancestry of both sides of family
— Recommended order of information placed below symbol (or to lower right)
  a) age; can note year of birth (e.g., b.1978) and/or death (e.g., d. 2007)
  b) evaluation (see Figure 4)
  c) pedigree number (e.g., I-1, I-2, I-3)
  d) limit identifying information to maintain confidentiality and privacy

	Male	Female	Gender not specified	Comments
1. Individual	□ b. 1925	○ 30y	◇ 4 mo	Assign gender by phenotype (see text for disorders of sex development, etc.). Do not write age in symbol.
2. Affected individual	■	●	◆	Key/legend used to define shading or other fill (e.g., hatches, dots, etc.). Use only when individual is clinically affected.
	▨	◕		With ≥2 conditions, the individual's symbol can be partitioned accordingly, each segment shaded with a different fill and defined in legend.
3. Multiple individuals, number known	□ 5	○ 5	◇ 5	Number of siblings written inside symbol. (Affected individuals should not be grouped).
4. Multiple individuals, number unknown or unstated	□ n	○ n	◇ n	"n" used in place of "?".
5. Deceased individual	⊠ d. 35	⊘ d. 4 mo	◇ d. 60's	Indicate cause of death if known. Do not use a cross (†) to indicate death to avoid confusion with evaluation positive (+).
6. Consultand	□↗	○↗		Individual(s) seeking genetic counseling/ testing.
7. Proband	■ P↗	● P↗		An affected family member comming to medical attention independent of other family members.
8. Stillbirth (SB)	⊠ SB 28 wk	⊘ SB 30 wk	◇ SB 34 wk	Include gestational age and karyotype, if known.
9. Prefnancy (P)	▨ P LMP: 7/1/2007 47,XY,+21	○ P 20 wk 46,XX	◇ P	Gestational age and karyotype below symbol. Light shading can be used for affected; define in key/legend.

Pregnancies not carried to term	Affected	Unaffected	
10. Spontaneous abortion (SAB)	▲ 17 wks female cystic hygroma	△ < 10 wks	If gestational age/gender known, write below symbol. Key/legend used to define shading.
11. Termination of pregnancy (TOP)	▲ 18 wks 47,XY,+18	⧄	Other abbreviations (e.g., TAB, VTOP) not used for sake of consistency.
12. Ectopic pregnancy (ECT)		⧄ ECT	Write ECT below symbol.

Fig. 20.1 Common standardized pedigree symbols. Reprinted with permission from Bennett et al. [9]

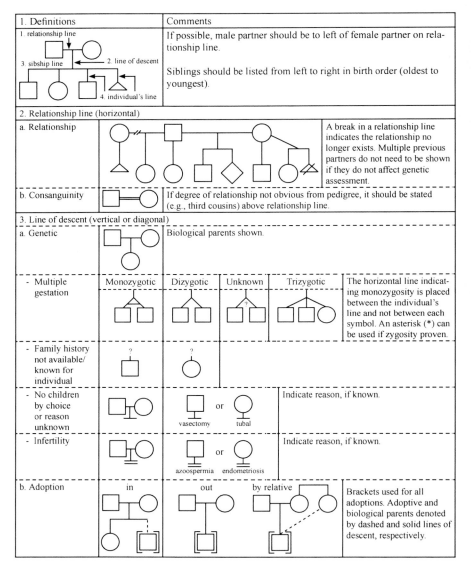

Fig. 20.2 Standard pedigree symbols for common relationships (e.g., twins, adoption, siblings). Reprinted with permission from Bennett et al. [9]

initiating sexual relationships. Chronic pain and fatigue may also contribute to sexual difficulties and problems with intimacy [14]. Chronic pain may even alter the ability to hold hands [5]. Erectile dysfunction can occur in association with Fabry disease, therefore urological consultation is important.

Instructions:
— E is used for evaluation to represent clinical and/or test information on the pedigree
  a. E is to be defined in key/legend
  b. If more than one evaluation, use subscript (E_1, E_2, E_3) and define in key
  c. Test results should be put in parentheses or defined in key/legend
— A symbol is shaded only when an individual is clinically symptomatic
— For linkage studies, haplotype information is written below the individual. The haplotype of interest should be on left and appropriately highlighted
— Repetitive sequences, trinucleotides and expansion numbers are written with affected allele first and placed in parentheses
— If mutation known, identify in parentheses

Definition	Symbol	Scenario	
1. Documented evaluation (*) Use only if examined/evaluated by you or your research/clinical team or if the outside evaluation has been reviewed and verified.	*	Woman with negative echocardiogram.	* E– (echo)
2. Carrier—not likely to manifest disease regardless of inheritance pattern		Male carrier of Tay-Sachs disease by patient report (* not used because results not verified).	
3. Asymptomatic/presymptomatic carrier—clinically unaffected at this time but could later exhibit symptoms		Woman age 25 with negative mammogram and positive BRCA1 DNA test.	* 25 y E_1– (mammogram) E_2+ (5385insC BRCA1)
4. Uninformative study (u)	Eu	Man age 25 with normal physical exam and uninformative DNA test for Huntington disease (E_2).	* 25 y E_1– (physical exam) E_2u (36n/18n)
5. Affected individual with positive evaluation (E+)	E+	Individual with cystic fibrosis and positive mutation study; only one mutation has currently been identified.	E+(ΔF508) Eu * E+(ΔF508/u)
		10 week male fetus with a trisomy 18 karyotype.	P * 10wk E+(CVS) 47, XY,+18

Fig. 20.3 How to document results of medical evaluations and genetic testing on a pedigree. Reprinted with permission from Bennett et al. [9]

20.6 Influence on Family

When a genetic disease is identified in a family it is common to have guilt feelings for passing the condition on to the next generation. Of course the shuffle of genes is random, and it is no one's fault that Fabry disease is passed in the family. It is important for the health professional to acknowledge feelings of *parental guilt* and emphasize that the disease is no one's fault.

Survivor guilt is another strong emotion that should be acknowledged. This is the feeling that can occur when a relative has conflicting emotions about not having the disease in the family while other relatives have been less fortunate. Clues from the family history may help the clinician further anticipate the likelihood of this occurring (for example, if the person is the only sibling to test negative for the *GLA* mutation).

If a person has a result opposite of what he or she believed would be the result (for example assuming that her or she is affected and finding out that he or she is unaffected), it may take time to readjust to a new sense of self [15]. A 'sick role' may have been unconsciously 'assigned' to a family member (*preselection*), thereby creating the illusion of control over the randomness of gene transmission [10]. A person with diagnostic results that are opposite of his or her preconceived notion of affected status may be at higher risk for adverse psychological consequences [10].

20.7 Trust in Health Professionals

Unfortunately, a person with Fabry disease may see multiple health professionals before a diagnosis is finally made. For many, the average number of years from symptom onset to diagnosis may be more than 10 years, with affected individuals typically seeing ten specialists before diagnosis [16, 17]. For females a diagnosis may be delayed by more than 16 years from the onset of symptoms [17]. Because of this experience, the person may lack trust in a health care system that has failed to recognize the diagnosis particularly if the person with Fabry disease has been made to feel that he or she has somaticized the symptoms and thus the problems were 'all in your head.' In a study of women with Fabry disease, Gibas et al. [5] quote female participants who say: 'They [healthcare professionals] think we're crazy' or 'Over the years I have been called a hypochondriac a psychotic woman, and many other titles.'

20.8 Reproductive Options

Once a diagnosis of Fabry disease is made, genetic counseling is important to discuss reproductive options for persons of childbearing age. There may be challenges to religious and ethical belief systems between couples and their extended families as couples wrestle with core values of biological parenting and views on prenatal diagnosis, assistive reproductive technologies, and potential adoption [1]. Genetic counseling should be supportive to the couple in making a choice that is best for them; they should not be coerced into a decision.

Any prenatal diagnosis or preimplanatation diagnosis would require genotyping of the person with Fabry disease so that mutational analysis can be done, and therefore ideally this should be done in advance of conception.

20.8.1 Gamete Donation

For a man who has Fabry disease who is concerned about passing Fabry disease to all of his daughters, there is the option of using a donor sperm. For a woman who has Fabry disease, she may choose to use a donor egg.

20.8.2 Preimplantation Diagnosis

Preimplantation diagnosis allows a couple where a woman has Fabry disease to test the developing blastocyst at a few cell stage to determine if the embryo has a *GLA* mutation for Fabry disease and then only implanting embryos that do not have the mutation.

Preimplantation diagnosis could be performed for a couple where the man has Fabry disease by only implanting male embryos (which will all receiving the Y chromosome and therefore not be at risk for Fabry disease). All female embryos conceived from a man with Fabry disease would be obligate heterozygotes with the potential to have manifestations of Fabry disease.

20.8.3 Prenatal Diagnosis

Both amniocentesis and chorionic villus sampling are options for prenatal diagnosis for a woman who has Fabry disease. Amniocentesis involves analysis of DNA from cultured amniocytes from the amniotic fluid at 12–16 weeks in pregnancy. Chorionic villus sampling, either transabdominal or transcervical, is done at approximately 10–12 weeks in pregnancy and involves testing DNA from the chorionic villus.

20.9 Potential Teratogenic Effects on Pregnancy

A careful medication history should be taken for a woman with Fabry disease of childbearing age, or if she is pregnant or planning a pregnancy to determine if any of the medications she is taking are teratogenic. Dilantin, carbamazepine, and gapabentin (neurontin) are commonly used for pain symptoms; their potential teratogenic effects should be reviewed with the client [18]. Ideally monotherapy is preferred over using multiple medications to control seizures during pregnancy, and if she has been seizure free for 2–5 years, then weaning off of medications may be appropriate.

Because of the association with an increased risk for neural tube defects associated with dilantin and carbamazepine, preconception use of folate supplements, 4 mg/day, for prevention of neural tube defects is important. Maternal serum screening for alpha-fetoprotein levels for screening for neural tube defects, as well as level 2 ultrasound is warranted. Because of the association with cardiac defects with some seizure medications, a fetal echo is also important [18].

Women with Fabry disease may use a variety of supplements and alternative medicine for management of their symptoms [19], so it is important to specifically ask about these potential teratogens as well.

Limited information exists about pregnancy outcomes in women with Fabry disease who are on enzyme replacement therapy, but there has not been any teratogenic effects demonstrated.

20.10 Summary

The diagnosis of Fabry disease not only has important health consequences for the person, but the ramifications of the disease may affect multiple relatives. A team of health professionals is important for the care of a person with Fabry disease which should include specialists in genetics to provide support for the person with Fabry disease and the family. In particular it is important that the medical and psychosocial needs of both men and women in the family are considered; women in families with Fabry disease have traditionally been informed that they are unlikely to have symptoms, when in fact they often have similar complications as their male relatives. In a family with Fabry disease, the needs for genetic counseling can change over time; genetic counseling is often not just a one-time encounter. The needs change based on the age of the client, changes in management options, and reproductive decision-making. A family history in the form of a pedigree can be an important multifunctional tool used for diagnosis and clinical decision making, risk assessment and identification of relatives with possible Fabry disease, patient education. and psychosocial assessment.

References

1. Bennett RL (2006) Genetic counseling. In: Runge MS, Patterson C (eds) Principles of molecular medicine, 2nd edn. Human Press, Totowa, pp 46–52
2. Resta RG, Beisecker BB, Bennett RL et al (2006) A new definition of genetic counseling. National Society of Genetic Counselor's Task Force Report. J Genet Couns 15(2):77–83
3. Bennett RL (2010) The practical guide to the genetic family history, 2nd edn. Wiley-Blackwell, Hoboken
4. Peters FP, Sommer A, Vermeulean A, Cheriex EC, Kho TL (1997) Fabry's disease: a multidisciplinary disorder. Postgrad Med J 73:710–712
5. Gibas AL, Klatt R, Johnson J, Clarke JTR, Katz J (2008) Disease rarity, carrier status, and gender: a triple disadvantage for women with Fabry disease. J Genet Couns 17:528–537
6. Bennett RL, Hart KA, O'Rourke EO et al (2002) Fabry disease in genetic counseling practice: recommendations of the National Society of Genetic Counselors. J Genet Couns 11(2): 121–146
7. Rodriquez-Mari A, Coll MJ, Chabas A (2003) A molecular analysis in Fabry disease in Spain: fifteen novel *GLA* mutations and identification of a homozygous female. Hum Mutat 22(3):258

8. Bennett RL, Steinhaus KA, Uhrich SB et al (1995) Recommendations for standardized pedigree nomenclature. Am J Hum Genet 56:745–752
9. Bennett RL, Steinhaus KA, Resta RG, Doyle DL (2008) Standardized human pedigree nomenclature: update and assessment of the recommendations of the National Society of Genetic Counselors. J Genet Couns 7(5):424–433
10. Resta RG (ed) (2000) Psyche and Helix. Psychological aspects of genetic counseling. Essays by Seymour Kessler, PhD. Wiley-Liss, New York
11. Weil J (2000) Psychosocial genetic counseling. Oxford University Press, Oxford
12. Uhlmann WR, Schuette JL, Yashar B (2009) A guide to genetic counseling, 2nd edn. Wiley-Blackwell, Hoboken
13. MacDermot KD, Holmes A, Miners AH (2001) Anderson Fabry disease: clinical manifestations and impact of disease in a cohort of 98 hemizygous males. J Med Genet 38:750–760
14. Stryker VL, Kreps C (2001) Fabry disease. Amer J Neurol 101:39–44
15. Williams JK, Schutte DL, Evers C, Holkup PA (2000) Redefinition. Coping with normal results from predictive gene testing for neurodegenerative disorders. Res Nurs Health 23:260–269
16. Morgan SH, d'A Crawford M (1988) Anderson-Fabry disease: a commonly missed diagnosis. Br Med J 297:872–873
17. Mehta A, Ricci R, Widmer U et al (2004) Fabry disease defined: baseline clinical manifestations of 366 patients in the Fabry outcome survey. Eur J Clin Invest 34(3):236–242
18. Caughey AB. Seizure disorders in pregnancy. eMedicine http://emedicine.medscape.com/article/272050-overview, update 4/20/2009. Accessed 26 Oct 2009
19. Balwani M, Fuerstman L, Desnick RJ, Buckley B, McGovern MM (2009) Use of complementary and alternative medicine by patients with lysosomal storage diseases. Genet Med 11(10):722–727
20. Marymee K, Dolan CR, Pagon RA, Bennett RL, Coe S, Fisher N (1998) Development of the critical elements of genetic evaluation and genetic counseling for genetic professionals and perinatologists in Washington State. J Genet Couns 6:133–165
21. National Society of Genetic Counselors (2007) Scope of practice, June 2007. Available at http://www.nsgc.org/client_files/SOP_final_060.pdf. Accessed 2009 Oct 30

Chapter 21
Fabry Disease in Females

D.A. Hughes

Abstract Anderson-Fabry disease is an X-linked lysosomal storage disorder resulting from deficiency of alpha galactosidase A and accumulation of globotriaosyl ceramide (Gb3) in cells throughout the body. Despite X-linked inheritance, females with Fabry disease may manifest significant multi-system pathology with effects on organ function, physical symptoms, quality of life and survival. Lyonisation within the peripheral blood results in some females exhibiting normal plasma or leucocyte enzyme activities which can lead to difficulties in diagnosis. Evidence of Gb3 storage has been found in urine and plasma and by histological analysis of renal and cardiac biopsies. However the disease causing mechanisms, given the presence of some enzyme activity from the normal alpha galactosidase A gene are not clear. Therapeutic effects of alpha galactosidase A have been demonstrated in the clinical trials, registries and case studies of females with documented improvements in pain, quality of life, left ventricular cardiac mass, and stabilised renal function. The optimum timing for initiation of enzyme replacement therapy nor its role in pregnancy and lactation is unknown. There is a necessity to develop strategies to identify which females are most like to benefit from Fabry specific therapy.

Keywords Female · Fabry · Therapy · Heterogeneity · Lyonisation

21.1 Introduction

Fabry disease is an X-linked lysosomal storage disorder. As a consequence of deficiency of the hydrolytic enzyme alpha galactosidase A [1] accumulation of globotrioasoyl ceramide (Gb3) occurs in cells throughout the body of both males and females. Although X-linked, Fabry disease has significant multi-system pathology and clinical manifestations in females and these may be as severe as males

D.A. Hughes (✉)
Lysosomal Storage Disorders Unit, Department of Academic Haematology, Royal Free Hospital and University College Medical School, London, UK
e-mail: d.hughes@medsch.ucl.ac.uk

D. Elstein et al. (eds.), *Fabry Disease*, DOI 10.1007/978-90-481-9033-1_21,
© Springer Science+Business Media B.V. 2010

[2–4]. The clinical features result in impaired quality of life and reduced life expectancy.

The pathophysiology underlying these manifestations in females is not entirely clear and may relate not only to skewed lyonisation but also to effects of the stored substrate on normal as well as abnormal cells. That females may manifest significant clinical features even though their peripheral blood enzyme activity may be in the normal range presents problems not only in the understanding of disease mechanisms but also for the diagnosis of females who could be overlooked if only enzyme activity is considered. Specific algorithms for the diagnosis of females should therefore be considered.

Evidence from case reports, observational studies, and clinical trials support the use of enzyme replacement therapy (ERT) in females with Fabry disease [5, 6]. Improvements include reduction in left ventricular cardiac mass, stabilised renal function, and improvements in pain and quality of life; however, an international consensus on which females to treat and when therapy should begin is lacking.

21.2 Pathology of Fabry Disease in Females

The alpha galactosidase A gene is differentially expressed within the cells of a female according to the principles of random X inactivation [7]. This results in a mosaic with some cells exhibiting normal expression and others little or no expression [8].

The local level of enzyme activity will depend on the balance between normal and mutant X inactivation in a given tissue and will vary from organ to organ i.e., skewing of X-inactivation. If skewing of X-inactivation in peripheral blood leucocytes and clinical expression of Fabry disease were the only factor, one might predict a straightforward relationship between enzyme activity and disease severity. The contribution of alpha galactosidase A activity from normal cells may result in an overall enzyme activity in the normal range, however that these patients still manifest substrate storage and clinical features implies that in vivo cross complementation by enzyme from normal cells is unlikely. The reason for this is unclear but may relate to inability of native exogenous enzyme to penetrate the abnormal cells or toxic effect of substrate or its metabolites in both normal and abnormal cells.

The biochemical consequences of alpha galactosidase A deficiency in males include cellular accumulation of Gb3 [9]. In females, elevated Gb3 has been detected in urine but not consistently in plasma [10, 11]. Gupta et al. also found no significant deposition of Gb3 in the capillary endothelium of females and no significant relationship to clinical features [11]. Conversely, a female patient with Fabry disease was found to have renal tubular and glomerular deposits on renal biopsy [12] and the endomyocardial biopsy of a female patient with late-onset disease and concentric left ventricular (cardiac) hypertrophy also showed Gb3 storage [13].

The finding of elevated deacylated globotriaosylsphingosine (lyso-Gb3) an inhibitor of alpha-galactosidase A, in plasma of classically affected male patients with Fabry may have some relevance to the pathology in females [14]. Lyso-Gb3 tended to be higher in female heterozygote patients, increasing with age and with severity. Inhibition of normal alpha galactosidase A by lyso-GB3 may reduce the efficacy of cross correction by enzyme from normal cells.

21.3 Diagnosis of Fabry Disease in Females

Pedigree analysis of an X-linked disorder predicts approximately twice the female to male prevalence of this condition; however, data from observational studies such as the Fabry Outcome Survey (FOS) suggest almost parity of ascertainment implying that many Fabry females remain undiagnosed or unreported [15]. This may reflect the heterogeneity of manifestations in females with some young heterozygotes being essentially asymptomatic, lack of awareness of female presentation among physicians, or more worryingly, misdiagnosis due to problems with the interpretation of biochemical data.

Depending on the skewing of lyonisation, the activity of alpha galactosidase A in peripheral blood leucocytes or plasma is variable in females. Activities may be low in the equivalent range to hemizygotic males, moderately reduced, or even within the normal range [16, 17]. For this reason, definitive diagnosis of females requires genetic analysis of the alpha galactosidase A gene. This is straightforward where a family history and knowledge of the mutation facilitates targeted assessment, but does present possible difficulties for female index cases and screening studies where full sequence analysis is necessary. In some instances despite clinical features, borderline low enzyme activity, and perhaps even evidence of substrate storage suggest a diagnosis of Fabry disease, mutation analysis fails to reveal an exonic mutation. In these cases Multiplex Ligation-dependent Probe Amplification (MLPA) should be performed to exclude exonic deletions, and if necessary, alpha galactosidase A mRNAs on the patient's fibroblasts should be examined for evidence of transcriptional regulation defects.

Other methodologies such as urinary globotriaosylceramide/creatinine ratios are being validated for high throughput screening of males and females.

21.4 Prenatal Diagnosis

In an early paper intimating that women may be severely affected by Fabry disease, prenatal diagnosis of enzyme deficiency by chorionic villus sampling (CVS) was described [18]. It has been suggested that prenatal screening should be offered to all families with an enzymatic and/or molecular diagnosis of Fabry disease [19]. Currently, prenatal diagnosis of Fabry disease can be performed by analysis of alpha galactosidase A activity and/or mutation on cultured amniocytes or cultured CVS or directly on chorionic villi. Due to the variability of symptoms in heterozygotes, the American Society of Genetic Counsellors has recommended fetal sex determination as the first diagnostic step [20]. However, some clinicians feel that since heterozygous women who carry a mutation in the alpha galactosidase A gene are at risk of developing full-blown Fabry disease, genetic counselling for heterozygous women should include discussion of the option of prenatal molecular analysis in female fetuses [21]. Pre-implantation diagnosis (PGD) on blastomeres has been performed and should be confirmed by subsequent CVS or amniocentesis.

21.5 Clinical Manifestations of Fabry Disease in Females

Until recently, disease-specific symptoms in females with Fabry disease were said to be the exception [22, 23] (Table 21.1). With the emergence of ERT and an increased necessity to clinically characterise patients with this condition, manifestations of disease in female heterozygotes have been well described [2–4, 24]. It is now widely accepted that females may express a range of clinical features including life threatening manifestations such as cardiomyopathy and stroke [13, 25]. Disease expression is heterozygous and the strongest correlation with this heterogeneity is with age, with the proportion of women suffering from a particular symptom reflecting that found in males approximately a decade previously [3]. In a recent study of 1,077 female patients from the Fabry Registry, the median age at onset of symptoms in females was 13 years, compared to 9 years in males ($P < 0.0001$) with the median age of diagnosis 24 years and females at 31 years, respectively [24]. Only 82 females (7.6%) had been diagnosed prior to symptom onset, largely due to screening of family members of an index patient. This is comparable to recent data from FOS (unpublished; personal communication) where currently 902 of 1,692 patients are females with the median age of symptom onset 14 years and diagnosis 31 years; 43% of these females are receiving ERT with median age of initiation 44.8 years.

21.6 Pain

Acral pain is a common and often severe feature in females occurring as early as 4 years of age [4] and impacting significantly on quality of life. Like males, females may experience exacerbations with fever and activity. In a recent study of 1,077 female patients from the Fabry Registry [24] female patients reported less pain (i.e., lower mean Brief Pain Inventory scores) than males. With increasing age, female patients reported increasing 'worst pain' symptoms.

21.7 Dermatological and Ophthalmological Findings

Angiokeratoma have been reported in up to 55% of females with Fabry disease [26] but are usually less extensive and more dispersed than in males. Cornea verticillata

Table 21.1 Clinical features of Fabry disease in females

	MacDermot et al. [2]	Whybra et al. [26]	Galanos et al. [27]	Mehta et al. [32]	Deegan et al. [3]	Wilcox et al. [24]
n	60	20	38	165	248	1,077 (1,055 analysed)
Mean age	44.9	NR	NR	41±17	38.2±18	40.5±17.4
Angiokeratoma (%)	35	55	13	50	40	17.8
Acroparasthesia (%)	70	90	53	64	77	43.3
Eye changes (%)	NR	70	76	53	50	12.5 at presentation
Sweating abnormality (%)	32	NR	11	NR	NR	NR
Gastrointestinal symptoms (%)	58.3	60	11	50	50	21.4
Left ventricular hypertrophy (%)	19	55	5 (cardiomyopathy)	28	26	18.2
Proteinuria (%)	35%	NR	21	33	35	39
Renal failure	3.3%- ESRF	55%	NR	1%-ESRF	1% transplant	2.2%-ESRF
Cerebrovascular disease	21%	85%	5%	27%	25%	3.9% TIA 4.2% CVA
Vertigo/tinnitus/hearing loss (%)	25	85	NR	47	48	NR
Lymphoedema (%)	8.3	50	2.6	NR	NR	NR

are also found in females: up to 76% in one study [27]; when present, this can be helpful in suggesting the diagnosis.

21.8 Gastrointestinal Manifestations

Gastrointestinal symptoms are common and often debilitating in females with Fabry disease. Diarrhea, abdominal pain, constipation, and vomiting have been described in 50–60% of females. In the Fabry registry, a higher percentage of female patients reported abdominal pain and diarrhea than males [24].

21.9 Cardiac Manifestations

Description of cardiac manifestations in females includes symptoms such as palpitations (in approximately 30% of women; [27]); structural disease including septal hypertrophy, cardiomyopathy, and mitral insufficiency; and symptomatic conduction disease, including requirement for pacemaker insertion [28]. There has been a report of a female with restrictive cardiomyopathy requiring cardiac transplantation [29]. Wilcox et al. describe the cardiovascular involvement exhibited by females to occur at approximately the same rate as in males, but at later age [24]. Left ventricular hypertrophy (LVH) was detected in 18.2% of females at an average age of 49.81 ± 12.4 years compared to 21.6% of male patients at 41.6 ± 10.9 years ($P < 0.0001$). Uncontrolled hypertension has been found in 57% of men and 47% of women [30].

21.10 Renal Failure

Despite a frequent finding of proteinuria [31] e.g., 39% of patients in the Fabry registry, progression to end-stage renal failure appears to be infrequent in females with Fabry disease with only 1–2% females requiring dialysis or transplantation [2, 24, 32].

21.11 Neurovascular Complications

Cerebrovascular complications of stroke and transient ischemic attacks (TIA) have been documented in significant but widely ranging proportions, e.g., 4.2% stroke in the Fabry registry [24] and up to 85% stroke and TIA from a large clinical experience [4]. Memory loss, dizziness, ataxia, hemiparesis, loss of consciousness, and hemi-sensory disturbance have all been reported in female heterzygotes [33]. MRI appearances include white matter changes and evidence of infarction [34].

Vertigo, tinnitus, hearing loss, and hypohidrosis can also be present in females.

21.12 Quality of Life, Fatigue, and Depression

Compared to the general population, both females and males with Fabry disease show consistently impaired quality of life (QoL). The greatest differences between males and females were observed for the social functioning and mental health subscales with females scoring higher than males in the social functioning subscale [24]. In the general population, females are twice as likely to suffer from symptoms of depression as males; however, in males with Fabry, the depression score has been found to be higher than in females. Male patients reported more symptoms of severe depression than females (36 and 22%, respectively), and were more affected by symptoms of Fabry disease [35]. Wang et al. have investigated fatigue and its relationship to oxygen consumption in patients with Fabry disease [36]. Fatigue was present in 59% of female patients studied, and associated with reduced maximum oxygen consumption ($P=0.049$); exercise intolerance, present in 83%, was associated with reduced maximal heart rate ($P=0.0089$). Fatigue correlated with the result of exercise testing: the measured VO_{2max} in women complaining of fatigue was a lower proportion of their predicted VO_{2max} than that in the 11 women without fatigue ($P = 0.049$) and the maximum heart rate attained during exercise testing was significantly lower in those who complained of exercise intolerance versus those who did not ($P = 0.0089$) [36].

21.13 Survival

In men, cardiac failure, renal failure, and stroke result in death approximately 20 years earlier than the general male population [37]. In female patients, reports suggest that cardiac disease and cerebrovascular disease are the most frequent causes of death [6, 32, 38] occurring on average 15 years earlier in females than in the general female population [2, 3]. A recent study has found the mean age at death was 51.8 years and 64.4 years for males and females, respectively. The primary cause of death in both was cardiac disease [15].

21.14 Enzyme Replacement Therapy (ERT) for Females with Fabry Disease

Two preparations of alpha galactosidase A received marketing approval by the EMEA in 2001: agalsidase beta (Genzyme Corporation, Cambridge MA, USA) and agalsidase alfa (Shire HGT Inc, Cambridge MA, USA) [39, 40]. Clinical trials and observational studies have provided evidence for efficacy of ERT with alpha galactosidase A in terms of symptoms of pain, gastrointestinal disturbance hypohidrosis, organ dysfunction including left ventricular mass index, and glomerular filtration rate (GFR), and quality of life in men [41–50]. The effects of ERT on females have been noted both in clinical trials and outcome surveys [48].

21.15 Clinical Trials

In a trial of 15 severely affected females treated with agalsidase alfa for 55 weeks, Baehner et al. [5] noted mean urine sediment and plasma Gb3 levels decreased from baseline, significant decreases in left ventricular mass from baseline at weeks 27 ($P=0.003$) and 41 ($P=0.039$), and a significant reduction in QRS durations at week 27 ($P=0.007$). Renal function remained stable. There was also significant improvement in quality of life. No antibody formation to agalsidase alfa was detected during the course of this trial in these females. More recently, the same group has published a longer term (4 year) study in 36 symptomatic females. Total disease burden, was significantly reduced after 12 months of treatment and continuously improved over 4 years. Pain was reduced after 12 months ($P=0.001$) and remained reduced throughout the study. Mean left ventricular (cardiac) mass decreased from 89.4 ± 29.3 g/m$^{2.7}$ at baseline to 66.5 ± 29.3 g/m$^{2.7}$ after 12 months ($P<0.001$) and again remained reduced. Average kidney function remained constant. The authors concluded that ERT with agalsidase alfa was safe and effective in female patients heterozygous for Fabry disease [6].

A number of trials of agalsidase beta have included female subjects however no exclusively female trial has been performed. In a placebo-controlled trial and its extension study, of 58 patients demonstrating clearance of microvascular endothelial deposits of Gb3 from the kidneys, heart, and skin, two of 29 patients receiving the active agent were female [39, 50]. In a phase IV placebo-controlled trial of 82 patients showing that agalsidase beta therapy reduced the likelihood of any clinical event in patients with advanced Fabry disease, eight female patients received agalsidase beta five of these females remaining seronegative [51].

21.16 Observational Studies

Other trials and observational studies have included small numbers of females in the study population; however, few provide specific details of the female response. For example, in a study of agalsidase alfa on hearing improvement, 18 patients were male (median age $= 30.1$ years, range 3.4–54.8 years) and eight patients were female (median age $= 41.0$ years, range 10.0–62.8 years). But the data on the females could not be separated from the group response [52].

Two larger studies from the FOS by Hoffman et al. [53, 54] demonstrate positive effects of agalsidase alfa on gastrointestinal disturbance and pain in females. Female patients were found to be more frequently affected by gastrointestinal symptoms than male patients. ERT with agalsidase alfa reduced the prevalence of abdominal pain, with a statistically significant decrease in male patients and in children after 12 months of treatment [53].

In terms of pain, the prevalence in female patients was 65.3% [54]. Mean age at onset of pain was 19.8 ± 1.4 years and was most frequently reported in the hands and feet but often affected the whole body. Interference of pain with daily life was higher in females than in males. At 24 and 36 months of ERT, pain became less severe ($P<0.05$) with similar mean changes in males and females, except for pain at its worst where the change was greater in females [54].

21.17 ERT During Pregnancy and Lactation

There is one published report of a female patient with Fabry receiving ERT during pregnancy [55]. The 34-year old female patient requested ERT to continue during pregnancy and accepted responsibility for the outcome. The dose and frequency of ERT were unchanged throughout and the patient remained stable, giving birth to a healthy boy at 37 weeks. The authors concluded that pregnancy should not be a contraindication for ERT. Currently, the summary of product characteristics (SMPC) for agalsidase alfa states that 'very limited clinical data on pregnancies exposed to agalsidase alfa ($n=4$) have shown no adverse effects on the mother and newborn child' (SMPC Replagal). Clearly, any decision to continue ERT during pregnancy should be taken jointly with the patient after full discussion of the potential and unquantifiable risks and benefits to the patient, the pregnancy, and the fetus. Similarly, it is not know if exogenously replaced enzyme is excreted into breast milk and no data is available on neonates exposed to recombinant alpha galactosidase A via breast milk.

21.18 Antibody Responses in Females

Given the preservation of enzyme activity from the normal X chromosome, albeit at varying levels in affected females, the prevalence of an immune response to infused alpha galactosidase A would be expected to be lower in females than in males. In the two trials of agalsidase alfa mentioned above there were no reports of anti-agalsidase alfa antibodies at any time during this treatment period [5, 6]. In trial reports of agalsidase beta, a low level of sero-conversion was noted [39, 51]. A retrospective analysis of IgG antibodies to agalsidase beta during placebo-controlled clinical trials and their open label follow-up studies demonstrated that half of the females seroconverted and that peak titres for the seropositive females were comparable to the lowest-titre sub-group of males. Over time, titres declined for most seropositive patients: 83% females tolerized [56]. No correlation between anti-alpha galactosidase A IgG titres and the onset of clinical events or elevations in plasma Gb3 was found although a significant association was detected between anti- alpha galactosidase A IgG titres and Gb3 deposition in the dermal capillary endothelium of males [56]. In an independent study of effects on antibody formation of algalsidase alpha and agalsidase beta, no antibody formation was detected in 24 females [57]. Despite the low prevalence of antibodies, it is possible for women to experience infusion reactions characterized by fever and chills which are unrelated to immune status.

21.19 Which Females Should Receive ERT and When

The use of ERT in females with Fabry disease varies by practitioner and region. In some countries no females receive treatment, in others only those with advanced clinical consequences of their disease; [58]. Guidelines published by US and UK groups of physicians suggest females should be offered ERT for Fabry disease if they manifest significant symptoms or show evidence of progressive end organ involvement. Features for consideration include pain unresponsive to conventional therapy, persistent proteinuria (>300 mg/24 h), GFR <80 ml/min/1.73 m^2, clinically significant cardiac or neurovascular involvement, or gastrointestinal dysfunction affecting quality of life [59, 60].

It would be anticipated that early specific therapy in females might prevent or stabilise clinical manifestations which result in significant morbidity and mortality and reduction in quality of life. However, even relatively late in life, there is a proportion of females who remain essentially asymptomatic [3]. Therefore, before treatment of females without significant symptoms is considered, not only will clinical trials assessing the preventative effects of ERT be needed, but it will also be essential to develop a means to identify which females are likely to go on to develop quality or quantity of life-limiting manifestation later in life. Prevention of the clinical and biochemical consequences of alpha galactosidase A deficiency by early intervention with ERT should be shown to have net benefit on quality of life and be cost efficient [61].

21.20 Conclusions

There is evidence that females heterozygotic for mutations in the alpha galactosidase A gene can manifest biochemical and clinical consequences of alpha galactosidase A deficiency in vital organs despite often borderline normal levels of enzyme activity in the peripheral blood due to lyonisation. It is important that clinicians be aware that normal plasma and leucocyte enzyme activity do not preclude the diagnosis of Fabry disease in a female which therefore mandates genetic testing. Females diagnosed with this condition should be thoroughly assessed as they may exhibit clinical features of the same range and severity as males albeit some years later. Two therapeutic trials, registries, and case series support the beneficial effects of ERT in females although longer follow-up is necessary to demonstrate an effect on the survival of females with Fabry disease, which untreated appears to be reduced. However, females with Fabry disease are not simply males with an attenuated version of the disease. There are unanswered questions as to the pathophysiology of the condition in females, optimum strategies for diagnosis, the effect of hormonal changes throughout the females life cycle on Fabry symptoms, the effects of ÉRT in pregnancy, the psychological burden of transmission of the gene to sons and the label 'carrier'. Above all, physicians treating patients with Fabry disease should be mindful that it is a heterogeneous condition and each patient, male or female, must be assessed and treated as an individual.

References

1. Kint JA (1970) Fabry's disease: alpha-galactosidase deficiency. Science 167:1268–1269
2. MacDermot KD, Holmes A, Miners AH (2001) Anderson-Fabry disease: clinical manifestations and impact of disease in a cohort of 60 obligate carrier females. J Med Genet 38:769–775
3. Deegan PB, Baehner AF, Barba Romero MA, Hughes DA, Kampmann C, Beck M (2006) Natural history of Fabry disease in females in the Fabry Outcome Survey. J Med Genet 43:347–352
4. Whybra C, Kampmann C, Willers I et al (2001) Anderson-Fabry disease: clinical manifestations of disease in female heterozygotes. J Inherit Metab Dis 24:715–724
5. Baehner F, Kampmann C, Whybra C, Miebach E, Wiethoff CM, Beck M (2003) Enzyme replacement therapy in heterozygous females with Fabry disease: results of a phase IIIB study. J Inherit Metab Dis 26:617–627
6. Whybra C, Miebach E, Mengel E et al (2009) A 4-year study of the efficacy and tolerability of enzyme replacement therapy with agalsidase alfa in 36 women with Fabry disease. Genet Med 11:441–449
7. Lyon MF (1961) Gene action in the X-chromosome of the mouse (Mus musculus L.). Nature 190:372–373
8. Happle R (2006) X-chromosome inactivation: role in skin disease expression. Acta Paediatr Suppl 95:16–23
9. Mills K, Morris P, Lee P et al (2005) Measurement of urinary CDH and CTH by tandem mass spectrometry in patients hemizygous and heterozygous for Fabry disease. J Inherit Metab Dis 28:35–48
10. Cable WJ, McCluer RH, Kolodny EH, Ullman MD (1982) Fabry disease: detection of heterozygotes by examination of glycolipids in urinary sediment. Neurology 32:1139–1145
11. Gupta S, Ries M, Kotsopoulos S, Schiffmann R (2005) The relationship of vascular glycolipid storage to clinical manifestations of Fabry disease: a cross-sectional study of a large cohort of clinically affected heterozygous women. Medicine (Baltimore) 84:261–268
12. Osunkoya AO, Agte SD, Laszik ZA (2006) 67-year-old woman with chronic proteinuria. Focal segmental and global glomerulosclerosis with light microscopic and ultrastructural features consistent with Fabry disease. Arch Pathol Lab Med 130:e93–e95
13. Chimenti C, Pieroni M, Morgante E et al (2004) Prevalence of Fabry disease in female patients with late-onset hypertrophic cardiomyopathy. Circulation 110:1047–1053
14. Aerts JM, Groener JE, Kuiper S et al (2008) Elevated globotriaosylsphingosine is a hallmark of Fabry disease. Proc Natl Acad Sci USA 105:2812–2817
15. Mehta A, Clarke JT, Giugliani R et al (2009) Natural course of Fabry disease: changing pattern of causes of death in. J Med Genet 8:548–552
16. Ashton-Prolla P, Ashley GA, Giugliani R, Pires RF, Desnick RJ, Eng CM (1999) Fabry disease: comparison of enzymatic, linkage, and mutation analysis for carrier detection in a family with a novel mutation (30delG). Am J Med Genet 84:420–424
17. Desnick RJ, Bernstein HS, Astrin KH, Bishop DF (1987) Fabry disease: molecular diagnosis of hemizygotes and heterozygotes. Enzyme 38:54–64
18. Kleijer WJ, Hussaarts-Odijk LM, Sachs ES, Jahoda MG, Niermeijer MF (1987) Prenatal diagnosis of Fabry's disease by direct analysis of chorionic villi. Prenat Diagn 7:283–287
19. Desnick RJ (2007) Prenatal diagnosis of Fabry disease. Prenat Diagn 8:693–694
20. Bennett RL, Hart KA, O'rourke E et al (2002) Fabry disease in genetic counseling practice: recommendations of the National Society of Genetic Counselors. J Genet Couns 11: 121–146
21. Raas-Rothschild A, Lacombe D (2008) Fabry disease prenatal diagnosis. Prenat Diagn 28:268
22. Nakao S, Takenaka T, Maeda M et al (1995) An atypical variant of Fabry's disease in men with left ventricular hypertrophy. N Engl J Med 3(333):288–293
23. Redonnet-Vernhet I, Ploos van Amstel JK, Jansen RP, Wevers RA, Salvayre R, Levade T (1996) Uneven X inactivation in a female monozygotic twin pair with Fabry disease and

discordant expression of a novel mutation in the alpha-galactosidase A gene. J Med Genet 33:682–688

24. Wilcox WR, Oliveira JP, Hopkin RJ et al (2008) Females with Fabry disease frequently have major organ involvement: lessons from the Fabry Registry. Mol Genet Metab 93:112–128

25. Giacomini PS, Shannon PT, Clarke JT, Jaigobin C (2004) Fabry's disease presenting as stroke in a young female. Can J Neurol Sci 31:112–114

26. Whybra C, Wendrich K, Ries M, Gal A, Beck M (2001) Clinical manifestation in female Fabry disease patients. Contrib Nephrol 136:245–250

27. Galanos J, Nicholls K, Grigg L, Kiers L, Crawford A, Becker G (2002) Clinical features of Fabry's disease in Australian patients. Intern Med J 32:575–584

28. Nakayama Y, Tsumura K, Yamashita N, Yoshimaru K (1999) Dynamic left ventricular arterial pressure gradient and sick sinus syndrome with heterozygous Fabry's disease improved following implantation of a dual chamber pacemaker. Pacing Clin Electrophysiol 22:1114–1115

29. Cantor WJ, Daly P, Iwanochko M, Clarke JT, Cusimano RJ, Butany J (1998) Cardiac transplantation for Fabry's disease. Can J Cardiol 14:81–84

30. Kleinert J, Dehout F, Schwarting A et al (2006) Prevalence of uncontrolled hypertension in patients with Fabry disease. Am J Hypertens 19:782–787

31. Yuen NW, Lam CW, Chow TC, Chiu MC (1997) A characteristic dissection microscopy appearance of a renal biopsy of a Fabry heterozygote. Nephron 77:354–356

32. Mehta A, Ricci R, Widmer U et al (2004) Fabry disease defined: baseline clinical manifestations of 366 patients in the Fabry Outcome Survey. Eur J Clin Invest 34:236–242

33. Mitsias P, Levine SR (1996) Cerebrovascular complications of Fabry's disease. Ann Neurol 40:8–17

34. Grewal RP, McLatchey SK (1992) Cerebrovascular manifestations in a female carrier of Fabry's disease. Acta Neurol Belg 92:36–40

35. Cole AL, Lee PJ, Hughes DA, Deegan PB, Waldek S, Lachmann RH (2007) Depression in adults with Fabry disease: a common and under-diagnosed problem. J Inherit Metab Dis 30:943–951

36. Wang RY, Lelis A, Mirocha J, Wilcox WR (2007) Heterozygous Fabry women are not just carriers, but have a significant burden of disease and impaired quality of life. Genet Med 9:34–45

37. MacDermot KD, Holmes A, Miners AH (2001) Anderson-Fabry disease: clinical manifestations and impact of disease in a cohort of 98 hemizygous males. J Med Genet 38:750–760

38. Linhart A, Kampmann C, Zamorano JL et al (2007) Cardiac manifestations of Anderson-Fabry disease: results from the international Fabry outcome survey. Eur Heart J 28: 1228–1235

39. Eng CM, Banikazemi M, Gordon RE et al (2001) A phase 1/2 clinical trial of enzyme replacement in fabry disease: pharmacokinetic, substrate clearance, and safety studies. Am J Hum Genet 68:711–722

40. Schiffmann R, Kopp JB, Austin HA III et al (2001) Enzyme replacement therapy in Fabry disease: a randomized controlled trial. J Am Med Assoc 285:2743–2749

41. West M, Nicholls K, Mehta A et al (2009) Agalsidase alfa and kidney dysfunction in Fabry disease. J Am Soc Nephrol 20:1132–1139

42. Hughes DA, Elliott PM, Shah J et al (2007) Effects of enzyme replacement therapy on the cardiomyopathy of Anderson-Fabry disease: a randomized, double-blind, placebo-controlled clinical trial of agalsidase-alfa. Heart 94:153–158

43. Moore DF, Altarescu G, Herscovitch P, Schiffmann R (2002) Enzyme replacement reverses abnormal cerebrovascular responses in Fabry disease. BMC Neurol 2:4

44. Schiffmann R, Floeter MK, Dambrosia JM et al (2003) Enzyme replacement therapy improves peripheral nerve and sweat function in Fabry disease. Muscle Nerve 28: 703–710

45. Hoffmann B, Garcia dL, Mehta A, Beck M, Widmer U, Ricci R (2005) Effects of enzyme replacement therapy on pain and health related quality of life in patients with Fabry disease: data from FOS (Fabry Outcome Survey). J Med Genet 42:247–252

46. Hoffmann B, Reinhardt D, Koletzko B (2004) Effect of enzyme-replacement therapy on gastrointestinal symptoms in Fabry disease. Eur J Gastroenterol Hepatol 16:1067–1069

47. Hajioff D, Goodwin S, Quiney R, Zuckerman J, MacDermot KD, Mehta A (2003) Hearing improvement in patients with Fabry disease treated with agalsidase alfa. Acta Paediatr Suppl 92:28–30

48. Beck M, Ricci R, Widmer U et al (2004) Fabry disease: overall effects of agalsidase alfa treatment. Eur J Clin Invest 34:838–844

49. Banikazemi M, Ullman T, Desnick RJ (2005) Gastrointestinal manifestations of Fabry disease: clinical response to enzyme replacement therapy. Mol Genet Metab 85:255–259

50. Germain DP, Waldek S, Banikazemi M et al (2007) Sustained, long-term renal stabilization after 54 months of agalsidase beta therapy in patients with Fabry disease. J Am Soc Nephrol 18:1547–1557

51. Banikazemi M, Bultas J, Waldek S et al (2007) Agalsidase-beta therapy for advanced Fabry disease: a randomized trial. Ann Intern Med 146:77–86

52. Hajioff D, Hegemannn S, Conti G et al (2006) Agalsidase alpha and hearing in Fabry disease: data from the Fabry Outcome Survey. Eur J Clin Invest 36:663–667

53. Hoffmann B, Schwarz M, Mehta A, Keshav S (2007) Gastrointestinal symptoms in 342 patients with Fabry disease: prevalence and response to enzyme replacement therapy. Clin Gastroenterol Hepatol 5:1447–1453

54. Hoffmann B, Beck M, Sunder-Plassmann G, Borsini W, Ricci R, Mehta A (2007) Nature and prevalence of pain in Fabry disease and its response to enzyme replacement therapy–a retrospective analysis from the Fabry Outcome Survey. Clin J Pain 23:535–542

55. Wendt S, Whybra C, Kampmann C, Teichmann E, Beck M (2005) Successful pregnancy outcome in a patient with Fabry disease receiving enzyme replacement therapy with agalsidase alfa. J Inherit Metab Dis 28:787–788

56. Benichou B, Goyal S, Sung C, Norfleet AM, O'Brien F (2009) A retrospective analysis of the potential impact of IgG antibodies to agalsidase beta on efficacy during enzyme replacement therapy for Fabry disease. Mol Genet Metab 96:4–12

57. Vedder AC, Breunig F, Donker-Koopman WE et al (2008) Treatment of Fabry disease with different dosing regimens of agalsidase: effects on antibody formation and GL-3. Mol Genet Metab 94:319–325

58. Whybra C, Kampmann C, Krummenauer F et al (2004) The Mainz severity score index: a new instrument for quantifying the Anderson-Fabry disease phenotype, and the response of patients to enzyme replacement therapy. Clin Genet 65:299–307

59. Eng CM, Germain DP, Banikazemi M et al (2006) Fabry disease: guidelines for the evaluation and management of multi-organ system involvement. Genet Med 8:539–548

60. Hughes DA, Ramaswami U, Elliott P et al. Guidelines for the diagnosis and management of Anderson-Fabry Disease. Publications and statistics 2005. Available from http://www.dh.gov.uk/en/Publicationsandstatistics/Publications/PublicationsPolicyAndGuidance/DH_4118404

61. Connock M, Juarez-Garcia A, Frew E et al (2006) A systematic review of the clinical effectiveness and cost-effectiveness of enzyme replacement therapies for Fabry's disease and mucopolysaccharidosis type 1. Health Technol Assess 10:iii–113

Chapter 22
Fabry Disease in Pediatric Patients

Maryam Banikazemi

Abstract Fabry disease, α-galactosidase A (α-Gal A) deficiency, is an X-linked lysosomal storage disease resulting in the progressive accumulation of globotriaosylceramide (GL-3) in the lysosomes of endothelial cells, as well as epithelial, perithelial and smooth muscle cells throughout the body. Classically affected males (<1% α-Gal A activity) present in childhood with acroparesthesias, hypohidrosis, angiokeratomas, corneal/lenticular opacities, and abdominal pain. With advancing age, renal failure and cerebrovascular and cardiovascular complications lead to early demise. Manifestations of disease in heterozygotes for the classic phenotype are variable due to Lyonization [1–7, 8]. In children and adolescence unusual signs and symptoms, and/or clusters of relatively common signs and symptoms should direct the physicians toward further investigations. In such cases, additional clinical signs of disease and a detailed family history can be helpful. Eventually, definitive diagnosis is relatively simple through enzyme activity assay, and DNA testing [5, 9, 10]. Here we focus on clinical presentation in pediatric and adolescent age groups. We will discuss the signs and symptoms unique in Fabry disease, as well as clusters of common signs and symptoms, which are suggestive of Fabry disease in this age group.

Keywords Children · Adolescents · Neuropathic pain · Post-prandial abdominal pain · Hypohidrosis · Quality of life · Family history

22.1 Introduction

Fabry disease is a progressive, debilitating disease, affecting multiple organ-systems with an increasing chance of significant morbidity and mortality over time. The primary pathology is lysosomal accumulation of GL-3 and resulting cell and tissue

M. Banikazemi (✉)
Columbia University School of Medicine, New York, NY, USA
e-mail: mb3186@columbia.edu

damage. Today, disease-specific treatment has become a reality for Fabry disease [11, 12–14]. Therefore, early diagnosis of affected individuals is essential, as the degree of success of treatment for these patients depends on the extent and length of cell and tissue damage at the time of initiation of treatment.

The diagnosis of Fabry, as for many other lysosomal storage disorders (LSD), remains challenging. Despite sometimes obvious clinical signs and symptoms, parents of children with Fabry disease often embark on a 'diagnostic odyssey' before the diagnosis is made. During this diagnostic process patients may see several specialists and the diagnosis is often delayed for several years [9, 12, 15].

Unusual signs and symptoms, and/or clusters of relatively common signs and symptoms should direct the physicians toward further investigation. In such cases, additional clinical signs of disease and a detailed family history can be helpful. Eventually, definitive diagnosis is relatively simple through enzyme activity assay, and DNA testing.

The clinical manifestation of Fabry disease can be reviewed under two main periods; early disease manifestation and late disease manifestation. The latter will be discussed elsewhere in this book.

22.2 Fabry Disease Clinical Manifestation

Early symptoms in children and adolescents suffering from Fabry disease include acroparesthesia, angiokeratoma, hypohydrosis, gastrointestinal symptoms, ocular findings, poor heat and exercise tolerance, and psychosocial difficulties (primarily frequent absences from school, poor participation especially in physical activity, and behavioral problems mostly related to chronic pain and gastrointestinal symptoms). Several studies of presenting features in pediatric patients who have Fabry's disease show onset of symptoms in boys as young as 2 years, with an average age of onset of 5–6 years. Girls report first symptoms at an average age of 9 years [16, 15, 17].

22.3 Fabry Pain and Acroparesthesis

The most common initial symptom of Fabry disease reported by patients is pain. It usually occurs within the first 10 years of life, and tends to be intermittent. Pain is most often noted in fingers and toes, or the hands or feet, and may be excruciating. The pain is often described as having a burning sensation and there may be associated acroparesthesias. Pain is typically the most disabling consequence of Fabry disease for patients, especially during the first two decades of life [15, 17].

The pain in Fabry disease is recurrent in nature and may occur on daily basis with some variability in severity. The pain may radiate to the proximal extremities and other parts of the body [9, 18, 19]. Pain attacks may be brief or may last for days or even weeks, and are experienced by 80–90% of male patients. With time, the intensity of chronic pain might increase or decrease. For some patients it persists throughout life [13, 15].

Extreme pain attacks, referred to as 'Fabry pain crises' are mostly experienced by male patients with classic Fabry disease. A Fabry pain crisis can last several hours to days (Table 22.1).

Table 22.1 Fabry pain and acroparesthesis; comparison between male and females

	Male	Female
Percentage of patients	Almost All	Variable
Frequency	Daily → Weekly	Occasional
Intensity	Mild → Severe	Mild → Moderate
	Excruciating pain crises	
Percentage of patients	Almost all	Rare
Frequency	Frequent	Infrequent
Intensity	Excruciating; Incapacitating	Mild → Severe

Fabry pain crises can be a component of a cascade of events such as fever of unknown origin, body pains, fatigue, and in some cases high sedimentation rate of erythrocytes (ESR). Although, pain associated with Fabry disease is generally not accompanied by any physical findings such as swelling, erythema, or even tenderness.

Factors triggering these episodes can be identified in some patients, including emotional stressors, febrile illnesses, rapid environmental change of temperature and humidity, physical activity and fatigue. Direct or indirect increase of core body temperature is the common consequence of these triggering factors. The regulation of core temperature is achieved through physiologic responses such as vasodilatation and/or sweating and these are greatly compromised in this disease.

The pathophysiology of pain is not fully understood. However, multiple mechanisms have been identified that play a role in pain and acroparesthesia in Fabry disease.

Acroparesthesias most probably result from transitory ischemia and prolonged small fiber dysfunction. The glycosphingolipid, GL-3 deposition in the small vessels narrows the vascular lumen and decreases blood supply to the peripheral nerves. The endothelial glycosphingolipid accumulation, and vessel spasms or frank infarction can initiate the excruciating pain [18].

Spontaneous pain and spontaneous remission is characteristic of neuropathic pain due to small fiber neuropathy. It has been documented that in Fabry disease, prominent small fiber dysfunction and high vulnerability of small-diameter nerve fibers, specifically unmyelinated C and thinly myelinated A δ fibres resulting in small fiber neuropathy (SFN) occurs [8, 20, 21, 22, 23].

In addition, Peripheral vascular autonomic dysfunction is also a common finding in patients with small fiber neuropathy that can contribute to poor regulatory respond to temperature changes.

22.4 Gastrointestinal Symptoms

Gastrointestinal (GI) symptoms, most commonly abdominal cramps and diarrhea, are often an early and prominent manifestation of Fabry disease. These typically begin in childhood and adolescence and may worsen with age. Patients of both sexes are affected [24]. Generally, symptoms are more frequent and appear earlier in life in males than in heterozygote females, with males reporting symptoms as early as 5–6 years of age. Abdominal cramps and diarrhea are regarded as the second most common presentation of this disease in children and young adults and can be the presenting symptoms of Fabry disease. Although gastrointestinal problems are generally not life threatening, they do have a substantial impact on the individuals' quality of life [25, 24].

Most prominently, the GI symptoms are experienced as post-prandial abdominal pain and bloating followed by multiple bowel movements and diarrhea. Patients often fail to identify a relationship between discrete episodes and ingestion of specific foods. The modification of timing, amount, or type of food intake has limited impact on symptoms [24].

Other gastrointestinal symptoms include nausea, vomiting, early satiety, poor weight gain, and weight loss. Gastrointestinal symptoms may continue into adulthood and in severe cases may progress to complete intolerance of oral intake. Additionally, achalasia (failure of the lower esophageal sphincter to relax) and jejunal diverticulosis, which may lead to perforation of the small bowel, have been described.

The complaints of post-prandial abdominal pain and diarrhea leading to sitophobia are suggestive of intestinal ischemia. It is generally accepted that abdominal angina develops when gastrointestinal vasculature (splanchnic and mesenteric arteries) exhibit a critical obstruction. The GI manifestations of Fabry disease are suggested to be a consequence of GL-3 deposition in endothelial of intestinal vasculature and compromised mesenteric circulation. Compromised circulation in intestinal mesenteric vasculature can also present as thromboangiitis obliterans and may progress to unpredictable acute episodes of gangrene [24].

22.5 Dermatological Findings

Dermatological disturbances in Fabry disease include the cutaneous vascular lesions (angiokeratomas) and anhidrosis, or more commonly hypohidrosis. Consistently reported poor heat and exercise tolerance among classical Fabry disease is thought to be in large due to accumulation of GL-3 in skin vascular endothelium, smooth muscle, fibroblasts, perineurium, and eccrine sweat glands cell, which presents as angiokeratomas [3, 4, 26] and impaired sweating [27].

22.6 Angiokeratomas

The main dermatologic manifestation of Fabry disease is angiokeratomas [3, 4, 26]. These cutaneous lesions are one of the earliest clinical signs of Fabry disease and are seen in most male patients with classic Fabry disease (Figs. 22.1 and 22.2). They usually appear between 5 and 13 years of age, but may be present as early as infancy. They initially appear as small, slightly raised, purplish-red, nonblanching angiectases (Fig. 22.1). With age, there is progressive increase in the number and size of these lesions [15, 17]. Among individuals, there is a wide variation in the pattern of distribution and density of the lesions. The clusters of lesions are most dense between the umbilicus and the knees and have a tendency toward bilateral symmetry. The hips, back, thighs, buttocks, penis, and scrotum are commonly affected (Fig. 22.2). Involvement of the oral mucosa and conjunctiva is common, and involvement of other mucosal areas may also occur. Among female carriers, 10–35% develop angiokeratomas generally beginning in adolescence. In female carriers, the lesions usually present as isolated, small macules on the breasts, groin, or flanks at a later age.

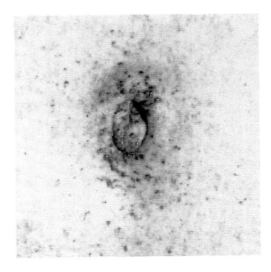

Fig. 22.1 Angiokeratoma is the small punctate *reddish-to-bluish* angiectases on the umbilicus

The large genital lesions are particularly susceptible to thrombosis and bleeding. In female carriers, the lesions usually present as isolated, small macules on the breasts, groin, or flank (Fig. 22.2).

Angiokeratomas are caused by weakness of the capillary wall due to GL-3 accumulation and vascular ectasia within the epidermis and dermis. The accumulation of

Fig. 22.2 Angiokeratomas are commonly observed as dense cluster of lesions on the flank and private areas

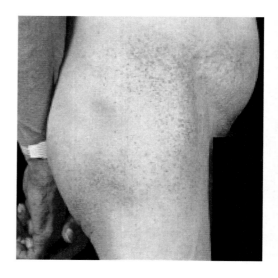

GL-3 in dermal tissue has been demonstrated in vascular endothelial cells, smooth muscle, fibroblasts, perineurium, and eccrine sweat glands in Fabry patients. In rare cases, even though the skin biopsy is positive for GL-3 deposits in vascular endothelial cells, no visual lesions can be identified [28].

In histopathology analysis of skin biopsy samples using light microscopy, the GL-3 deposits appear as small, dense, beaded, perinuclear cytoplasmic inclusions in the endothelial cells. On electron microscopy, many of these granules appear as dense and laminated 'myelin figures'. Biochemical confirmation of Fabry diagnosis is critical because angiokeratomas are also present in other enzyme deficiencies such as alpha-L- fucosidase, neuraminidase, C-mannosidase, and aspartylglycosaminidase deficiencies [4].

In addition to its diagnostic value, skin biopsy in patients with classic Fabry disease can offers a valuable and reliable method for monitoring efficacy of treatment [21, 29, 11].

22.7 Sweating Deficit

In patients with Fabry disease involvement of the skin thermoregulatory system manifests itself as poor heat and exercise tolerance. The sweating deficiency (hypohidrosis or anhidrosis) is an early manifestation of classical Fabry disease. Decrease in sweat gland function might be evident at infancy or develop during childhood. The reported poor heat and exercise tolerance among classical Fabry disease is thought to be in large due to accumulation of GL-3 in skin vascular endothelium, smooth muscle, fibroblasts, perineurium, and eccrine sweat glands cell. This symptom may presents in varying degree in female heterozygotes [30, 27, 28]. An ultrastructural study of Fabry skin pathology demonstrated narrowing of small blood vessels around the eccrine sweat glands due to heavy endothelial cell inclusions. GL-3 deposits also have been observed in eccrine sweat gland epithelium.

22.8 Eye Findings

Ocular manifestation of Fabry disease is well recognized. These findings are mostly unique to Fabry disease. The whorl-like or starburst pattern on the cornea, which is only visible through slit-lamp examination, is found almost universally among males and most of females with classic Fabry disease. This finding can be the earliest and only finding in these patients (Fig. 22.3).

Fig. 22.3 Corneal verticillata, commonly seen in patients with Fabry disease, detectable by slit lamp examination

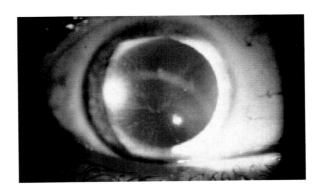

Other segments of eye also can be involved as retinal and conjunctival vascular tortuosity is documented in large number of patients as aneurysmal dilatation of these vessels. The prevalence of tortuous vessels in males increased with age. Lenticular change also is typical and include opacity with a 'spore-like' pattern at the level of posterior capsule, as referred to as 'Fabry cataract'. Confocal microscopy has demonstrated structural alterations throughout the entire ocular surface epithelia. None of these findings has impact on vision.

Fabry Disease-related cornea verticillata is attributable to glycosphingolipids accumulation. The earliest corneal verticillata is documented in male at age 3 years. However, this finding is marked in literature as early as few month of age and even in fetus. Therefore, finding of characteristic corneal whirling is diagnostic in young patients.

The fact that the ocular findings in female can be seen in slit-lamp exam in over 80% in female heterozygotes, slit-lamp eye examinations can be used as a diagnostic screening tool for Fabry disease in females who are at risk or who may have clinical manifestations suggestive of Fabry disease.

No clear relationship between ocular manifestations and organ involvement in Fabry patients has been appreciated [13, 15, 17, 31].

22.9 Psycho-Social Issues

Fabry-related symptoms have significant negative effect on quality of life in children and adolescents as well as their families. Young Fabry disease patients are chronically distressed by disease symptoms and physical limitations brought in by these symptoms.

Here we review the psychological consequences/impact of Fabry disease in young patients and their families in two major categories, each category is well recognized and studied by health care professionals [32, 23, 16, 15].

1. Impact of Chronic, debilitating and progressive disease on individuals mental health

    In these patients pain attacks, poor exercise and heat tolerance significantly limits the patient's physical capabilities during their first two decade of life. Recurrent gastrointestinal symptoms impact maybe prominent in ones daily life activity. The psychosocial impact of genital lesions in a young male can be also significant and often becomes a major source of primary concern in this age group as has impact in their self-esteem and fitness in the society.

    Never the less these symptoms consequences become more significant if the individual fail to adapt healthy coping skills or offered alternative choices. That may explain for increase rate of depression, narcotic dependence, alcoholism, marital problems, unemployment, and suicide among male with Fabry disease.

2. Social and psychological consequences related to genetic disease diagnosis

    The spectrum of psychological issues related to genetic diagnosis such as denial, anxiety, anger, grief, survivor and parental guilt, blame, depression, isolation, inability to cope, hopelessness, damage to self-esteem, changed relationship with family of origin, change sense of identity might be seen among these patients and their families.

Fabry disease is an X-Linked inherited lysosomal storage disorder. Even though heterozygotes females may experience varying degrees of disease symptoms, the disease is almost always more severe and progressive in affected males. Therefore it is no surprise that pschycological pressure; namely parental guilt and blame being prominent team in these families. The mothers frequently neglect themselves and their care in regard to Fabry disease.

If the disease is diagnosed in the family, it is not uncommon that families would face dilemma in regard to testing their young children. They would be conflicted in respect to the potential adverse consequences of testing for minors at risk, such as affecting family's perception of the child, loss of future adult autonomy, affecting future relationships of the child, fear/guilt in family planning, possible discriminations, increased medical surveillance, damage to self-esteem.

However, there are major potential benefits of testing for minors at risk that has to be discussed with family including; resolution of the parents concerns/anxiety, providing time to adjust to the status, planning physical activities and occupation, health status acceptance, making informed reproductive decisions, benefiting from available medical intervention.

Understanding all the issues that families are going through is essential, as counseling is provided to these families.

22.10 Renal Disease

Progressive renal disease is the prominent feature and main cause of premature death in classical Fabry disease. Microalbuminuria, proteinuria, and high filtration rate may be apparent in late childhood and adolescence [12, 16, 23, 15]. Even in affected males the progression of proteinuria, impairment of renal function, and the subsequent increase in serum creatinine levels and reduction GFR is not expected before the third decade of life. However, a case of early progressive renal failure requiring renal transplant at age 15 years with concomitant IgA nephropathy has been documented.

22.11 Cardiac Disease

Cardiac bradycardia and valvular regurgitation, the earliest manifestations of cardiac involvement, might be present as early as second decade of life [6, 12, 16, 23, 15]. Hypertrophic cardiomyopathy is not expected at a young age, and presence of such findings should warrant for further work up.

22.12 CNS/TIAs

Stroke and transient ischemic attack are a common and serious late manifestation of Fabry disease. Occasionally, CNS abnormalities in the first two decades of life have been reported, and in such cases other contributing factors should be investigated [12, 16, 23, 15].

22.13 Growth and Development

Slow growth and sexual maturation in affected males has been observed. However, there is no documented evidence of significant impact of Fabry disease on final growth potential and physical or mental development of in these patients. Difficulties with weight gain, and even weight loss, at all ages may be an issue for individuals with substantial gastrointestinal involvement [12, 16, 23, 15].

22.14 Others

Sensorineural hearing loss and tinnitus are infrequent symptoms of Fabry disease. When they occur, they often begin after the second decade of life [12].

Paroxysmal attacks of rotational vertigo independent from hearing loss or tinnitus occur in large groups of patients. Even though these episodes are most commonly experienced in more advance stages of disease, health care providers should be questioning patients in this regard. It has been suggested that these attacks most likely result from megadolichobasilar compression of the vestibulocochlear nerve, although other causes of vertigo occur in Fabry disease [12].

Lymphedema of the legs is a poorly described and less common manifestation of Fabry disease that is more likely to be experienced later in life. However, early and severe cases, often asymmetric, have been reported during the second decade of life. This manifestation presumably reflects the progressive glycosphingolipid deposition in the lymphatic vessels and lymph nodes, compromising lymphatic circulation [12].

Patients may complain of generalized fatigue and weakness.

22.15 Family History

A carefully obtained family history, including a detailed pedigree, may reveal an X-linked pattern of relatives with kidney failure, heart disease, stroke, or other signs and/or symptoms of Fabry disease.

22.16 Discussion

Patients may see many different specialists for specific organ-system symptoms such as Pediatrician, rheumatologists, dermatologists, ophthalmologists, nephrologists or cardiologists.

Observation of unusual signs and symptoms such as angiokeratomas and ocular findings should increase suspicious for specific disease diagnosis. In such suspected cases, obtaining family history and detail medical history and finally referral of patient to a metabolic disorders specialty center would be appropriate.

On the other hands, clusters of relatively common diseases signs and symptoms should direct the pediatricians and generalists toward further investigation. In such cases, obtaining additional clinical signs and a detailed family history can be helpful. In all cases, definitive diagnosis is possible by simple enzyme assay, and DNA testing.

Frequently seen early symptoms of Fabry disease that are mistaken for other more common disorders and making early diagnosis of these patients challenging, is summarized below;

- Pain in the joints or elevated erythrocyte sedimentation rate may be misdiagnosed as juvenile rheumatoid arthritis, Raynaud's Syndrome
- Pain accompanied by fever and an elevated erythrocyte sedimentation rate may be misdiagnosed as rheumatic fever.
- Acute pain in the extremities may be mislabeled as growing pain or erythromelalgia.
- Acute pain with no apparent cause often is labeled as neurosis.
- Angiokeratomas may be misdiagnosed as petechiae or lupus.
- Severe abdominal pain episode may be misdiagnosed as food allergy, acute Inflammatory Bowel Syndrome (IBD), and in acute and severe pain episode as appendicitis.
- Issues resulting from Fabry pain, poor heat and exercise tolerance often is interpreted as Gym and school avoidance, Depression, Isolation

References

1. Sweeley CC, Klionsky B (1963) Fabry's disease: classification as a sphingolipidosis and partial characterization of a novel glycolipid. J Biol Chem 238:3148–3150
2. Colombi A, Kostyal A, Bracher R, Gloor F, Mazzi R, Tholen H (1967) Angiokeratoma corporis diffusum – Fabry's disease. Helv Med Acta 34(1):67–83
3. Van Mullem PJ, Ruiter M (1970) Fine structure of the skin in angiokeratoma corporis diffusum (Fabry's disease). J Pathol 101(3):221–226
4. Van Mullem PJ (1972) Ultrastructure of lipid bodies and lysosomes in the skin in Fabry's disease (angiokeratoma corporis diffusum). Arch Belg Dermatol Syphiligr 28(1): 41–49
5. Bishop DF, Calhoun DH, Bernstein HS et al (1986) Human alpha-galactosidase A: nucleotide sequence of a cDNA clone encoding the mature enzyme. Proc Natl Acad Sci USA 83(13):4859–4863
6. Goldman ME, Cantor R, Schwartz MF et al (1986) Echocardiographic abnormalities and disease severity in Fabry's disease. J Am Coll Cardiol 7(5):1157–1161
7. Morgan SH, Crawfurd MA (1988) Anderson-Fabry disease. BMJ 297:872–873
8. Desnick RJ, Ioannou YA, Eng CM (2001) a-Galactosidase A deficiency: Fabry disease. In: Scriver CR, Beaudet AL, Sly WS (eds) Metabolic and molecular bases of inherited disease, 8th edn. McGraw-Hill Professional, New York, pp 3733–3774
9. Shelley ED, Shelley WB, Kurczynski TW (1995) Painful fingers, heat intolerance and telangiectases of the ear: easily ignored childhood signs of Fabry disease. Pediatr Dermatol 12(3):215–219
10. Linthorst GE, De Rie MA, Tjiam KH, Aerts JM, Dingemans KP, Hollak CE (2004) Misdiagnosis of Fabry disease: importance of biochemical confirmation of clinical or pathological suspicion. Br J Dermatol 150(3):575–577
11. Turberg BL, Randolph Byers H, Granter SR, Phelps RG, Gordon RE, O'Callaghan M (2004) Monitoring the 3-Year efficacy of enzyme replacement therapy in Fabry disease by repeated skin biopsies. J Invest Dermatol 122(4):900–908
12. Eng CM, Germain DP, Banikazemi M et al (2006) Fabry disease: guidelines for the evaluation and management of multi-organ system involvement. Genet Med 8(9):539–548
13. Banikazemi M, Desnick RJ (2006) Does enzyme replacement therapy improve symptoms of Fabry disease in patients undergoing dialysis? Nat Clin Pract Nephrol 2(2):72–73
14. Schiffmann R (2006) Neuropathy and Fabry disease: pathogenesis and enzyme replacement therapy. Acta Neurol Belg 106(2):61–65

15. Hopkin RJ, Bissler J, Banikazemi M et al (2008) Characterization of Fabry disease in 352 pediatric patients in the Fabry Registry. Pediatr Res 64(5):550–555
16. Ramaswami U, Whybra C, Parini R et al (2006) Clinical manifestations of Fabry disease in children: data from the Fabry Outcome Survey. FOS european investigators. Acta Paediatr 95(1):86–92
17. Zarate YA, Hopkin RJ (2008) Fabry's disease. Lancet 372(9647):1427–1435
18. Morgan SH, Rudge P, Smith SJ et al (1990) The neurological complications of Anderson-Fabry disease (α-galactosidase A deficiency)—investigation of symptomatic and pre-symptomatic patients. Q J Med 75:491–507
19. Morgan SH, Rudge P, Smith SJ et al (1990) The neurological complications of Anderson-Fabry disease (alpha-galactosidase A deficiency)—investigation of symptomatic and pre-symptomatic patients. Q J Med 75(277):491–507
20. Hilz MJ, Stemper B, Kolodny EH et al (2000) Lower limb cold exposure induces pain and prolonged small fiber dysfunction in Fabry patients. Pain 84(2–3):361–365
21. Brady RO, Schiffmann R (2000) Clinical features of and recent advances in therapy for Fabry disease. J Am Med Assoc 284(21):2771–2775
22. Hilz MJ, Brys M, Marthol H (2004) Enzyme replacement therapy improves function of C-, Adelta-, and Abeta-nerve fibers in Fabry neuropathy. Neurology 62(7):1066–1072
23. Ries M, Gupta S, Moore DF et al (2005) Pediatric Fabry disease. Pediatrics 115(3):e344–e355
24. Banikazemi M, Ullman T, Desnick RJ (2005) Gastrointestinal manifestations of Fabry disease: clinical response to enzyme replacement therapy. Mol Genet Metab 85(4):255–259
25. Hoffmann B, Reinhardt D, Koletzko B (2004) Effect of enzyme-replacement therapy on gastrointestinal symptoms in Fabry disease. Eur J Gastroenterol Hepatol 16(10):1067–1069
26. Schiller PI, Itin PH (1996) Angiokeratomas: an update. Dermatology 193:275–282
27. Lao LM, Kumakiri M, Mima H et al (1998) The ultrastructural characteristics of eccrine sweat glands in a Fabry disease patient with hypohidrosis. J Dermatol Sci 18(2):109–117
28. Desnick RJ, Banikazemi M (2003) Fabry disease: α-Galactosidase A deficiency (Angiokeratoma Corporis Diffusum Universale). In: Freedberg IM, Eisen AZ, Wolff K, Austen KF, Goldsmith LA, Katz SI (eds) Fitzpatrick's dermatology in general medicine, Chapter 151. McGraw Hill, New York, pp 1474–1486
29. Desnick RJ, Brady R, Barranger J, Collins AJ, Germain DP, Goldman M et al (2003) Fabry disease, an under-recognized multisystemic disorder: expert recommendations for diagnosis, management, and enzyme replacement therapy. Ann Intern Med 138(4):338–346
30. Yamamoto K, Sobue G, Iwase S et al (1996) Possible mechanism of anhidrosis in a symptomatic female carrier of Fabry's disease: an assessment by skin sympathetic nerve activity and sympathetic skin response. Clin Auton Res 6:107–110
31. Fumex-Boizard L, Cochat P, Fouilhoux A, Guffon N, Denis P (2005) Relation between ocular manifestations and organ involvement in ten patients with Fabry disease. J Fr Ophtalmol 28(1):45–50
32. Bennett RL, Hart KA, O'Rourke E et al (2002) Fabry disease in genetic counseling practice: recommendations of the National Society of Genetic Counselors. J Genet Couns 11(2):121–146

Chapter 23
Experimental Studies in Mice on the Vasculopathy of Fabry Disease

James A. Shayman

Abstract Understanding the basis for the vasculopathy associated with Fabry disease is an important challenge. The α-galactosidase A (Gla) knockout mouse has provided an important tool for the identification of experimental models that may phenocopy the human disease. Specifically, three in vivo models of vascular disease have been identified in the Gla null mouse. These models include oxidant induced thrombosis, accelerated atherogenesis, and impaired vascular reactivity. Aberrant endothelial cell function underlies the basis for these abnormalities. The characterization of these models has led to the identification of the uncoupling of endothelial nitric oxide synthase within the endothelium with the subsequent generation of reactive oxidant species as a likely mechanism underlying the vasculopathy of Fabry disease. More recent work in the exploration of the nexus between Gla deficiency and vasculopathy has followed from the establishment of an in vitro model of Fabry disease. In this chapter the development and characterization of these models is discussed and a model tying glycosphingolipid accumulation to eNOS uncoupling is proposed.

Keywords Fabry disease · Globotriaosylceramide · D-*threo*-ethylenedioxylphenyl-2-palmitoylamino-3-pyrrolidino-propanol · Endothelial nitric oxide synthase · Endothelium

23.1 Introduction

Significant interest has been generated in Fabry disease following the development, approval, and generalized use of recombinant α-galactosidase A (Gla). Enzyme replacement therapy presents specific challenges since it is highly expensive, and the important clinical outcomes, viz. stroke, heart disease, and renal failure are

J.A. Shayman (✉)
Department of Internal Medicine, University of Michigan, Ann Arbor, MI, USA
e-mail: jshayman@umich.edu

D. Elstein et al. (eds.), *Fabry Disease*, DOI 10.1007/978-90-481-9033-1_23,
© Springer Science+Business Media B.V. 2010

difficult to follow in the limited numbers of patients available for study. Because vascular complications are difficult to measure in small numbers of patients, the clinical benefits of recombinant Gla for Fabry disease have been difficult to prove. A particular challenge is establishing a benefit of enzyme replacement therapy for the vascular complications of Fabry disease because of a generally poor understanding of the mechanisms responsible for the vasculopathy resulting from Gla deficiency. Additionally, Gla deficiency, although rare, may provide a window on the basis for vascular disease that occurs in more common clinical settings.

Therefore, establishing the mechanistic basis for the vascular abnormalities in Fabry disease is a useful goal. The Gla knockout mouse has proven to be a useful model for probing the basis of the vascular defect associated with Gla deficiency. However, when initially described, the Gla knockout mouse had no obvious vascular phenotype. Recent studies have been reported demonstrating that this mouse has a number of inducible forms of vascular abnormalities. In this chapter, these studies are reviewed and a model explaining the vasculopathy associated with globotriaosylceramide (Gb3) accumulation is proposed.

23.2 Vascular Disease and Dysregulation in Humans with Fabry Disease

Vascular disease has long been recognized as an important complication of Fabry disease. In 2007 the baseline characteristics of 1,765 male and female patients in the Fabry disease registry were reported [1]. Cardiovascular events (arrhythmias, myocardial infarction, angina, congestive heart failure, and significant cardiac procedures) occurred in 19% of male patients and 14% of female patients with a mean age of onset of 39.0 and 47.6 respectively. Cerebrovascular events (stroke) were observed in 7% of male and 5% of female patients with a mean age of onset of 38.6 and 43.2. Viewed differently, the incidence of Fabry disease in patients under the age of 55 presenting with cryptogenic strokes is approximately 4%.

In theory the vasculopathy could be due to abnormalities in the coagulation system, blood components, or the vessel walls. For example, DeGraba and colleagues reported that Fabry patients are characterized by increased soluble sICAM-1, sVCAM-1, P-selectin, plasminogen activator inhibitor, and decreased thrombomodulin consistent with a prothrombotic state [2]. A number of studies by Moore, Schiffmann and colleagues have identified increased in cerebral perfusion, cerebral blood flow velocity, and cerebral vascular reactivity in Fabry disease [3–5]. Coronary vascular flow was measured by two groups using echocardiography and PET scanning and demonstrated to be significantly reduced in the Fabry population [6, 7]. Abnormalities in post-ischemia peripheral blood flow have also been reported [8].

The Schiffmann group has proposed that these abnormalities may be the result of excess reactive oxygen species (ROS) generation since both superoxide and peroxynitrite may cause dilation of the cerebral vasculature [3]. Because eNOS can be both the source and target of ROS, the mechanisms responsible for increased oxidant formation in Fabry disease remain unclear. Because Fabry disease has a low incidence, because the occurrence of vascular complications is rare, and because patients with Fabry disease have a heterogeneous clinical phenotype, clinical studies are limited in their ability to provide insight into the mechanisms responsible for the vasculopathy. Several years ago, our group began an effort to discern the basis for vascular abnormalities in Fabry disease. However, the Gla knockout mouse, although characterized by the age dependent accumulation of Gb3 in the vasculature, lacked a spontaneous vascular phenotype. We therefore asked whether inducible forms of vasculopathy may be associated with Gla deficiency.

23.3 Models of Vasculopathy in the Gla Knockout Mouse

23.3.1 Accelerated Thrombosis

A photochemical injury model was applied to Gla–/0 mice bred on a C57BL6/J background [9]. In this model the photochemical rose bengal is injected into the tail vein while the right carotid artery is exposed to a green laser light. Upon activation, toxic reactive oxygen species are released. The ensuing endothelial damage results in the formation of a platelet and thrombin rich thrombus at the site of injury. By continuous monitoring of the arterial flow, the time to occlusive thrombosis is measured. When Gla–/0 were compared to Gla+/0 mice no differences in baseline carotid blood flow were noted. However, a marked age dependent shortening of the time to occlusion was observed. This thrombosis correlated with the age dependent accumulation of Gb3 within the vascular wall (Fig. 23.1).

Because blood cells, including platelets express glycosphingolipids with terminal gal-α 1,4-gal linkages, we wished to ascertain whether the pro-thrombotic defect was due to a change in the vascular wall or to a circulating blood element. Bone marrow transplantation was performed on Gla+/0 and Gla–/0 mice. Each group of recipients received Gla+/0 or Gla–/0 bone marrow. Six weeks after transplantation and following engraftment, the mice were studied for rose bengal induced carotid occlusion. It was observed that the host retained the thrombotic phenotype regardless of the source of the bone marrow. In other words, the Gla–/0 mice displayed markedly reduced time to thrombosis regardless of whether they received Gla–/0 or Gla+/0 bone marrow. We concluded that the pro-thrombotic phenotype was based on a change in the vascular wall and was not due to an abnormality in circulating cells.

The possibility that Gla deficiency could interact with other genetic predispositions to thrombosis was also considered. Factor V Leiden (FVL) deficiency is a common genetic factor in the propensity to stroke. When Gla–/0 mice were bred on a FVL null background, fibrin deposition was noted to be markedly increased

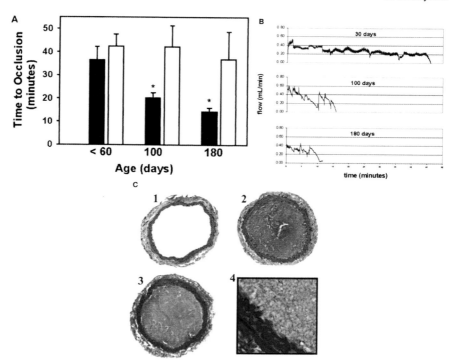

Fig. 23.1 Effect of age on thrombosis in Fabry mice. (**a**) With increasing age, the time to occlusive carotid thrombosis progressively shortens in Fabry mice (*filled bar*); $n = 12, 8$, and 6 for ages <60, 100, and 180 d, respectively (*$p < 0.05$ compared with age-matched wild-type mice), whereas occlusion times in wild-type mice (*open bar*) are not affected by age; $n = 8, 4$, and 4 respectively. (**b**) Representative compressed carotid blood flow tracings from Fabry mice of various ages. (**c**) Histology of carotid artery. Sections harvested from perfusion fixed mouse carotid arteries 50 min after the onset of photochemical injury. *Panel 1* is a Masson trichrome stain demonstrating the widely patent uninjured left carotid artery (×200). *Panel 2* is a Masson trichrome stain demonstrating occlusive thrombosis in the injured right carotid artery (×200). *Panels 3* and *4* are low-power (×200) and high-power (x1,000) views of an injured section stained with Carstairs stain. No differences were noted in the appearance of the cross-sections between the groups (Reprinted with the permission of the American Society of Nephrology)

[10]. While only a limited number of mice were bred and followed, spontaneous thrombosis did occur in a Gla–/–, FVL–/– mouse.

23.3.2 Atherogenesis

To ascertain whether Gla null were more susceptible to atherogenesis, Gla–/0 and Gla+/0 mice were bred on an ApoE–/– background [11]. Forty-one week old mice were then subjected to 4 weeks of feeding with Western chow. At 45 weeks of age the mice were euthanized and their thoracic and abdominal aortas along with the major arterial branches were dissected. The lesion areas of the arterial trees were measured following staining with oil red O. Under these conditions, both male and female Gla null, ApoE null mice (*Gla–/0, ApoE–/–* and *Gla–/–, ApoE–/–*) had significantly greater lesion areas than did normal mice on the ApoE null background (*Gla+/0, ApoE–/–* and *Gla+/+, ApoE–/–*). Gla heterozygous mice displayed and intermediary phenotype. Aortic staining for iNOS and nitrotyrosine was marked increased in the *Gla–/0* and *Gla–/–* mice, consistent with the increased production of ROS.

23.3.3 *Impaired Vasoreactivity*

The inducible models of thrombosis and atherogenesis were consistent with Gla deficient abnormalities localized to the arterial wall. To ascertain whether the defects were attributable to global vascular abnormalities or confined to the endothelium, another model of vascular function was evaluated [12]. Isometric force measurements were conducted in either carotid or aortic vascular rings of Gla+/+ and Gla–/0 mice to assess responsiveness to known vasoconstrictors and vasodilators. A complex pattern of responsiveness was observed in this model. When vasocontractility was measured in response to a series of agonists, Gla–/0 aortic rings were observed to have impaired responsiveness to phenylephrine and serotonin as measured by both the half maximal effective concentration ($-\log EC_{50}$) and maximal contraction (E_{max}). By contrast, contraction to the thromboxane receptor agonist U46619 was minimally different between the Gla+/+ and Gla–/0 aortic rings. The differences in responses to these agonists was blunted but not abolished by preincubation with the nitric oxide synthase inhibitor N^G-nitro-L-arginine. However, the differences were largely abolished in endothelium denuded rings.

When aortic rings were precontracted to 80% of maximum with phenylephrine and then exposed to acetylcholine, the relaxation response was markedly impaired in the Gla–/0 rings compared to those from Gla+/0 mice. The relaxation response was eliminated with N^G-nitro-L-arginine pretreatment or in endothelium denuded rings. These observations were consistent with impaired nitric oxide generation from the endothelium of the Gla–/0 mice. When exposed to sodium nitroprusside, no difference in vasorelaxation was observed, consistent with the interpretation that this difference was secondary to a change in nitric oxide generation (Fig. 23.2).

To further confirm that this was a plasma membrane, endothelium dependent phenomenon, ionomycin induced vasorelaxation was studied by infusing the calcium ionophore into the luminal area of the rings. Under these conditions only the endothelial cells are exposed to the calcium flux and an observed calcium stimulated vasorelaxation can be observed. Ionomycin induced calcium relaxation was no different between the Gla+/0 and Gla–/0 mice suggesting that the acetylcholine based difference was plasma membrane based (Fig. 23.3).

Fig. 23.2 Acetylcholine-mediated endothelium dependent relaxation in endothelium. Intact aortic rings from wild type (Gla+/0, *closed symbols*) or knockout (Gla–/0, *open symbols*) mice were studied. Data are expressed as a percentage of the contraction elicited by the EC80 for phenylephrine and show the mean +/– SEM for five to seven animals. *denotes $p < 0.05$ compared with Gla+/0 using two way ANOVA followed by Bonferoni's post hoc test. (**a**) Rings treated alone without any pharmacologic intervention, (**b**) rings treated in the presence of 10^{-4} mol/l N^G-nitro-L-arginine. (**c**) Endothelium denuded rings (Reprinted with the permission of John Wiley and Sons, Ltd.)

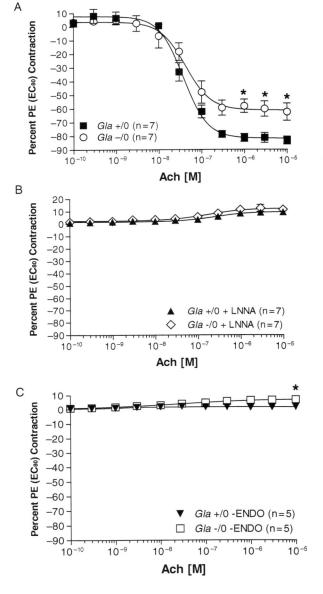

23.3.4 eNOS Dysregulation as the Common Link in the Three Models of Vasculopathy

Three independent models of vasculopathy have thus been identified in the Gla null mouse but each may arise from a common mechanism. Based on the bone

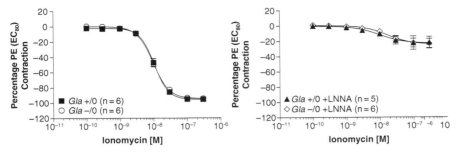

Fig. 23.3 Ionomycin-induced endothelial nitric oxide dependent relaxation in endothelium intact rings. Studied were aortic rings from Gla+/0 (*closed symbols*) and Gla–/0 (*open symbols*) mice. The rings were precontracted with and EC80 concentration of phenylephrine. (**a**) Alone without pharmacologic intervention. (**b**) In the presence of 10^{-4} mol/l N^G-nitro-L-arginine. Data represent the mean +/– SEM (Reprinted with the permission of John Wiley and Sons, Ltd.)

marrow transplantation studies in the rose bengal model and the observed atherogenesis, these models are consistent with a blood vessel based defect. Based also on the endothelium dependent abnormalities in vasorelaxation and vasoconstriction, these abnormalities are in large part secondary to an endothelium based defect. Finally, based on the ability to abolish the differences in the vasorelaxation response with either sodium nitroprusside or ionomycin, the defect appears to be plasma membrane based.

The accelerated thrombosis, enhanced atherogenesis, and impaired vasorelaxation are each potentially explainable based on dysregulation of endothelial nitric oxide synthase (eNOS) with impaired in nitric oxide generation. Thrombosis, atherogenesis, and impaired relaxation responses are each associated with eNOS uncoupling. But under basal conditions, eNOS is localized to the plasma membrane. How could the lysosomal accumulation result in a loss of eNOS activity?

23.4 Glycolipid Localization in Endothelial Cells

To further understand the role of Gb3 accumulation in the dysregulation of signaling at the endothelial cell plasma membrane, a model endothelial cell system was established [13]. Conditions for the establishment of mouse aortic endothelial cells were determined, and these cells were characterized and compared between Gla+/0 and Gla–/0 mice. The cultured cells retained an endothelial phenotype with prolonged culture (e.g. acetylated-LDL binding) and the Gla–/0 cells were characterized by persistently elevated Gb3 levels. The Gb3 content increased as a function of the age of the Gla–/0 mice from which they were derived.

Using this model we then assessed whether the content of Gb3 and of other globo series glycosphingolipids was increased in the plasma membrane in addition to the lysosomes [14]. Gb3 and Gb4 levels increased in both the plasma membrane and caveolar fractions of the Gla–/0 endothelial cells as a function of the age.

A corresponding decrease in caveolar cholesterol was measured in parallel with the increase in these glycolipids. When the Gb3 depletion was measured following treatment with either recombinant Gla or the glucosylceramide synthase inhibitor D-*threo*-ethylenedioxyphenyl-P4 [15–17], a difference in the degree of depletion and persistence with the removal of the agents was noted. The synthase inhibitor induced a greater and more persistent degree of Gb3 depletion.

Thus there were three noteworthy findings in this study. First, Gb3 and G4 accumulation in the Gla–/0 endothelial cells was present in the plasma membrane and caveolar fractions in addition to the plasma membrane. Second, the content of other caveolar lipids changed as Gb3 levels increased. Specifically, caveolar cholesterol was displaced. Third, changes in caveolar glycolipids and cholesterol during and following depletion with a synthase inhibitor of catabolic enzyme were highly dynamic. These data supported the concept that endothelial dysfunction in the setting of Gla deficiency might result from changes within the plasma and caveolar membranes.

23.5 eNOS Activity and Regulation in Fabry Endothelia

23.5.1 Treatment of Gla–/0 Mice with D-Threo-Ethylenedioxyphenyl-P4

With these tools in hand a more detailed study of the basis for decreased nitric oxide bioavailability in the Gla null mouse was pursued [18]. Two common causes of decreased bioavailability are changes in the expression or activity of eNOS and eNOS uncoupling. To determine whether aortic Gb3 depletion in the Gla null mice would reverse the defect in vasoregulation, Gla–/0 mice were treated with 10 mg/kg D-*threo*-ethylenedioxyphenyl-P4 daily for 28 days. Aortic Gb3 levels were normalized following treatment as assessed by biotinylated shigatoxin binding and staining. However, the impaired responsiveness of the aortic rings to acetylcholine was only partially reversed.

23.5.2 Decreased eNOS and Caveolin-1 in Gla Null Mouse Aortas

The expression of caveolin-1 and eNOS was next studied in the aortas of Gla+/0 and Gla–/0 mice. An age dependent decrease in both caveolin-1- and eNOS was observed in the Gla–/0 mice. In particular, the levels of high molecular weight caveolin-1 oligomers was markedly decreased in 8, 12, and 16 month old Gla null compared to wild type aortas. Co-immunoprecipitation studies of caveolin-1 and eNOS demonstrated that the interactions between the two proteins was preserved raising the possibility that the decrease in eNOS was secondary to lower levels of caveolin-1.

23.5.3 *Impaired eNOS Activity*

Direct measurements of eNOS expression and activity were next made utilizing the aortic endothelial cell system. Consistent with the immunoblotting studies in whole aorta, a marked decrease in eNOS levels was noted in the cultured cells. This decrement was reversed, albeit partially following Gb3 depletion with inhibition of glucosylceramide synthase. A concomitant decrease in insulin stimulated eNOS activity as measured by tritiated citrulline formation was observed which also was only partially reversed by use of the inhibitor. Caveolin-1 monomers and high molecular weight oligomers were then measured. Although monomeric caveolin-1 was not significantly lower in the cultured cells, the 250 and 400 kDa oligomeric forms of caveolin-1 were decreased in the Gla–/0 cells. Gb3 depletion with D-*threo*-ethylenedioxyphenyl-P4 only partially restored the high molecular weight caveolin-1.

Caveolar eNOS and caveolin-1 levels were next measured. High molecular weight oligomeric and monomeric caveolin-1 was reduced in the caveolar fractions and was again only partially restored with Gb3 depletion. By contrast, eNOS was undetectable in the Gla–/0 caveolae and was persistent absent even with the restoration of normal Gb3 levels. Thus the decrease in nitric oxide bioavailability could be explained in part based on the low expression of eNOS at it normal site of activity.

23.5.4 *Oxidant Formation Secondary to eNOS Uncoupling*

We next sought to determine whether the alteration in eNOS activity is accompanied by an uncoupling of the enzyme. Uncoupling of eNOS results in formation of the highly reactive oxidant peroxynitrite, a compound that forms when nitric oxide reacts with superoxide. Previous studies have demonstrated that *ortho*-tyrosine and nitrotyrosine are markers of peroxynitrite mediated oxidation. To determine whether proteins from endothelial cells contain oxidized amino acid products of peroxynitrite oxidation, we isolated endothelial cells from Gla+/0 and Gla–/0 mice. After delipidating the cells and hydrolysis with acid, amino acids were isolated as described in the proposal. We then determined the content of the two oxidized amino acids, *ortho*-tyrosine and 3-nitrotyrosine. These are 'molecular signatures' characteristic of peroxynitrite mediated oxidation by isotope dilution liquid chromatography tandem mass spectrometry. The samples from the endothelial cells of Gla–/0 animals contained 90% more *ortho*-tyrosine than those from the control animals (Gla–/0, 63.8 ± 8.6 μmol/mol phenylalanine (the precursor of *ortho*-tyrosine); control, 33.7 ± 3 μmol/mol phenylalanine; $n = 3$ per group). Similarly, levels of nitrotyrosine were 72% greater in the Gla–/0 endothelial cells (Gla–/0, 93.7 ± 18.6 μmol/mol tyrosine (the precursor of nitrotyrosine); control, 54.37 ± 1.4 μmol/mol tyrosine; $n = 3$ per group). The marked elevation of both of these oxidized amino acids is consistent with peroxynitrite oxidation of proteins in the endothelial cells. We also demonstrated that the increase in *ortho*-tyrosine and nitrotyrosine were not corrected when cells Gb3 levels in the cells are normalized with treatment with D-*threo*-ethylenedioxyphenyl-P4. These observations strongly support the hypothesis that the eNOS becomes uncoupled in this model.

23.6 A Proposed Model for eNOS Uncoupling

Caveolae are small, uncoated pits in the plasma membrane. They are an abundant feature of endothelial cells. Caveolae are defined by the presence of caveolins. They are considered to be a form of lipid raft. Cholesterol and sphingolipids are critical components of lipid rafts and at least the former lipid is believed to be critical for caveolus formation. Caveolin-1 is clearly critical for caveolus formation since the expression of caveolin-1 in cells normally lacking the protein results in the formation of caveolae. Similarly, the experimental loss of caveolin-1 results in the loss of caveolae. Approximately 100–200 caveolin molecules are present in each caveolus, most in an oligomeric form [19]. Caveolins are synthesized on the rough endoplasmic reticulum and transit through the Golgi complex prior to trafficking to the plasma membrane. At some point during this synthetic route, caveolins change from a monomeric form to an oligomeric form. Studies utilizing a caveolin-1-GFP fusion construct are consistent with the formation of the caveolae in the Golgi complex [20]. Cholesterol appears to be important for this process [21]. The addition of cholesterol appears to decrease the transit time through the Golgi complex [22]. Cholesterol binds directly to caveolin-1 as demonstrated by photoactivatable crosslinking studies, plasma membrane cholesterol enrichment in cells expressing caveolin-1, and numerous structural studies defining cholesterol binding motifs.

The association of eNOS through palmitoylation and myristoylation sites appears to depend on the lipid composition of the caveolae [23, 24]. The importance of caveolar lipid is based on studies restricted to evaluating the role of cholesterol in caveolae. Cholesterol depletion with cyclodextrin or HDL or cholesterol displacement with oxidized LDL lowers eNOS activity by redistribution of eNOS from caveolae [25]. However, the role of other caveolar lipid components in eNOS redistribution, most notably sphingomyelin and glycosphingolipids such as Gb3, is unknown.

Based on the known properties of caveolae and the observed dysregulation of eNOS in the Gla null mouse, a testable model of relating the accumulation of Gb3 to aberrant eNOS regulation can be proposed (Fig. 23.4). In this model the co-assembly of caveolin oligomers and eNOS is dependent upon the appropriate molar ratio of cholesterol and other sphingolipids including Gb3. Under conditions of excess Gb3 proper assembly does not occur and eNOS is not appropriately trafficked to the caveolar lipid raft domain of the endothelial cells. Improper eNOS localization results in both a decrement in nitric oxide production in addition to eNOS uncoupling. The former change results in impaired vasorelaxation and increased risk of thrombosis and atherogenesis. The latter change leads to the formation of ROS including peroxynitrite with secondary changes due to the oxidation of important target proteins and cofactors within the endothelium.

GLA+/0 CAVEOLAE   GLA-/0 CAVEOLAE

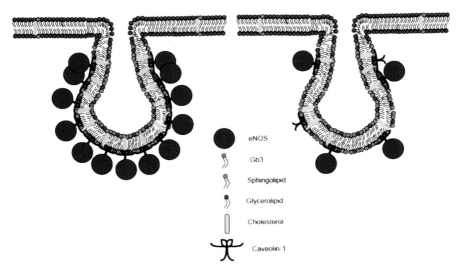

eNOS

Gb3

Sphingolipid

Glycerolipid

Cholesterol

Caveolin-1

Fig. 23.4 A proposed model for eNOS uncoupling in the presence of Gla deficiency. Under conditions where Gb3 metabolism is normal, endothelial cell caveolar lipid content is characterized by a high molar ratio of cholesterol and sphingolipids and low molar content of glycerophospholipids. Caveolin-1 oligomerization is present due to caveolin-1 cholesterol and/or caveolin-1 glycosphingolipid interactions and eNOS binding is intact. Under conditions of Gla deficiency and increased cellular Gb3, endothelial cell caveolar lipid content is characterized by a high molar ratio of Gb3 with secondary displacement of cholesterol and other glycosphingolipids. Under these conditions caveolin-1 oligomerization is impaired resulting in the presence of monomeric caveolin-1 with secondary loss of eNOS binding

23.7 Future Directions and Challenges

The Gla knockout mouse provides a potentially valuable portal to understanding the basis of vasculopathy in Fabry disease. Although three primary models of vasculopathy have been identified in this model, others are undoubtedly yet to be discovered. While a decrease in nitric oxide bioavailability may partly account for the differences in the Gla–/0 and Gla+/0 mice, other mechanisms are likely to be important as well. For example, impaired nitric oxide formation alone can not account for the differences in responses to vasoconstrictive agonists.

Several mechanisms can account for eNOS uncoupling. These include loss of (6R)-5,6,7,8-tetrahydro-L-biopterin (BH4) due to its oxidation or dihydrofolate reductase deficiency. The latter is observed in the setting of angiotensin II overproduction. In addition, eNOS itself can be the target of oxidants resulting from excess superoxide production from mitochondria and NADPH oxidase. These alternative causes of eNOS uncoupling have yet to be studied.

While impaired eNOS expression and trafficking to caveolae in addition to eNOS uncoupling may explain much of the loss of nitric oxide, other causes of decreased NO bioavailability have yet to be explored. These include the enhanced breakdown of nitric oxide and impaired transmission of nitric oxide signaling.

The precise mechanisms whereby changes in membrane lipid content and more specifically caveolar lipid content result in loss of eNOS activity remain to be elucidated. Presently, we do not know whether it is the excess presence of Gb3 or a related lipid or the displacement of other lipids such as cholesterol that accounts for the pathophysiology. Undoubtedly these lipids are important for the structural and functional basis of cell signaling at the level of the caveolus either through appropriate assembly and trafficking or the dynamic regulation of signaling molecules. The Fabry mouse should provide fertile ground for the study of these mechanisms.

References

1. Eng CM, Fletcher J, Wilcox WR, Waldek S, Scott CR, Sillence DO, Breunig F, Charrow J, Germain DP, Nicholls K, Banikazemi M (2007) Fabry disease: baseline medical characteristics of a cohort of 1765 males and females in the Fabry Registry. J Inherit Metab Dis 30:184–192
2. DeGraba T, Azhar S, Dignat-George F, Brown E, Boutiere B, Altarescu G, McCarron R, Schiffmann R (2000) Profile of endothelial and leukocyte activation in Fabry patients. Ann Neurol 47:229–233
3. Moore DF, Scott LT, Gladwin MT, Altarescu G, Kaneski C, Suzuki K, Pease-Fye M, Ferri R, Brady RO, Herscovitch P, Schiffmann R (2001) Regional cerebral hyperperfusion and nitric oxide pathway dysregulation in Fabry disease: reversal by enzyme replacement therapy. Circulation 104:1506–1512
4. Moore DF, Herscovitch P, Schiffmann R (2001) Selective arterial distribution of cerebral hyperperfusion in Fabry disease. J Neuroimaging 11:303–307
5. Altarescu G, Moore DF, Pursley R, Campia U, Goldstein S, Bryant M, Panza JA, Schiffmann R (2001) Enhanced endothelium-dependent vasodilation in Fabry disease. Stroke 32:1559–1562
6. Elliott PM, Kindler H, Shah JS, Sachdev B, Rimoldi OE, Thaman R, Tome MT, McKenna WJ, Lee P, Camici PG (2006) Coronary microvascular dysfunction in male patients with Anderson-Fabry disease and the effect of treatment with alpha galactosidase A. Heart 92:357–360
7. Dimitrow PP, Krzanowski M, Undas A (2005) Reduced coronary flow reserve in Anderson-Fabry disease measured by transthoracic Doppler echocardiography. Cardiovasc Ultrasound 3:11
8. Stemper B, Hilz MJ (2003) Postischemic cutaneous hyperperfusion in the presence of forearm hypoperfusion suggests sympathetic vasomotor dysfunction in Fabry disease. J Neurol 250:970–976
9. Eitzman DT, Bodary PF, Shen Y, Khairallah CG, Wild SR, Abe A, Shaffer-Hartman J, Shayman JA (2003) Fabry disease in mice is associated with age-dependent susceptibility to vascular thrombosis. J Am Soc Nephrol 14:298–302
10. Shen Y, Bodary PF, Vargas FB, Homeister JW, Gordon D, Ostenso KA, Shayman JA, Eitzman DT (2006) Alpha-galactosidase A deficiency leads to increased tissue fibrin deposition and thrombosis in mice homozygous for the factor V Leiden mutation. Stroke 37:1106–1108
11. Bodary PF, Shen Y, Vargas FB, Bi X, Ostenso KA, Gu S, Shayman JA, Eitzman DT (2005) Alpha-galactosidase A deficiency accelerates atherosclerosis in mice with apolipoprotein E deficiency. Circulation 111:629–632

12. Park JL, Whitesall SE, D'Alecy LG, Shu L, Shayman JA (2008) Vascular dysfunction in the alpha-galactosidase A-knockout mouse is an endothelial cell-, plasma membrane-based defect. Clin Exp Pharmacol Physiol 35:1156–1163
13. Shu L, Murphy HS, Cooling L, Shayman JA (2005) An in vitro model of Fabry disease. J Am Soc Nephrol 16:2636–2645
14. Shu L, Shayman JA (2007) Caveolin-associated accumulation of globotriaosylceramide in the vascular endothelium of alpha-galactosidase A null mice. J Biol Chem 282:20960–20967
15. Lee L, Abe A, Shayman JA (1999) Improved inhibitors of glucosylceramide synthase. J Biol Chem 274:14662–14669
16. Abe A, Arend LJ, Lee L, Lingwood C, Brady RO, Shayman JA (2000) Glycosphingolipid depletion in fabry disease lymphoblasts with potent inhibitors of glucosylceramide synthase. Kidney Int 57:446–454
17. Abe A, Gregory S, Lee L, Killen PD, Brady RO, Kulkarni A, Shayman JA (2000) Reduction of globotriaosylceramide in Fabry disease mice by substrate deprivation. J Clin Invest 105:1563–1571
18. Shu L, Park JL, Byun J, Pennathur S, Kollmeyer J, Shayman JA (2009) Decreased nitric oxide bioavailability in a mouse model of Fabry disease. J Am Soc Nephrol 20(9):1975–1985
19. Parton RG, Hanzal-Bayer M, Hancock JF (2006) Biogenesis of caveolae: a structural model for caveolin-induced domain formation. J Cell Sci 119:787–796
20. Tagawa A, Mezzacasa A, Hayer A, Longatti A, Pelkmans L, Helenius A (2005) Assembly and trafficking of caveolar domains in the cell: caveolae as stable, cargo-triggered, vesicular transporters. J Cell Biol 170:769–779
21. Monier S, Dietzen DJ, Hastings WR, Lublin DM, Kurzchalia TV (1996) Oligomerization of VIP21-caveolin in vitro is stabilized by long chain fatty acylation or cholesterol. FEBS Lett 388:143–149
22. Pol A, Martin S, Fernandez MA, Ingelmo-Torres M, Ferguson C, Enrich C, Parton RG (2005) Cholesterol and fatty acids regulate dynamic caveolin trafficking through the Golgi complex and between the cell surface and lipid bodies. Mol Biol Cell 16:2091–2105
23. Liu J, Garcia-Cardena G, Sessa WC (1996) Palmitoylation of endothelial nitric oxide synthase is necessary for optimal stimulated release of nitric oxide: implications for caveolae localization. Biochemistry 35:13277–13281
24. Robinson LJ, Michel T (1995) Mutagenesis of palmitoylation sites in endothelial nitric oxide synthase identifies a novel motif for dual acylation and subcellular targeting. Proc Natl Acad Sci USA 92:11776–11780
25. Shaul PW (2002) Regulation of endothelial nitric oxide synthase: location, location, location. Annu Rev Physiol 64:749–774

Part III
Management

Chapter 24
Overview

Michael Beck

Abstract In the last years, much progress has been achieved in the field of lysosomal storage disorders. In the past no specific treatment was available for the affected patients, management mainly consisted of supportive care and treatment of complications. The situation promptly changed, however, when so-called orphan drug regulations, at first in the United States, thereafter also in Europe, heartened the pharmaceutical industry to develop drugs for rare disorders by providing the companies with commercial benefits, for example by giving marketing exclusivity for 10 years. And thereafter within a few years enzyme replacement therapy became available for the lysosomal storage disorders Gaucher disease, Fabry disease, mucopolysaccharidoses type I, II and VI and Pompe disease. In addition, new therapeutic drugs such as substrate inibitors and chaperones have been developed. This review will summarize the efficacy and limitations of enzyme replacement in Fabry disease. New therapeutic perspectives currently under preclinical investigations such as chaperone-mediated and gene therapy will also be discussed.

Keywords Chaperone · Enzyme replacement therapy · Gene therapy · Limitation

24.1 Enzyme Replacement Therapy

24.1.1 Clinical Trials

The pathophysiology of Fabry disease is very different from that of Gaucher disease although it belongs to the group of glycosphongolipidoses. In Gaucher disease, the accumulation of the storage material is restricted to macrophages that are easily accessible to intravenously administered enzyme. However, in Fabry disease

M. Beck (✉)
Children's Hospital, University of Mainz, Mainz, Germany
e-mail: Dr.M.Beck@t-online.de

D. Elstein et al. (eds.), *Fabry Disease*, DOI 10.1007/978-90-481-9033-1_24,
© Springer Science+Business Media B.V. 2010

multiple cell types are affected leading to clinical manifestation of several organs. Although the storage process in endothelial cells plays an essential role in the pathophysiology of Fabry disease, the clinical picture cannot be explained solely by the accumulation of Gb3 in this cell type. And as enzyme replacement therapy should reach also the kidney, heart and other target organs to be successful, the pharmacodynamics of ERT for Fabry disease differ significantly from those for Gaucher disease. This was one of the reasons why it has been difficult to create study protocols that would enable to examine the efficacy of a study drug in a small number of patients within a relatively short time frame. And in addition, as onset and severity of signs and symptoms are quite variable in Fabry disease, one would need many years and a large number of patients in order to prove the efficacy of a newly developed enzyme preparation by using these clinical signs as an endpoint for clinical trials.

As an alternative to a clinical parameter a biomarker may be used in clinical trials. Biomarkers are analytical tools that reflect the presence of a given disease (diagnostic biomarker). The concentration of a biomarker should also correlate directly with disease severity and should indicate the response to treatment. Two types of biomarkers have to be differentiated in lysosomal storage disorders: The first group is comprised of those substances that show an increased concentration as a result of the underlying defective lysosomal function. Examples are the increased urinary excretion of glycosaminoglycans (GAGs) in mucopolysaccharidoses or of globotriaosylceramide (Gb_3) in Fabry disease. The second group includes biomarkers that are related to the lysosomal defect in an indirect way: These biomarkers reflect the effects of the primary metabolic defect on cell, tissue or organ function. An example is the increased activity of the enzyme chitotriosidase in patients with Gaucher disease. As in Fabry disease the concentration of globotriaosylceramide (Gb3) is elevated in plasma and urine of affected patients, this glycolipid may be used as a diagnostic tool, particularly in hemizygote males.

The usefulness of a biomarker as an alternative for a clinical parameter has been shown in the study that has been performed by Eng et al. [1]: The clearance of microvascular endothelial deposits of storage material Gb3 from the kidney, heart, and skin served as a biomarker: Those patients, who were treated with the recombinant enzyme agalsidase beta did not show any microvascular endothelial deposits of globotriaosylceramide in renal biopsies after treatment, as compared with none of the 29 patients in the placebo group ($P < 0.001$). Patients in the treatment group also had decreased microvascular endothelial deposits of globotriaosylceramide in the skin and heart. The clinical efficacy of recombinant α-galactosidase has been demonstrated in clinical trials and observational studies [2–4].

In a double-blind, placebo-controlled clinical trial, performed by Schiffmann and colleagues, the level of pain was chosen as a clinical endpoint in order to prove the efficacy of the recombinant enzyme agalsidase alfa. In this study it could be demonstrated that in patients treated with the enzyme mean neuropathic pain, measured by the Brief Pain Inventory (BPI), significantly declined from 6.2 to 4.3, whereas no significant change was seen in the placebo group ($P = 0.02$) [5]. The analysis of the latest reports regarding the clinical efficacy and tolerability of agalsidase alfa in patients with Fabry disease have demonstrated that this enzyme preparation is effective in treating pain and to improve hearing, sweating and quality of life [6]. It is able reduce left ventricular mass index and to stabilize kidney function and slow down progression of renal failure in patients with endstage renal disease [7, 8].

24.1.2 Limitations

In spite of the encouraging clinical results that have been observed in clinical trials of enzyme replacement therapy, it has become clear very soon that this therapeutic approach has some limitations and is not able to treat all aspects of the disorders equally. The efficacy of enzyme replacement therapy is partially reduced for example by the fact that exogenously administered enzymes lead to the formation of antibodies that may be followed by different responses: Hypersensitivity reactions may occur, but are very rare. The antibody may lead to reduced bioavailability of the enzyme or finally may neutralize the activity of the protein abolishing the clinical efficacy [9].

In some lysosomal storage disorders enzyme replacement therapy does not have an effect anymore as specific organs are irreversibly damaged, for example the kidney in the late stage of Fabry disease: Schiffmann et al. have reported that Fabry patients with stage III renal disease showed a decline of glomerular filtration rate despite long term enzyme replacement therapy [10].

Some limitations of enzyme replacement therapy are possibly due to the timing of therapy, and early therapeutic intervention may be more efficient [4]. In order to start treatment as soon as possible newborn screening programmes for lysosomal storage disorder have been developed [11, 12]. However, as for most of these conditions a strict genotype-phenotype correlation does not exist, the screening programmes will probably not be generally introduced until the phenotype from the newborn result can be exactly predicted.

Finally, it should be mentioned that the availability of the enzyme preparations is limited as not both drugs have got marketing approval in all countries. For example, in the United States until now only Fabrazyme, and not Replagal is available. This situation implies a vulnerable position for some patients with Fabry disease as they had to be withdrawn from therapy if the only drug that they can get in their country cannot be supplied anymore due to production problems. And West and LeMoine [13] have shown that withdrawal of ERT from patients with Fabry disease for 9 months leads to a significant decline in renal function.

24.2 Chaperones

To become active, each newly synthesized enzyme has to be folded in a very specific manner. The correct folding is controlled by a machinery that involves the ubiquitin system, proteosomes and so-called chaperones. Under physiological conditions, chaperones restore the native confirmation of misfolded proteins. It has been estimated that up to 30% of normal proteins do not become functionally active, but misfold and/or aggregate and are rapidly (within minutes) degraded by the cell's quality control machinery [14]. In genetic disorders, certain missense mutations and some small in-frame deletions may cause polypeptide misfolding, but may not (or only slightly) impair the functionally essential domains of the mutant protein (the active site, receptor-binding site, etc.). And it could be demonstrated that pharmacological chaperones, such as substrate analogues, are able to stabilize misfolded proteins and to increase enzyme activity.

Considering that galactose, a nontoxic reversible competitive inhibitor of α-galactosidase may enhance the residual activity of a mutant enzyme, Frustaci et al. conducted a study in a male Fabry patient with predominant cardiac manifestation. After it has been observed that three daily galactose infusions increased α-galactosidase activity in the patient's lymphocytes and endomyocardial cells, galactose infusions were given every other day. The infusions were well tolerated, and a reduction in cardiac mass and an improvement in cardiac function were documented after 2 years of treatment [15].

In the last years it has been found that imino-sugars such as deoxynojirimycin-analogues do not only act as enzyme inhibitors but also serve as a chemical chaperone. Yam et al. have added 1-deoxygalactonojirimycin (DGJ, migalastat hydrochloride, AT1001) to Fabry fibroblast cell lines with missense mutations (R301Q and Q357X) which showed extensive lysosomal Gb3 accumulation. After treatment for up to 100 days a significant reduction or even a disappearance of lysosomal Gb3 was observed [16].

Ishii et al. studied the preclinical efficacy and safety of 1-deoxygalactonojirimycin (DGJ) in a mouse model of Fabry disease. After 2 weeks of treatment the activity of mutant α-galactosidase increased in heart, kidney, spleen and liver. Globotriaosylceramide storage was reduced in kidney. No change in life span was observed during a 2-year period of continuous administration of 1-Deoxygalactonojirimycin at the effective dosage [17].

The effect of 1-deoxygalactonojirimycin (DGJ) on α-galactosidase levels was analyzed in cultured lymphoblasts and fibroblasts from males with Fabry disease in order to identify DGJ-responsive mutant forms of α-galactosidase [18]. After continuous DGJ incubation for 5 days a significant in enzyme levels was seen for 49 different missense mutant forms. In responsive fibroblasts elevated Gb3 levels were reduced after 1-deoxygalactonojirimycin (DGJ) incubation.

After animal studies have provided promising results, a clinical trial of the chaperone AT1001 has been initiated. First results of this trial were reported at the 58th Annual Meeting of the American Society of Human Genetics [19]: The drug was generally well-tolerated, 24 of the 26 patients (males and females) have shown an increase in α-galactosidase level in several cells and tissues. Urinary Gb3 decreased in subjects who demonstrated a significant increase in enzyme activity. Also an improvement of renal and heart function was observed. Based on these data, further investigations of AT1001 as a potential therapy are planned.

24.3 Gene Therapy

As described above, enzyme replacement therapy has become a therapeutic option for some lysosomal storage disorders, but has been shown to be of limited efficacy, especially regarding the effect on kidney and central nervous system manifestation. Furthermore, recurring administration of an exogenous protein bears the risk of inducing an immune response that may interfere with the therapeutic enzyme or even neutralize its activity. Gene-based therapy may overcome this problem, as it may allow constant delivery of a therapeutic protein to the whole body or to targeted organs. Lysosomal storage disorders are excellent candidates for therapy by gene transfer for several reasons [20]. First of all, they represent generally well-characterized single gene disorders. Furthermore they are not subject to complex regulation mechanisms, and an enzyme activity of only 15–20% of the normal level is sufficient for clinical efficacy.

There are two ways to deliver a gene into the organism, the in-vivo and the ex-vivo technique.

24.3.1 In Vivo Gene Therapy

As a depot organ the lung or liver have been used to establish a sustained source of therapeutic enzyme within the body for metabolic correction in peripheral organs. In animal experiments several vehicles such as adenoviral adeno-associated, retroviral and lentiviral vectors were used for efficient organ transduction. By this strategy, the transduced organs produced large amounts of therapeutic enzyme that was secreted into the bloodstream and recaptured by the target organs by the mannose-6-phosphate receptor. The efficacy of this technique has been demonstrated in several animal models. In the mouse model of Fabry disease it could be demonstrated that biochemical and functional abnormalities can be corrected by gene therapy using various delivery systems. The therapeutic efficay, however, is influenced by factors such as route of vector administration, choice of the vector and promotor and the sex of the mice.

Li and co-workers used the lung as a depot organ for delivering α-galactosidase into the heart and kidney of mice affected by Fabry disease [21]. Long-term analysis of several gene transfer experiments has shown the occurrence of immune response leading to clearance of the transduced cells and/or loss of enzyme activity [22]. However, it could be demonstrated that the immune response may be prevented by using hepatocyte-specific promoters that restrict transgene expression to parenchymal cells of the liver and avoid transgene expression within antigen-presenting cells [23].

Considering that early therapeutic intervention may be more effective than delayed treatment of older patients with advanced clinical symptoms Ogawa et al. examined the possibility of gene therapy in neonatal animals [24]. AAV vector carrying human α-galactosidase cDNA was intravenously administered into neonatal

M. Beck

(2 days old) and adult (12 weeks old) Fabry mice. Several investigations were made 25 weeks after the injection. AAV vector preferentially transduced the liver, and in male adults high levels of α-galactosidase were found in heart, liver and plasma. In female adult animals, however, AAV-mediated gene expression was suppressed. When the vector was administered to neonates, enzyme activity was found for many weeks in plasma and in the heart, independently from the gender of the mice. From these animal studies it can be concluded that by treatment in the early life major organ failure may be prevented.

24.3.2 Ex Vivo *Gene Therapy*

Based on the positive clinical experience with bone marrow transplantation in some lysosomal storage disorders, hematopoietic stem cell-mediated gene therapy was considered as an attractice alternative for the treatment of LSDs. Gene transfer strategies aimed at correcting the genetic defect in the hematopoietic stem cells has some advantages compared with conventional allogeneic stem cell transplantation. As autologous cells are used for gene therapy, transplant-related morbidity and mortality are reduced because there is no risk of graft-versus-host disease. In addition, genetically modified cells most likely express higher levels of the therapeutic enzyme and become more effective than wild-type cells.

For *ex vivo* therapy stem cells of the patient are transfected with the gene and thereafter returned to the body. The efficacy of this procedure has been demonstrated in many experiments on LSD animals, for example in the mouse model of Fabry disease [25]. Bone marrow mononuclear cells from these animals were transduced with a retrovirus encoding α-galactosidase and transplanted into irradiated α-galactosidase deficient mice. Bone marrow mononuclear cells were then transplanted into secondary recipients. Increased enzyme activity and decreased Gb3 accumulation were found in all organs of all recipient groups. These results indicate that correction of bone marrow cells transduced with the α-galactosidase gene via a vector may be able to correct the metabolic defect in Fabry patients.

Although gene therapy studies performed in animal models are rather promising, many important issues regarding safety and efficacy of this therapeutic strategy need to be addressed before clinical trials can be initiated on a large scale. It has to be considered that translation of cell culture and animal studies in clinical trials requires development of large-scale manufacturing and quality assays, rigorous demonstration of safety and efficacy of new gene therapy protocols, and last but not least the assurance of the consensus and approval of the scientific and biomedical communities.

References

1. Eng CM, Guffon N, Wilcox WR et al (2001) Safety and efficacy of recombinant human alpha-galactosidase A replacement therapy in Fabry's disease. N Engl J Med 345(1):9–16

2. Banikazemi M, Bultas J, Waldek S et al (2007) Agalsidase-beta therapy for advanced Fabry disease: a randomized trial. Ann Intern Med 146(2):77–86
3. Wilcox WR, Banikazemi M, Guffon N et al (2004) Long-term safety and efficacy of enzyme replacement therapy for Fabry disease. Am J Hum Genet 75(1):65–74
4. Weidemann F, Niemann M, Breunig F et al (2009) Long-term effects of enzyme replacement therapy on Fabry cardiomyopathy: evidence for a better outcome with early treatment. Circulation 119(4):524–529
5. Schiffmann R, Kopp JB, Austin HA III et al (2001) Enzyme replacement therapy in Fabry disease: a randomized controlled trial. J Am Med Assoc 285(21):2743–2749
6. Beck M (2009) Agalsidase alfa for the treatment of Fabry disease: new data on clinical efficacy and safety. Exp Opin Biol Ther 9(2):255–261
7. West M, Nicholls K, Mehta A et al (2009) Agalsidase alfa and kidney dysfunction in Fabry disease. J Am Soc Nephrol 20(5):1132–1139
8. Mehta A, Beck M, Elliott P et al (2009) Enzyme replacement therapy with agalsidase alfa in patients with Fabry's disease: an analysis of registry data. Lancet 374(9706):1986–1996
9. Wang J, Lozier J, Johnson G et al (2008) Neutralizing antibodies to therapeutic enzymes: considerations for testing, prevention and treatment. Nat Biotechnol 26(8):901–908
10. Schiffmann R, Ries M, Timmons M, Flaherty JT, Brady RO (2006) Long-term therapy with agalsidase alfa for Fabry disease: safety and effects on renal function in a home infusion setting. Nephrol Dial Transplant 21(2):345–354
11. Zhang XK, Elbin CS, Chuang WL et al (2008) Multiplex enzyme assay screening of dried blood spots for lysosomal storage disorders by using tandem mass spectrometry. Clin Chem 54(10):1725–1728
12. Spada M, Pagliardini S, Yasuda M et al (2006) High incidence of later-onset Fabry disease revealed by newborn screening. Am J Hum Genet 79(1):31–40
13. West M, Le Moine K (2007) Effect of withdrawal of enzyme replacement therapy in Fabry disease. Acta Paediatrica 96(s455):105
14. Bernier V, Lagace M, Bichet DG, Bouvier M (2004) Pharmacological chaperones: potential treatment for conformational diseases. Trends Endocrinol Metab 15(5):222–228
15. Frustaci A, Chimenti C, Ricci R et al (2001) Improvement in cardiac function in the cardiac variant of Fabry's disease with galactose-infusion therapy. N Engl J Med 345(1):25–32
16. Yam GH, Zuber C, Roth J (2005) A synthetic chaperone corrects the trafficking defect and disease phenotype in a protein misfolding disorder. FASEB J 19(1):12–18
17. Ishii S, Chang HH, Yoshioka H et al (2009) Preclinical efficacy and safety of 1-deoxygalactonojirimycin in mice for Fabry disease. J Pharmacol Exp Ther 328(3): 723–731
18. Benjamin ER, Flanagan JJ, Schilling A et al (2009) The pharmacological chaperone 1-deoxygalactonojirimycin increases alpha-galactosidase A levels in Fabry patient cell lines. J Inherit Metab Dis 32(3):424–440
19. Schiffmann R, Germain DP, Castelli J, Shenker A, Lockhart DJ (eds) (2008) Phase 2 clinical trials of the pharmacological chaperone AT1001 for the treatment of Fabry disease. 58th annual meeting American Society of Human Genetics, Philadelphia, 11–15 Nov 2008
20. Sands MS, Davidson BL (2006) Gene therapy for lysosomal storage diseases. Mol Ther 13(5):839–849
21. Li C, Ziegler RJ, Cherry M et al (2002) Adenovirus-transduced lung as a portal for delivering alpha-galactosidase A into systemic circulation for Fabry disease. Mol Ther 5(6): 745–754
22. Di Domenico C, Villani GR, Di Napoli D et al (2005) Gene therapy for a mucopolysaccharidosis type I murine model with lentiviral-IDUA vector. Hum Gene Ther 16(1):81–90
23. Follenzi A, Battaglia M, Lombardo A, Annoni A, Roncarolo MG, Naldini L (2004) Targeting lentiviral vector expression to hepatocytes limits transgene-specific immune response and establishes long-term expression of human antihemophilic factor IX in mice. Blood 103(10):3700–3709

24. Ogawa K, Hirai Y, Ishizaki M et al (2009) Long-term inhibition of glycosphingolipid accumulation in Fabry model mice by a single systemic injection of AAV1 vector in the neonatal period. Mol Genet Metab 96(3):91–96
25. Takenaka T, Murray GJ, Qin G et al (2000) Long-term enzyme correction and lipid reduction in multiple organs of primary and secondary transplanted Fabry mice receiving transduced bone marrow cells. Proc Natl Acad Sci USA 97(13):7515–7520

Chapter 25
Agalsidase Alfa in the Treatment of Anderson-Fabry Disease

Gregory M. Pastores

Abstract Agalsidase alfa is a formulation of the human enzyme α-galactosidase A (AGAL), generated by activation of the encoding gene in a continuous human cell line. The regular infusion of agalsidase alfa into patients with Anderson-Fabry disease (AFD), in whom AGAL deficiency can lead to multi-organ system failure, has been demonstrated to be safe. By facilitating the clearance of the substrate globotriaosylceramide, which accumulates in tissues of affected individuals, agalsidase alfa treatments have resulted in a modification of disease course. These developments are anticipated to lead to improvement in the patient's health-related quality of life and delay or prevent the development of morbidity related to renal, cardiac and cerebrovascular disease associated with AFD. Therapeutic outcome appears to be influenced by disease stage, and possibly by antibody formation and a putative problem in the intracellular trafficking of the infused enzyme. These premises have led to the recommendation of early intervention, prior to established organ dysfunction.

Keywords Agalsidase alfa · Anderson-Fabry disease · Enzyme replacement therapy · Mainz Severity Score Index

25.1 Introduction

Enzyme replacement therapy (ERT) has been demonstrated to be a safe and effective means of managing patients with lysosomal storage disorders caused by a deficiency of a soluble hydrolase [1]. Agalsidase alfa, a formulation of the human enzyme α-galactosidase A (AGAL), was developed specifically for regular intravenous

G.M. Pastores (✉)
Departments of Neurology and Pediatrics, New York University School of Medicine, New York, NY, USA
e-mail: gregory.pastores@nyumc.org

D. Elstein et al. (eds.), *Fabry Disease*, DOI 10.1007/978-90-481-9033-1_25,
© Springer Science+Business Media B.V. 2010

administration into patients with Anderson-Fabry disease (AFD), an X-linked disorder caused by AGAL deficiency. In clinical trials, agalsidase alfa has been demonstrated to be safe and effective; and met with regulatory approval of the product in 2001 in member countries of the European Union and other states, except for the United States [2, 3]. Additional information regarding the use of agalsidase alfa has derived from the Fabry Outcome Survey (FOS), a post-marketing surveillance program which collects data on treated and untreated patients with AFD [4].

25.2 Agalsidase Alfa: Product Characteristics and Pharmacology

Agalsidase alfa is a human AGAL produced by a stably transfected human cell line. The mature enzyme is a glycoprotein consisting of a 100 kD homodimer of two approximately 50 kD subunits, which has been modified by cleavage of a signal peptide sequence and the addition of 3 N-linked oligosaccharides [2]. Molecular masses from 46 to 55 kD are found by mass spectrometry, indicating heterogeneous glycosylation, which is necessary for enzyme internalisation and localisation to lysosomes. The specific activity of agalsidase alfa is approximately 3.9×10^6 U/mg protein.

The pharmacokinetics of varying doses of agalsidase alfa (0.1, 0.2, or 0.4 mg/kg weekly; and 0.2 or 0.4 mg/kg every other week) and the effect of enzyme dose and frequency of administration on plasma Gb3 levels were examined in a 10-week study involving 18 adult male patients with AFD [5]. The mean half-life was 56–76 min, and the mean volume of distribution at steady state was 17–18% of body weight, with no significant associations between dose and half-life, clearance, or volume of distribution at steady state. The area under the curve was linearly proportional to the dose from 0.1 to 0.4 mg/kg. Average plasma Gb3 levels were significantly reduced by about 50% in each of the treated patients, with no statistically significant differences between dose groups (Fig. 25.1). Similar pharmacokinetic

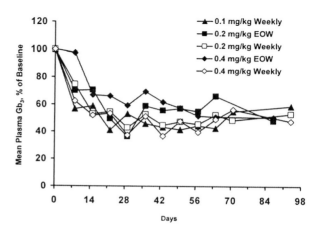

Fig. 25.1 Agalsidase alfa: Changes in mean plasma Gb3 in male AFD patients on five different dosing regimens. Clarke et al. [5]

results were reported in separate groups of adult men ($n = 18$) and women ($n = 15$), who were treated with 0.2 mg/kg agalsidase alfa, although clearance tended to be slightly lower in these groups (2.5 ± 0.7 ml/min/kg in men and 2.1 ± 0.6 ml/min/kg in women) and t½ tended to be longer (112 ± 25 min in men and 89 ± 28 in women) [6].

The pharmacokinetics of agalsidase alfa (0.2 mg/kg every other week) was examined separately in patients with AFD and end-stage renal disease (ESRD); a major disease-related complication. Analysis of pharmacokinetic parameters in 22 patients (20 males and two females) on dialysis or post-kidney transplantation, treated with agalsidase alfa (0.2 mg/kg every other week), revealed measurements that were comparable to that observed in the patients without ESRD [7].

The pharmacokinetics and pharmacodynamics of agalsidase alpha (0.2 mg/kg every other week) were also examined in pediatric patients (19 boys, five girls, 6–18 years old; mean age, 11.8 years) [8]. In children, serum clearance (2.0–9.4 ml/min/kg) tended to decrease with increasing age. The average clearance in children, 3.7 ± 1.5 ml/min/kg (mean +/– SD), was significantly greater than that measured in 33 adults (2.3 ± 0.7 ml/min/kg). Mean terminal elimination half-life of agalsidase alfa was found to be prolonged at week 25 compared with baseline (150 vs. 66 min) in eight of 19 male children. The magnitude of the reduction of plasma Gb3 was similar in all age groups and was independent of area under the curve and other pharmacokinetic parameters. Thus, except for clearance in younger patients, agalsidase alfa appears to have comparable pharmacokinetic and pharmacodynamic profiles in pediatric and adult AFD patients of both genders.

25.3 The Use of Agalsidase Alfa in Clinical Trials

The initial clinical trials with agalsidase alfa were conducted at a single center, the National Institutes of Health (NIH). The NIH investigators showed that a single administration of agalsidase alfa (with doses ranging from 0.007 to 0.1 mg/kg) to patients ($N = 10$) with AFD resulted in a reduction of the substrate globotriaosylceramide (Gb3) levels in the liver and in shed renal tubular epithelial cells in the urine sediment [2]. Liver biopsies taken 44 h after the enzyme infusion showed that approximately 8–32% of the total administered AGAL dose was still present; indicating a tissue half-life in the liver >24 h. Interestingly, 28 days after treatment mean Gb3 levels in urine had decreased by 38% from baseline. No drug-related adverse events were observed and none of the patients exhibited any antibodies against agalsidase alfa.

The clinical efficacy of agalsidase alfa (at 0.2 mg/kg q 2 weeks) was subsequently demonstrated in a double-blind placebo-controlled trial, which was also conducted at the NIH. The main outcome measure was the effect on neuropathic pain determined by question 3 ('pain at its worst' item) of the Brief Pain Inventory (BPI) while without neuropathic pain medication, which declined significantly (from

6.2 ± 0.46 at baseline to 5.3 ± 0.73 after 24 weeks, $p = 0.02$) in the agalsidase alfa group ($N = 14$) compared to the group on placebo ($N = 14$) [3]. This trial was followed by an extension phase which lasted for another 6 months during which time all patients received agalsidase alfa. Stabilization in renal function (based on creatinine clearance) was also noted among the treated patients; associated with a significant and persistent decrease in plasma and urine sediment Gb3 levels (by approximately 20–50% at 6 months and by approximately 50–80% after 12–18 months of treatment).

25.4 The Use of Agalsidase Alfa in Postmarketing Studies

Several reports describe various observations in AFD patients treated with agalsidase alfa, including a reduction in plasma and urine sediment Gb3 on the recommended dose of 0.2 mg/kg q 2 weeks. In general, these studies have indicated that disease expression among symptomatic females which is similar to that seen among male patients with AFD is equally response to treatment with agalsidase alfa.

Data from FOS on patients, mainly on adult males with AFD, treated with agalsidase alfa (0.2 mg/kg q 2 weeks), in the majority of cases for a period of 1–2 years, has revealed the following observations:

- Renal: stabilization of renal function (based on estimated GFR) or a decline in the rate of deterioration in patients with mild (GFR between 60 and 90 ml/min/ 1.73 m^2) or moderate (GFR: 30 and 60 ml/min/1.73 m^2) reduction in renal function at baseline (Fig. 25.2) [9–13]. Several studies suggest the magnitude of

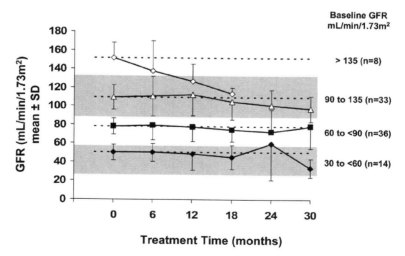

Fig. 25.2 Agalsidase alfa: GFR patterns in treated male patients with AFD, grouped according to baseline GFR. West et al. [13]

proteinuria (≥ 1 g/d) at baseline is a strong predictor of the rate of loss of GFR during ERT [13].

- Cardiac: reduction in left ventricular (LV) size (based on echocardiography) in patients with an enlarged heart (mean LV wall thickness >11 mm and left ventricular mass >50 g/m$^{2.7}$) at baseline; with a significant reduction in QRS duration at week 27 ($N = 15$ female patients) [9]. In one placebo-controlled trial, a mean reduction (20%) in myocardial Gb3 content (as assessed by serial transvenous endomyocardial biopsies) was demonstrated over the 6 months of agalsidase alfa; whereas a mean increase (10%) was observed in patients receiving placebo [14]. In a separate study, involving 29 patients (mean age 37 ± 13 years) with a median follow-up of 37 months, there was a small improvement in diastolic function (29% decrease of E/Ea); although the incidence of LV wall thickness was unchanged and an increase in interventricular septal wall thickness was observed [15].
- Neurologic: improvement in the clinical manifestations of the small fiber neuropathy, including pain relief, reduction in the threshold for warm and cold sensation in the foot and increased sweat excretion (based on quantitative sudomotor axon reflex testing and confirmed by thermoregulatory sweat testing) at 36 months [9, 16–18].
- Pains and quality of life measures: improvements in pain scores and quality of life (based on responses to the BPI and European Quality of Life Questionnaire EQ-5D) [9, 19, 20].
- Gastrointestinal system: relief of gastrointestinal symptoms (primarily abdominal pain and diarrhea) following 6 months of treatment ($n = 11$) [21].
- Audiologic: gradual improvement in hearing (by 4.0 dB) at 42 months ($n = 15$) [22].

Some of the reports on the effect of agalsidase alfa describe changes in disease severity, as measured with the Mainz Severity Score Index (MSSI); a scoring system composed of four sections that cover the general, neurological, cardiovascular, and renal signs and symptoms of AFD [23]. In one study, improvements were noted in 39 AFD patients (including 24 males and 15 females) following 1 year of agalsidase alfa treatment [24]. In a separate study, involving female patients only ($N = 36$) MSSI was significantly reduced after 12 months of agalsidase alfa treatment and continuously improved over 4 years (Fig. 25.3) [25]. Additional findings in this study included: a reduction in BPI 'pain at its worst' score (from 4.6 ± 2.9 at baseline to 3.3 ± 2.9); decrease in mean left-ventricular mass (from 89.4 ± 29.3 g/m at baseline to 66.5 ± 29.3 g/m); and stable kidney function (based on eGFR and proteinuria) [25]. These observations confirm earlier findings in a cohort of symptomatic females treated with agalsidase alfa for up to 55 weeks [6].

With respect to the use of agalsidase alfa (0.2 mg/kg q 2 weeks) in children, the study by Ramaswami and colleagues involving nine boys and four girls (Median age 11.0 years; range 3.5–18) showed two of the boys and the one girl on regular pain medication at baseline could stop taking analgesics [26]. Also, BPI scores decreased and pain-related quality of life (QoL) scores improved in most patients

Fig. 25.3 Agalsidase alfa in women with AFD ($N = 36$), *MSSI profile*. Whybra et al. [25]

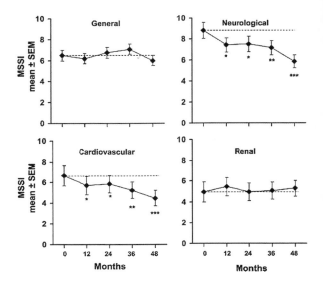

by week 12 and the benefits were sustained until the end of the 6-months study. The observed change in BPI scores was greater in the boys, who had higher (or worse) BPI scores at baseline. Increases in sweat volume were recorded in three out of five boys and in one of two girls tested after 23 weeks of treatment. These observations were confirmed in the study by Ries et al. (which was an open label, 6-month trial involving 19 boys and five girls) which revealed that three patients with anhidrosis developed sweating, and six of 11 patients could reduce or cease their use of antineuropathic analgesics [27]. The latter study also showed an improvement in heart rate (HR) variability, as determined by 2-h ambulatory monitoring; which was decreased in the boys compared with the girls at baseline [The abnormality in HR variability seen in AFD patients has been hypothesized to be caused by autonomic dysfunction. Decreased HR variability has been associated with an increase in cardiac mortality, possibly related to sudden death [28]. The significance of the changes in HR variability in AFD patients treated with agalsidase alfa remains to be established].

Although agalsidase alfa treatment has been shown to reverse or lead to the resolution of cerebrovascular hyperdynamicity, a finding in untreated AFD patient, it is not certain that enzyme therapy reduces the risk of stroke [29–31]. Despite the significant improvement in the function of the cerebral vasculature, four of 25 (16%) patients, followed for 4.5 years on therapy, developed non-debilitating strokes and one patient had a transient ischemic attack [32].

25.5 Agalsidase Alfa: Safety Considerations

During the clinical trials and in the post-marketing phase, several adverse events (AE) were observed in patients with AFD on agalsidase alfa [3, 9]. However, the majority of these AEs was not infusion-related and likely represents AFD-related disease complications. In patients with infusion related adverse-events, these appeared to occur primarily in patients who have developed antibodies against the infused enzyme. These occurrences could be mitigated by a reduction in the rate of enzyme infusion or the use of appropriate medication.

Antibodies against agalsidase alfa are seen is about 55% of treated male patients, but in none of the treated females so far [3, 9]. The antibodies are primarily of the IgG class, and none of the infused patients have developed IgE antibodies. A proportion of the antibodies appear to exhibit neutralizing properties, which has been associated with an increase in urinary Gb3 level [32]. There are no clearcut effects of antibody formation on therapeutic outcome, perhaps because antibody titers tend to decline with on-going treatment; however, further studies are necessary to clarify this point [33, 34].

The relative safety profile of agalsidase alfa has enabled its home administration, as opposed to infusions delivered in an ambulatory or hospital-based facility [32].

25.6 Summary and Final Comments

In patients with AFD, the use of agalsidase alfa, when administered at 0.2 mg/kg of body weight every 2 weeks, appears to halt and possibly reverse disease progression [35]. However, the extent to which treatment modifies the natural history of the disease and the magnitude of the resulting improvement in patients' quality of life remain to be determined. Examination of deaths among 181 affected relatives of patients in FOS, the majority of whom had died before 2001, revealed that renal failure in males (42%) and cerebrovascular disease in females (25%) as a principal cause. In contrast, among the 42 patients enrolled in FOS whose deaths were reported between 2001 and 2007, cardiac disease was the main cause of death in both males (34%) and females (57%) [36]. As enzyme therapy may stabilize or improve renal and cardiac disease related to AFD, we may see a reduction of sentinel clinical events and an increase in patient survival; although this remains to be established.

As most studies have examined a singular dosing schedule, it is also not certain whether certain aspects of the disease may have a better response profile on an alternative enzyme dose/frequency regimen. Indeed, one study has examined weekly infusion of agalsidase alfa in adult male patients ($N = 11$) who have demonstrated a continuing decline in renal function (≥ 5 ml/min per 1.73 m^2/year) despite 2–4 year of conventional treatment (Fig. 25.4) [37]. The results revealed an improvement in the slope of decline on a weekly agalsidase alfa dose of 0.2 mg/kg. In light of current observations and given the costs of enzyme therapy, the issue of optimal dosing needs to be examined in greater detail [37].

The major determinants of response to enzyme therapy also need to be established, and the influence of antibodies formed against the infused enzyme requires further delineation. The wide variability in clinical presentation among patients with

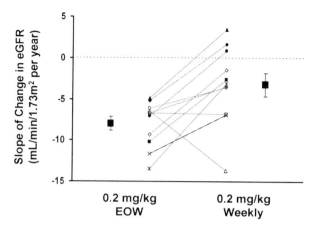

Fig. 25.4 Agalsidase alfa: from every other week to weekly in patients whose eGFR declined at >5 ml/min per 1.73 m²/year. *11/41 (27%) of 41 adult male patients treated for 2–4 years on the recommended schedule. Schiffmann et al. [36]

AFD and heterogeneity in clinical response are major confounding factors. Apart from the issue of antibody formation, enzyme access to certain sites of tissue substrate storage may be another limiting factor. Investigations of the relative tissue and cellular distribution of agalsidase alfa, following a single intravenous injection in a mouse knockout model of AFD has revealed a very heterogeneous systemic distribution [38]. The implications of this findings in human is not known. It is possible serial infusions of the enzyme may address some of the unevenness in enzyme-tissue distribution, but more studies are required to clarify this point.

It is likely that disease stage impacts therapeutic outcome and that increasing proteinuria can have an adverse influence on renal response to enzyme therapy. These observations, together with identification of patients in 'at-risk' populations (i.e., those with cryptogenic stroke or hypertrophic cardiomyopathy, or on dialysis or post-kidney transplant), have led to advocacy for screening and early detection programs [39]. Treatment of pauci-symptomatic AFD children with agalsidase alfa appears to be safe, and there are indications of potential benefit. However, longterm studies are necessary to ascertain the degree to which enzyme therapy delays the onset or prevents the development of renal, cardiac and cerebrovascular disease, when treatment is commenced in childhood or the teenage years.

There is a paucity of biomarkers and validated measures of disease severity, which limits our ability to predict disease course. Uromodulin (UMOD), a protein selectively expressed in the thick ascending limb of Henle's loop, the macula densa segment and distal convoluted tubule has been observed to be decreased or absent in some patients with AFD; this abnormality has been shown to be corrected by enzyme therapy [40]. The significance of these observation remains to be established, but UMOD abnormalities may prove to be a surrogate marker of disease, and which can be serially monitored in treated patients to examine dose-response relationship and the impact of antibody formation. Another interesting finding is the presence of elevated levels of endothelial cell membrane-derived microparticles (EMP, specifically, CD144+CD105+) in peripheral venous blood samples of 10 pediatric Fabry patients (9 males and 1 female) [41]. A decrease in EMP levels was observed after 6 months of agalsidase alfa treatment [41]. As the patients involved in the study were children, without significant cardiac and renal disease, monitoring EMP-levels may be useful in determination of the optimal time to initiate therapy; but this matter requires further investigation.

Currently, it is felt that adjunctive measures, such as use of aspirin for stroke prevention and ACE-inhibitors or sartans for its renoprotective properties, should remain part of the treatment armamentarium [42]. Meanwhile, other therapeutic strategies, including the use of pharmacologic chaperones and substrate synthesis inhibitors, are being actively explored [43]. It is possible therapeutic response may be optimized by using a combination of approaches.

References

1. Burrow TA, Hopkin RJ, Leslie ND, Tinkle BT, Grabowski GA (2007) Enzyme reconstitution/replacement therapy for lysosomal storage diseases. Curr Opin Pediatr 19(6):628–635
2. Schiffmann R, Murray GJ, Treco D et al (2000) Infusion of alpha-galactosidase A reduces tissue globotriaosylceramide storage in patients with Fabry disease. Proc Natl Acad Sci USA 97(1):365–370
3. Schiffmann R, Kopp JB, Austin HA III et al (2001) Enzyme replacement therapy in Fabry disease: a randomized controlled trial. J Am Med Assoc 285(21):2743–2749
4. Mehta A, Ricci R, Widmer U et al (2004) Fabry disease defined: baseline clinical manifestations of 366 patients in the Fabry Outcome Survey. Eur J Clin Invest 34(3):236–242
5. Clarke JT, West ML, Bultas J, Schiffmann R (2007) The pharmacology of multiple regimens of agalsidase alfa enzyme replacement therapy for Fabry disease. Genet Med 9(8):504–509
6. Baehner F, Kampmann C, Whybra C, Miebach E, Wiethoff CM, Beck M (2003) Enzyme replacement therapy in heterozygous females with Fabry disease results of a phase IIIB study. J Inherit Metab Dis 26(7):617–627
7. Pastores GM, Boyd E, Crandall K, Whelan A, Piersall L, Barnett N (2007) Safety and pharmacokinetics of agalsidase alfa in patients with Fabry disease and end-stage renal disease. Nephrol Dial Transplant 22(7):1920–1925
8. Ries M, Clarke JT, Whybra C et al (2007) Enzyme replacement in Fabry disease: pharmacokinetics and pharmacodynamics of agalsidase alpha in children and adolescents. J Clin Pharmacol 47(10):1222–1230
9. Beck M, Ricci R, Widmer U et al (2004) Fabry disease: overall effects of agalsidase alfa treatment. Eur J Clin Invest 34(12):838–844
10. Dehout F, Schwarting A, Beck M et al (2003) Effects of enzyme replacement therapy with agalsidase alfa on glomerular filtration rate in patients with Fabry disease: preliminary data. Acta Paediatr Suppl 92(443):14–15
11. Schwarting A, Dehout F, Feriozzi S et al (2006) Enzyme replacement therapy and renal function in 201 patients with Fabry disease. Clin Nephrol 66(2):77–84
12. Feriozzi S, Schwarting A, Sunder-Plassmann G, West M, Cybulla M (2009) International Fabry Outcome Survey Investigators. Agalsidase alfa slows the decline in renal function in patients with Fabry disease. Am J Nephrol 29(5):353–361
13. West M, Nicholls K, Mehta A et al (2009) Agalsidase alfa and kidney dysfunction in Fabry disease. J Am Soc Nephrol 20(5):1132–1139
14. Hughes DA, Elliott PM, Shah J et al (2008) Effects of enzyme replacement therapy on the cardiomyopathy of Anderson-Fabry disease: a randomised, double-blind, placebo-controlled clinical trial of agalsidase alfa. Heart 94(2):153–158

15. Kovacevic-Preradovic T, Zuber M, Attenhofer Jost CH et al (2008) Anderson-Fabry disease: long-term echocardiographic follow-up under enzyme replacement therapy. Eur J Echocardiogr 9(6):729–735

16. Schiffmann R, Hauer P, Freeman B et al (2006) Enzyme replacement therapy and intraepidermal innervation density in Fabry disease. Muscle Nerve 34(1):53–56

17. Gupta SN, Ries M, Murray GJ et al (2008) Skin-impedance in Fabry Disease: a prospective, controlled, non-randomized clinical study. BMC Neurol 8:41

18. Schiffmann R, Floeter MK, Dambrosia JM et al (2003) Enzyme replacement therapy improves peripheral nerve and sweat function in Fabry disease. Muscle Nerve 28(6):703–710

19. Hoffmann B, Garcia de Lorenzo A, Mehta A et al (2005) Effects of enzyme replacement therapy on pain and health related quality of life in patients with Fabry disease: data from FOS (Fabry Outcome Survey). J Med Genet 42(3):247–252

20. Hoffmann B, Beck M, Sunder-Plassmann G et al (2007) Nature and prevalence of pain in Fabry disease and its response to enzyme replacement therapy-a retrospective analysis from the Fabry Outcome Survey. Clin J Pain 23(6):535–542

21. Hoffmann B, Schwarz M, Mehta A, Keshav S (2007) Fabry Outcome Survey European Investigators. Gastrointestinal symptoms in 342 patients with Fabry disease: prevalence and response to enzyme replacement therapy. Clin Gastroenterol Hepatol 5(12): 1447–1453

22. Hajioff D, Hegemann S, Conti G et al (2006) Agalsidase alpha and hearing in Fabry disease: data from the Fabry Outcome Survey. Eur J Clin Invest 36(9):663–667

23. Whybra C, Kampmann C, Krummenauer F et al (2004) The Mainz Severity Score Index: a new instrument for quantifying the Anderson-Fabry disease phenotype, and the response of patients to enzyme replacement therapy. Clin Genet 65(4):299–307

24. Parini R, Rigoldi M, Santus F et al (2008) Enzyme replacement therapy with agalsidase alfa in a cohort of Italian patients with Anderson-Fabry disease: testing the effects with the Mainz Severity Score Index. Clin Genet 74(3):260–266

25. Whybra C, Miebach E, Mengel E et al (2009) A 4-year study of the efficacy and tolerability of enzyme replacement therapy with agalsidase alfa in 36 women with Fabry disease. Genet Med 11(6):441–449

26. Ramaswami U, Wendt S, Pintos-Morell G et al (2007) Enzyme replacement therapy with agalsidase alfa in children with Fabry disease. Acta Paediatr 96(1):122–127

27. Ries M, Clarke JT, Whybra C et al (2006) Enzyme-replacement therapy with agalsidase alfa in children with Fabry disease. Pediatrics 118(3):924–932

28. Lauer MS (2009) Autonomic function and prognosis. Cleve Clin J Med 76(Suppl 2): S18–S22

29. Moore DF, Altarescu G, Herscovitch P, Schiffmann R (2002) Enzyme replacement reverses abnormal cerebrovascular responses in Fabry disease. BMC Neurol 2:4

30. Moore DF, Altarescu G, Ling GS et al (2002) Elevated cerebral blood flow velocities in Fabry disease with reversal after enzyme replacement. Stroke 33(2):525–531

31. Moore DF, Scott LT, Gladwin MT et al (2001) Regional cerebral hyperperfusion and nitric oxide pathway dysregulation in Fabry disease: reversal by enzyme replacement therapy. Circulation 104(13):1506–1512

32. Schiffmann R, Ries M, Timmons M, Flaherty JT, Brady RO (2006) Long-term therapy with agalsidase alfa for Fabry disease: safety and effects on renal function in a home infusion setting. Nephrol Dial Transplant 21(2):345–354

33. Linthorst GE, Hollak CE, Donker-Koopman WE, Strijland A, Aerts JM (2004) Enzyme therapy for Fabry disease: neutralizing antibodies toward agalsidase alpha and beta. Kidney Int 66(4):1589–1595

34. Hollak CE, Linthorst GE (2009) Immune response to enzyme replacement therapy in Fabry disease: impact on clinical outcome? Mol Genet Metab 96(1):1–3

35. Beck M (2009) Agalsidase alfa for the treatment of Fabry disease: new data on clinical efficacy and safety. Expert Opin Biol Ther 9(2):255–261

36. Schiffmann R, Askari H, Timmons M et al (2007) Weekly enzyme replacement therapy may slow decline of renal function in patients with Fabry disease who are on long-term biweekly dosing. J Am Soc Nephrol 18(5):1576–1583
37. Mehta A, Clarke JT, Giugliani R et al (2009) Natural course of Fabry disease: changing pattern of causes of death in FOS – the Fabry Outcome Survey. J Med Genet 46(8):548–552
38. Murray GJ, Anver MR, Kennedy MA, Quirk JM, Schiffmann R (2007) Cellular and tissue distribution of intravenously administered agalsidase alfa. Mol Genet Metab 90(3):307–312
39. Auray-Blais C, Millington DS, Young SP, Clarke JT, Schiffmann R (2009) Proposed high-risk screening protocol for Fabry disease in patients with renal and vascular disease. J Inherit Metab Dis 32(2):303–308
40. Vylet'al P, Hůlková H, Zivná M et al (2008) Abnormal expression and processing of uromodulin in Fabry disease reflects tubular cell storage alteration and is reversible by enzyme replacement therapy. J Inherit Metab Dis 31(4):508–517
41. Gelderman MP, Schiffmann R, Simak J (2007) Elevated endothelial microparticles in Fabry children decreased after enzyme replacement therapy. Arterioscler Thromb Vasc Biol 27(7):e
42. Wanner C, Breunig F (2007) Fabry nephropathy and the case for adjunctive renal therapy. J Am Soc Nephrol 18(9):2426–2428
43. Pastores GM (2008) Therapeutic options for childhood-onset lysosomal storage disorders. Pediatr Health 2(1):21–32

Chapter 26
Agalsidase Beta Clinical Trials and Long Term Experience

Carlos E. Prada and Robert J. Hopkin

Abstract There have been phase I/II and III clinical trials of agalsidase beta infusions for treatment of Fabry disease. The phase I/II trial demonstrated that agalsidase beta infusions were well tolerated, and that globotriaocylceramide (GL-3) clearance was dose dependent. A phase III trials demonstrated clearance of GL-3 on a tissue level. A separate study demonstrated decreased risk of renal progression with therapy in a population with advanced disease. There is evidence of benefit for the renal, cardiac, and quality of life manifestations. Additional studies are needed to address cerebrovascular disease, life expectancy, and other problems related to Fabry disease. Enzyme replacement therapy with agalsidase beta has been a major advance in the care of patients with this disorder.

Keywords Enzyme replacement therapy (ERT) · Agalsidase beta · Clinical trials · Clinical endpoints · Proteinuria · Left heart ventricular function

26.1 Introduction

Life expectancy of patients with Fabry disease is decreased by 2 decades compared with unaffected males. Treatment by replacing the deficient enzyme was proposed decades ago. A method for large scale production of human α-galactosidase A was developed using a distinct construct to overproduce the enzyme in CHO cells. This method was suitable for commercial production and is now marketed as agalsidase beta or Fabrazyme®. Enzyme Replacement Therapy has now been available for several years. It received approval in Europe in 2001 and in the USA in 2003 [1]. Historically the leading cause of death was renal failure. More recently cardiac complications have emerged as an important source of morbidity and mortality. It

R.J. Hopkin (✉)
Division of Human Genetics, Cincinnati Children's Hospital Medical Center, University of Cincinnati College of Medicine, Cincinnati, OH, USA
e-mail: rob.hopkin@cchmc.org

D. Elstein et al. (eds.), *Fabry Disease*, DOI 10.1007/978-90-481-9033-1_26,   401
© Springer Science+Business Media B.V. 2010

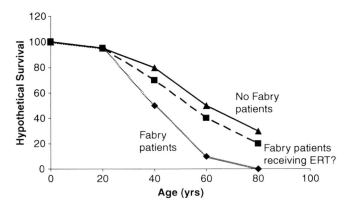

Fig. 26.1 Hypothetical survival curve for Fabry disease. Fabry patients life expectancy is decreased by two decades compared with unaffected males. Survival data from Fabry patients receiving enzyme replacement therapy (ERT) has not been published but literature supports benefit in affected patients

is therefore not surprising that renal and cardiac measures have been the primary focus of clinical studies with enzyme replacement therapy (ERT). Figure 26.1 shows a hypothetical improvement of survival with ERT, although there is evidence that ERT is beneficial to patients with Fabry disease, there are no studies published that analyze survival with therapy. More experience will be required to clearly answer this important question.

26.2 Clinical Trials Agalsidase Beta

Preclinical models do not always predict the risk of adverse reactions and hence the importance of well designed phase I, II and III clinical trials. We will now summarize and review the results of these studies for agalsidase beta.

A single center, open label phase I/II clinical trial by Eng et al. studied five dosing regimens of agalsidase beta replacement therapy in 15 male patients with Fabry disease to evaluate safety, pharmacokinetics and efficacy [2]. Three patients were enrolled in each of five regimens and all received a total of 5 doses of enzyme. Mean plasma concentration reached 80% of peak values 60 min into the infusion for the 0.3 mg/kg dose and 90 min for the 1 and 3 mg/kg dose. Clearance was biphasic for all biweekly dosing groups with a rapid elimination phase lasting 1–2 h post-infusion and a dose-dependent clearance rate of 4 mg/kg/min to 1 mg/kg/min with increasing dose. Terminal half-life was not affected by dose.

Tissue clearance was dose and organ dependent, hepatic globotriaocylceramide (GL-3) measured by ELISA was reduced by an average of 84% after infusion 5. There was marked reduction in all treatment groups. The patients receiving 3 mg/kg every 14 days had the most profound response (clearance 92%). Sinusoid endothelial cells and kupffer cells on histological analyses showed a decrease of GL-3 scores from 2.4 to 2.8 at baseline to 0.5 and 1 after infusion 5, respectively.

Endomyocardial biopsies were obtained in seven patients with a GL-3 level mean of 21,400 ng/mg tissue and after treatment, GL-3 level decreased 15.6% to an average of 18,300 ng/mg tissue in four patients. Histological scores for the capillary endothelium were decreased in all seven patients with mean scores of 1.75 at baseline to 0.57 after treatment. GL-3 storage remained unchanged in the cardiomyocytes, pericytes, and vascular smooth muscle. Kidney biopsies were obtained in five patients with a GL-3 mean average of 5,530 ng/mg tissue at baseline to 1,790 ng/mg tissue after treatment (clearance 67.6%). There was one patient in whom the GL-3 level was doubled compared to baseline. This discrepancy was attributed to sampling variability. GL-3 accumulation in the endothelium of interstitial capillaries declined in four of five patients and increased in one. GL-3 in the glomerular capillary area decreased in two patients, there was marked response in mesangial and in cortical interstitial cells. GL-3 storage was most prominent in the distal convoluted tubules, collecting ducts and the glomerular podocytes. The GL-3 deposits in the glomerular podocytes were unchanged after treatment.

Thirteen patients completed all five α-galactosidase A infusions. The infusions were well tolerated. The most common adverse reaction was transient increased blood pressure during the infusion that did not required therapy and returned to normal after infusion. One patient had a pulmonary embolus at the end of the trial secondary to stopping anticoagulant therapy for lower extremity deep venous thrombosis. Eight patients developed IgG antibodies specific to α-galactosidase A and four patients developed hypersensitivity type reactions like transient fever, chills, and tachycardia. One patient developed hives. Most of the patients developed antibodies after the second and third infusion. The antibodies did not affect the pharmacokinetic profile. This suggests that the antibodies were not neutralizing at the dose used. Treatment with antipyretics and antihistamines helped to prevent infusion reactions.

This study was important as proof of principle for ERT by reduction of GL-3 storage in multiple cell types. Liver tissue showed the most marked response to therapy. Cardiomyocytes were resistant to treatment at all doses. This lack of response in cardiomyocytes could be secondary to the short duration of treatment. One patient in the 3 mg/kg every 48 h group had increased sinusoid and kupffer cell GL-3 scores and was not included in the histological analyses. The authors did not explain the reason for this result. In the kidneys the total GL-3 was reduced after treatment but the GL-3 in podocytes was unchanged. A goal of phase II trials is dose optimization and this study suggests that the biweekly regimen cleared more substrate and the 1 and 3 mg/kg doses were the most effective. Weaknesses of this study were the small sample size and the lack of clinical endpoints or validated measures for the outcomes. Still the study reached its goal of demonstrating that ERT was feasible for clearance of GL-3 deposits associated with Fabry disease.

A phase III study enrolled 58 patients in a placebo controlled trial [3]. The initial period was 20 weeks followed by an open label extension in which all participants received agalsidase beta. The primary endpoint for the study was clearance of GL-3 from the capillary endothelium of the kidneys. Secondary endpoints included clearance of GL-3 from the vascular endothelium of skin and cardiac tissues. All of these were met with a near complete clearance from the majority of treated patients and no clearance from those who received placebo. In the extension period all patients showed clearance of the microvasculature. A few clinical endpoints were evaluated but no significant differences were identified between treated patients and controls. This study demonstrated that ERT was very effective in improving the histological abnormalities seen in Fabry disease. This was the basis for FDA approval of agalsidase beta. The FDA recognized that the results of this study demonstrated proof that the enzyme could be delivered and function in the target organs, but requested additional studies to demonstrate clinical utility.

A separate phase III multicenter, randomized, double blind, placebo controlled clinical trial was reported by Banikazemi et al. to determine whether treatment with agalsidase beta could delay the onset of clinical events and death in patients with advanced Fabry disease [4]. The study enrolled 82 eligible patients from 41 referral centers from nine different countries. All patients received intravenous infusions of agalsidase beta for up to 35 months. Patients were randomized 2:1 treatment to placebo ratio to give more patients access to treatment. The study allowed patients to transition to open label agalsidase beta therapy after a primary endpoint event had occurred.

The primary endpoint of the study was the time to first clinical event. A significant limitation for the group analysis was that not all patients completed the study, 71 patients were active at the end of the study, eight withdrew and three died. In the agalsidase beta group one patient died of multiple pulmonary emboli and one patient died of cardiac arrest; and in the placebo group one patient died of cardiac arrest. All three patients had significantly advanced disease and because of this the authors did not attribute any deaths to the treatment. Six patients withdrew before the end. The treatment was generally well tolerated. Most of the adverse events were rhinitis, cough and headache with similar frequency in both groups. Fever and chills occurred in 55% of patients in the agalsidase group and 23% of patients in the placebo group. These symptoms were generally mild and not associated with significant health problems or complications.

About one third of the participants experienced one of the predefined clinical endpoints, 14/51 (27%) patients in the agalsidase beta group and 13/31 (42%) controls. Most of the events were renal consisting of increased of serum creatinine level and progression to end stage renal disease. Patients with estimated glomerular filtration rates (GFRs) greater than 55 ml/min per 1.73 m^2 and creatinine levels less than 1.5 mg/dL at baseline had a greater response to enzyme replacement than patients with lower GFRs and greater creatinine levels. More patients with elevated proteinuria at baseline were in the agalsidase beta group. This became an important confounder in the analyses of clinical endpoints. Additional analysis demonstrated that when primary intention to treat was adjusted by the Cox proportional hazard model for imbalanced proteinuria, the agalsidase beta group showed delayed time to first clinical event (hazard ratio of 0.47). Secondary analyses in protocol adherent patients showed similar, but more significant results (hazard ratio 0.39) compared with placebo. This suggests that therapy reduced the likelihood of any clinical event in patients with advanced Fabry disease indicating slower disease progression with treatment.

It is important that the study showed no changes in proteinuria with ERT, and that the therapeutic effect of ERT was not significant until adjustments were made to control for the degree of proteinuria. This highlights the importance of well controlled trials, and demonstrates that there is a point in progression after which the process is no longer reversible. In fact, it seems likely that there is a point in progression beyond which renal disease will continue to progress even with aggressive therapy.

26.2.1 Cardiac Function in Response to Agalsidase Beta

A study conducted by Imbriaco et al. is one of the few studies published that assess the effects of agalsidase beta therapy on left ventricular function by cardiac Magnetic Resonance Imaging (MRI) [5]. Eleven patients were enrolled, eight male and three female. They were treated with standard dose of agalsidase beta for a total of 45 months. In spite of the small sample, this study was able to detect statistically significant differences of the left ventricular functional parameters (left ventricular mass, septum, apex and lateral wall thickness) and myocardial T2 relaxation times after a mean of 45 months of treatment. Interestingly there was no significant change in the left ventricular ejection fraction after therapy with agalsidase beta. This was a promising result but the study design lacked clinical correlation endpoints, histology and more time points for analysis of the heart function. Prior histological studies have showed reduction of GL-3 in the myocardium after therapy with agalsidase beta [3]. Additional studies have showed some mild improvement of the left ventricular parameters after 6 months and 2 years of therapy [6, 7]. In a recent study performed in nine adult patients with advanced heart disease, agalsidase beta showed a minimal increase in stroke volume (15%) and slightly positive change in ejection fraction but this was not statistically significant [7]. Larger studies will be necessary to determine cardiac function improvement over time. Controlling for the stage of disease at the initiation of therapy will be critical to interpretation of these studies.

GL-3 accumulation in the microvasculature from patients with Fabry disease can alter the homeostasis of the endothelium and favor atherosclerosis [8]. A study conducted by Thurberg et al. [9] proposed that microvascular GL-3 clearance with ERT will restore normal endothelial function and prevent adverse effects associated with endothelial dysfunction. The results of the cardiac biopsies from the pivotal phase III trial study showed that 72% of the patients treated with agalsidase beta had decreased GL-3 in the microvasculature compared with only 3% of the placebo patients [3]. The placebo group had similar results during the open label extension. Only eight patients consented for biopsy at the end of the treatment. Six patients remained GL-3 free in the capillary endothelium at that point. There was no change in the GL-3 levels in the myocardium during this study including analysis by electron microscopy. The findings of this study suggest that long-term therapy with agalsidase beta will slow down the progression of the microvascular disease and may prevent clinical manifestations. The original report did not include clinical information in the analysis however long-term follow up of this cohort has been published [10]. A study of 23 patients with Fabry disease that were treated with ERT for 443 days reported no significant change in lipid profile [11].

The data on ERT with agalsidase beta appears to support a likely beneficial effect on the heart. However, additional studies are needed that include clinical endpoints and are long enough to determine if the improved histology and other changes truly result in better cardiac health by reduced incidence of life-threatening complications. It appears that there are irreversible changes associated with advanced heart disease and that response to therapy will be better with early treatment to prevent progression rather than later treatment to reverse or stabilize cardiac function.

26.2.2 Kidney Function in Response to Agalsidase Beta

Storage of GL-3 occurs throughout the nephrons and kidney vasculature, leading to progressive glomerular injury associated with mesangial widening and segmental and diffuse glomerulosclerosis. Advanced kidney disease is a common complication of patients with Fabry disease [12]. Studies have shown that early enzyme therapy initiation can stabilize renal function in adults with mild to moderate nephropathy through clearance of GL-3 from kidney cells [13]. As a part of the phase III clinical trial kidney biopsies were analyzed by three different pathologists at week 20. An average of 233 capillaries in each renal biopsy was assessed by each renal pathologist. The primary efficacy end point of the study required more than 50% of the renal interstitial capillaries in each specimen to have a score of 0 (normal or near normal), less than 5% to have a score of 1 or greater (multiple granules leading to distortion of the luminal endothelial cells), and the remainder would be designated as having trace evidence of endothelial deposits of GL-3. A majority score was determined from the review of three pathologists. At baseline the composite score for endothelial GL-3 in the agalsidase beta group was 1.9 ± 0.8 and the placebo group 2.2 ± 0.7, these values were not statistically different. At week 20 the agalsidase beta group had a composite score of 0.4 ± 0.7 which was statistically significant improvement. No differences were seen in the placebo group. The endpoint was reached by 20 of the 29 patients (69%) in the Fabrazyme® group compared with none of the 29 patients in the placebo group. This study was well designed and provides strong evidence of decreased storage of GL-3 in the kidney vasculature after therapy with agalsidase beta. It would be of interest to know the individual results from the three renal pathologists in addition to the composite score.

Patients with advanced nephropathy will need a combination of ERT and antiproteinuric therapy to prevent further decline in kidney function. A study reported by Tahir et al. [14] demonstrated that treatment with angiotensin-converting enzyme inhibitors (ACEI) and/or angiotensin receptor blocker (ARB) therapy in conjunction with agalsidase beta; resulted in sustained reductions in proteinuria with stabilization of kidney function in a group of six patients with severe Fabry nephropathy. This study included eight males and three females with Fabry disease, the majority of these patients were receiving treatment with antiproteinurics for 7 ± 6 months before starting ERT. Some patients received both ACEI and ARB; the dosages were different depending on proteinuria and antihypertensive effects. Kidney biopsies were obtained in eigt of the 12 patients; all had Fabry nephropathy. The blood pressure remained high in patients with severe nephropathy despite the use of ERT and more aggressive ACEI/ARB therapy. The average progression of estimated glomerular filtration rate (eGFR) rate for patients with severe nephropathy was 0.23 ± 1.12 ml/min per 1.73 m²/year within 30 months of follow-up. This study suggests that the combination of ERT and antiproteinurics has a high impact in slowing progression of Fabry nephropathy. This study has some limitations including small sample, single center, non blinded controls and short duration of follow-up.

The evidence of tissue level improvement from treatment with agalsidase beta infusions is strong. In addition there is clinical evidence of benefit to support use of ERT in patients advanced and early disease. It is likely that the earlier treatment is started the greater the impact will be on the progression of renal disease. Studies are needed to document the impact of treatment on renal manifestation of Fabry disease in pediatric patients. Because there is no overt renal dysfunction in this population it is likely this will require renal biopsies to provide interpretable data. It is also important to note that ERT did not clear the storage in podocytes even with long-term treatment [10]. The importance of this finding remains controversial.

26.2.3 Cerebrovascular Function in Response to Agalsidase Beta

Cerebrovascular events including transient ischemic attacks and stroke occur in Fabry disease patients at an early age. Cerebral manifestations are likely due mainly to progressive cerebrovascular dysfunction. These are a major and often life threatening manifestations of Fabry disease [15, 16]. A recent study of 721 patients with cryptogenic stroke showed a high prevalence of Fabry disease 4.9% of males and 2.4% females. Brain magnetic resonance shows white matter lesions that are frequently found in patients with Fabry disease, and recent studies suggest that male and female are equally affected [17]. There are no studies documenting outcomes of therapy on risk for stroke or other CNS manifestations of Fabry disease.

26.2.4 Gastroenterology Function in Response to Agalsidase Beta

Gastrointestinal complaints are a common and early manifestation of Fabry disease which worsens with age. The most common symptoms are postprandial abdominal pain and bloating followed by multiple bowel movements and diarrhea. Banikazemi et al. [18] reported four patients with severe gastrointestinal symptoms that significantly improved after treatment with agalsidase beta. At baseline all patients experienced postprandial abdominal pain and severe diarrhea with 6–10 bowel movements per day. After 6–7 months of treatment all patients reported no pain or occasional abdominal pain or diarrhea, all have discontinued gastrointestinal medications, had no food restrictions and had gained 3–8 kg.

Although the number of patients in this study was low and the lack of comparison to a placebo makes the interpretation of results difficult, the marked improvement of symptoms in these four patients is an early favorable outcome with significant implications for the quality of life of patients with Fabry disease. Larger studies will be needed to corroborate these results and to provide insights into the pathophysiology of this symptomatology.

26.2.5 *Pain and Quality of Life After Agalsidase Beta*

Pain is a significant problem and greatly impacts the quality of life of patients with Fabry disease. Chronic pain can be the most debilitating symptom experienced by Fabry disease patients.

Pain response to ERT is difficult to evaluate because of variability at base line, medication management independent of ERT, and placebo response. This is further complicated by use of different outcome questionnaires. A secondary endpoint of the multicentric double blind study conducted by Eng et al. was measurement of pain as an outcome. Pain measurements were done at the beginning and end of the study. All patients remained on their baseline medications throughout the study. The authors reported improved pain and quality of life in both treatment and placebo groups. It was impossible to differentiate treatment related benefits from a placebo effect.

An open label extension study by Wilcox et al. [19], reported that patients treated with agalsidase beta therapy for 30 months for the original placebo group and 36 months for the original enzyme treated group experienced a slight improvement for most of the SF-36 scale but these changes were not statistically significant.

A study by Konskenvuo et al. analyzed the quality of life as a secondary endpoint using the SF-36 scale in patients with advanced heart disease after treatment with agalsidase for 2 years [7]. Two out of eight patients reported exercising more and six reported no change in their physical activity. Four patients reported a reduced number of acroparesthesias with therapy.

Accumulation of GL-3 in the peripheral nervous system induces small nerve fiber dysfunction. Early ERT may improve small fiber function. In 22 patients with Fabry disease who underwent biweekly treatment with agalsidase beta showed a significant improvement in small fiber function after 18–23 months [20]. Few patients had abnormal cold detection thresholds and heat pain perception after the use of ERT. The authors attributed the lack of recovery in some patients to the late onset of ERT and irreversible nerve fiber loss. In spite of multiple clinical outcome studies that have included measures of pain and quality of life there is no clear demonstration a dramatic improvement with therapy. This may be due in part to the fact that most studies have enrolled primarily adult men with relatively advanced disease. Studies of earlier treatment and of treatment outcomes in females are clearly needed.

Other autonomic or sensory problems associated with Fabry disease include hearing loss, hot and cold sensation, and decreased sweating. The severity of hearing loss and tinnitus did not improve after short-term agalsidase [21]. There are few reports that suggest that long-term ERT appears to reverse sensorineural hearing loss [22]. Several studies have reported that treatment improves sweating, hearing and sensation but the evidence is not strong enough to clearly show long term benefit for these problems [18, 23, 24].

26.2.6 Pulmonary Function in Response to Agalsidase Beta

A case report in a 38 year old female with symptomatic pulmonary disease underwent treatment with agalsidase beta. The authors reported significant improvement of symptoms, pulmonary function test and computer tomography findings after 10 months of treatment [24].

26.3 Agalsidase Beta in Pediatric Patients with Fabry Disease

Most of the current literature on therapy for Fabry disease has ignored the pediatric and the female patients. Figure 26.2 is a schematic representation of Fabry disease clinical manifestations. Under-represented study groups are noted in a blue color. One of the challenges in the treatment of Fabry disease is that in adults the damage present at the time of treatment initiation is often irreversible. Obvious

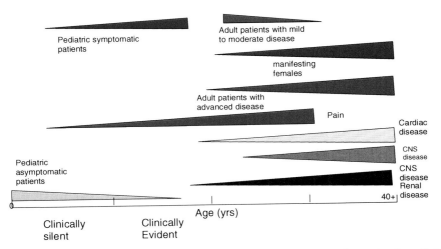

Fig. 26.2 Schematic model of the progression of Fabry disease. Fabry disease is often clinically silent during childhood with no obvious organ dysfunction. Symptomatic females, pediatric patients, and adults with mild disease are under-represented in clinical studies. Fabry patients have renal, cardiac, and central nervous system (CNS) disease at time of diagnosis and treatment initiation

organ dysfunction is uncommon in childhood. A recent natural history study of pediatric patients by Hopkin et al. [25] reported the characteristics of Fabry disease in 352 children and adolescents enrolled in the Fabry registry. The most frequent symptom was neuropathic pain which was present in 59% of males and 41% of females. Gastrointestinal symptoms were reported by 18% of children. Chronic renal disease (stage 2 and 3) was seen in three patients and left ventricular hypertrophy in three. This suggests that many pediatric patients report early symptoms, impaired quality of life and some children can experience major complications of the disease [25]. Studies suggest that early initiation of ERT treatment in pediatric patients will be important to achieve the best possible outcomes for these patients [26].

A recently published open label multicenter study of symptomatic pediatric patients treated with agalsidase beta showed improvement of symptoms with early therapy [27]. This study enrolled 14 male and two female patients between 8 and 15 years of age. One of the major limitations of this study is that the primary efficacy or end-point was not defined. Children were infused with agalsidase beta for 48 weeks. Before treatment 12 male patients showed moderate or severe GL-3 accumulation in dermal capillary endothelial cells, after treatment these cells were completely clear of GL-3 at week 24 and no re-accumulation was seen at week 48. Plasma GL-3 levels decreased from 15.9 μg/ml to a 6.3 μg/ml by week 4 of treatment. Gastrointestinal symptoms significantly decreased in incidence by week 24 of the study. Patient diaries documented significant reduction in school absences due to sickness. Noninvasive studies of renal function similar to those commonly used for adults were collected. Not surprisingly these were normal in all patients. These results are quite promising, but are not sufficient to state that there is clear benefit from initiation of ERT with agalsidase beta in pediatric patients with Fabry disease. The next steps will include a trial of ERT in asymptomatic pediatric patients. Future studies of cardiac and renal function in pediatric patients are clearly needed these will require sensitive measures for early signs of organ damage. It seems likely that tissue biopsies will be required to assess early renal involvement. Other important studies will include comparisons of different dose regimens in pediatric patients.

26.4 Agalsidase Beta in Women with Fabry Disease

The clinical manifestations of Fabry disease in females range from asymptomatic to severe symptoms of Fabry disease. A study from the Fabry registry enrolled 1,077 female patients and reported that 69.4% had symptoms and signs of Fabry disease [28]. Females with Fabry disease had a significant risk for major complications. This supports the rationale for more clinical studies that will evaluate the response of women to ERT. There are several studies that compared the pharmacokinetic and pharmacodynamics of ERT in female and male patients. No significant differences have been identified. Base line studies on manifestations of Fabry disease in women have clearly documented females are frequently symptomatic and that the disease has a significant impact [28, 29].

In spite of the number of symptomatic females there are no published studies that document treatment outcomes of significant numbers of female patients with agalsidase beta. Small numbers of females have been included in clinical trials, but not enough to allow for separate analysis. Because this is an X-linked disease there may be significant differences in optimal dosing of ERT, reversibility of organ damage, and/or response of symptoms to therapy. This highlights the need for studies focused on treatment of female patients. It is not safe to assume that treatment response will be similar to that seen in hemizygous men.

26.4.1 Immune Response to Agalsidase Beta

Antibody formation in response to ERT raises serious concerns about potential impact on the treatment efficacy in Fabry disease. The antibodies can bind to the infused enzyme and modify tissue distribution, clearance, subcellular trafficking, and catabolic activity. IgG antibodies against α-galactosidase A develop in the majority of patients upon repeated infusion. Bénichou et al. conducted a retrospective study on 134 adult male and female patients with Fabry disease who were treated with agalsidase beta for 5 years [30]. Blood samples were obtained pre-treatment and every 2 weeks prior to enzyme infusion. Anti-α-galactosidase A IgG titers were assessed by ELISA and confirmed by radioimmunoprecipitation assay. Patients were stratified in this study as seronegatives and seropositives. The seropositives were divided in lowest, intermediate and highest titer categories.

This study suggested that there are important differences in between male and female patients. The majority of male subjects seroconverted and only half of the females seroconverted. Peak titers for the seropositive females were in the range of the lowest subgroup of males. Rate of tolerization was also higher in females. The peak titers of anti-α-galactosidase A IgG in the patients who experienced a clinical event during agalsidase beta treatment were similar to the event free population. No statistical differences between titer subgroups were found. There was no correlation between anti-α-galactosidase A IgG titers and the onset of clinical events or the rate of change in estimated GFR during treatment. There was no statistical association between anti-α-galactosidase A IgG titers and elevation of plasma GL-3 during treatment. Patients with high anti-α-galactosidase A IgG titers had increased GL-3 deposition in the dermal capillary endothelial cells of skin, suggesting that GL-3 clearance may be impaired in patients with high antibody titers [30].

Occurrence of clinical endpoints may take years in Fabry disease which makes it difficult to assess the clinical importance of antibody formation. Earlier studies have shown that reappearance GL-3 in urine may occur as a result of the development of an antibody response [31]. Antibodies may also impact the recurrence of storage in skin capillaries, although no relation between antibody formation and plasma GL-3 response or clinical outcomes has been established.

A recent report by Lubanda et al. investigated the utility of low dose agalsidase beta at 0.3 mg/kg every 2 weeks after treatment with standard dose of 1 mg/kg suggested that there maybe a benefit in terms of frequency of infusion adverse reactions, optimizations of time and conditions of infusion and use of prophylactic medications [32]. This study raised several intriguing questions about current treatment options, patient risk stratification, antibody formation and the need for larger study groups, longer periods of observation and better clinical biomarkers to optimize the current treatment management with ERT. The study suggested that lower dose of agalsidase beta may maintain GL-3 clearance in some patients with Fabry disease, but other patients seem to require a higher dose to prevent GL-3 re-accumulation in skin and kidney cells.

26.4.2 *Comparison Between Recombinant Forms of* α-gal A

One of the major limitations in the direct comparison in between Fabrazyme® (agalsidase beta) and Replagal (agalsidase alpha) is that the dosing regimen is very different. The study design and analysis of data in clinical trials have also been different. There are limited published data about the pharmacodynamics and pharmacokinetics of the two recombinant forms of α-galactosidase A [33]. The Replagal trials were conducted with a dose of 0.05–0.2 mg/kg and the Fabrazyme® trials were conducted with 0.3–3 mg/kg. Thus, the dosing in these studies may differ by an order of magnitude. The clearance of both drugs was approximately 1–3 ml/kg/min, and the disappearance values $t\frac{1}{2}$ were about the same. In general, Replagal levels were approximately 50% of Fabrazyme® levels in all tissues after injection equivalent doses with the exception of the liver where nearly identical levels were achieved and maintained.

There are few direct comparisons between the two different enzymes preparations. The studies that are available include a biochemical and pharmacological comparison that demonstrated no significant differences in structure, activity, or immunogenicity when the same mass of enzyme was used [34]. A clinical study published by Vedder and colleagues found no significant differences between the two drugs with the same dose (0.2 mg/kg every 2 weeks) [35]. This issue is reviewed in detail in the chapter by Burrow and Grabowski. Our conclusion is that Fabrazyme and Replagal are functionally equivalent drugs. Any differences in response to these medications are likely to be due to either the difference in recommended dosing or to differences in study design and data interpretation.

26.5 Summary

The evidence supports a beneficial effect of agalsidase beta in decreasing concentrations of globotriaocylceramide in plasma and several tissues, but there is lack of clear documentation that these changes correlate with clinical outcomes. The clinical endpoints that have been studied indicate beneficial effects in the stabilization of creatinine, slowing progression to end stage renal disease, improved cardiac measures and heart function, decreased gastrointestinal complaints and improved quality of life. Nevertheless there is a critical need for longer follow up of larger populations. Well designed investigation into a number of clinical outcomes are essential to optimize the treatment of Fabry disease. The Fabry registries funded by Genzyme and Shire will play an important role in this effort but are unlikely to provide clear answers to all of the remaining questions. There appears to be no significant differences between agalsidase beta and agalsidase alpha. However, there is significant controversy regarding optimal dosing of enzyme therapy for Fabry disease. In addition, there is a particular need for studies of treatment outcomes including studies focused specifically on pediatric and female populations.

Disclosure C.E.P declares no competing financial interests. R.J.H. has done consulting work with Genzyme and Shire. He has been an investigator on clinical trials funded by Genzyme and Amicus. He serves on the medical advisory board for the Fabry Registry which is funded by Genzyme. He does not hold a financial interest in any company that produces treatments for Fabry disease or other lysosomal diseases, and does not receive salary support from any pharmaceutical company.

References

1. Zarate YA, Hopkin RJ (2008) Fabry's disease. Lancet 372(9647):1427–1435
2. Eng CM, Banikazemi M, Gordon RE, Goldman M, Phelps R, Kim L et al (2001) A phase 1/2 clinical trial of enzyme replacement in fabry disease: pharmacokinetic, substrate clearance, and safety studies. Am J Hum Genet 68(3):711–722
3. Eng CM, Guffon N, Wilcox WR, Germain DP, Lee P, Waldek S et al (2001) Safety and efficacy of recombinant human alpha-galactosidase A–replacement therapy in Fabry's disease. N Eng J Med 345(1):9–16
4. Banikazemi M, Bultas J, Waldek S, Wilcox WR, Whitley CB, McDonald M et al (2007) Agalsidase-beta therapy for advanced Fabry disease: a randomized trial. Ann Intern Med 146(2):77–86
5. Imbriaco M, Pisani A, Spinelli L, Cuocolo A, Messalli G, Capuano E et al (2009) Effects of enzyme-replacement therapy in patients with Anderson-Fabry disease: a prospective long-term cardiac magnetic resonance imaging study. Heart (Br Cardiac Soc) 95(13):1103–1107
6. Weidemann F, Breunig F, Beer M, Sandstede J, Turschner O, Voelker W et al (2003) Improvement of cardiac function during enzyme replacement therapy in patients with Fabry disease: a prospective strain rate imaging study. Circulation 108(11):1299–1301
7. Koskenvuo JW, Hartiala JJ, Nuutila P, Kalliokoski R, Viikari JS, Engblom E et al (2008) Twenty-four-month alpha-galactosidase A replacement therapy in Fabry disease has only minimal effects on symptoms and cardiovascular parameters. J Inherit Metabol Dis 31(3):432–441
8. DeGraba T, Azhar S, Dignat-George F, Brown E, Boutiere B, Altarescu G et al (2000) Profile of endothelial and leukocyte activation in Fabry patients. Ann Neurol 47(2):229–233
9. Thurberg BL, Fallon JT, Mitchell R, Aretz T, Gordon RE, O'Callaghan MW (2009) Cardiac microvascular pathology in Fabry disease: evaluation of endomyocardial biopsies before and after enzyme replacement therapy. Circulation 119(19):2561–2567
10. Germain DP, Waldek S, Banikazemi M, Bushinsky DA, Charrow J, Desnick RJ et al (2007) Sustained, long-term renal stabilization after 54 months of agalsidase beta therapy in patients with Fabry disease. J Am Soc Nephrol 18(5):1547–1557
11. Cartwright DJ, Cole AL, Cousins AJ, Lee PJ (2004) Raised HDL cholesterol in Fabry disease: response to enzyme replacement therapy. J Inherit Metabol Dis 27(6):791–793
12. Schiffmann R, Warnock DG, Banikazemi M, Bultas J, Linthorst GE, Packman S et al (2009) Fabry disease: progression of nephropathy, and prevalence of cardiac and cerebrovascular events before enzyme replacement therapy. Nephrol Dial Transplant 24(7):2102–2111
13. Ortiz A, Oliveira JP, Wanner C, Brenner BM, Waldek S, Warnock DG (2008) Recommendations and guidelines for the diagnosis and treatment of Fabry nephropathy in adults. Nat Clin Pract 4(6):327–336

14. Tahir H, Jackson LL, Warnock DG (2007) Antiproteinuric therapy and fabry nephropathy: sustained reduction of proteinuria in patients receiving enzyme replacement therapy with agalsidase-beta. J Am Soc Nephrol 18(9):2609–2617

15. Fellgiebel A (2007) Stroke and brain structural alterations in Fabry disease. Clin Ther 29(Suppl A):S

16. Sims K, Politei J, Banikazemi M, Lee P (2009) Stroke in Fabry disease frequently occurs before diagnosis and in the absence of other clinical events: natural history data from the Fabry Registry. Stroke; a journal of cerebral circulation 40(3):788–794

17. Fellgiebel A, Muller MJ, Mazanek M, Baron K, Beck M, Stoeter P (2005) White matter lesion severity in male and female patients with Fabry disease. Neurology 65(4):600–602

18. Banikazemi M, Ullman T, Desnick RJ (2005) Gastrointestinal manifestations of Fabry disease: clinical response to enzyme replacement therapy. Mol Genet Metabol 85(4): 255–259

19. Wilcox WR, Banikazemi M, Guffon N, Waldek S, Lee P, Linthorst GE et al (2004) Long-term safety and efficacy of enzyme replacement therapy for Fabry disease. Am J Hum Genet 75(1):65–74

20. Hilz MJ (2007) Peripheral nervous system involvement in Fabry disease: role in morbidity and mortality. Clin Ther 29(Suppl A):S

21. Choi JH, Cho YM, Suh KS, Yoon HR, Kim GH, Kim SS et al (2008) Short-term efficacy of enzyme replacement therapy in Korean patients with Fabry disease. J Korean Med Sci 23(2):243–250

22. Hajioff D, Enever Y, Quiney R, Zuckerman J, Mackermot K, Mehta A (2003) Hearing loss in Fabry disease: the effect of agalsidase alfa replacement therapy. J Inherit Metabol Dis 26(8):787–794

23. Schiffmann R, Floeter MK, Dambrosia JM, Gupta S, Moore DF, Sharabi Y et al (2003) Enzyme replacement therapy improves peripheral nerve and sweat function in Fabry disease. Muscle Nerve 28(6):703–710

24. Kim W, Pyeritz RE, Bernhardt BA, Casey M, Litt HI (2007) Pulmonary manifestations of Fabry disease and positive response to enzyme replacement therapy. Am J Med Genet 143(4):377–381

25. Hopkin RJ, Bissler J, Banikazemi M, Clarke L, Eng CM, Germain DP et al (2008) Characterization of Fabry disease in 352 pediatric patients in the Fabry Registry. Pediatric Res 64(5):550–555

26. Ries M, Clarke JT, Whybra C, Timmons M, Robinson C, Schlaggar BL et al (2006) Enzyme-replacement therapy with agalsidase alfa in children with Fabry disease. Pediatrics 118(3):924–932

27. Wraith JE, Tylki-Szymanska A, Guffon N, Lien YH, Tsimaratos M, Vellodi A et al (2008) Safety and efficacy of enzyme replacement therapy with agalsidase beta: an international, open-label study in pediatric patients with Fabry disease. J Pediatr 152(4). 563–570, 570.e1

28. Wilcox WR, Oliveira JP, Hopkin RJ, Ortiz A, Banikazemi M, Feldt-Rasmussen U et al (2008) Females with Fabry disease frequently have major organ involvement: lessons from the Fabry Registry. Mol Genet Metabol 93(2):112–128

29. Street NJ, Yi MS, Bailey LA, Hopkin RJ (2006) Comparison of health-related quality of life between heterozygous women with Fabry disease, a healthy control population, and patients with other chronic disease. Genet Med 8(6):346–353

30. Benichou B, Goyal S, Sung C, Norfleet AM, O'Brien F (2009) A retrospective analysis of the potential impact of IgG antibodies to agalsidase beta on efficacy during enzyme replacement therapy for Fabry disease. Mol Genet Metabol 96(1):4–12

31. Hollak CE, Linthorst GE (2009) Immune response to enzyme replacement therapy in Fabry disease: impact on clinical outcome? Mol Genet Metabol 96(1):1–3

32. Lubanda JC, Anijalg E, Bzduch V, Thurberg BL, Benichou B, Tylki-Szymanska A (2009) Evaluation of a low dose, after a standard therapeutic dose, of agalsidase beta during enzyme replacement therapy in patients with Fabry disease. Genet Med 11(4):256–264

33. Schiffmann R, Murray GJ, Treco D, Daniel P, Sellos-Moura M, Myers M et al (2000) Infusion of alpha-galactosidase A reduces tissue globotriaosylceramide storage in patients with Fabry disease. Proc Natl Acad Sci USA 97(1):365–370

34. Lee K, Jin X, Zhang K, Copertino L, Andrews L, Baker-Malcolm J et al (2003) A biochemical and pharmacological comparison of enzyme replacement therapies for the glycolipid storage disorder Fabry disease. Glycobiology 13(4):305–313

35. Vedder AC, Linthorst GE, Houge G, Groener JE, Ormel EE, Bouma BJ et al (2007) Treatment of Fabry disease: outcome of a comparative trial with agalsidase alfa or beta at a dose of 0.2 mg/kg. PLoS ONE 2(7):e598

Chapter 27
Analyses of Agalsidase Alfa and Agalsidase Beta for the Treatment of Fabry Disease

T. Andrew Burrow and Gregory A. Grabowski

Abstract Within the past decade, two recombinant α-galactosidase A replacement products have been developed for Fabry disease treatment: Agalsidase alfa (Replagal®, Shire TKT Pharmaceuticals, Cambridge, MA, USA) and agalsidase beta (Fabrazyme®, Genzyme Corp., Cambridge, MA, USA). Agalsidase alfa and beta are licensed in Europe, Canada, Australia, and the countries of the Pacific Rim (including Japan) at doses of 0.2 and 1.0 mg/kg body weight, respectively, whereas only agalsidase beta is licensed in the United States. The biological and therapeutic equivalency of these two recombinant alfa-galactosidase A preparations has been the subject of debate. The purpose of this chapter is to compare the available efficacy and safety data on agalsidase alfa and beta, and to provide suggestions for future comparative studies.

Keywords Comparison · Agalsidase alfa · Agalsidase beta · Recombinant alfa-galactosidase A · Enzyme replacement therapy

27.1 Biochemical/Pharmacokinetic Properties

Two enzyme preparations have been developed for the treatment of patients with Fabry disease. Using the human gene or cDNA that encode α-galactosidase A (EC 3.2.1.22), the enzyme is over-expressed in either a human fibrosarcoma cell line (agalsidase alfa) or in Chinese hamster ovary cells (CHO, agalsidase beta). The enzymes secreted into the media surrounding these cells are purified and formulated for use by intravenous injection.

Agalsidase alfa uses 'gene activation' to achieve α-galactosidase A over-expression by inserting regulatory sequences in specific regions of the genome upstream of the endogenous α-galactosidase A gene in a human fibrosarcoma cell

G.A. Grabowski (✉)
Division of Human Genetics, Cincinnati Children's Hospital Medical Center, Cincinnati, OH, USA; Department of Pediatrics, University of Cincinnati College of Medicine, Cincinnati, OH, USA
e-mail: greg.grabowski@cchmc.org

D. Elstein et al. (eds.), *Fabry Disease*, DOI 10.1007/978-90-481-9033-1_27,
© Springer Science+Business Media B.V. 2010

line [1]. In comparison, agalsidase beta is derived by transfection into CHO cell and amplification of the integrated α-galactosidase A cDNA [2]. The final formulations are Agalsidase alfa (Replagal®, Shire TKT Pharmaceuticals, Cambridge, MA, USA), and agalsidase beta (Fabrazyme®, Genzyme Corp., Cambridge, MA, USA). Agalsidase alfa and agalsidase beta are licensed in Europe, Canada, Australia, and the countries of the Pacific Rim (including Japan) at doses of 0.2 mg/kg and 1.0 mg/kg body weight, respectively; only agalsidase beta is licensed in the United States.

The recombinant α-galactosidase As from either system have similar amino acid sequences and exist as 100,000 molecular weight (MW) homodimers consisting of two ~51,200 MW glycosylated subunits [3]. Differences in post-translational modification of the alfa and beta variant preparations exist and result in differences in C-terminal amino acid sequences and glycosylation patterns.

From the cDNA, the predicted C-terminal sequence of α-galactosidase A is LKDLL [3]. However, differential post-translational proteolytic modification occurs, resulting in the presence of truncated polypeptide species (i.e., LKD and LKDL) in addition to the full length protein with LKDLL [3]. The amounts of these polypeptide species differ between the agalsidases with ~70% full-length (LKDLL) and 30% LKD and LKDL for agalsidase beta compared to ~94% LKD and LKDL for agalsidase alfa [3]. The functional or biological consequences of these differences are not known.

N-glycosylation occurs at asparagines 108, 161, and 184 on either enzyme, but the glycosylation structures differ. Complex oligosaccharides are present at Asn 108 for both preparations, although significant differences in the degree of sialyation are observed (35% vs. 85%, agalsidase alfa vs. beta, respectively). Phosphorylated oligomannose residues are the predominant species at Asn 161 and 184, but the percentage of complex oligosaccharides varies between the two preparations. Agalsidase alfa contains more complex oligosaccharides (i.e., fucose, N-acetylglucosamine, and galactose) at Asn 161 and 184 than agalsidase beta as follows: At Asn 161, 52% of the oligosaccharides chains were complex in alfa vs. 25% in beta; at Asn 184, 34% were complex in alfa vs. 4% in beta [3]. Overall the beta form has higher degrees of sialyation (total sialic acid: galactose ratio, 0.88 vs. 0.56) and mannose-6-phosphorylation (total, 3.1 ± 0.1 mol/mol protein vs. 1.8 ± 0.0) than the alfa form [3]. Sakuraba and colleagues found similar oligosaccharide characteristics except for lower levels of N-acetylglucosamine; sialic acid content was not determined for either enzyme preparation [4].

Given the greater degree of mannose-6-phosphate levels of agalsidase beta, this preparation might be expected to be more effectively taken up by mannose-6-phosphate receptors, and therefore have increased cellular/tissue activity. Indeed, enhanced binding of agalsidase beta to mannose-6-phosphate receptors of Fabry fibroblasts and higher intracellular α-galactosidase A activity is obtained when compared to agalsidase alfa up to saturating concentrations of both enzymes [4]. In vivo α-galactosidase A activity in the organs of α-galactosidase A knock out mice increased in a dose dependent manner following bolus intravenous administrations of agalsidase alfa and beta. The amount of enzyme activity was greater with beta in kidneys, heart, and spleen after administration of equal doses of agalsidase beta or alfa. Little differences were observed in the liver [3, 4], since the majority of either enzyme preparation (~65–70%) was recovered in the liver [3]. Evidently, several different oligosaccharide receptors participate in the hepatocellular, endothelial, and Kupffer cell uptake in the liver [3–5].

These differences in oligosaccharide and amino acid characteristics of the two preparations have no significant effect in the in vitro kinetics of either enzyme. For the pure alfa and beta forms, the final specific activities (64.0 ± 3.0 vs. 65.0 ± 3.0 μmol/min/mg), K_m (2.0 vs. 2.0 ± 0.2 mM), and V_{max} (79.5 ± 2.2 vs. 80.5 ± 0.7 μmol/min/mg), respectively, were identical using 4-methylumbelliferyl-α-D-galactopyranoside as a substrate [3]. The pharmacokinetics of these preparations in humans are also quite similar [2, 6–11]. The peak plasma concentration (C_{max}) of both preparations occurs at the end of the infusion and elimination from plasma occurs in a biphasic manner. The area under the curve (AUC) for agalsidase alfa was proportional to dose, whereas agalsidase beta was not. This suggests that agalsidase beta was administered at saturating doses, whereas agalsidase alfa was not. Furthermore, clearance decreases from 4 ml/min/kg to ~1 ml/min/kg with increasing doses of agalsidase beta. Given this information, agalsidase beta appears to be cleared from the circulation by saturable and nonsaturable pathways. Despite this, the clearance of both preparations at standard doses (0.2–1 mg/kg, agalsidase alfa and beta, respectively) occurs at approximately 1–4 ml/min/kg and $t_{1/2}$ are similar. Similar Vss values of ~1–4 blood volumes are noted for both preparations [12]. There does not appear to be a significant difference in pharmacokinetics between men and women. The pharmacokinetics of these preparations are also similar in children, except for serum clearance, which is slightly increased in children; however, this was suggested to be related to increased uptake into tissues and organs (increased organ/body weight ratios in children compared to adults) in children [13].

27.2 Analysis of Previous Clinical Trial Designs

Direct comparisons of the clinical results for these two preparations are complicated by variations in design and analyses of studies for agalsidase alfa and beta. A major challenge in such comparisons is that different doses were/are used: agalsidase alfa, 0.2 mg/kg/2 weeks vs. agalsidase beta, 1.0 mg/kg/2 weeks. Only one study has directly compared the efficacy and safety of agalsidase alfa and beta at identical doses (See below) [14].

Furthermore, the pivotal trials involve relatively small numbers of participants, because of the rarity of Fabry disease. Many other reports are anecdotal since they are not well controlled and contain only a few patients. The phase III trials of agalsidase alfa and beta involved 26 and 58 patients, respectively: Two patients in the agalsidase beta and none in the agalsidase alfa study were females [9, 11]. The rarity of Fabry disease makes the registries crucial to obtaining larger patient data sets to determine the comparative efficacy of enzyme replacement therapy (ERT) and long-term outcomes. However, data from the different Fabry registries must be interpreted carefully as data collection is voluntary at each participating center, and fully standardized monitoring protocols are not currently used. Furthermore, the baseline characteristics of participants, i.e., age, race, and degree of disease involvement, vary significantly among various therapeutic trials. Such intrinsic variability in the patient populations renders interpretation of the comparative efficacy of ERT very difficult. Additionally, relatively few studies have focused on women and children with Fabry disease [6, 10, 15]. The significant clinical involvement of heterozygous females indicates a major risk of complications from Fabry disease that may benefit from ERT. But this female population has clearly different dynamics of α-galactosidase A expression that varies between tissue and differential dosing may depend on knowledge of this variation.

The results of various studies are also confounded by differences in patient assessment tools and controls. In studies evaluating response of pain to ERT, different pain scales were used, i.e., BPI-3 or the McGill Pain Questionnaire and Body Pain SF-36 component score [16, 17]. Other studies have relied solely on patient self-reporting in pain diaries [18]. Importantly, these pain scales may not adequately or accurately reflect and evaluate the pain experienced by individuals with Fabry disease [12]. Quantifying patients' clinical response to pain is also confounded by their frequent use of pain medications (i.e., neuroleptics, narcotics, and anti-inflammatory agents), potentially falsely exaggerating the role of ERT in alleviating pain. This confounder was highlighted in the phase III trial of agalsidase alfa in which patients self-adjusted pain medications. This study concluded that pain decreased with the length of therapy. This was indeed observed, but the non-ERT control population maintained a parallel decrease in pain. This result showed that the test group had more perceived pain than the controls, and that the difference was maintained over the course of the trial. These results appear to support an equal effect on pain for both groups just by participating in the trial. In several clinical trials, patients discontinued all pain medications for a period of time (i.e., 1 week) prior to completing a pain scale, which can also alter a patient's perception of pain intensity [11, 19].

Variation in technique used to assess therapeutic effects, e.g., echocardiogram and cardiac magnetic resonance imaging (MRI), complicate comparative analyses [20–22] as do non-standardized cutoffs defining the degree of cardiac involvement. While ECHO and MRI provide accurate measures of cardiac structure and function, ECHO is particularly subject to inter/intra-technician and interpreter variability, making quantitative conclusions difficult. This is particularly relevant when studies have shown conflicting results – some identifying improvements in cardiac disease and others not [20–23]. Such non-standardized assessments also complicate the histopathological analyses of various organs. The phase III trials for agalsidase alfa and beta used renal histology as end points [9, 11]. In the alfa trial, the reported degree of renal involvement might lead to the conclusion of more pervasive and severe histological involvement, because of the focus on glomerulosclerosis and mesangial disease [11]. In the beta trial, interstitial capillary enthothelial cell globotriaocylceramide (GL-3) inclusions were the primary end point and the degree of glomerular disease was not [16]. In the alfa trial no specific improvements were apparent, whereas in the beta trial dramatic improvements were documented. However, the focus on sclerotic glomeruli (irreversible) or endothelial cell GL-3 (reversible) clearly prejudice interpretation.

Significant differences have been reported in IgG antibody sensitization to agalsidase alfa and beta with antibody positivity rates ranging between 56 and 86% in the agalsidase alfa groups, and up to 88% in the agalsidase beta groups [2, 9, 11, 24]. These discrepancies could be based on differential immunogenicity, in the compositions of the two enzymes, or in the differential dosing (0.2 vs. 1.0 mg/kg/2 weeks) [25, 26]. Non-standardized methods and sensitivities for anti-α-galactosidase A (e.g., Enzyme-linked immunosorbent assay (ELISA) and immunoprecipiation) contribute to difficulties in making direct [2, 11]. In a direct comparison, the antigenicity of agalsidase alfa and beta was analyzed in 18 patients and no differences were found. Also, the antibodies induced with agalsidase alfa or beta cross-reacted with either enzyme, indicating that antigenicity of these enzymes is likely caused by common epitopes [27]. In addition, the nature and amount of residual α-galactosidase A in the genetically heterogeneous Fabry population is likely to be of major importance in determining antibody sensitization rate. For example, females, having significant amounts of normal α-galactosidase A expressed in various tissues, have very low antibody positivity rates [6, 28].

To place these disparate studies and results in context, an optimal trial design can be developed conceptually for comparison of the efficacy of agalsidase alfa and beta in treating Fabry disease. Three treatment groups would include 0.2, 1.0 mg/kg/2 weeks, and 0.3–0.5 mg/kg/2 weeks of either drug. This protocol design would be particularly useful in comparing the efficacy of 0.2 and 1 mg/kg/2 weeks, in light of the study by Lubanda and colleagues, which suggested a lower maintenance dose may be effective in certain patients [29]. A placebo group would not be included as ERT is generally accepted to be beneficial in patients with Fabry disease and many would consider withholding treatment to this group unethical. The study would ideally be double blinded, although this would be challenging given the different doses and adverse event profile related to dose.

Sufficient patient numbers would be needed to provide adequate power to identify differences in standardized primary and secondary endpoints among the treatment groups. The baseline characteristics of participants, i.e., age, sex, ethnicity, and genotype, would need to be matched among the treatment groups – for example, randomization of extended families of affected males all with the same genotype. More importantly, a standardized protocol or scale to match the degrees of disease involvement would be needed and importantly these clinical parameters would need to be responsive to therapy (i.e., reversible). One to one assignment of matched patients with similar degrees of disease severity to agalsidase alfa and beta would be important to insure that variability was not a result of differences in baseline disease characteristics. This would be challenging given the broad degree of severity in patients with Fabry disease. A validated Fabry disease severity scoring system would be essential for this type of study. While many centers utilize the Mainz Severity Score Index (MSSI) for this purpose; it has not been formally validated in Fabry disease [30].

The variable rates of progression of Fabry disease tissue involvement implies the need for specific organ severity ratings independent of age, and that matched cohorts be evaluated for sufficient time assess changes in progressivity. Failing a formal randomized trial, registry data using combined data on 0.2 or 1 mg/kg/2 weeks could be analyzed using propensity score matching with agreed severity indices to compare the two drugs on a large cohort as has been done with Gaucher disease type 1 [31]. Data obtained from the Fabry disease registries will need to be more rigorously standardized.

Secondary markers (i.e., tissue, urine, and plasma GL-3) may prove useful, but they have not been shown to correlate with disease severity and progression. Consequently, direct evaluations of progression of renal (e.g., >25% worsening in renal function and/or renal failure), cardiovascular (e.g., progression of left ventricular hypertrophy and/or occurrence of myocardial infarction), and cerebrovascular disease (occurrence of transient ischemic attacks (TIAs) and/or stroke) would be superior. Other secondary endpoints, including evaluation of changes in pain/requirements for pain medication, gastrointestinal symptoms, sweating, and auditory/vestibular function would be reasonable to evaluate, given the uncertainty documented quantitative measures of therapeutic efficacy of ERT for these manifestations.

27.3 Direct Comparisons of Agalsidase Alfa and Beta

One study has directly compared the efficacy and safety of agalsidase alfa and beta [14] using a fix dose (0.2 mg/kg) of either drug. The change in the primary endpoint from improvements in renal function to reduction in left ventricular mass midway through the study complicates the analyses. Other endpoints included the occurrence of treatment failure (progression of cardiac, renal, or cerebral disease), glomerular filtration rate, pain, urine and plasma GL-3 levels, and the development of antibodies to α-galactosidase A.

After 12 and 24 months of either drug, no significant differences in median left ventricular mass were identified in either treatment group. Additional analysis of the data show that poor renal function (i.e., GFR <60 ml/min) correlated with increased left ventricular mass during the study (4/34 patients). When this sub group was removed, a significant reduction ($\sim$14%) in left ventricular mass was identified only in the combined (but not separate) treatment groups after 12 months. The individual treatment groups were separately underpowered.

Baseline median GFR was similar between the two treatment groups (agalsidase alfa, 99 ml/min; agalsidase beta, 109 ml/min, $p = 0.50$) as was proteinuria (data available for Dutch patients only; agalsidase alfa, 0.25 g/24 h; agalsidase beta 0.24 g/24 h, $p = 0.59$). No effect on renal function (glomerular filtration rate (GFR) or proteinuria) was present in either treatment group after 12 or 24 months. Two patients receiving agalsidase alfa showed progression of renal disease (>33% increase in creatinine) during the study, but these patients had significantly impaired (GFRs ≤ 30 ml/min) baseline renal function. No reduction in pain scores (BPI-3) were identified after 12 and 24 months and no differences in the incidence of treatment failure were detected among the two groups.

Anti-agalsidase antibodies were identified in 10/16 males (4/8 agalsidase alfa, 6/8 agalsidase beta; $p = 0.3$), but no females. This finding, based upon similar ELISA techniques for both preparations, is quite different from previous studies that have suggested an increased frequency of antibodies produced to agalsidase beta. Significantly, in antibody positive males, urine GL-3 levels failed to decline. In plasma, the GL-3 level rate of decline decreased in patients with antibodies to either enzyme preparation after 12 and 24 months compared to antibody negative males.

Although the study design had its weaknesses, several findings warrant attention. First, these data suggest that the presence of antibodies may have a significant inhibitory effect on the efficacy of ERT in Fabry disease. Although development of antibodies did not necessarily correlate with treatment failure in males, a majority of males experiencing treatment failure were antibody positive (6/10 antibody positive vs. 2/6 antibody negative). Disease progression (i.e., MRI brain abnormalities) continued despite switching patients from 0.2 to 1 mg/kg/2 weeks dosing of agalsidase beta. Second, no difference was found in the efficacy of the two preparations at similar doses. This is not surprising given the similar biochemical and kinetic properties of each preparation. It is unclear if patients receiving agalsidase beta would have experienced an improved therapeutic effect and avoided the effects resulting from seroconversion had they received the standard dose (1 mg/kg/2 weeks) of agalsidase beta.

Whether low doses (0.2 mg/kg/2 weeks) of agalsidase beta are as efficacious as the higher dose (1.0 mg/kg/2 weeks) is uncertain. To further address this issue, Lubanda and colleagues evaluated clearance of GL-3 in renal and skin biopsies in patients treated with agalsidase beta at a dose of 1.0 mg/kg/2 weeks for 24 weeks followed by 0.3 mg/kg/2 weeks for 72 weeks, for a total of 96 weeks [29]. Clearance of GL-3 from interstitial capillary endothelium, the primary endpoint, increased from 14% at baseline to 100% of fields in patients treated with 1.0 mg/kg/2 weeks after 24 weeks ($p < 0.001$). This degree clearance was maintained in 90% of fields in patients treated with 0.3 mg/kg/2 weeks after 96 weeks ($p = 0.25$). A significant increase in clearance of GL-3 from other renal cell types (except podocytes and non-capillary smooth muscle cells) occurred after 24 weeks at 1.0 mg/kg/2 weeks, but no increased difference was observed from weeks 24–96. Furthermore, the mean composite GL-3 score for all renal cell types improved significantly ($p < 0.001$) from baseline through the 1.0 mg/kg/2 weeks dose period (24 weeks), and did not change ($p = 0.06$) during the 0.3 mg/kg/2 weeks period (through week 96).

Similarly, clearance of GL-3 from superficial dermal capillary endothelial cells increased from 24% at baseline to 95% after 24 weeks of treatment at 1.0 mg/kg/2 weeks, but decreased to 70–80% during the remaining study period of 96 weeks. At one or more points during the 0.3 mg/kg/2 weeks dose treatment period, seven of 21 patients had increased histological GL-3 scores in the dermal capillary endothelium compared to those at the end of the 1 mg/kg/2 weeks treatment period. Two patients developed new angiokeratomas during this time.

Mean plasma GL-3 levels decreased to normal levels during the 1 mg/kg/2 weeks period. Although no significant change was observed in plasma GL-3 levels during the 0.3 mg/kg/2 week period, 10/21 patients exhibited increased plasma GL-3 levels on at least one occasion during this time. Mean urine GL-3 levels also decreased significantly from baseline during the 1 mg/kg/2 weeks period, but increased significantly during the 0.3 mg/kg/2 week period. Higher GL-3 levels were in urine sediment of seropositive (IgG) patients. Significant deterioration in renal function was noted in four patients during the 0.3 mg/kg/2 weeks period; two of these patients had clinically significant proteinuria (>3.0 g protein/g creatinine) at baseline.

These data suggest that after initial treatment with 1 mg/kg/2 weeks of agalsidase beta, 0.3 mg/kg/2 weeks may be sufficient in selected patients at maintaining clearance of GL-3 in certain cells types of renal tissue. This study was not designed to address the question of dose equivalency, since it was a maintenance study. In this regard, a subset of patients showed that the lower dose was insufficient in preventing GL-3 re-accumulation in the selected cells. Indeed, only patients with intermediate to high titers of antibodies had recurrence of GL-3 accumulation in the renal capillary endothelial cells. However, clearance of GL-3 from tissues has not been shown to predict long-term outcome, and the present study was conducted over too short of a period to address this question (see below) [29].

The overall conclusion indicates that a subset of individuals with Fabry disease could be maintained on lower doses of agalsidase beta, once therapeutic goals have been achieved. Indeed, in individuals without major preexisting irreversible tissue damage, e.g., young males, might have good therapeutic response (lack of progression), with low dose ERT. Certainly, experience with ERT in Gaucher disease has demonstrated that dosage may be adjusted in each individual [32]. For example, initiation of individuals on higher doses of enzyme and then decreasing the dose as tolerated once improvement/stabilization of the disease manifestations has been achieved is commonplace, particularly in adults. However, unlike Gaucher disease in which putative biomarkers (e.g., ACE, Tartrate Resistant Alkaline Phosphatase, and Chitrotriosidase), blood counts, and spleen and liver volume can assist in medical decision making for adjusting dosage, similar biomarkers for Fabry disease are not available. For example, chitotriosidase, which is elevated in several lysosomal storage diseases, particularly Gaucher disease, is not elevated in patients with Fabry disease [33].

Globotriaocylceramide (GL-3) accumulation in tissue, plasma, and urine have has been used for this purpose. Indeed, treatment with agalsidase alfa and beta effectively reduces GL-3 levels in plasma and urine sediment within 6 months of initiating therapy and maintains such levels for up to 54 months [9, 10, 14, 16, 18, 28, 34]. Likewise, decreased accumulation of GL-3 can be identified to varying degrees within tissues (i.e., kidney, heart, and skin) in patients treated with ERT [9]; however, this finding has not been shown to clinically correlate with disease severity/progression in patients.

Symptomatic/subjective data, i.e., pain, gastrointestinal symptoms, sweating, might facilitate dosing decisions, but no clear evidence is available that ERT consistently impacts these signs/symptoms. Also, these signs/symptoms do not correlate directly with the manifestations associated with the greatest risk of morbidity and mortality and potentially clinically significant progressive renal, cardiovascular, and cerebrovascular disease.

Certainly, selected disease manifestations (e.g., proteinuria) can be detected long before overt organ dysfunction (decreased GFR). While ERT appears to slow the progression of renal and cardiovascular complications, particularly in individuals in whom ERT is initiated early, there are no ERT prevention studies to verify this assertion. Importantly, once a disease damage threshold is surpassed, progression appears to continue independent of ERT.

Using ERT at individualized doses in Fabry disease, as in Gaucher disease, will require identification of markers that correlate with tissue disease activity, and prior to irreversible organ damage. In this respect, important lessons can be drawn from renal disease in children with Fabry disease. Namely, light microscopic evidence of glomerular, interstitial, and vascular changes and electron micrographic inclusions in podocytes, mesangial cells, and glomerular endothelial cells are present in children at the time that microalbuminuria is detected, and long before detection of clinically overt renal disease [35].

This highlights the importance of early treatment of patients with Fabry disease, prior to the onset of symptoms and development of a threshold of disease after which progression is inevitable.

27.3.1 Differential Clinical Effects of Agalsidase Alfa and Beta

Direct comparisons of the therapeutic efficacy of each of these two preparations are confounded by differences in patient characteristics (i.e., gender, severity, age, etc), dosing guidelines for the two drugs, endpoints, and methods in clinical studies. However, some conclusions can be gleaned.

27.3.1.1 Cardiac

Conflicting results have been reported of the effects of either drug on cardiac parameters, e.g., cardiac structure, function, and conduction [20–22, 36, 37]. Review of the Fabry Outcome Survey (FOS) data suggested that patients do experience improvements in cardiac structure and function [38]; however, there is significant inter-study variability in participant populations, study techniques (i.e., Echocardiogram vs. Cardiac MRI) and measures of cardiac structure/function, thereby making comparisons difficult. Decreased widening of the QRS-complex duration has resulted from ERT in affected adults [11, 20], but such effects on the frequency of arrhythmias or the likelihood of a cardiac event (i.e., heart attack, symptomatic arrhythmia, unstable angina) are uncertain. Such events have continued in adults with advanced disease who are treated with agalsidase beta [23, 39]. Cardiac disease also appears to progress in Fabry patients with multi organ involvement, particularly those with significant renal impairment [14, 23, 39].

Few data are available on affected females or children. Baehner and colleagues evaluated cardiac response to agalsidase alfa in 15 females (mean age 45.3 years) and identified statistically significant and continuous decline in left ventricular mass index from a baseline of 148.1 ± 10.17 g/m^2 after 27 (-23.0 ± 5.78 g/m^2, $p = 0.003$) and 41 weeks (-25.2 ± 8.12 g/m^2, $p = 0.039$) in 11/15 and 7/15 females, respectively. Similarly, there was a significant reduction in QRS duration at week 27 ($p = 0.007$) [6].

A 48 week open- label study of agalsidase beta in affected boys demonstrated stable cardiac conduction, and cardiac structure and function in 15/16 patients. The exception was a child with left ventricular hypertrophy at baseline and no change at 24 weeks [18]. Interestingly, normal left ventricular mass and mean ejection fraction were observed in 24 pediatric patients (19 males and five females) prior to ERT with agalsidase alfa. However, heart rate variability in the boys was significantly reduced compared to the girls (normal variability) and age-matched normal controls. This variability became more normal after 24 weeks of agalsdiase alfa ERT. This result was attributed to improved autonomic function in the boys treated with ERT [10]. This cardiac variability abnormality may be the harbinger of clinically significant adult cardiac disease, but actual data is needed to confirm this concept.

27.3.1.2 Renal

The effects of ERT (agalsidase beta) on mild to moderate Fabry disease were assessed by the time to a clinical event. These included renal events of 33% increase in serum creatinine or development of end-stage kidney disease requiring long-term dialysis or transplantation. Over a 35 month period worsening renal function was the most frequently identified clinical event in the treated and placebo groups. The significantly greater baseline proteinuria in the treatment group confounded the results. When adjusted for proteinuria a significant treatment effect was observed (hazard ratio, 0.39; $p = 0.034$). Furthermore, proteinuria was strongly associated with any clinical event (hazard ratio 1.3; $p = 0.005$) and any renal event (hazard ratio, 1.4; $p < 0.001$). These data provided highlight the need to carefully match patient groups and to develop technologies or markers for assessments of independent disease progression. Furthermore, these results emphasize the need to move beyond the monotherapy approaches that rely only on ERT and aggressively institute renoprotective medications (angiotensin converting enzyme inhibitor and angiotensin receptor blockers) [23].

The above study and registry data provide evidence that ERT slows and, possibly, prevents or reverses the progression of renal disease in Fabry patients prior to overt manifestations [6, 10, 16, 18, 24, 38, 40, 41]. Indeed, there appears to be a threshold of renal disease that includes (GFR <59 ml/min) (stage III renal disease), significant proteinuria (>1 g/24 h), and/or renal pathologic histological changes (>50% glomerulosclerosis), which if exceeded, will lead to continued renal deterioration despite ERT or other intervention [16, 24, 39]. This self-propagation of end-stage pathology is evident in many other diseases and represents irreversible disease pathway [42].

27.3.1.3 Gastrointestinal

The use of agalsidase alfa or beta leads to improved gastrointestinal signs/symptoms. Three clinical trials and one review from the Fabry Outcome Survey (FOS) documented significant relief of frequency and severity of abdominal pain, decreased frequency of diarrhea and vomiting, and decreased reliance on gastrointestinal medications occurs within 6 months of ERT initiation [18, 43–45]. These improvements persisted for over 3 years of treatment [43]. The degrees of improvement with agalsidase alfa or beta are difficult to compare since gastrointestinal problems were assessed differently, and there is heavy reliance on reporting. Such assessment methods are inherently flawed, as patient recall of symptoms is inaccurate. Irrespective of these issues, a large number of patients report improvements in gastrointestinal signs/symptoms with ERT [45, 46].

27.3.1.4 Central Nervous System Disease

Few studies have focused on the effects of ERT on the central nervous system (CNS) involvement in Fabry disease. Although neither enzyme variant crosses the blood-brain-barrier in significant amounts, delivery to the involved microvasculature in the brain might be expected to decrease the propensity to cerebrovascular events. With agalsidase beta, stroke or transient ischemic attacks were used as clinical events in a double-blind, placebo-controlled trial. Two Fabry patients in the placebo group experience cerebrovascular events near the beginning of the trial, whereas no events occurred in the treated group [23]. Thus, it is unclear if this represents a treatment effect [23].

MRI angiography (MRA) and brain proton magnetic resonance spectroscopy (MRS) were used to evaluate the effects of ERT on cerebral blood flow [47]. At baseline, four of eight patients had asymmetric widespread patterns of deep white matter hyperintense lesions on T2 and FLAIR-weighted images. After 12 months of receiving agalsidase alfa, the MRIs obtained in 7/8 patients remained normal in 3/7, showed no change in white matter lesions in 2/7, and showed worsening of these lesions in 2/7 patients. Abnormal MRS metabolite ratios were detected in 5/6 patients that showed improvement with ERT in two patients, but one had progression of white matter lesions [47]. Also, abnormal cerebral blood flow in patients with Fabry disease improved in those treated with agalsidase alfa [48, 49]. No comparative CNS imaging studies have been done with the two drugs.

27.3.1.5 Pain and Quality of Life

In the only direct comparative study of agalsidase alfa and beta (0.2 mg/kg/2 weeks) no significant reduction in pain score (BPI-3) was evident after 12 and 24 months of either therapy [14]. Several retrospective analyses from the Fabry Outcome Survey (agalsidase alfa) report improvements in degree of pain based upon an improved score on individual questions in the BPI after up to 3 years of treatment with agalsidase alfa [17, 38, 50]. Studies evaluating pain in boys treated with agalsidase alfa have been relatively short-term (6 months), potentially too short to show a clinical effect [10, 15]. Also, the pain surveys used in these studies have not been validated in children.

The subjective nature of pain, make for significant difficulties in quantitating changes. Inter-patient variability in scoring secondary to differences in pain tolerance and placebo effects are significant concerns as is the perception of pain following withdrawal of medications. While the various pain scales used are validated measures of pain in adults, such pain scales may not adequately or accurately evaluate the various types of pain that individuals with Fabry disease experience. Importantly some of these pain experiences are responsive to treatments and others are not [12].

As alternatives, quantitative objective sensory testing has been used in Fabry disease to evaluate large and small fiber function, dysfunction in the latter may be associated with neuropathic pain [51]. In ERT treated patients, quantitative sensory testing have shown improvements in small nerve fiber function, i.e., improved vibratory, cold, and heat-pain detection threshold, providing evidence of improvements in the peripheral nervous system disease [11, 52].

27.4 Conclusions

To date evidence shows that agalsidase alfa and beta have therapeutic effects on several of the clinical features of Fabry disease, but the degree to which the manifestations are stabilized or improved remains unclear. Certainly, renal and cardiac function progression is slowed. The long term outcome effects, particularly in affected children treated prior to the onset of overt multi-organ involvement, needs to be addressed.

Despite the many similarities of the two recombinant alfa-galactosidase A preparations, a significant amount of controversy exists regarding the clinical equivalency of the preparations. Comparisons of the two drugs have been complicated by differences in the clinical trials (i.e., different patient populations, primary endpoints, assessment tools, etc). Of major importance is the dosing differences – 0.2 mg/kg vs. 1 mg/kg every 2 weeks for agalsidase alfa and beta, respectively. Therefore, while it appears that one could use either preparation in patients, and switch between preparations as the need arises (in countries in which both preparations are licensed for use) maintaining equivalent dosing would be a particular challenge. Thus, more uniform collaborative and standardized cross-platform studies of various doses are needed to directly address this important question.

Significant differences exist in the cost of these two drugs. While both enzyme products are very expensive, the average wholesale price of agalsidase beta (1.0 mg/kg EOW) is approximately $112,320 for a 30 kg child, compared to

$132,129 for agalsidase alfa (0.2 mg/kg/2 weeks [53]). Comparing the two preparations, gram per gram of drug, agalsidase alfa is approximately 5.9 times as expensive as agalsidase beta. This annual cost calculation does not account for other fees, including markup on the drug from hospitals, private offices, and infusion centers, and cost of supplies, among others.

In conclusion, controversies regarding the comparability of agalsidase alfa and beta remain and further studies must be performed to further clarify this issue. Furthermore, the long term efficacy of these preparations in preventing disease manifestations, particularly in children, must be further addressed.

References

1. Enzyme Replacement Therapy with Replagal [Internet]. Shire human genetic therapies (updated April 29, 2009). Available from http://www.replagal.com/hcp_replagal.aspx. Accessed 3 Sept 2009
2. Eng CM, Banikazemi M, Gordon RE, Goldman M, Phelps R, Kim L et al (2001 Mar) A phase 1/2 clinical trial of enzyme replacement in fabry disease: pharmacokinetic, substrate clearance, and safety studies. Am J Hum Genet 68(3):711–722
3. Lee K, Jin X, Zhang K, Copertino L, Andrews L, Baker-Malcolm J et al (2003 Apr) A biochemical and pharmacological comparison of enzyme replacement therapies for the glycolipid storage disorder Fabry disease. Glycobiology 13(4):305–313
4. Sakuraba H, Murata-Ohsawa M, Kawashima I, Tajima Y, Kotani M, Ohshima T et al (2006) Comparison of the effects of agalsidase alfa and agalsidase beta on cultured human Fabry fibroblasts and Fabry mice. J Hum Genet 51(3):180–188
5. Bijsterbosch MK, Donker W, van de Bilt H, van Weely S, van Berkel TJ, Aerts JM (1996 Apr 15) Quantitative analysis of the targeting of mannose-terminal glucocerebrosidase. Predominant uptake by liver endothelial cells. Eur J Biochem 237(2): 344–349
6. Baehner F, Kampmann C, Whybra C, Miebach E, Wiethoff CM, Beck M (2003) Enzyme replacement therapy in heterozygous females with Fabry disease: results of a phase IIIB study. J Inherit Metab Dis 26(7):617–627
7. Beck M (2009 Feb) Agalsidase alfa for the treatment of Fabry disease: new data on clinical efficacy and safety. Expert Opin Biol Ther 9(2):255–261
8. Clarke JT, West ML, Bultas J, Schiffmann R (2007 Aug) The pharmacology of multiple regimens of agalsidase alfa enzyme replacement therapy for Fabry disease. Genet Med 9(8):504–509
9. Eng CM, Guffon N, Wilcox WR, Germain DP, Lee P, Waldek S et al (2001 Jul 5) Safety and efficacy of recombinant human alpha-galactosidase A–replacement therapy in Fabry's disease. N Engl J Med 345(1):9–16
10. Ries M, Clarke JT, Whybra C, Timmons M, Robinson C, Schlaggar BL et al (2006 Sep) Enzyme-replacement therapy with agalsidase alfa in children with Fabry disease. Pediatrics 118(3):924–932
11. Schiffmann R, Kopp JB, Austin HA III, Sabnis S, Moore DF, Weibel T et al (2001 Jun 6) Enzyme replacement therapy in Fabry disease: a randomized controlled trial. J Am Med Assoc 285(21):2743–2749
12. Hopkin RJ, Bissler J, Grabowski GA (2003) Comparative evaluation of alpha-galactosidase A infusions for treatment of Fabry disease. Genet Med 5(3):144–153
13. Ries M, Kim HJ, Zalewski CK, Mastroianni MA, Moore DF, Brady RO et al (2007 Jan) Neuropathic and cerebrovascular correlates of hearing loss in Fabry disease. Brain 130(Pt 1):143–150

14. Vedder AC, Linthorst GE, Houge G, Groener JE, Ormel EE, Bouma BJ et al (2007) Treatment of Fabry disease: outcome of a comparative trial with agalsidase alfa or beta at a dose of 0.2 mg/kg. PLoS ONE 2(7):e598

15. Ramaswami U, Wendt S, Pintos-Morell G, Parini R, Whybra C, Leon Leal JA et al (2007 Jan) Enzyme replacement therapy with agalsidase alfa in children with Fabry disease. Acta Paediatr 96(1):122–127

16. Germain DP, Waldek S, Banikazemi M, Bushinsky DA, Charrow J, Desnick RJ et al (2007 May) Sustained, long-term renal stabilization after 54 months of agalsidase beta therapy in patients with Fabry disease. J Am Soc Nephrol 18(5):1547–1557

17. Hoffmann B, Beck M, Sunder-Plassmann G, Borsini W, Ricci R, Mehta A (2007) Nature and prevalence of pain in Fabry disease and its response to enzyme replacement therapy–a retrospective analysis from the Fabry Outcome Survey. Clin J Pain 23(6):535–542

18. Wraith JE, Tylki-Szymanska A, Guffon N, Lien YH, Tsimaratos M, Vellodi A et al (2008) Safety and efficacy of enzyme replacement therapy with agalsidase beta: an international, open-label study in pediatric patients with Fabry disease. J Pediatr 152(4). 563–570, 570.e1

19. Schiffmann R, Floeter MK, Dambrosia JM, Gupta S, Moore DF, Sharabi Y et al (2003 Dec) Enzyme replacement therapy improves peripheral nerve and sweat function in Fabry disease. Muscle Nerve 28(6):703–710

20. Hughes DA, Elliott PM, Shah J, Zuckerman J, Coghlan G, Brookes J et al (2008 Feb) Effects of enzyme replacement therapy on the cardiomyopathy of Anderson-Fabry disease: a randomised, double-blind, placebo-controlled clinical trial of agalsidase alfa. Heart 94(2):153–158

21. Imbriaco M, Pisani A, Spinelli L, Cuocolo A, Messalli G, Capuano E et al (2009) Effects of enzyme replacement therapy in patients with Anderson-Fabry disease: a prospective long term cardiac magnetic resonance imaging study. Heart 95(13):1103–1107

22. Weidemann F, Breunig F, Beer M, Sandstede J, Turschner O, Voelker W et al (2003 Sep 16) Improvement of cardiac function during enzyme replacement therapy in patients with Fabry disease: a prospective strain rate imaging study. Circulation 108(11):1299–1301

23. Banikazemi M, Bultas J, Waldek S, Wilcox WR, Whitley CB, McDonald M et al (2007 Jan 16) Agalsidase-beta therapy for advanced Fabry disease: a randomized trial. Ann Intern Med 146(2):77–86

24. Schiffmann R, Ries M, Timmons M, Flaherty JT, Brady RO (2006 Feb) Long-term therapy with agalsidase alfa for Fabry disease: safety and effects on renal function in a home infusion setting. Nephrol Dial Transplant 21(2):345–354

25. Beck M (2002 Jun) Agalsidase alfa–a preparation for enzyme replacement therapy in Anderson-Fabry disease. Expert Opin Investig Drugs 11(6):851–858

26. Pastores GM, Thadhani R (2001 Aug 25) Enzyme-replacement therapy for Anderson-Fabry disease. Lancet 358(9282):601–603

27. Linthorst GE, Hollak CE, Donker-Koopman WE, Strijland A, Aerts JM (2004 Oct) Enzyme therapy for Fabry disease: neutralizing antibodies toward agalsidase alpha and beta. Kidney Int 66(4):1589–1595

28. Vedder AC, Breunig F, Donker-Koopman WE, Mills K, Young E, Winchester B et al (2008 Jul) Treatment of Fabry disease with different dosing regimens of agalsidase: effects on antibody formation and GL-3. Mol Genet Metab 94(3):319–325

29. Lubanda JC, Anijalg E, Bzduch V, Thurberg BL, Benichou B, Tylki-Szymanska A (2009 Apr) Evaluation of a low dose, after a standard therapeutic dose, of agalsidase beta during enzyme replacement therapy in patients with Fabry disease. Genet Med 11(4):256–264

30. Beck M (2006 Apr) The Mainz Severity Score Index (MSSI): development and validation of a system for scoring the signs and symptoms of Fabry disease. Acta Paediatr Suppl 95(451): 43–46

31. Grabowski GA, Kacena K, Cole JA, Hollak CE, Zhang L, Yee J et al (2009 Feb) Dose-response relationships for enzyme replacement therapy with imiglucerase/alglucerase in patients with Gaucher disease type 1. Genet Med 11(2):92–100

32. Andersson HC, Charrow J, Kaplan P, Mistry P, Pastores GM, Prakash-Cheng A et al (2005 Feb) Individualization of long-term enzyme replacement therapy for Gaucher disease. Genet Med 7(2):105–110

33. Isman F, Hobert JA, Thompson JN, Natowicz MR (2008 Jan) Plasma chitotriosidase in lysosomal storage diseases. Clin Chim Acta 387(1–2):165–167

34. Schiffmann R, Murray GJ, Treco D, Daniel P, Sellos-Moura M, Myers M et al (2000 Jan 4) Infusion of alpha-galactosidase A reduces tissue globotriaosylceramide storage in patients with Fabry disease. Proc Natl Acad Sci U S A 97(1):365–370

35. Tondel C, Bostad L, Hirth A, Svarstad E (2008 May) Renal biopsy findings in children and adolescents with Fabry disease and minimal albuminuria. Am J Kidney Dis 51(5):767–776

36. Koskenvuo JW, Hartiala JJ, Nuutila P, Kalliokoski R, Viikari JS, Engblom E et al (2008 Jun) Twenty-four-month alpha-galactosidase A replacement therapy in Fabry disease has only minimal effects on symptoms and cardiovascular parameters. J Inherit Metab Dis 31(3):432–441

37. Kovacevic-Preradovic T, Zuber M, Jost CH, Widmer U, Seifert B, Schulthess G et al (2008 Nov) Anderson-Fabry disease: long-term echocardiographic follow-up under enzyme replacement therapy. Eur J Echocardiogr 9(6):729–735

38. Beck M, Ricci R, Widmer U, Dehout F, de Lorenzo AG, Kampmann C et al (2004 Dec) Fabry disease: overall effects of agalsidase alfa treatment. Eur J Clin Invest 34(12):838–844

39. Breunig F, Weidemann F, Strotmann J, Knoll A, Wanner C (2006 Apr) Clinical benefit of enzyme replacement therapy in Fabry disease. Kidney Int 69(7):1216–1221

40. Feriozzi S, Schwarting A, Sunder-Plassmann G, West M, Cybulla M (2009) Agalsidase alfa slows the decline in renal function in patients with Fabry disease. Am J Nephrol 29(5):353–361

41. Schwarting A, Dehout F, Feriozzi S, Beck M, Mehta A, Sunder-Plassmann G (2006 Aug) Enzyme replacement therapy and renal function in 201 patients with Fabry disease. Clin Nephrol 66(2):77–84

42. Marinides GN (1993) Progression of chronic renal disease and diabetic nephropathy: a review of clinical studies and current therapy. J Med 24(4–5):266–288

43. Banikazemi M, Ullman T, Desnick RJ (2005 Aug) Gastrointestinal manifestations of Fabry disease: clinical response to enzyme replacement therapy. Mol Genet Metab 85(4):255–259

44. Dehout F, Roland D, Treille de Granseigne S, Guillaume B, Van Maldergem L (2004) Relief of gastrointestinal symptoms under enzyme replacement therapy [corrected] in patients with Fabry disease. J Inherit Metab Dis 27(4):499–505

45. Hoffmann B, Schwarz M, Mehta A, Keshav S (2007 Dec) Gastrointestinal symptoms in 342 patients with Fabry disease: prevalence and response to enzyme replacement therapy. Clin Gastroenterol Hepatol 5(12):1447–1453

46. Hoffmann B, Keshav S (2007 Apr) Gastrointestinal symptoms in Fabry disease: everything is possible, including treatment. Acta Paediatr Suppl 96(455):84–86

47. Jardim L, Vedolin L, Schwartz IV, Burin MG, Cecchin C, Kalakun L et al (2004) CNS involvement in Fabry disease: clinical and imaging studies before and after 12 months of enzyme replacement therapy. J Inherit Metab Dis 27(2):229–240

48. Moore DF, Altarescu G, Herscovitch P, Schiffmann R (2002 Jun) Enzyme replacement reverses abnormal cerebrovascular responses in Fabry disease. BMC Neurol 18(2):4

49. Moore DF, Altarescu G, Ling GS, Jeffries N, Frei KP, Weibel T et al (2002 Feb) Elevated cerebral blood flow velocities in Fabry disease with reversal after enzyme replacement. Stroke 33(2):525–531

50. Hoffmann B, Garcia de Lorenzo A, Mehta A, Beck M, Widmer U, Ricci R (2005) Effects of enzyme replacement therapy on pain and health related quality of life in patients with Fabry disease: data from FOS (Fabry Outcome Survey). J Med Genet 42(3):247–252

51. Dutsch M, Marthol H, Stemper B, Brys M, Haendl T, Hilz MJ (2002 Dec) Small fiber dysfunction predominates in Fabry neuropathy. J Clin Neurophysiol 19(6):575–586

52. Hilz MJ, Brys M, Marthol H, Stemper B, Dutsch M (2004 Apr 13) Enzyme replacement therapy improves function of C-, Adelta-, and Abeta-nerve fibers in Fabry neuropathy. Neurology 62(7):1066–1072

53. Burrow TA, Hopkin RJ, Leslie ND, Tinkle BT, Grabowski GA (2007 Dec) Enzyme reconstitution/replacement therapy for lysosomal storage diseases. Curr Opin Pediatr 19(6):628–635

Chapter 28
Enzyme Replacement Therapy in Children with Fabry Disease

Uma Ramaswami

Abstract Anderson-Fabry Disease (FD) is an X-linked glycosphingolipid storage disorder caused by a deficiency of α-galactosidase A. This deficiency results in a slowly progressive disease due to the accumulation of globotriaosylceramide (Gb3) in cells of various tissues and occurs in both males and females. The early non specific gastrointestinal symptoms and unexplained pain of this progressive condition often results in a delay in diagnosis by up to a decade. The safety and efficacy of treatment with Enzyme Replacement Therapy (ERT) with both agalsidase alfa and agalsidase beta has been well documented in adults. More recent studies have also shown the response to ERT in adults to be less effective when started in the later stages of disease progression. The optimal timing and dosing of ERT to delay or stop cardiac and renal complications of FD is currently unknown. The early clinical presentation of FD is heterogeneous with life threatening complications seen in adults being uncommon in children. The published literature of studies in children is currently limited but demonstrates safety and encouraging early efficacy data. Long term follow up data on the safety and efficacy of ERT in children is essential and this emphasizes the importance of accurate and meticulous data collection, both as individual treating clinicians and also for collating data on such rare diseases using the disease-specific global registries.

Keywords Enzyme replacement therapy · Fabry Disease · Safety · Efficacy · Infusion associated reaction · Agalsidase alfa · Agalsidase beta

Abbreviations

α-Gal A	α-galactosidase A
BPI	Brief pain inventory
CTH	Ceramidetrihexoside
eGFR	Estimated glomerular filtration rate
ERT	Enzyme replacement therapy

U. Ramaswami (✉)
Department of Paediatrics, Addenbrooke's Hospital, Cambridge, UK
e-mail: uma.ramaswami@addenbrookes.nhs.uk

D. Elstein et al. (eds.), *Fabry Disease*, DOI 10.1007/978-90-481-9033-1_28,
© Springer Science+Business Media B.V. 2010

FD	Fabry disease
Gb3	Globotriaosylceramide
GI	Gastrointestinal
IAR	Infusion associated reaction
IgE	Immunoglobulin E
IgG	Immunoglobulin G
LVM/h	Left ventricular mass indexed for height
Lyso Gb3	Globotriaocylsphingosine
MSSI	Mainz Severity Score Index
pNN50	Square root of the mean of the sum of squares of differences between adjacent filtered RR intervals that are >50 ms for the whole analysis
QoL	Quality of life
QSART	Quantitative sudomotor axon reflex test
QST	Quantitative sensory testing
RR	Inter-beat
SDNN	Standard deviation of the normal beat to normal beat intervals over the length of the analysis
SDNN-i	Mean of the standard deviation of all of the filtered RR intervals for all of the 5 min segments of the analysis
SDANN-i	Standard deviation of the mean of all filtered RR intervals for all of the 5 min segments of the analysis

Anderson-Fabry Disease, also known as Fabry Disease (FD) is a rare X-linked glycosphingolipid storage disorder caused by a deficiency of lysosomal enzyme α-galactosidase A (α-Gal A) [1] (OMIMM Number 301500). This deficiency results in a slowly progressive disease due to the accumulation of globotriaosylceramide (Gb3) in cells of various tissues and organs [2–4] in both males and females [5, 6]. Lysosomal accumulation of Gb3 begins in utero [7–9], and signs and symptoms of Fabry Disease emerge in childhood and adolescence [10, 11]. Common early symptoms in children include pain, hypohidrosis, gastrointestinal manifestations, acroparaesthesiae and cornea verticillata; symptoms can interfere with well being, school attendance and daily activities [12, 13]. Life threatening complications such as stroke, end stage renal failure and cardiomyopathy, often seen in adult patients with FD, are rare in children as is angiokeratoma [12]. However, early signs of renal dysfunction detected through microalbuminuria and Fabry specific renal histological changes [14, 15], left ventricular hypertrophy [16] and subclinical white matter changes on MRI scans [17] have been reported in childhood. Although the beneficial effects of enzyme replacement therapy (ERT) have been demonstrated in both male and female adults with Fabry Disease [18–23], it has also been shown that there is less benefit if ERT is commenced once there is evidence of significant or irreversible organ damage [24–27]. However data on the safety and efficacy of ERT in children are limited, with studies being short term and having small sample sizes [12, 28–31]. This chapter will address the available evidence on ERT with agalsidase alfa and agalsidase beta in children with Fabry Disease.

The incidence of Fabry Disease is approximately 1 in 117,000 [32] although in a recent Italian report, the prevalence of FD by newborn screening is estimated at 1 in 3,100 [33]. The deficiency of α-Gal A results in the accumulation of a neutral glycosphingolipid, ceramide trihexosidase (also known as globotriaosylceramide or Gb3 or GL3). Accumulation of this GSL substrate results in significant accumulation of ceramidetrihexoside (CTH) in various tissues and organs, including vascular endothelium, cardiac myocytes, neurons and dorsal root ganglia and renal cells including glomerular and tubular epithelium [34–38]. The progressive accumulation of CTH results in life threatening renal, cardiac and neurological complications in the third to fifth decades in adult males, with similar presentation in females but a later onset [39–43].

Although life threatening complications are rare in children, the onset of symptoms with significant disease burden in children occurs in the first decade of life with acroparaesthesiae, fever pain crisis, gastrointestinal manifestations, decreased sweating, lethargy and eye findings such as cornea verticillata seen on slit lamp examination [10, 44].

Two forms of ERT are currently available – agalsidase alfa, Replagal® (Shire Human Genetics Therapies, Inc., Cambridge, MA, USA) and agalsidase beta, Fabrazyme® (Genzyme Corporation, Cambridge, MA, USA.) Replagal is licensed for children over the age of 7 years and the current recommended dose is 0.2 mg/kg biweekly given as a 40 min infusion (for a summary of the product characteristics see: http://emc.medicines.org.uk/medicine/19760/SPC/Replagal). The recommended dose for Fabrazyme is 1 mg/kg given biweekly as an infusion over 2–3 h but in some cases up to 4 h (for a summary of the product characteristics see: http://emc.medicines.org.uk/medicine/18404/SPC/Fabrazyme).

The safety and efficacy of ERT in adults have been well described [19, 21, 26, 45–48]. Clinically significant efficacy data on the use of Replagal or Fabrazyme in patients with Fabry Disease show an improvement or stabilization of organ function including an improvement in pain [19], reduction in left ventricular mass index in adult males [49], improvement in quality of life [21] and gastrointestinal [50] and renal manifestations [51, 52]. Similar studies showing the efficacy of stabilization of organ function using Fabrazyme have been reported [24–26, 53–56].

Data on the effects of ERT in children are limited. There have so far been four publications of the results of clinical trials of ERT in children [28–31].

Ries and colleagues conducted an open label study of agalsidase alfa at 0.2 mg/kg given every other week [29]. The pharmacokinetics of this study showed similar results to those in adults; serum clearance of agalsidase alfa was slightly faster in children than as seen in some adults, but with no clinical consequences.

Ries et al. and Ramaswami et al. further reported the safety and efficacy of ERT with agalsidase alfa in children with Fabry Disease [28, 30]. In their earlier study, Ries and colleagues reported on 19 boys and five girls aged 6.5–18 years of age with Replagal 0.2 mg/kg biweekly [28]. Infusions were well tolerated with mild to moderate infusion associated reactions (IARs) such as fever, rigors, nausea and vomiting noted in 29% of infusions. Treatment of one patient was stopped due to the severity of the IARs, although premedication with antipyretic and antihistamine and/or steroids prevented further IARs. No immunoglobulin E (IgE) antibodies were detected during the study period and only one patient seroconverted with IgG positivity. This patient continued on ERT with no clinical consequences. Several exploratory efficacy end points were measured including plasma Gb3, which halved by 10 weeks (baseline 7.91 ± 0.71 nmol/ml; normal range <3 nmol/ml) and remained below half baseline value at 6 months but still above the normal range. In girls the baseline and 6 month plasma Gb3 results were within the normal range. A similar reduction in urinary Gb3 was noted in the 19 boys; overall there was a 78% decrease in urinary Gb3 over the course of the trial. A smaller but significant decrease in urinary Gb3 was noted in the girls.

Left ventricular mass indexed for height (LVM/h) was within the normal range at baseline with a non-significant decrease at 25 weeks. Only three children (two girls and one boy) had an increased LVM/h at baseline over 40 $g/m^{2.7}$ and demonstrated a 15% decrease in LVM/h at 25 weeks.

Heart rate variability parameters determined by 2 h ambulatory blood pressure monitoring was abnormal in all 19 boys at baseline. After 6 months of ERT, mean inter-beat (RR) intervals improved slightly. The other parameters including standard deviation of the normal beat to normal beat intervals over the length of the analysis (SDNN), mean of the standard deviation of all of the filtered RR intervals for all of the 5 min segments of the analysis (SDNN-i), standard deviation of the mean of all filtered RR intervals for all of the 5 min segments of the analysis (SDANN-i) and square root of the mean of the sum of squares of differences between adjacent filtered RR intervals that are >50 ms for the whole analysis (pNN50) showed significant improvement in all boys (see Table 28.1). Heart rate variability parameters in the girls were normal at baseline and at 25 weeks.

Most of the patients had a normal estimated Glomerular Filtration Rate (eGFR) at baseline and after 6 months of ERT. However, in seven patients who had an eGFR >135 ml/min per 1.73 m^2 (hyperfiltration) eGFR normalized within the first

Table 28.1 Heart rate variability parameters from 2-h ambulatory recordings in 23 paediatric fabry patients at baseline and after 25 weeks of agalsidase alfa therapy (from Ries et al. [28])

	Boys ($n = 18$)		Girls ($n = 5$)	
Variable	Baseline	25 week	Baseline	25 week
Mean RR, ms	627 ± 19	641 ± 26	794 ± 90	675 ± 53
SDNN, ms	75.5 ± 5.3	95.9 ± 7.8[a]	138.6 ± 23.1	102.6 ± 8.3
SDNN-I, ms	57.6 ± 4.1	69.2 ± 5.1[b]	105.2 ± 18.8	85.6 ± 9.0
SDANN-i, ms	46.7 ± 3.8	65.0 ± 6.3[b]	78.5 ± 23.3	52.8 ± 4.9
r-MSSD, ms	32.9 ± 4.1	45.7 ± 4.4[b]	91.9 ± 21.3	72.7 ± 17.9
pNN50, %	10.8 ± 2.5	18.3 ± 2.8[b]	39.9 ± 8.7	28.3 ± 7.1

[a]$p < 0.02$

[b]$p < 0.01$, Wilcoxon signed-rank test

3 months and remained within the normal range for the rest of the study period. In two patients who had stage 2 kidney disease as noted by an eGFR between 60 and 89 ml/min per 1.73 m^2, this appeared to improve by week 17 and then stabilized thereafter until the end of the study period at 26 weeks as shown in Fig. 28.1

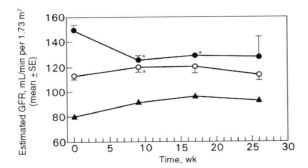

Fig. 28.1 Kidney function in 24 paediatric patients with FD by baseline chronic kidney disease stages. • Patients with FD with eGFR > 135 ml/min per 1.73 m^2 ($n = 7$); ○ Patients with normal renal function (National Kidney Foundation stage 1) with baseline eGFR 90–135 ml/min per 1.73 m^2 ($n = 15$); ▲ Patients with evidence of renal dysfunction (chronic kidney disease stage 2) at baseline with eGFR 60–89 ml/min per 1.73 m^2 ($n = 2$). eGFR was estimated in paediatric patients using the Counahan–Barratt equation [84]. $^{a}p < 0.05$ vs. baseline (time 0; Wilcoxon signed-rank test). From Ries et al. [28]

Although scores on the Brief Pain Inventory appeared to improve in all the boys and girls after 25 weeks of ERT, this did not achieve statistical significance. 6/11 patients (55%) who were on analgesics including gabapentin no longer needed pain medication after 25 weeks of treatment with ERT ($p = 0.12$).

Sweating was assessed using quantitative sudomotor axon reflex test (QSART) in 13 patients (12 males and one female). Interestingly, three patients who had anhidrosis defined as sweat volume using QSART of less than 0.1 μL/mm^2 had measurable sweating after 25 weeks of ERT and the mean increase in sweat volumes from baseline to 25 weeks in the whole cohort was statistically significant ($p = 0.06$).

A similar study on safety and efficacy of agalsidase alfa was reported by Ramaswami et al. and this was the first study to evaluate the safety of agalsidase alfa in children below the age of 7 years [30]. 13 children, aged between 3.5 and 18 years were treated with 0.2 mg/kg agalsidase alfa biweekly for 23 weeks. This was primarily a safety study with exploratory efficacy parameters including the Brief Pain Inventory, scores on which improved between baseline and 6 months in all patients with significant improvements in two patients who had pain scores of over seven (on a scale of one to ten) at baseline. Agalsidase alfa was well tolerated in all patients with one boy developing IgG antibodies during the study period with no impairment in clinical improvement. No patients developed IgE antibodies during the study period.

A study of the safety and efficacy of agalsidase beta (Fabrazyme) in children with Fabry Disease was reported by Wraith and colleagues [31] in 14 boys and two girls aged between 8 and 16 years. Following an initial period of 12 weeks of observation, patients were treated with the standard dose of Fabrazyme of 1 mg/kg biweekly for 48 weeks. All patients had routine pre-medication with an antipyretic ± an antihistamine. Plasma Gb3 halved over the study period and, more importantly, complete clearance of vascular endothelial GL3 in skin biopsies was noted within 24 weeks of treatment with no further accumulation noted at the end of the study. IgG agalsidase beta antibodies were detected in 11/16 patients, with reductions in antibody titer during the study period. One patient withdrew from the study due to severe infusion associated reactions.

Published short term studies have provided only limited information on the improvements in the gastrointestinal (GI) manifestations of treatment of Fabry Disease with ERT. Studies by three European centers have demonstrated interesting results with significant improvements in GI manifestations over a period of 24 months (Parini R, Ramaswami U, Pintos G: unpublished data courtesy Dr. Parini). The number and frequency of GI symptoms were analyzed in 41 patients (20 males and 21 females) less than 21 years of age. 17/41 patients (13 males and four females) were treated with agalsidase alfa at a dose of 0.2 mg/kg biweekly and at the time of analysis of this data, had been receiving treatment for at least 1 year.

29/41 patients (70%) had GI symptoms more than once a week. The most frequent GI symptoms were abdominal pain [27], diarrhoea [13], constipation [11], nausea [8], bloating [9] and vomiting [5]. Two patients had all six symptoms while 19/29 patients (65%) had more than one symptom.

In the treated subgroup at baseline, 12/17 (70%) had GI symptoms and 11/12 (92%) had symptoms more than once a week. Data after 12 and 24 months of ERT showed a reduction in the frequency of GI symptoms. The number of patients with GI symptoms fell from 12 at baseline to nine and five at 12 and 24 months respectively (see Figs. 28.2 and 28.3). The number of patients with GI symptoms more

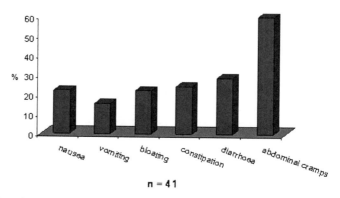

n = 41

Fig. 28.2 Prevalence of gastrointestinal manifestations in children with Fabry disease. Data from three centers in the UK, Italy and Spain

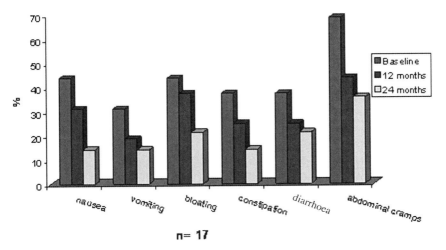

Fig. 28.3 Effects of agalsidase alfa on gastrointestinal manifestations in children with Fabry Disease. Data from three centers in the UK, Italy and Spain

than once per week fell from 11 at baseline to three and one at 12 and 24 months. It appeared that 70% of children with Fabry Disease had GI symptoms, which is a similar figure to previously published data [10, 30]. This cohort of patients clearly and quickly benefited from treatment with ERT with regards to their GI symptoms (Table 28.2).

Current studies in children with Fabry Disease are limited by the heterogeneity in clinical presentation and the short term nature of the studies, from 6 months to 1 year. The clinical presentation in children can be non specific with gastrointestinal symptoms, decreased sweating, hearing impairment and lethargy. Acroparaesthesia, which often goes unrecognized for up to 5 years [44] is common in children with Fabry Disease with 58% of children reporting acroparaesthesia by the first decade of life (see Fig. 28.4).

28.1 Usefulness of Disease Severity Scores in Children

The Mainz Severity Score Index (MSSI) [57] is a useful clinical scoring tool to assess the severity of disease and to monitor progression and treatment effects in adults with Fabry Disease. However, the use of this tool is currently limited in children due to the nature of the clinical presentation. Although Fabry Disease causes significant disease burden, often it cannot be truly represented by MSSI due to the nature of the weighting used and a bias towards increased scores for more life threatening complications such as renal failure, stroke and cardiac disease, which are well-recognized complications in adults but not children with Fabry Disease. The MSSI is divided into four categories: general, neurological, cardiovascular

Table 28.2 Abnormal clinical findings at baseline and improvement at end of study. Results from Ries et al. [28], Ramaswami et al. [30] and Wraith et al. [31]

Study	Ries et al. [28]		Ramaswami et al. [30]		Wraith et al. [31]	
Mean or median age (range)[a]	M: $n = 19$; 11.5 years (6.5–18 years)[a] F: $n = 5$; 13.5 years (8–17 years) No asymptomatic patients		M: $n = 9$; 10.4 years (3.5–18 years)[a] F: $n = 4$; 14.5 years (4.4–17.4 years) No asymptomatic patients		M: $n = 14$; 12.2 years (8.5–16 years)[a] F: $n = 2$; 11.4 years (11.1–11.7 years) No asymptomatic patients	
Enzyme treatment	Agalsidase alfa		Agalsidase alfa		Agalsidase beta	
Symptom/outcome	Baseline	6 months	Baseline	6 months	Baseline	12 months
Gastrointestinal	NR	NR	8	4 improved; 2 worsened	11/16 (68/8%)	Improvement in post-prandial pain ($p = 0.031$) and vomiting ($p = 0.008$)
Pain	24	24 (non-significant improvements)	10	6	NR	NR
Pain medication	11	5	0	0	NR	NR
Heart rate variability	19	Significant improvement in all patients	NR	NR	NR	NR
Increased left ventricular mass index	3	3 (15% improvement)	0	0	1	No data available
Measures of renal dysfunction						
Hyperfiltration	7	0	0	0	3	Improvement at 24 weeks[b]
Microalbuminuria	4	3	0	0	Mild proteinuria in 8/15 patients	Mild proteinuria in 3/8 patients

Table 28.2 (continued)

Study	Ries et al. [28]		Ramaswami et al. [30]		Wraith et al. [31]	
Mean or median age (range)[a]	M: n = 19; 11.5 years (6.5–18 years)[a] F: n = 5; 13.5 years (8–17 years) No asymptomatic patients		M: n = 9; 10.4 years (3.5–18 years)[a] F: n = 4; 14.5 years (4.4–17.4 years) No asymptomatic patients		M: n = 14; 12.2 years (8.5–16 years)[a] F: n = 2; 11.4 years (11.1–11.7 years) No asymptomatic patients	
Enzyme treatment	Agalsidase alfa		Agalsidase alfa		Agalsidase beta	
Symptom/outcome	Baseline	6 months	Baseline	6 months	Baseline	12 months
Abnormal sweating (QSART)	3	0	NR	NR	NR	NR
Central nervous system	Yes [1]	Yes [1]	No	No	No	No
Plasma Gb3	M: all abnormal F: all normal	M: all significant improvement F: unchanged	M: all abnormal F: all normal	M: all significant improvement F: unchanged	M: all abnormal F: all normal	M: all significant improvement ($p < 0.001$) F: unchanged
Urinary Gb3	M: all abnormal F: all normal	M: improvement in 13; overall 78% decrease F: unchanged	M: all abnormal F: abnormal in 2	M: improvement in 6 F: improvement in both	NR	NR
GL3 deposits in skin dermal capillary endothelium	NR	NR	NR	NR	12/16 data available – abnormal in all 12 patients	General improvement[c]
Quality of life	Normal at baseline (Health Utility Index)	Remained stable (Health Utility Index)	6 patients had reduced QoL scores due to pain	2 patients had reduced QoL scores due to pain	Days off school 12%; difficulty with low energy activities 12%	Days off school 7% ($p = 0.04$); difficulty with low energy activities 3% ($p < 0.001$)

Numbers represent the number of patients with results reported at baseline and after 6 or 12 months of treatment with ERT

NR: Not reported

[a]Ries et al. [28]: mean age reported; Ramaswami et al. [30]: median age reported; Wraith et al. [31]: mean age reported

[b]At 12 months, eGFR within the normal range in one patient; hyperfiltration but improved from baseline in second patient; data not available in third patient

[c]At 24 weeks, complete clearance in all 12 patients for whom data was available. At 48 weeks, sustained clearance in 5/12

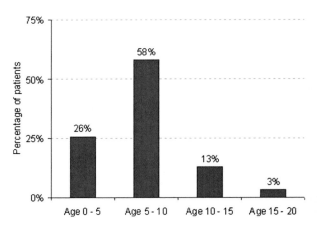

Fig. 28.4 Age at onset of acroparaesthesia. Data from Fabry Outcome Survey (unpublished)

and renal, with the sum of all four scores giving a total MSSI score. The severity score is categorized as follows: Mild <20; Moderate 20–40; Severe >40. Recently Parini and colleagues reported on the use of the MSSI to monitor treatment effects of ERT with agalsidase alfa in 30 Italian patients for a median treatment period of 2.9 years (range 1–6.2 years). They demonstrated that total MSSI scores were significantly lower than those at baseline ($p < 0.001$) [58]. An increase in the MSSI score over time can be demonstrated even in children as shown in Fig. 28.5 [10] but will not be sensitive enough to be used as a tool to monitor the effects of ERT in children.

Pain is an early symptom of Fabry Disease and has a significant impact on quality of life. However the published literature has a limited number of patients, with many patients either being too young to complete the Brief Pain Inventory (BPI) or no significant changes being noted at the end of 6–12 months treatment with

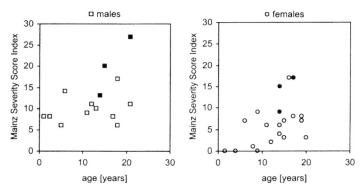

Fig. 28.5 Disease severity in males (*squares*) and females (*circles*) shown as a function of age. *Open symbols* represent patients without renal involvement and *solid symbols* those with renal involvement. A general increase in MSSI scores with age in children with Fabry Disease can be seen

ERT. The BPI is a validated tool to measure pain and quality of life in patients with chronic disease [59] and was used to demonstrate the effectiveness of ERT [19] and to monitor treatment effects of agalsidase alfa in adult patients with Fabry Disease [21]. Ramaswami and colleagues set out to quantify the extent of pain in 69 adolescents with Fabry Disease aged 10–20 years (29 males, mean age 14.9 years, SD 3) enrolled in the Fabry Outcome Survey [60]. Mean BPI scores at baseline were 2.2 ± 2.6 for pain and 2.6 ± 3.1 for pain at its worst; 39 of the 69 patients were receiving pain medication. Not surprisingly, patients who started ERT with agalsidase alfa were more severely affected than those who were not treated; mean BPI scores for pain were 3.0 ± 2.8 in the treated group and 1.5 ± 2.2 in the non-treated group (see Figs. 28.6 and 28.7).

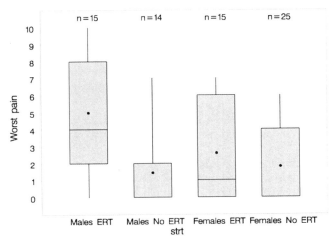

Fig. 28.6 Brief pain inventory: pain at its worst at baseline in adolescents with Fabry Disease. Data from the Fabry Outcome Survey (Ramaswami et al. [60])

Similarly, BPI scores for pain at its worst were 3.8 ± 3.4 in treated and 1.7 ± 2.5 in non-treated patients. The effect of pain in the patients' quality of life scores was significant (data not shown). Data on 21 of these patients treated with agalsidase alfa for 12 months showed a beneficial effect of ERT, with scores for pain at its worst and pain on average decreasing by 0.8 ± 0.8 and 0.5 ± 0.6, respectively (Figs. 28.8 and 28.9). These data illustrate the burden of pain in adolescents with FD and suggest an improvement after early ERT with agalsidase alfa.

28.2 Home Therapy

There is no doubt that the burden of disease and treatment with biweekly infusions has an impact on adults and children with Fabry Disease. To limit the disruption to daily living, some countries have successfully managed with ERT given at home either by a home care nurse, a carer or the patient themselves. This has also been successfully carried out for children receiving ERT (author's personal experience).

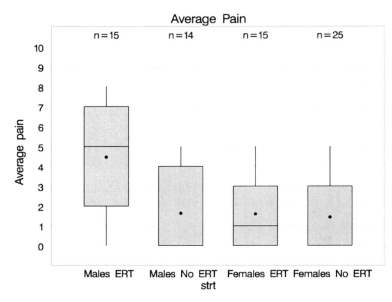

Fig. 28.7 Brief pain inventory: pain on average at baseline in adolescents with Fabry Disease. Data from the Fabry Outcome Survey (Ramaswami et al. [60])

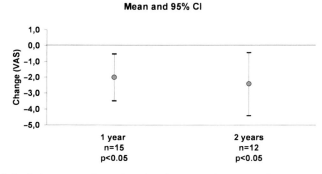

Fig. 28.8 Brief pain inventory: change in pain at its worst after 1 year of treatment with agalsidase alfa in adolescents with Fabry Disease

Milligan et al. reported on a questionnaire sent to 34 adult patients with Fabry Disease and 49 patients with type I Gaucher Disease, who were on home treatment with agalsidase alfa ERT or cerezyme respectively [61]. Of the 45 returned questionnaires were 20 patients with Fabry Disease. Just under half (45%) reported that infusions given at the hospital were stressful and 60% (12/20) reported that it had affected their family life. In contrast, only 10% of patients (2/20) found home infusions stressful with 90% (18/20) preferring to have their ERT in the comfort of their own homes. A quarter (5/20) felt that home infusions affected their family life but 75% (15/20) reported that home therapy improved the quality of their family life.

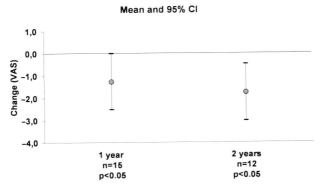

Fig. 28.9 Change in pain on average after 1 year of treatment with agalsidase alfa in adolescents with Fabry Disease

In the UK, children with lysosomal storage disorders (Gaucher, Fabry, MPS I, MPS II, Pompe) requiring ERT can also have home infusions. This is usually considered once ERT is established in the hospital and the child is deemed safe to transfer to home therapy. The number of hospital infusions vary between patient groups and indeed from patient to patient. Careful consideration also needs to be given to family circumstances. A recent patient satisfaction survey in May 2009 in the Pediatric Lysosomal Storage Disorders Unit at Addenbrooke's University Teaching Hospital in Cambridge UK revealed that families preferred ERT given at home and they were satisfied with the support provided by the hospital team and the home care service provided (unpublished, personal data, Dr Ramaswami). In order for 'hospital to home care' services to work effectively, the home care services, the family, the child receiving the treatment and hospital services must work in close partnership. The hospital clinicians caring for these children must have individual written and agreed management plans, not only for administering ERT but also a clear plan for infusion associated reactions, premedication and management of emergencies, including providing contact details of the hospital teams to both the home care teams and families. Patients who develop moderate to severe infusion associated reactions are usually brought back in to the hospital for infusions; transferring back to home therapy would depend on resolution of IARs with premedication. Commonly used drugs for premedication include paracetamol and hydroxyzine ± piriton which are best given 1 h prior to the infusion; steroids are rarely indicated as premedication (author's personal experience).

28.3 Dosing Studies: Agalsidase Alfa and Agalsidase Beta

Currently there is little information available regarding the optimal timing or indeed the dosing of ERT in children with FD. Dosing studies and the successful use of low dose cerezyme for adults with Gaucher disease is well established. In adults with Fabry Disease, dosing studies have been reported for both agalsidase alfa [27] and agalsidase beta [62].

Schiffmann et al. compared the efficacy of standard to weekly dosing of ERT in patients who demonstrated a continued worsening of renal function despite 2–4 years of standard treatment with agalsidase alfa at a dose of 0.2 mg/kg biweekly. This was a prospective open label study of 11/41 adults males with FD who had previously participated in long term clinical trials of agalsidase alfa who met the inclusion criteria of a decline in renal function by >5 ml/min per 1.73 m²/year. These patients were switched from biweekly to weekly infusions of agalsidase alfa, hence doubling the dose, and were followed up for a further 24 months. Improvements in eGFR were noted in 3/11 patients and stabilization in 6/11 patients while two patients showed ongoing worsening of renal function (see Fig. 28.10) [27]. Multiple regression analysis confirmed that the weekly dosing regimen was the most significant explanatory factor ($p = 0.0008$) with a weaker correlation being shown with the concomitant use of angiotensin converting enzyme inhibitors (ACE) or angiotensin receptor blockers ($p = 0.02$). The authors recommend consideration of weekly ERT with agalsidase alfa in patients who have worsening renal function with 2 years of standard treatment (0.2 mg/kg biweekly).

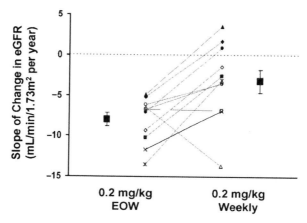

Fig. 28.10 The effect of changing the dosing frequency of agalsidase alfa from every other week (EOW) to weekly in patients whose estimated GFR (eGFR) declines at >5 ml/min per 1.73 m²/year during long-term EOW therapy. Each *symbol* represents an individual patient, and the *squares* represent the mean ± SEM during EOW and weekly dosing. From Schiffmann et al. [27]

Lubanda et al. considered a different treatment approach and evaluated dose reduction following a standard dose of agalsidase beta in patients with Fabry Disease [62]. This was an open label single-arm study over a period of 96 weeks. Twenty-one adult male patients first received 12 infusions at a standard dose of agalsidase beta (1 mg/kg biweekly) over a 6 month period followed by agalsidase beta at a dose of 0.3 mg/kg biweekly over the next 18 months. The primary end point was defined as the percentage of patients who had maintained GL3 clearance from kidney interstitial cells at the lower dose of agalsidase beta compared to the standard dose. GL3 accumulation was scored on a scale of 0–3; 0 = clear or trace, 1 = mild, 2 = moderate, 3 = severe. The primary end point of interstitial cell clearance during the study period showed an increase from 14% at baseline to 100% of patients on the standard regimen and 90% of patients on the reduced dosing schedule. A composite score, derived when all eight cell types were included, showed a significant improvement from baseline to week 24 ($p < 0.001$) with no further changes from week 24 to week 96 in most patients with only three patients showing a worsening of the composite scores at the end of the study.

28.4 Discussion

This chapter addresses the safety and efficacy parameters of ERT in children with Fabry Disease from currently available published literature.

Safety: A reduction in plasma GB3 was documented for both agalsidase alfa and beta. Urinary Gb3 reductions were documented for agalsidase alfa. Infusion associated reactions were noted in similar frequencies in the two clinical trials with agalsidase alfa [28, 30] and one study on agalsidase beta [31] (22%, 29% and 17% respectively). In all three studies, the IARs were mostly mild, the common symptoms being fever and rigor, which were managed effectively with pre-medication. Seroconversion rates of 11.1% and 5.3% with positive IgG antibodies were reported by Ramaswami et al. and Ries et al. respectively for agalsidase alfa. Seroconversion with agalsidase beta was however significantly higher at 69% as reported by Wraith and colleagues [31]. In both the Ramaswami et al. and Wraith et al. studies, the authors reported that the development of antibodies did not impair the efficacy of enzyme replacement therapy. No patients on agalsidase alfa developed IgE antibodies. No patients were reported to have IgE antibodies in the agalsidase beta study although one patient had withdrawn from this study due to severe infusion associated reactions. A review paper by Pintos et al. states that this patient who had been reported to have withdrawn from the agalsidase beta study had subsequently developed IgE antibodies whilst on commercial treatment [63]. The significance of developing high IgG antibody titers is currently uncertain. However, Benichou et al. have recently shown in adult patients on Fabrazyme that developing IgG titers in moderate amounts did not affect the clinical efficacy parameters [64].

In the absence of a robust biomarker to monitor disease progression or assess treatment effects, plasma and urinary Gb3 have been used as surrogate biomarkers. An elegant study by Auray-Blais et al. showed a clear correlation between urinary Gb3 excretion and types of mutations, with the highest excretion of urinary Gb3 being noted in patients with a nonsense mutation Q386X [65]. The authors showed that urinary Gb3 excretion was however variable in patients with missense mutations. Furthermore the authors also concluded that the sex of the patient was the most important parameter that influenced Gb3 levels, which therefore raises the question of the use of urinary Gb3 as a biomarker in heterozygotes. Over half of the patients with mutations in the GLA gene have missense mutations [66] and in addition Vedder et al. reported the lack of correlation between urinary/plasma Gb3 and clinical manifestations of Fabry Disease [67]. The negative effects of antibodies with increased excretion of urinary Gb3 in patients on ERT who developed IgG antibodies was shown by Whitfield et al. [68]. More recently, Aerts et al. have shown that deacylated Gb3, globotriaocylsphingosine (lyso Gb3) is significantly increased in Fabry Disease [69]. The authors demonstrated that lyso GB3 inhibits alpha galactosidase A activity and also that levels of lyso Gb3 seen in affected Fabry patients result in proliferation of smooth muscles in vitro. The authors therefore speculate that the vessel changes observed in Fabry Disease maybe due to an increase in lyso Gb3. Further studies are required to establish the role of plasma lyso Gb3 as a robust biomarker to monitor disease progression and treatment effects in both adults and children.

Efficacy: The primary endpoints in children consist of improvements in pain and gastrointestinal symptoms which, although considered to be subjective endpoints, have a significant impact on the day to day quality of life in children. End stage renal disease, cardiomyopathy and strokes are rare in childhood. The effects of ERT on quality of life assessments showed it either to improve [30, 31] or stabilize [28] in children with Fabry Disease. The Mainz Severity Score has been shown to be a useful tool in assessing the efficacy of ERT in adults with Fabry Disease [58]. This study included four children under the age of 16 years. As discussed previously, the MSSI score is divided into three severities (scores): mild (<20); moderate [20–40]; severe (>40). The MSSI scores in all four children were classified as mild (<20) and remained <20 after 1 year of ERT. In two children the scores worsened but were still in the mild category with a total score of less than 10. The weighting of MSSI scores relies on higher scores for renal, cardiac and central nervous system involvement with lower scores for manifestations such as gastrointestinal symptoms, which are more common in children. The original study by Whybra et al. had validated the MSSI scores for adults [57]. There are currently no specific disease severity scores that are sensitive enough to address small but significant efficacy measures in children with Fabry Disease receiving treatment with ERT.

Decreased sweating is a well recognized manifestation of Fabry Disease in both adults and children [44]. The quantitative sudomotor axon reflex testing (QSART) is a well known method that has been used in various studies to measure sweating [70]. Improvements in sweating using QSART were demonstrated by Ries et al. [28]. The involvement of the peripheral nervous system affecting mainly small Adelta and C fibers has been described and may be causally related to the autonomic dysfunction and neuropathic pain seen in patients with Fabry Disease [71]. Small fiber neuropathy has also been described in heterozygote females when tested using quantitative sensory testing (QST) [72]. However, reproducibility of QSART and QST was considered unacceptable for use as a secondary endpoint measure in clinical research trials in a study by Peltier et al. in patients with neuropathy and impaired glucose tolerance [73]. Moreover the equipment is expensive and not widely available for use in standard practice for the investigation and monitoring of patients with Fabry Disease.

Subjective improvements in gastrointestinal symptoms, improvements in quality of life and pain scores have been reported in studies on children for both agalsidase alfa and beta. It is therefore important that age-related disease severity scores are developed and suitable biomarkers are evaluated in children.

The impact of pain on quality of life in children is underestimated. The Brief Pain Inventory (BPI) is a validated tool to assess chronic pain. It measures the effect of pain on daily activity, quality of life and also defines the location of pain the effectiveness of treatments such as pain medication [59, 74, 75]. The BPI has been used to monitor the treatment effects of ERT in pivotal studies [19].

The impact of pain on QoL in patients with Fabry Disease and other conditions is well documented in the literature [21, 24, 47, 76, 77]. Improvements in BPI whilst on ERT has been demonstrated in children with FD [30]. Although scores on the BPI improved in all patients after ERT, the result did not reach statistical significance due to the small sample. BPI is also not a reliable tool in very young children and therefore it is not always possible to use BPI as a sufficiently sensitive tool to assess pain in children.

Despite the limitations in available tools to evaluate disease burden in children with Fabry Disease, the impact of FD on affected children cannot be underestimated; several authors have attempted to evaluate this in children and have shown a reduction in QoL in children with Fabry Disease [24, 77, 78]. Hopkin et al. in a study of 352 children from the Fabry Registry also showed impairment in QoL in children with FD [79]. The psychological impact of Fabry Disease and the under-recognition of significant depression in adults with Fabry Disease was shown in a study by Cole et al. [80]. Data on the psychosocial impact of Fabry Disease on children is currently not available and remains an urgent unmet need.

Dworkin et al. report on assessing the effectiveness of pain medication for chronic illness, by publishing recommendations by the Initiative on Methods, Measurement and Pain Assessment in Clinical Trials (IMMPACT) committee. This includes assessing pain using four core criteria:

- Pain intensity, assessed by 0–10 numerical rating scale
- Physical functioning, assessed by the Multidimensional Pain Inventory and Brief Pain Inventory interference scales
- Emotional functioning, assessed by the Beck Depression Inventory and Profile of Mood States
- Participant ratings of overall improvement, assessed by the Patient Global Impression of Change scale.

It was recommended that two or more different methods be used to evaluate the clinical importance of improvement or worsening for chronic pain clinical trial outcome measures [81]. Debilitating chronic pain is a hallmark of Fabry Disease with fever pain crisis and acroparaesthesiae being well recognized features in young children with Fabry Disease. Mehta et al. reported that these clinical manifestations are often misdiagnosed and the average time between onset of symptoms and diagnosis in males and females was reported as 13.7 and 16.3 years respectively [77]. It is important that meticulous attention is paid in the future to assessing the burden of pain with the use of methods which are appropriate and validated for children.

Currently there are no broadly accepted pediatric guidelines for treatment with enzyme replacement therapy; decisions on treatment are based on national guidelines and the criteria to treat can vary. An example of such a guideline is the UK National Guideline for the Management of Fabry Disease [82].

The current available literature on ERT in children with Fabry Disease does demonstrate that it is safe and early efficacy data is also promising. As widespread histologic changes in the kidneys, heart and brain may be seen in children and adolescents with Fabry Disease, before clinical evidence of significant complications become apparent, early initiation of ERT may prove essential for obtaining the best possible therapeutic benefit. However the most advantageous dose and age at which therapy should be initiated are as yet unknown. This is currently being evaluated in a study of lower dose Fabrazyme in males naïve to treatment aged 5–18 years with mild symptoms [83]. This study may prove valuable in understanding the disease progression and also providing guidance on the optimum timing of ERT in children with Fabry Disease to delay progression of or avoid the life threatening complications that are well recognized in later years of life. Long term follow up data on the safety and efficacy of ERT in children is essential and this emphasizes the importance of accurate and meticulous data collection, both as individual treating clinicians and also for collating data on such rare diseases using the disease-specific global registries.

References

1. Brady RO (1967 Jul) Enzymatic abnormalities in diseases of sphingolipid metabolism. Clin Chem 13(7):565–577
2. Desnick RJ, Banikazemi M, Wasserstein M (2002 Jan) Enzyme replacement therapy for Fabry disease, an inherited nephropathy. Clin Nephrol 57(1):1–8
3. Desnick RJ, Brady R, Barranger J, Collins AJ, Germain DP, Goldman M et al (2003 Feb 18) Fabry disease, an under-recognized multisystemic disorder: expert recommendations for diagnosis, management, and enzyme replacement therapy. Ann Intern Med 138(4):338–346
4. Desnick RJ, Schuchman EH (2002 Dec) Enzyme replacement and enhancement therapies: lessons from lysosomal disorders. Nat Rev Genet 3(12):954–966
5. MacDermot KD, Holmes A, Miners AH (2001 Nov) Anderson-Fabry disease: clinical manifestations and impact of disease in a cohort of 60 obligate carrier females. J Med Genet 38(11):769–775
6. MacDermot KD, Holmes A, Miners AH (2001 Nov) Anderson-Fabry disease: clinical manifestations and impact of disease in a cohort of 98 hemizygous males. J Med Genet 38(11):750–760
7. Vedder AC, Strijland A, vd Bergh Weerman MA, Florquin S, Aerts JM, Hollak CE (2006) Manifestations of Fabry disease in placental tissue. J Inherit Metab Dis 29(1):106–111
8. Tsutsumi O, Sato M, Sato K, Sato K, Mizuno M, Sakamoto S (1985 Mar) Early prenatal diagnosis of inborn error of metabolism: a case report of a fetus affected with Fabry's disease. Asia Oceania J Obstet Gynaecol 11(1):39–45
9. Tsutsumi A, Uchida Y, Kanai T, Tsutsumi O, Satoh K, Sakamoto S (1984 Dec) Corneal findings in a foetus with Fabry's disease. Acta Ophthalmol (Copenh) 62(6):923–931

10. Ries M, Ramaswami U, Parini R, Lindblad B, Whybra C, Willers I et al (2003 Nov) The early clinical phenotype of Fabry disease: a study on 35 European children and adolescents. Eur J Pediatr 162(11):767–772

11. Lidove O, Ramaswami U, Jaussaud R, Barbey F, Maisonobe T, Caillaud C et al (2006 Sep) Hyperhidrosis: a new and often early symptom in Fabry disease. International experience and data from the Fabry Outcome Survey. Int J Clin Pract 60(9):1053–1059

12. Ramaswami U (2008 Apr) Fabry disease during childhood: clinical manifestations and treatment with agalsidase alfa. Acta Paediatr Suppl 97(457):38–40

13. Zarate YA, Hopkin RJ (2008) Fabry's disease. Lancet 372(9647):1427–1435

14. Tondel C, Bostad L, Hirth A, Svarstad E (2008) Renal biopsy findings in children and adolescents with Fabry disease and minimal albuminuria. Am J Kidney Dis 51(5):767–776

15. Tondel C, Bostad L, Laegreid LM, Houge G, Svarstad E (2008) Prominence of glomerular and vascular changes in renal biopsies in children and adolescents with Fabry disease and microalbuminuria. Clin Ther 30(Suppl B):S42

16. Kampmann C, Wiethoff CM, Whybra C, Baehner FA, Mengel E, Beck M (2008 Apr) Cardiac manifestations of Anderson-Fabry disease in children and adolescents. Acta Paediatr 97(4):463–469

17. Cabrera-Salazar MA, O'Rourke E, Charria-Ortiz G, Barranger JA (2005 Jul) Radiological evidence of early cerebral microvascular disease in young children with Fabry disease. J Pediatr 147(1):102–105

18. Eng CM, Banikazemi M, Gordon RE, Goldman M, Phelps R, Kim L et al (2001 Mar) A phase 1/2 clinical trial of enzyme replacement in fabry disease: pharmacokinetic, substrate clearance, and safety studies. Am J Hum Genet 68(3):711–722

19. Schiffmann R, Kopp JB, Austin HA III, Sabnis S, Moore DF, Weibel T et al (2001 Jun 6) Enzyme replacement therapy in Fabry disease: a randomized controlled trial. J Am Med Assoc 285(21):2743–2749

20. Schiffmann R, Floeter MK, Dambrosia JM, Gupta S, Moore DF, Sharabi Y et al (2003 Dec) Enzyme replacement therapy improves peripheral nerve and sweat function in Fabry disease. Muscle Nerve 28(6):703–710

21. Hoffmann B, Garcia de Lorenzo A, Mehta A, Beck M, Widmer U, Ricci R (2005 Mar) Effects of enzyme replacement therapy on pain and health related quality of life in patients with Fabry disease: data from FOS (Fabry Outcome Survey). J Med Genet 42(3):247–252

22. Mehta A (2002 Jun) Agalsidase alfa: specific treatment for Fabry disease. Hosp Med 63(6):347–350

23. Whybra C, Miebach E, Mengel E, Gal A, Baron K, Beck M et al (2009 Jun) A 4-year study of the efficacy and tolerability of enzyme replacement therapy with agalsidase alfa in 36 women with Fabry disease. Genet Med 11(6):441–449

24. Banikazemi M, Ullman T, Desnick RJ (2005 Aug) Gastrointestinal manifestations of Fabry disease: clinical response to enzyme replacement therapy. Mol Genet Metab 85(4):255–259

25. Banikazemi M, Desnick RJ (2006 Feb) Does enzyme replacement therapy improve symptoms of Fabry disease in patients undergoing dialysis? Nat Clin Pract Nephrol 2(2):72–73

26. Banikazemi M, Bultas J, Waldek S, Wilcox WR, Whitley CB, McDonald M et al (2007 Jan 16) Agalsidase-beta therapy for advanced Fabry disease: a randomized trial. Ann Intern Med 146(2):77–86

27. Schiffmann R, Askari H, Timmons M, Robinson C, Benko W, Brady RO et al (2007 May) Weekly enzyme replacement therapy may slow decline of renal function in patients with Fabry disease who are on long-term biweekly dosing. J Am Soc Nephrol 18(5):1576–1583

28. Ries M, Clarke JT, Whybra C, Timmons M, Robinson C, Schlaggar BL et al (2006 Sep) Enzyme-replacement therapy with agalsidase alfa in children with Fabry disease. Pediatrics 118(3):924–932

29. Ries M, Clarke JT, Whybra C, Mehta A, Loveday KS, Brady RO et al (2007 Oct) Enzyme replacement in Fabry disease: pharmacokinetics and pharmacodynamics of agalsidase alpha in children and adolescents. J Clin Pharmacol 47(10):1222–1230

30. Ramaswami U, Wendt S, Pintos-Morell G, Parini R, Whybra C, Leon Leal JA et al (2007 Jan) Enzyme replacement therapy with agalsidase alfa in children with Fabry disease. Acta Paediatr 96(1):122–127
31. Wraith JE, Tylki-Szymanska A, Guffon N, Lien YH, Tsimaratos M, Vellodi A et al (2008) Safety and efficacy of enzyme replacement therapy with agalsidase beta: an international, open-label study in pediatric patients with Fabry disease. J Pediatr 152(4). 563–570, 570.e1
32. Meikle PJ, Hopwood JJ, Clague AE, Carey WF (1999 Jan 20) Prevalence of lysosomal storage disorders. J Am Med Assoc 281(3):249–254
33. Spada M, Pagliardini S, Yasuda M, Tukel T, Thiagarajan G, Sakuraba H et al (2006 Jul) High incidence of later-onset fabry disease revealed by newborn screening. Am J Hum Genet 79(1):31–40
34. Desnick RJ (2001 Apr) Enzyme replacement and beyond. J Inherit Metab Dis 24(2):251–265
35. Sessa A, Toson A, Nebuloni M, Pallotti F, Giordano F, Battini G et al (2002) Renal ultrastructural findings in Anderson-Fabry disease. J Nephrol 15(2):109–112
36. Sessa A, Meroni M, Battini G, Righetti M, Nebuloni M, Tosoni A et al (2003) Evolution of renal pathology in Fabry disease. Acta Paediatr Suppl 92(443):6–8, discussion 5
37. Brady RO (2003 Dec) Gaucher and Fabry diseases: from understanding pathophysiology to rational therapies. Acta Paediatr Suppl 92(443):19–24
38. Gadoth N, Sandbank U (1983 Aug) Involvement of dorsal root ganglia in Fabry's disease. J Med Genet 20(4):309–312
39. Branton M, Schiffmann R, Kopp JB (2002 Jun) Natural history and treatment of renal involvement in Fabry disease. J Am Soc Nephrol 13(Suppl 2):S139–S143
40. Branton MH, Schiffmann R, Sabnis SG, Murray GJ, Quirk JM, Altarescu G et al (2002 Mar) Natural history of Fabry renal disease: influence of alpha-galactosidase A activity and genetic mutations on clinical course. Medicine (Baltimore) 81(2):122–138
41. Kampmann C, Baehner F, Whybra C, Martin C, Wiethoff CM, Ries M et al (2002 Nov 6) Cardiac manifestations of Anderson-Fabry disease in heterozygous females. J Am Coll Cardiol 40(9):1668–1674
42. Linhart A, Kampmann C, Zamorano JL, Sunder-Plassmann G, Beck M, Mehta A et al (2007 May) Cardiac manifestations of Anderson-Fabry disease: results from the international Fabry outcome survey. Eur Heart J 28(10):1228–1235
43. Rolfs A, Bottcher T, Zschiesche M, Morris P, Winchester B, Bauer P et al (2005 Nov 19) Prevalence of Fabry disease in patients with cryptogenic stroke: a prospective study. Lancet 366(9499):1794–1796
44. Ramaswami U, Whybra C, Parini R, Pintos-Morell G, Mehta A, Sunder-Plassmann G et al (2006 Jan) Clinical manifestations of Fabry disease in children: data from the Fabry Outcome Survey. Acta Paediatr 95(1):86–92
45. Eng CM, Guffon N, Wilcox WR, Germain DP, Lee P, Waldek S et al (2001 Jul 5) Safety and efficacy of recombinant human alpha-galactosidase A–replacement therapy in Fabry's disease. N Engl J Med 345(1):9–16
46. Schiffmann R (2007 Jan 16) Enzyme replacement in Fabry disease: the essence is in the kidney. Ann Intern Med 146(2):142–144
47. Beck M, Ricci R, Widmer U, Dehout F, de Lorenzo AG, Kampmann C et al (2004 Dec) Fabry disease: overall effects of agalsidase alfa treatment. Eur J Clin Invest 34(12):838–844
48. Hoffmann B, Beck M, Sunder-Plassmann G, Borsini W, Ricci R, Mehta A (2007) Nature and prevalence of pain in Fabry disease and its response to enzyme replacement therapy–a retrospective analysis from the Fabry Outcome Survey. Clin J Pain 23(6):535–542
49. Hughes DA, Elliott PM, Shah J, Zuckerman J, Coghlan G, Brookes J et al (2008 Feb) Effects of enzyme replacement therapy on the cardiomyopathy of Anderson-Fabry disease: a randomised, double-blind, placebo-controlled clinical trial of agalsidase alfa. Heart 94(2):153–158
50. Hoffmann B, Schwarz M, Mehta A, Keshav S (2007 Dec) Gastrointestinal symptoms in 342 patients with Fabry disease: prevalence and response to enzyme replacement therapy. Clin Gastroenterol Hepatol 5(12):1447–1453

51. Feriozzi S, Schwarting A, Sunder-Plassmann G, West M, Cybulla M (2009) Agalsidase alfa slows the decline in renal function in patients with Fabry disease. Am J Nephrol 29(5): 353–361

52. West M, Nicholls K, Mehta A, Clarke JT, Steiner R, Beck M et al (2009 May) Agalsidase alfa and kidney dysfunction in Fabry disease. J Am Soc Nephrol 20(5):1132–1139

53. Kovacevic-Preradovic T, Zuber M, Attenhofer Jost CH, Widmer U, Seifert B, Schulthess G et al (2008 Nov) Anderson-Fabry disease: long-term echocardiographic follow-up under enzyme replacement therapy. Eur J Echocardiogr 9(6):729–735

54. Imbriaco M, Pisani A, Spinelli L, Cuocolo A, Messalli G, Capuano E et al (2009 Jul) Effects of enzyme-replacement therapy in patients with Anderson-Fabry disease: a prospective long-term cardiac magnetic resonance imaging study. Heart 95(13):1103–1107

55. Tahir H, Jackson LL, Warnock DG (2007 Sep) Antiproteinuric therapy and fabry nephropathy: sustained reduction of proteinuria in patients receiving enzyme replacement therapy with agalsidase-beta. J Am Soc Nephrol 18(9):2609–2617

56. Wilcox WR, Banikazemi M, Guffon N, Waldek S, Lee P, Linthorst GE et al (2004 Jul) Long-term safety and efficacy of enzyme replacement therapy for Fabry disease. Am J Hum Genet 75(1):65–74

57. Whybra C, Kampmann C, Krummenauer F, Ries M, Mengel E, Miebach E et al (2004 Apr) The Mainz Severity Score Index: a new instrument for quantifying the Anderson-Fabry disease phenotype, and the response of patients to enzyme replacement therapy. Clin Genet 65(4):299–307

58. Parini R, Rigoldi M, Santus F, Furlan F, De Lorenzo P, Valsecchi G et al (2008 Sep) Enzyme replacement therapy with agalsidase alfa in a cohort of Italian patients with Anderson-Fabry disease: testing the effects with the Mainz Severity Score Index. Clin Genet 74(3):260–266

59. Cleeland CS, Ryan KM (1994 Mar) Pain assessment: global use of the Brief Pain Inventory. Ann Acad Med Singapore 23(2):129–138

60. Ramaswami U, Pintos G, Kalkim G, Parini R, Beck M (2006) Effect of agalsidase alfa on pain in adolescents with FD: Data from FOS- The Fabry outcome Survery. JIMD 29(Suppl 1):46

61. Milligan A, Hughes D, Goodwin S, Richfield L, Mehta A (2006) Intravenous enzyme replacement therapy: better in home or hospital? Br J Nurs 15(6):330–333

62. Lubanda JC, Anijalg E, Bzduch V, Thurberg BL, Benichou B, Tylki-Szymanska A (2009 Apr) Evaluation of a low dose, after a standard therapeutic dose, of agalsidase beta during enzyme replacement therapy in patients with Fabry disease. Genet Med 11(4):256–264

63. Pintos-Morell G, Beck M (2009 Feb) Fabry disease in children and the effects of enzyme replacement treatment. Eur J Pediatr 168(11):1355–1363

64. Benichou B, Goyal S, Sung C, Norfleet AM, O'Brien F (2009 Jan) A retrospective analysis of the potential impact of IgG antibodies to agalsidase beta on efficacy during enzyme replacement therapy for Fabry disease. Mol Genet Metab 96(1):4–12

65. Auray-Blais C, Cyr D, Ntwari A, West ML, Cox-Brinkman J, Bichet DG et al (2008 Mar) Urinary globotriaosylceramide excretion correlates with the genotype in children and adults with Fabry disease. Mol Genet Metab 93(3):331–340

66. Schafer E, Baron K, Widmer U, Deegan P, Neumann HP, Sunder-Plassmann G et al (2005 Apr) Thirty-four novel mutations of the GLA gene in 121 patients with Fabry disease. Hum Mutat 25(4):412

67. Vedder AC, Linthorst GE, van Breemen MJ, Groener JE, Bemelman FJ, Strijland A et al (2007 Feb) The Dutch Fabry cohort: diversity of clinical manifestations and Gb3 levels. J Inherit Metab Dis 30(1):68–78

68. Whitfield PD, Calvin J, Hogg S, O'Driscoll E, Halsall D, Burling K et al (2005) Monitoring enzyme replacement therapy in Fabry disease–role of urine globotriaosylceramide. J Inherit Metab Dis 28(1):21–33

69. Aerts JM, Groener JE, Kuiper S, Donker-Koopman WE, Strijland A, Ottenhoff R et al (2008 Feb 26) Elevated globotriaosylsphingosine is a hallmark of Fabry disease. Proc Natl Acad Sci U S A 105(8):2812–2817

70. Jaradeh SS, Prieto TE (2003 May) Evaluation of the autonomic nervous system. Phys Med Rehabil Clin N Am 14(2):287–305

71. Schiffmann R, Scott LJ (2002) Pathophysiology and assessment of neuropathic pain in Fabry disease. Acta Paediatr Suppl 91(439):48–52

72. Laaksonen SM, Roytta M, Jaaskelainen SK, Kantola I, Penttinen M, Falck B (2008 Jun) Neuropathic symptoms and findings in women with Fabry disease. Clin Neurophysiol 119(6):1365–1372

73. Peltier A, Smith AG, Russell JW, Sheikh K, Bixby B, Howard J et al (2009 Apr) Reliability of quantitative sudomotor axon reflex testing and quantitative sensory testing in neuropathy of impaired glucose regulation. Muscle Nerve 39(4):529–535

74. Cleeland CS (2002) Pain assessment: the advantages of using pain scales in lysosomal storage diseases. Acta Paediatr Suppl 91(439):43–47

75. McDermott AM, Toelle TR, Rowbotham DJ, Schaefer CP, Dukes EM (2006 Feb) The burden of neuropathic pain: results from a cross-sectional survey. Eur J Pain (London, England) 10(2):127–135

76. Beck M (2009 Feb) Agalsidase alfa for the treatment of Fabry disease: new data on clinical efficacy and safety. Expert Opin Biol Ther 9(2):255–261

77. Mehta A, Ricci R, Widmer U, Dehout F, Garcia de Lorenzo A, Kampmann C et al (2004) Fabry disease defined: baseline clinical manifestations of 366 patients in the Fabry Outcome Survey. Eur J Clin Invest 34(3):236–242

78. Ries M, Gupta S, Moore DF, Sachdev V, Quirk JM, Murray GJ et al (2005) Pediatric Fabry disease. Pediatrics 115(3):e344–e355

79. Hopkin RJ, Bissler J, Banikazemi M, Clarke L, Eng CM, Germain DP et al (2008 Nov) Characterization of Fabry disease in 352 pediatric patients in the Fabry Registry. Pediatr Res 64(5):550–555

80. Cole AL, Lee PJ, Hughes DA, Deegan PB, Waldek S, Lachmann RH (2007 Nov) Depression in adults with Fabry disease: a common and under-diagnosed problem. J Inherit Metab Dis 30(6):943–951

81. Dworkin RH, Turk DC, Wyrwich KW, Beaton D, Cleeland CS, Farrar JT et al (2008 Feb) Interpreting the clinical importance of treatment outcomes in chronic pain clinical trials: IMMPACT recommendations. J Pain 9(2):105–121

82. Hughes DA, Ramaswami U, Elliott P, Deegan P, Lee P, Waldek S, Apperley G, Cox T, Mehta AB (2004) UK National guidelines for the diagnosis and management of Anderson-Fabry Disease. http://wwwncgnhsuk/documents/lsd_guidelines_for_anderson-fabry_disease-010805pdf

83. Genzyme (2009) A study of two Fabrazyme Dosing Regimens in Treatment-naïve, Male Pediatric Patients Without Severe Symptoms (FIELD). http://clinicaltrialsgov/ct2/show/NCT00701415

84. Counahan R, Chantler C, Ghazali S, Kirkwood B, Rose F, Barratt TM (1976 Nov) Estimation of glomerular filtration rate from plasma creatinine concentration in children. Arch Dis Child 51(11):875–878

Chapter 29
Pharmacological Chaperone Therapy for Fabry Disease

Jian-Qiang Fan and Satoshi Ishii

Abstract Pharmacological chaperone therapy is an emerging therapeutic treatment for genetic disorders resulting from the improper folding of proteins. A large set of disease-causing missense mutations in Fabry disease result in the synthesis of improperly folded α-galactosidase A that are retarded in the endoplasmic reticulum (ER) and degraded in the ER-associated degradation pathway, although these proteins may be enzymologically active, if they could be properly transported to the lysosomes. Pharmacological chaperones increase the residual enzyme activity in patients by acting as a folding template in the ER to facilitate proper folding of mutant proteins, hence accelerating their transport out from the ER and reach to lysosomes. 1-Deoxygalactonojirimycin (DGJ, migalastat, Amigal^{TM}) is a pharmacological chaperone for Fabry disease. This chapter describes the protein misfolding phenotype of Fabry disease, the mechanism of pharmacological chaperone therapy for Fabry disease, and the clinical development of DGJ for treating Fabry disease.

Keywords Pharmacological chaperone · Active-site-specific chaperone · Protein misfolding · Endoplasmic reticulum-associated degradation (ERAD) · 1-deoxygalactonojirimycin

29.1 Introduction

Currently, enzyme replacement therapy (ERT) is the only FDA-approved therapy for the treatment of Fabry disease. The strengths and limitations of the therapy have been detailed and discussed in the previous chapters by Pastores and Hopkin. Despite the success of ERT, emerging therapeutic strategies using small molecule drugs for treating the disease are on the horizon [1, 2]. Small molecule drugs are attractive as they can be administered orally and have more potential to gain access

J.-Q. Fan (✉)
Pfantastic Medical Research Institute, Cresskill, NJ, USA
e-mail: jfan@pfantastic.com

D. Elstein et al. (eds.), *Fabry Disease*, DOI 10.1007/978-90-481-9033-1_29,
© Springer Science+Business Media B.V. 2010

to most cell types and the central neuronal system compared to the replacement enzyme molecules. In addition, small molecule drugs have advantages over ERT, such as the convenience and possible lower cost for the treatment.

There are two small molecule drugs proposed and are under investigation for Fabry disease. Zavesca™ (N-butyldeoxynojirimycin, miglustat) is a FDA- and EMEA-approved drug for treating type I Gaucher disease. Zavesca™ is an inhibitor of glycosphingolipid biosynthesis. It has been evaluated in mouse models of various glycosphingolipidosis including Fabry disease [3, 4]. Despite the positive outcomes in Fabry mice, early clinical trials of Zavesca™ in Fabry disease were terminated as a result of untoward neurological toxicity [5]. Amigal™ (1-deoxygalactonojirimycin, DGJ, migalastat) is another small molecule drug being developed for the treatment of Fabry disease. The mechanism of the drug is based on that small molecule drugs can be a folding template for the conformational fragile mutant endogenous enzymes that otherwise would be degraded within the endoplasmic reticulum-associated degradation (ERAD), hence restoring the enzyme activity [6]. These drugs are often referred to as 'pharmacological chaperones', or 'active-site-specific chaperones' (ASSCs) as they are specifically targeting the catalytic active-site of the enzyme (for recent reviews of pharmacological chaperone therapy see [2, 7–9]). Currently, Amigal™ is under clinical phase III trials for the treatment of Fabry disease.

In this chapter, we will focus on the mechanism and development of pharmacological chaperone therapy (PCT) for Fabry disease. The results present here can also be useful for developing pharmacological chaperones for other glycosphingolipidosis and other protein deficiencies of metabolic enzymes, receptors, and channel proteins, etc.

29.2 Lysosomal Enzyme Biosynthesis and ERAD

Lysosomal enzymes are synthesized in the cytoplasm and then secreted into the lumen of the endoplasmic reticulum (ER) in a largely unfolded state (Fig. 29.1). In general, protein folding is governed by the principle of self-assembly [10]. Newly synthesized polypeptides fold into their native (active) conformation based on their amino acid sequences in a thermodynamic fashion with aids from the residual molecular chaperones (e.g., BiP, calnexin, HSPs, etc.). In order to monitor the in vivo folding process, the ER has evolved a cellular 'quality control' mechanism, termed ERAD, which uses molecular chaperones to bind and rescue unstable misfolded conformers to facilitate their proper folding and assembly, and to prevent aggregation of non-native forms [11, 12]. This cellular process ensures that only properly folded and assembled proteins are transported to the Golgi complex for further maturation. Improperly folded proteins are retained in the ER and then transported to the cytosol for ubiquitin-mediated degradation within the cytosolic proteasomes. In such a way, misfolded proteins are eliminated from the cells to maintain the integrity of the cells [12–15]. It is estimated that misfolding and aggregated proteins occur in up to 30% of

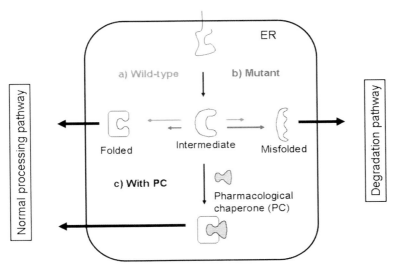

Fig. 29.1 Protein folding in the endoplasmic reticulum (ER) and pharmacological chaperone therapy (PCT). The initial protein folding process in the ER is based on thermodynamic equilibrium. Much of the folding preference is guided by the primary amino acid sequence coded by each gene (**a**) Wild-type proteins tend to gain their folded conformation based on their peptide sequence. These appropriately folded proteins are smoothly transported out of the ER for normal processing (**b**) On the other hand, folding preference of a mutant protein can be shifted in favor of a misfolded conformation. These proteins with misfolded/incorrect conformation are retarded by molecular chaperones, followed by either entering a refolding process or retro-translocation to the cytosolic proteasome-based degradation pathway (**c**) Interaction with pharmacological chaperone (PC) can dramatically change the folding equilibrium of mutant proteins toward the native-like folded conformation, and thus rescue the proteins from being degraded via ERAD and promoting safe exit from the ER for further processing. Because the binding of PC to the active-site of proteins is also thermodynamic, dissociation of PC from the mutant proteins can be accelerated based on many factors, including changing pH conditions, high concentration of substrates that compete with PCs for the active-site, and thereby allowing physiological functionality of the rescued mutant proteins (modified from Fan [2])

wild-type proteins even after interaction with molecular chaperones, and they are rapidly degraded within minutes of their synthesis by the cellular quality control machinery [16].

The consequences of genetic errors that lead to the dysfunction of coding proteins involved in genetic disorders can be various [17]. Nonsense and frame-shift mutations usually result in the premature termination of the biosynthesis, or dramatic alteration in the structure, thereby disabling the biological activity of the proteins. Splicing mutations cause abnormal translation, resulting in the synthesis of proteins with functionality at a totally or partially diminished level. Missense mutations involving the substitution of critical amino acids often result in the biosynthesis of mutant proteins that are nonfunctional. In many other cases, missense mutations or small in-frame deletions/insertions could have little or no impact on the biological activity of the mutant protein, but may lead to misfolding and an altered tertiary structure. These mutant proteins would be retained in the ER by molecular chaperones and further degraded by the ERAD, although they may become fully or partially functional if they could escape the cellular quality control machinery [18]. For example, the ΔF508 mutation in CFTR is fully functional if it is properly inserted into the cytoplasm membrane in vitro [19]. Retention of the mutant protein by CHIP along with Hsp70 in the ER, and subsequent degradation by the ubiquitin proteasome pathway, plays a direct role in the depletion of the protein in vivo [20].

In many lysosomal disorders, certain missense mutations produce mutant enzymes that retain a small amount of residual enzyme activity. The presence of residual enzyme activity presumably results from the small amount of the mutant polypeptide that is properly folded, assembled, normally matured and transported to the lysosomes. These mutations are often associated with the mild or late-onset disease phenotypes. This provides therapeutic optimism that rescuing a fraction of misfolded mutant proteins from the ERAD machinery may have significant clinical benefits for these diseases.

29.3 Misfolding Conformation in Missense α-Galactosidase a Mutant Enzymes

Fabry disease is an X-linked recessive disorder caused by the deficient activity of lysosomal α-galactosidase A (α-Gal A) [21]. The mature human α-Gal A enzyme is a homodimeric glycoprotein, each monomer containing 398 amino acid residues after cleavage of the signal peptide which has the first 30 amino acid residues (for detailed crystal structure of α-Gal A see chapter by Garman). To date, more than 500 mutations have been identified in the α-Gal A gene GLA (Human Gene Mutation Database Web site, http://www.hgmd.cf.ac.uk). More than 60% of mutations are missense, and the majority of mutations are private, occurring only in one or a few families. From the crystal structure, thirteen amino acid residues were predicted to be directly involved in the interaction with α-galactose. In addition, 30 residues of each monomer contribute to the dimer interface [22]. Garman et al. [22, 23]. mapped various missense mutations onto a model of human α-Gal A. The locations of the human α-Gal A point mutations reveal two major classes of Fabry disease protein defects: active-site mutations that reduce enzymatic activity by perturbing the active-site without necessarily affecting the overall α-Gal A structure; and folding mutations that reduce the stability of α-Gal A by disrupting its hydrophobic core. It is clear that the majority of amino acids that are replaced within missense mutant proteins do not directly contribute to the enzyme's catalytic function, but rather to the maintenance of the enzyme's tertiary structure.

During the course of examining the primary cause of deficient enzyme activity, Ishii et al. [24, 25]. examined the kinetic properties and stabilities of several mutant enzymes found in cardiac variants. Following the same approach, we further examined various disease-causing mutations that have been identified in patients who present with residual enzyme activity regardless of clinical phenotypes [26]. Sixteen mutant enzymes, including ten mutations identified in variant patients (A20P, E66Q,

M72V, I91T, R112H, F113L, N215S, Q279E, M296I, and M296V), four mutations found in classic patients (E59K, A156V, L166V, and R356W), and two mutations present in both variant and classic patients (A97V and R301Q) were efficiently purified from transfected COS-7 cells [27], and their enzymatic and biochemical properties were examined. Except for one mutation (E59K), all mutant proteins appeared to have normal kinetic properties, indicating that they retain full or partial catalytic activity. Although all the mutant enzymes examined showed the same optimal pH as the wild-type enzyme, the mutant enzymes were substantially less stable compared to the wild-type enzyme. Western blot analysis of mutant enzymes expressed in transfected COS-7 cells and patient fibroblasts demonstrated that most mutant enzymes had low protein yields, indicating that excessive degradation of the mutant enzyme could be directly responsible for deficient enzyme activity. Subcellular fractionations and metabolic labeling studies with the L166V and R301Q mutants indicated that the mutant proteins remained in unprocessed forms within the ER fractions and were eventually degraded without further processing and maturation.

The folding process of temporarily misfolded glycoproteins in the ER is subject to two dynamic competitive events, in which the calnexin calreticulin system and glucosidases I and II promote refolding, whereas ER α-mannosidases and the ER degradation enhancing α-mannosidase I-like protein are involved in retrotranslocation and degradation of misfolded proteins in the process of ERAD [28]. Removal of a mannose residue from Man9 N-linked oligosaccharides by ER α-mannosidase I is a critical luminal event for preventing proteins from reentering the refolding process, and serves as a signal for targeted ERAD. Inhibition of ER α-mannosidase I often delays the degradation of glycoproteins in the ERAD in favor of protein refolding. When kifunensine, a selective inhibitor of the ER α-mannosidase I, was added to the culture medium of transfected cells, the amount of all mutant proteins (except E59K) appeared to increase (Fig. 29.2), suggesting that the degradation of

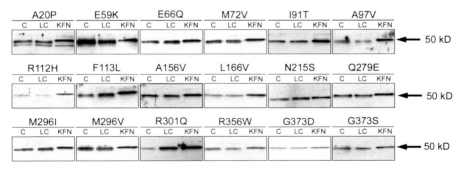

Fig. 29.2 Effects of ERAD inhibitors on the amount of mutant α-Gal A expressed in COS-7 cells. Wild-type or mutant α-Gal A enzymes were transiently expressed in COS-7 cells. Cells were treated with 2 mM lactacystin (LC) or 0.2 mM kifunensine (KFN) at the 5th h after transfection. Upon harvest, Western blot analyses of cell lysates from transfected COS-7 cells were performed. The 50 kDa band represents the unprocessed ER form of α-Gal A. (C), control (reproduced from Ishii et al. [26])

mutant enzymes was partially inhibited [26]. This result provided clear evidence that degradation of misfolded mutant α-Gal A enzymes occurred by the ERAD as the result of misfolding of mutant proteins.

Based on the results obtained from a large set of missense mutant α-Gal A, a large proportion of missense mutant enzymes in patients with residual enzyme activity could be kinetically active. Excessive degradation in the ER may be one of the most important causes responsible for the deficiency of enzyme activity in vivo.

29.4 Development of DGJ as a Pharmacological Chaperone for Fabry Disease

Despite the complexity of the initial protein folding process, there is ultimately only a small difference in energy that separates the proper functional fold from many of the folding intermediates (Fig. 29.1). Inclusion of a pharmacological chaperone that is capable of serving a folding template can dramatically shift the folding dynamics in favor of proper and native-like folding. In such a way, misfolded mutant proteins can be rescued from the degradation within the ERAD machinery and further preceded to the normal processing and trafficking pathways [2, 29]. Competitive enzyme inhibitors are effective pharmacological chaperones, because of their high affinity to the catalytic domain. Once the mutant enzyme/inhibitor complex is secreted out of the ER, the inhibitor at sub-inhibitory concentrations can be replaced by the highly concentrated substrate in lysosomes to allow the function of the enzyme, as the dynamic exchange of competitive inhibitor and substrate is dependent upon the relative concentrations of each.

In an attempt to rescue misfolded mutant enzymes from excessive degradation in the ER for the increase of the residual α-Gal A activity, Fan and colleagues evaluated a series of enzyme substrate analogues, and demonstrated that DGJ, a potent competitive inhibitor of α-Gal A, effectively increased α-Gal A activity in Fabry lymphoblasts derived from Fabry patients with the R301Q and Q279E mutations, when administered at concentrations lower than that usually required for intracellular inhibition of the enzyme [30, 31]. The residual enzyme activity in the R301Q or Q279E lymphoblasts increased 8- or 7-fold after incubation with DGJ for 4 days, respectively, and the increase was dose-dependent (Fig. 29.3). α-Gal A mRNA level was not changed, while the mutant protein amount was increased in the cells cultivated with DGJ, indicating that the action of DGJ is to prevent excessive intracellular degradation of the mutant protein [30]. Subcellular fractionation and metabolic labeling studies with COS-7 cells transfected with L166V and R301Q cDNA plasmids demonstrated that mutant enzymes were partially processed and trafficked to the lysosomal fractions in the cells cultured with DGJ [26].

DGJ was α-Gal A-specific and affects neither other lysosomal enzymes nor the ERAD machinery [31]. Immunoelectron microscopic study with transfected COS-7 cells revealed the presence of the mutant enzyme predominantly in the ER surrounding the nucleus (Fig. 29.4A–C) [32]. In contrast, the mutant enzyme was observed

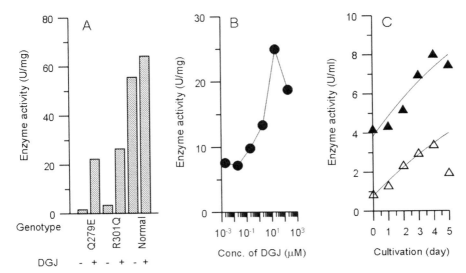

Fig. 29.3 Increase of α-Gal A in lymphoblasts from patients with Fabry disease. (**a**) α-Gal A activity in lymphoblasts (Q279E, R301Q and normal) cultured in the presence (+) or absence (−) of 20 μM DGJ (**b**) Effect of DGJ concentration on α-Gal A activity. Lymphoblasts (R301Q) were cultured with DGJ at various concentrations before collected for enzyme assay (**c**) Stablization of enhanced α-Gal A by DGJ. Lymphoblasts (R301Q) cultured with (▲) or without (△) 20 μM DGJ were washed and transferred to fresh medium. The cells in 2 ml of the medium were taken each day for enzyme assay. For (**a–c**), each value is an average of triplicate experiments, and standard deviation is less than 10% (reproduced from Fan et al. [30])

mainly in the lysosomes of the cells treated with DGJ (Fig. 29.4D–F). The ratio of the mutant enzyme localized in lysosomes and the ER was 6:94 in the absence of DGJ, but changed to 79:21 in the presence of DGJ which was similar to that of wild-type α-Gal A (82:18). Independent studies in transgenic mouse fibroblasts overexpressing human R301Q α-Gal A confirmed that the mutant enzyme was retained in the ER and not correctly folded, since it formed complex with BiP [32]. Incubation of the cells with DGJ significantly reduced the association with BiP, indicating that DGJ exerted a chaperone-like effect on the conformation of the enzyme.

DGJ is a small molecular iminosugar that resembles an α-galactose residue when bound to the active-site of α-Gal A. Based upon active-site interactions observed in the crystal structure of α-Gal A bound to α-galactose, a model of DGJ binding to α-Gal A shows many favorable interactions: the imino group on DGJ is expected to interact with D170; the hydroxyl groups of DGJ form hydrogen bounds with D92, D93, K168, E203, R227, and E231; and a hydrophobic surface on DGJ makes van der Waals interactions with W47 (Fig. 29.5). The binding between DGJ and the protein would fix the active-site involving the five loops β1-α1, β2-α2, β4-α4, β5-α5, and β6-α6. The initial folding process in the ER is a thermodynamic equilibrium based upon the amino acid sequence of the peptide. A firm binding between DGJ and the fragile enzyme could dramatically shift the folding process toward the

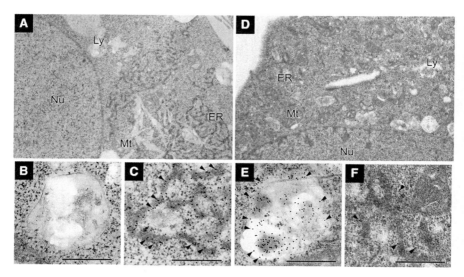

Fig. 29.4 Intracellular localization of R301Q. The intracellular localization of R301Q in COS-7 cells in the absence (**A–C**) or presence (**D–F**) of DGJ. COS-7 cells were transfected with pCXN2-GLA-R301Q and treated with 20 μM DGJ for 48 h, then cells were fixed and embedded. The ultrathin sections were incubated with an anti-α-Gal A antibody followed by immunogold labeling. Each thin section was examined with a transmission electron microscope (**B**) and (**E**) show the higher magnifications of the lysosome (**C**) and (**F**) show the higher magnifications of the ER. Scale bars represent 500 nm. Nu, nucleus; Mt, mitochondria; Ly, lysosomes. Typical gold particles are pointed by arrowhead (reproduced from Hamanaka et al. [32])

Fig. 29.5 Predicted interactions between DGJ and the active-site of α-Gal A. DGJ is a known active-site directed competitive inhibitor of α-Gal A. Interactions of α-Gal A with DGJ were modeled based upon the crystal structure of α-Gal A with bound α-galactose. The key interactions with the 2-, 3-, 4-, and 6-hydroxyls on the ligand are maintained when either α-galactose or DGJ bind to the active-site. One key interaction between E231 on the enzyme and the anomeric hydroxyl of α-galactose is lost when DGJ binds (modified from Ishii et al. [26])

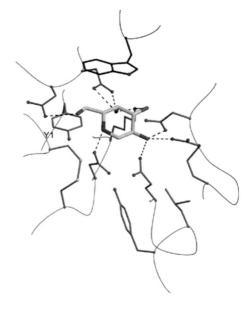

normal folding, conferring the correct conformation on mutant enzymes that would otherwise be largely misfolded.

Shin and colleagues have used a T cell based system to determine whether the activity of Fabry disease enzyme mutants can be enhanced using DGJ. When patient-derived T cells were grown in the presence of DGJ, α-Gal A activity increased to more than 50% of normal for several mutations, including A97V, R112H, R112C, A143T, and L300P [33, 34]. Ishii and colleagues recently tested DGJ enhancement in patient fibroblasts and lymphoblasts expressing a variety of disease-causing α-Gal A missense mutations. The results showed that residual enzyme activity could be specifically increased 20% above normal after incubating the cultured cells with DGJ at 20 μM for 5 days [26]. More recently, Benjamin and colleagues examined DGJ effect on cultured lymphoblasts from males with Fabry disease representing 75 different missense mutations [35]. Half of the missense mutant forms associated with classic Fabry disease and a majority mutants (90%) associated with later-onset Fabry disease were responsive to the DGJ treatment. In addition, elevated globotriaosylceramide (Gb3) levels in responsive Fabry fibroblasts were reduced after DGJ treatment, indicating that increased mutant α-Gal A can reduce the accumulated substrate. These results indicate that DGJ treatment may be broadly beneficial for Fabry patients with a variety of missense mutations.

29.5 Preclinical Efficacy and Safety of DGJ in Mice

Ishii and colleagues have developed suitable mouse models to evaluate efficacy and safety of DGJ in vivo. A transgenic mouse model (TgM) that expresses human mutant R301Q α-Gal A activity was initially generated [36]. Because these mice contained both the endogenous α-Gal A gene and the transgene, the α-Gal A activity measured in tissues was the combination of two enzymes. Ishii and colleagues further developed a mouse model (TgM/KO) exclusively expressing human mutant enzyme in tissues by crossbreeding the TgM mice with α-Gal A knockout (KO) mice [37]. Despite the transgene product being a mutant form of human α-Gal A, the tissue α-Gal A activity in heterozygous TgM/KO mice was found to be comparable or only slightly lower than that of wild-type mice, presumably because of the highly efficient β-actin promoter of the transgene. Although these mice do not present a clinical phenotype, they are an excellent biochemical animal model for in vivo evaluation of DGJ. In addition, because of the low level of α-Gal A activity in kidney of heterozygous TgM/KO mice, a small amount of accumulation of Gb3 was found in the kidney of such mice. These mice were particularly useful as a pathological animal model for evaluating efficacy of DGJ in vivo.

DGJ was orally administered ad libitum to the mice in drinking water. Upon administration of DGJ, α-Gal A activity responded to the treatment quickly, and a substantial increase in the enzyme activity could be observed in all major tissues within 3 days [38]. The increase of tissue α-Gal A activity was dose-dependent in mice treated with DGJ at 0.05–1 mM in drinking water (corresponds to daily dosage at 3–60 mg/kg body weight) for 1 week. Heart and kidney are main organs affected

Control   DGJ-treated

Heart

Kidney

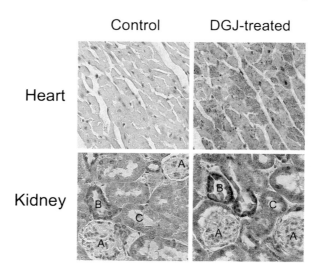

Fig. 29.6 Immunohistochemistry of heart and kidney of TgM/KO mice treated with DGJ. A TgM/KO male mouse was treated with 0.5 mM DGJ in drinking water ad libitum for 2 weeks. The estimated DGJ dosage was approximately 30 mg/kg body weight/day. α-Gal A activities in the heart from non-treated and DGJ-treated mice were 55 and 1,240 U/mg protein, respectively, and those in kidney were 9.5 and 79.0 U/mg protein, respectively. A, glomeruli; B, distal convoluted tubule; C, proximal convoluted tubule (reproduced from Ishii et al. [38])

by Fabry disease in patients. To determine whether DGJ treatment can affect these cell types, α-Gal A in the heart and kidney of TgM/KO mice treated with DGJ for 2 weeks was examined by immunohistochemical microscopic studies. A remarkable increase of α-Gal A was observed in the matrix of cardiomyocytes and distal convoluted tubules after the DGJ treatment (Fig. 29.6), although no clear change was found in endothelial and epithelial cells of glomerulus. These results indicate that DGJ can be physiologically effective in the increase of α-Gal A activity in such cell types. An additional administration of DGJ at 0.05 mM in drinking water to heterozygous TgM/KO mice was studied to examine whether DGJ treatment can reduce the Gb3 accumulation in kidney. After 4 weeks of treatment, Gb3 was substantially reduced to 54% of untreated mice in kidney (Fig. 29.7). This clearly indicates that a continuous dose of DGJ at approximately 3 mg/kg body weight/day cannot only increase tissue enzyme activity but also provide clinical benefit in mice for this mutation. Therefore, a daily dosage of 3 mg/kg body weight is considered to be the effective dosage in mice.

To examine the safety of DGJ in mice, blood biochemistry and hematological profiling, and pathological examination of tissues in TgM/KO mice treated with DGJ at a 10-fold higher dosage than the targeted effective dosage for 9 weeks were performed [38]. No abnormality in all tests and examinations was found at the end of treatment. Furthermore, no abnormality in appearance, growth retardation, fertility, and life span could be observed in mice treated with DGJ at approximately 3 mg/kg body weight/day for 2 years. These results indicate that DGJ is well tolerated in mice.

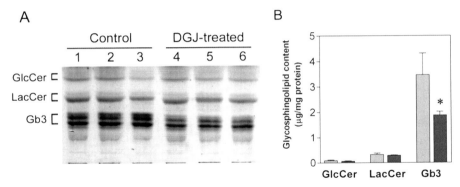

Fig. 29.7 Effect of DGJ treatment on Gb3 storage in kidney of TgM/KO mice. Ten-week-old female heterozygous TgM/KO mice were treated with a DGJ solution (0.05 mM) as drinking water (corresponding to a daily dosage of approximately 3 mg/kg body weight) for 4 weeks. A, HPTLC analysis of neutral glycosphingolipids extracted from kidney of mice. Lanes 1–3, untreated mice; lanes 4–6, DGJ treated mice. B, average concentrations of neutral glycosphingolipids from kidney of mice were determined from the band intensity of HPTLC based on standards. Light-colored bar, non-DGJ-treated group; dark-colored bar, DGJ-treated group. Glc-Cer, glucosylceramide; LacCer, lactosylceramide. The statistical significance of the difference was determined by Student's t test; *, $p < 0.05$ (reproduced from Ishii et al. [38])

29.6 Clinical Development of DGJ

DGJ (AT1001) is registered as migalastat (Amigal^{TM}) and developed by Amicus Therapeutics, Inc. The drug has been evaluated by the US FDA and the EMEA under the orphan drug regulatory procedures. It has been granted the orphan designation for the treatment of Fabry disease in February 2004 by the FDA and in May 2006 by the EMEA, respectively. Clinical Phase I and Phase II trials of Amigal^{TM} have been concluded. Currently, the drug is under clinical Phase III trial for Fabry disease.

In the Phase I studies, Amigal^{TM} was orally administered to 16 healthy volunteers and the results indicated high bioavailability and a favorable pharmacokinetic profile. Noticeably, administration of Amigal^{TM} also resulted in a statistically significant and dose-dependent increase in α-Gal A activity in each of the healthy volunteers. No drug related adverse events were reported in the Phase I trial. Subsequently, Phase II trials were conducted with the primary objective to be the evaluation of the safety and tolerability of the drug, and the secondary objective to be the evaluation of certain pharmacodynamic measurements, such as effects on α-Gal A and levels of Gb3 in cells and tissues. Four open-label, multi-national Phase II trials of Amigal^{TM} enrolled 18 men and nine women with Fabry disease between the ages of 17 and 65. These studies examined various dose levels and frequencies of Amigal^{TM} administration and had 12 or 24 week primary treatment arms with an optional treatment extension. Twenty-six subjects completed either 12 or 24 weeks of treatment during the Phase II studies. Twenty-three of the 26 subjects continue to receive treatment in an ongoing extension study designed to evaluate the long term safety and efficacy of Amigal^{TM}. Up to date, ten of the

23 subjects have been on treatment for at least 2 years and 4 subjects have been on treatment for more than 3 years. Patients identified as responders to Amigal™ at the completion of the Phase II trials continued to maintain elevated levels of α-Gal A activity in white blood cells, and reduced levels of Gb3 in urine. A reduction of Gb3 levels was also observed in interstitial capillary cells from kidney biopsies. Treatment with Amigal™ was generally well-tolerated, with no drug-related serious adverse events. The most common adverse events were headache, arthralgia and diarrhea.

In June of 2009, Amicus announced that the company reached an agreement with the US FDA on the key protocol design of its pivotal trial for Amigal™. The Phase III trial will evaluate the efficacy, safety and pharmacodynamics of Amigal™ in males and females with Fabry disease. The trial will consist of a 6-month double-blind, randomized, placebo-controlled treatment stage and will enroll approximately 60 subjects who are naive to ERT or who have not received ERT for at least 6 months prior to the start of treatment with Amigal™. The Amigal™ treatment arm dose and regimen will be 150 mg every other day. The primary endpoint will be the change in the amount of kidney interstitial capillary Gb3 as measured in kidney biopsies using histology. Secondary endpoints will include safety and tolerability, kidney Gb3 as measured in urine, and an assessment of renal function (including glomerular filtration rate and 24 h urine protein).

It should be noticed that the results of the clinical trials have not been peer reviewed. All the preliminary clinical results are based on the company's press release (www.amicustherapeutics.com), or US Securities and Exchange Commission filing documents (www.sec.gov).

29.7 Outlook of PCT for the Treatment of Fabry Disease

The expectation of PCT for Fabry disease is favorable, because of an early clinical proof-of-concept study with intravenous infusion of galactose to a cardiac Fabry patient [39]. Galactose is a weak inhibitor of α-Gal A. After a 3-month treatment period, remarkable improvements in the increase in the left ventricular ejection fraction (from 32 to 51%), and reduction in ventricular wall thickness (from 18 to 15 mm) were observed. DGJ is 120,000-fold more potent than galacotse and it is expected to be a more effective chaperone for the disease.

To date, ERT is the only available FDA-approved therapy for Fabry disease. ERT has clear advantages in that it can be administered to a full clinical spectrum of patients, including those with totally no functional enzyme activity. For them, DGJ alone would not be effective. On the other hand, DGJ is expected to be highly effective for patients who have missense mutations that primarily lead to misfolding of the mutant protein. Recently, Porto and colleagues provided evidence that the uptake of recombinant α-Gal A was increase in Fabry patient fibroblasts cultivated with DGJ, demonstrating a synergy between the pharmacological chaperone and the replacement enzyme [40]. DGJ may be useful as a combination therapy with ERT for patients whose residual enzyme activity cannot be increased by DGJ alone to a level that reverses disease development. This could potentially reduce the overall therapeutic cost and add convenience for patients. Compared to the protein macromolecule that is administered through intravenous infusion every other week, DGJ is an orally active small molecule drug. This would provide undeniable advantages of convenience, cost savings, and ease of accessibility by the drug to tissues, including the central neuronal system. Because a large proportion of mutant enzymes in Fabry patients with missense mutations are kinetically active, PCT using DGJ may be broadly applicable to Fabry patients with various missense mutations.

References

1. Brady RO (2006) Emerging strategies for the treatment of hereditary metabolic storage disorders. Rejuvenation Res 9(2):237–244
2. Fan JQ (2008) A counterintuitive approach to treat enzyme deficiencies: use of enzyme inhibitors for restoring mutant enzyme activity. Biol Chem 389(1):1–11
3. Platt FM, Jeyakumar M, Andersson U et al (2003) Substrate reduction therapy in mouse models of the glycosphingolipidoses. Philos Trans R Soc Lond B Biol Sci 358(1433):947–954
4. Abe A, Gregory S, Lee L et al (2000) Reduction of globotriaosylceramide in Fabry disease mice by substrate deprivation. J Clin Invest 105(11):1563–1571
5. Cox TM, Platt FM, Aerts JMFG (2007) Medicinal use of iminosugars. In: Compain P, Martin OR (eds) Iminosugars: from synthesis to therapeutic application. John Wiley & Sons Ltd, West Sussex, pp 295–326
6. Fan JQ, Ishii S (2007) Active-site-specific chaperone therapy for Fabry disease. Yin and Yang of enzyme inhibitors. Febs J 274(19):4962–4971
7. Conn PM, Janovick JA (2009) Drug development and the cellular quality control system. Trends Pharmacol Sci 30(5):228–233
8. Bernier V, Lagace M, Bichet DG et al (2004) Pharmacological chaperones: potential treatment for conformational diseases. Trends Endocrinol Metab 15(5):222–228
9. Cohen FE, Kelly JW (2003) Therapeutic approaches to protein-misfolding diseases. Nature 426(6968):905–909
10. Anfinsen CB, Scheraga HA (1975) Experimental and theoretical aspects of protein folding. Adv Protein Chem 29:205–300
11. Ellgaard L, Helenius A (2003) Quality control in the endoplasmic reticulum. Nat Rev Mol Cell Biol 4(3):181–191
12. Hartl FU, Hayer-Hartl M (2002) Molecular chaperones in the cytosol: from nascent chain to folded protein. Science 295(5561):1852–1858
13. Oda Y, Hosokawa N, Wada I et al (2003) EDEM as an acceptor of terminally misfolded glycoproteins released from calnexin. Science 299(5611):1394–1397
14. Fewell SW, Travers KJ, Weissman JS et al (2001) The action of molecular chaperones in the early secretory pathway. Annu Rev Genet 35:149–191
15. Schubert U, Anton LC, Gibbs J et al (2000) Rapid degradation of a large fraction of newly synthesized proteins by proteasomes. Nature 404(6779):770–774
16. Yewdell JW (2001) Not such a dismal science: the economics of protein synthesis, folding, degradation and antigen processing. Trends Cell Biol 11(7):294–297
17. Kuznetsov G, Nigam SK (1998) Folding of secretory and membrane proteins. N Engl J Med 339:1688–1695
18. Ellgaard L, Molinari M, Helenius A (1999) Setting the standards: quality control in the secretory pathway. Science 286(5446):1882–1888

19. Pasyk EA, Foskett JK (1995) Mutant (DF508) cystic fibrosis transmembrane conductance regulator Cl- channel is functional when retained in endoplasmic reticulum of mammalian cells. J Biol Chem 270:12347–12350

20. Meacham GC, Patterson C, Zhang W et al (2001) The Hsc70 co-chaperone CHIP targets immature CFTR for proteasomal degradation. Nat Cell Biol 3(1):100–105

21. Brady OR, Gal AE, Bradley RM et al (1967) Enzymatic defect in Fabry's disease: ceramide-trihexosidase deficiency. N Engl J Med 276:1163–1167

22. Garman SC, Garboczi DN (2004) The molecular defect leading to Fabry disease: structure of human alpha-galactosidase. J Mol Biol 337(2):319–335

23. Garman SC, Garboczi DN (2002) Structural basis of Fabry disease. Mol Genet Metab 77(1–2):3–11

24. Ishii S, Kase R, Sakuraba H et al (1993) Characterization of a mutant α-galactosidase gene product for the late-onset cardiac form of Fabry disease. Biochem Biophys Res Comm 197:1585–1589

25. Ishii S, Suzuki Y, Fan J-Q (2000) Role of Ser-65 in the activity of alpha-galactosidase A: characterization of a point mutation (S65T) detected in a patient with Fabry disease. Arch Biochem Biophys 377(2):228–233

26. Ishii S, Chang HH, Kawasaki K et al (2007) Mutant alpha-galactosidase A enzymes identified in Fabry disease patients with residual enzyme activity: biochemical characterization and restoration of normal intracellular processing by 1-deoxygalactonojirimycin. Biochem J 406(2):285–295

27. Yasuda K, Chang HH, Wu HL et al (2004) Efficient and rapid purification of recombinant human alpha-galactosidase A by affinity column chromatography. Protein Expr Purif 37(2):499–506

28. Helenius A, Aebi M (2004) Roles of N-linked glycans in the endoplasmic reticulum. Annu Rev Biochem 73:1019–1049

29. Fan J-Q (2003) A contradictory treatment for lysosomal storage disorders: inhibitors enhance mutant enzyme activity. Trends Pharmacol Sci 24(7):355–360

30. Fan J-Q, Ishii S, Asano N et al (1999) Accelerated transport and maturation of lysosomal α-galactosidase A in Fabry lymphoblasts by an enzyme inhibitor. Nat Med 59(1):112–115

31. Asano N, Ishii S, Kizu H et al (2000) In vitro inhibition and intracellular enhancement of lysosomal α-galactosidase A activity in Fabry lymphoblasts by 1-deoxygalactonojirimycin and its derivatives. Eur J Biochem 267:4179–4186

32. Hamanaka R, Shinohara T, Yano S et al (2008) Rescue of mutant alpha-galactosidase A in the endoplasmic reticulum by 1-deoxygalactonojirimycin leads to trafficking to lysosomes. Biochim Biophys Acta 1782(6):408–413

33. Shin SH, Murray GJ, Kluepfel-Stahl S et al (2007) Screening for pharmacological chaperones in Fabry disease. Biochem Biophys Res Commun 359(1):168–173

34. Shin SH, Kluepfel-Stahl S, Cooney AM et al (2008) Prediction of response of mutated alpha-galactosidase A to a pharmacological chaperone. Pharmacogenet Genomics 18(9):773–780

35. Benjamin ER, Flanagan JJ, Schilling A et al (2009) The pharmacological chaperone 1-deoxygalactonojirimycin increases alpha-galactosidase A levels in Fabry patient cell lines. J Inherit Metab Dis 32(3):424–440

36. Ishii S, Kase R, Sakuraba H et al (1998) α-Galactosidase transgenic mouse: heterogeneous gene expression and posttranslational glycosylation in tissues. Glycoconj J 15:591–594

37. Ohshima T, Murray GJ, Swaim WD et al (1997) α-Galactosidase A deficient mice: a model of Fabry disease. Proc Natl Acad Sci USA 94:2540–2544

38. Ishii S, Chang HH, Yoshioka H et al (2009) Preclinical efficacy and safety of 1-deoxygalactonojirimycin in mice for Fabry disease. J Pharmacol Exp Ther 328(3):723–731

39. Frustaci A, Chimenti C, Ricci R et al (2001) Improvement in cardiac function in the cardiac variant of Fabry's disease with galactose-infusion therapy. N Engl J Med 345(1):25–32

40. Porto C, Cardone M, Fontana F et al (2009) The pharmacological chaperone N-butyldeoxynojirimycin enhances enzyme replacement therapy in Pompe disease fibroblasts. Mol Ther 17(6):964–971

Chapter 30
Potential Factors Influencing Treatment Outcomes

G.E. Linthorst and C.E.M. Hollak

Abstract Treatment with enzyme replacement therapy in Fabry disease is successful in some, but not all patients. The presence of advanced disease, especially in the kidney or heart is associated with a less favorable outcome. Genetic and environmental factors that are known to play a role in the development of cardiovascular complications in the general population will probably put a patient with Fabry disease at a cumulative risk for disease progression. Apart from these patient related matters, the dose of enzyme as well as the formation of antibodies is discussed. Since antibodies interfere with surrogate markers such as levels of globotriaosylceramide in urine and endothelial cells in the skin, it is likely that they will affect clinical outcome. However, so far there is no evidence from clinical studies that this is the case.

Keywords Enzyme replacement therapy · Patient-related factors · Therapy-related factors · Antibody formation · Treatment efficacy

30.1 Introduction

In previous chapters the effects of enzyme replacement therapy have been extensively reviewed. In short, two enzyme replacement therapies have been developed: agalsidase-alfa (Replagal, Shire Human Genetic Therapies, Cambridge, MA, USA) and agalsidase-beta (Fabrazyme, Genzyme Corp., Cambridge, MA, USA). The pivotal trials with these enzymes were very different, using different endpoints and study populations [1, 2]. Subsequent long-term follow-up studies have shown clinical efficacy including improvement in quality of life, reduction or stabilization of cardiac mass and preservation of renal function for both of these enzymes [3–6].

G.E. Linthorst (✉)
Department of Internal Medicine/Endocrinology and Metabolism, Academic Medical Center, Amsterdam, The Netherlands
e-mail: g.e.linthorst@amc.nl

D. Elstein et al. (eds.), *Fabry Disease*, DOI 10.1007/978-90-481-9033-1_30,
© Springer Science+Business Media B.V. 2010

However, it has gradually become clear that not all patients improve and that progression of disease does occur in some. It has taken considerable time to become aware of this phenomenon, which is not surprising in light of the slowly progressive nature of the disease and the lack of sensitive biomarkers that relate to clinically important outcomes. The purpose of this chapter is to review patient as well as product related factors that may impact on the efficacy of treatment.

30.2 Patient Related Factors

30.2.1 General Patient Related Factors

The most prominent patient related factor that plays a role in the effect of ERT is obviously gender, because of the X-linked inheritance of the disease. The differences in phenotype between males and females are reviewed in Chapters 13 and 14. The current view is that a large proportion of carrier females may eventually develop identical clinical features compared to males, but at a later stage. It might be hypothesized that if early intervention would lead to a more favorable treatment outcome, females would respond better than males to enzyme therapy. To date, there are no studies to support this.

Since many of the symptoms in Fabry disease are presumably of vascular origin (renal insufficiency, cerebral infarctions, white matter lesions) it should be no surprise that factors known to result in vascular disease in the general population may contribute to the severity of the clinical picture. The most widely known risk factors are advanced age, smoking, hypertension, hypercholesterolemia, BMI >25 and diabetes. It seems reasonable to pay attention to these issues in order to try to optimize treatment outcome (e.g. weight reduction or smoking cessation programs). Again, there are no studies that systematically addressed the contribution of these common risk factors to the rate of disease progression. The influence of more circumscript genetic variations that have a relatively high prevalence in the general population and may induce a pro-thrombotic state have been studied by Schiffmann, Moore and co-workers. In one of their studies, they observed that a specific polymorphism of interleukin 6 (IL-6), endothelial nitric oxide synthase (eNOS), the factor V G1691A mutation as well as polymorphisms of protein Z were clearly associated with the presence of cerebral lesions on MRI [7]. Whether these polymorphisms may influence progression of renal disease and cardiac manifestations is not known. However, the general idea is that a cumulative risk for development of vascular lesions occurs when a subject carries both an α-galactosidase A (α-Gal A) mutation as well as one of these polymorphisms. This may open the possibility to identify patients most at risk for the development of vascular complications at an early stage. Whether earlier therapeutic intervention, such as ERT and/or anticoagulant therapy will slow down the rate of complications needs to be investigated. A trial that addresses the preventive effect of early ERT is now conducted. A similar influence could be expected from the newly discovered biochemical abnormality lyso-CTH (see Chapter 11).

It is possible that lyso-CTH, in combination with other determinants of disease severity such as age or the above mentioned polymorphisms, can to some extent predict the risk for future complications. Which genetic or environmental factors determine the levels of lyso-CTH is currently unknown.

Another genetic predisposition that was brought to attention a few years ago was the blood group B and secretor status of the patient. In a Fabry disease patient with blood group B and a positive secretor status, blood group B glycosphingolipids were shown to accumulate within the pancreas [8]. It was speculated that patients with blood group B (and a positive secretor status) had an additional accumulating glycosphingolipid compared to those with another blood group (or negative secretor status) and thus might suffer from more severe disease. An analysis of a large cohort, however, failed to demonstrate a correlation between blood group (and secretor) status and disease severity [9]. Most likely, blood group does not play a major role in severity of disease, or the effect of treatment.

A totally different and newly discovered phenomenon is the role of an isoform of alkaline phosphatase in human plasma that cleaves a phosphate-group from both agalsidases in vitro and in vivo and as such may influence uptake and kinetics of infused a-Gal A [10]. Additional studies will reveal if the presence and activity of this phosphatase has therapeutic implications.

30.2.2 Renal Disease

The initial short-term studies indicated that renal function could probably be preserved or even improved [1, 2]. In the study that investigated the effects of agalsidase-alfa, kidney biopsies showed improvement in histology, with a decrease in mesangial widening, a histological feature that is associated with glomerular damage. Also, renal function improved in the patients who switched from placebo to active treatment [1]. Longer term studies showed less favorable results, clearly depending on the degree of pre-treatment kidney failure. After 4–4.5 years of treatment with agalsidase-alfa, kidney function appeared to remain stable in the subgroups of patients with a GFR above 60 ml/min/1.73 m^2. In contrast, the patient subgroup with advanced renal disease at baseline (GFR < 60 ml/min) a mean rate of decline in eGFR of 5.2 ml/min/1.73 m^2 per year was observed [5]. In a recently published retrospective study it was reported that the natural course of decline in renal function in untreated patients with a GFR< 60 ml/min/1.73 m^2 was comparable [11], indicating that treatment does no longer have any effect in these cases. Similar results were observed for treatment with agalsidase-beta. The primary endpoint in the early agalsidase-beta trial was a decrease in globotriaosylceramide in the vascular endothelial cells of the kidney. Again, very positive results were noted, showing almost complete clearance in most cases. The renal function remained stable in this group of patients. However, treatment of Fabry patients for up to 36 months with agalsidase-beta at a dose of 1.0 mg/kg demonstrated that those who had a progression of renal failure had a baseline glomerular filtration rate (GFR) of < 60 ml/min or had proteinuria [3]. A follow up of this cohort, extending to 54 months of treatment, confirmed these findings [4]. Additional support for this observation is derived from the agalsidase-beta 1.0 mg/kg (phase IV) study, which specifically addressed disease progression in the more severely affected Fabry disease patients, treated with either agalsidase-beta or placebo [12]. The study failed to demonstrate benefit of treatment when analyzed by intention to treat analysis. Unfortunately, there was an imbalance of randomization concerning patients with proteinuria. When corrected for this imbalance, a positive effect of treatment (eg less disease progression) was found in favor of those treated. The effect was most prominent in those with a GFR > 55 ml/min/1.73 m^2. The overall conclusion of these observations is that preservation of renal function is probably the most optimal outcome of current ERT's, which means that therapy should be installed before the GFR has dropped below 55–70 ml/min/1.73 m^2.

Renal insufficiency, irrespective of its cause, poses by itself a risk factor for the development of vascular complications. It has become clear that in patients with Fabry disease, the occurrence of complications during treatment such as cardiac and cerebrovascular events is more likely to emerge in the presence of advanced renal failure. A 2 year follow-up in 25 agalsidase-beta treated patients showed 12 complications, including two deaths [13]. These events occurred only in the 16 patients with an impaired GFR (mean of 71 ml/min), while patients with a normal GFR exhibited no complications and had a better cardiac response. The role of proteinuria is less well established but is likely to be a harbinger of renal compromise as well, as it is a known risk factor for the development of renal failure in many renal diseases. A retrospective analysis of the effects of agalsidase-alfa on renal function showed that both GFR as well as proteinuria significantly predicted the rate of decline in renal function [14]. Positive effects of treatment with either Angiotensin Converting Enzyme inhibitors (ACEi) or Angiotensin II Receptor blockers (ARb) has first been demonstrated in proteinuric diabetics. Nowadays, in all patients with proteinuria, irrespective of the underlying (renal) disease, one of these drugs or its combination is prescribed [15]. In the aforementioned trials in Fabry disease the minority of patients were treated with these agents. The possible role of ACEi/ARb in preventing renal disease in Fabry disease is unknown, though it is prescribed routinely to those with micro-albuminuria or proteinuria in many treatment centers. A trial on the outcome of ACEi/ARB use and renal function in ERT treated Fabry disease patients is ongoing and will show results in the next year (NCT00343577).

30.2.3 Cardiac Disease

Left ventricular hypertrophy (LVH) is a significant feature of patients with Fabry disease. Initial studies of ERT showed reduction of globotriaosylceramide (GL-3) inclusions in cardiac tissue of biopsied patients [2], or reduction of left ventricular mass (LV mass) by the use of ultrasound [1] [16]. Additional studies with more sophisticated methods (such as MRI) showed a more heterogeneous picture.

In patients who are severely affected at baseline with extensive cardiac hypertrophy, the response is less robust [17]. The most plausible explanation for this, parallel to the observation in renal disease, is that the hypertrophy cannot be reversed once fibrosis occurs. This is supported by studies showing late enhancement in the ventricular wall after Gadolinium administration on cardiovascular magnetic resonance, which is indicative of fibrosis. It was shown that this phenomenon was specifically present in patients with more extensive hypertrophy, indicating that progressive hypertrophy coincides with irreversible interstitial collagen scarring [18]. Weideman and colleagues demonstrated a lack of response of ERT (defined as reduction in LVmass) in those with significant cardiac fibrosis as opposed to those without [19]. Thus, in order for ERT to be effective, patients should initiate treatment before the onset of fibrosis. One of the limitations of cardiac MRI as an imaging tool in Fabry disease is the fact that gadolinium cannot be applied in patients with severe renal impairment as well as in those with intracardial defibrillators (ICDs) or pacemakers. Of interest in this respect is a recently applied ultrasound technique that allows the detection of cardiac fibrosis as well [20].

30.2.4 Cerebral Disease

There is currently no study that specifically addressed the influence of ERT on the prevention of cerebrovascular accidents or white matter lesions in Fabry disease. White-matter lesions are small bright patches that show up on magnetic resonance imaging (MRI) of the brain. They can be found in elderly patients and probably reflect the normal aging process. When found at a younger age or in high amounts they presumably reflect small asymptomatic ischemic strokes. These white matter lesions can be found already at an early age in both males and female patients [21, 22]. During treatment with enzyme replacement therapy, variable responses have been reported. For example in the study by Jardim et al., in eight patients treated with agalsidase-alfa 0.2 mg/kg for 2 years, 4 lesions disappeared, whereas 8 appeared. The authors concluded that it was difficult to assess the role of enzyme therapy in this response pattern [23]. The agalsidase-beta phase IV study reported that 2/31 patients on placebo developed new strokes during the trial follow-up, as compared to 0/51 patients on ERT [12], which suggests a possible positive effect. Asymptomatic white matter lesions were not included in the endpoints of this study. In a comparative trial in which 0.2 mg/kg agalsidase-alfa was compared to equal dose of agalsidase-beta, white matter lesions were studied as a separate endpoint indicative of disease progression. In this trial, progressive disease was noted in 12 out of 34 patients, irrespective of product used [24]. The most frequent endpoint was the occurrence of new white matter lesions in the brain. According to the study protocol, these patients were switched to (1.0 mg/kg agalsidase-beta) on the assumption that a higher dose might abrogate the progression, assuming that both enzyme preparations appeared biologically equal. Despite this treatment switch, 7 of these patients demonstrated additional MRI abnormalities in the ensuing 12 months [24].

This in turn might suggest that apart from the kidney and the heart, cerebral involvement appears to have a point-of-no-return as well. To date, no stratifications are known to discern those with treatment amenable cerebral involvement and those without. Hopefully, more sensitive techniques to detect white matter lesions such as diffusion tensor imaging (DTI), a new structural MRI-technique that measures water diffusion characteristics, could be applied to use as a predictor for the occurrence of more severe brain injury [25].

30.3 Product Related Factors

30.3.1 Dose of Agalsidase-Alfa and Agalsidase-Beta

Several studies have addressed the influence of dose on clinical outcome. Agalsidase-alfa is used at a recommended dose of 0.2 mg/kg/biweekly. Following studies that showed that renal function might deteriorate despite treatment [3, 4, 6, 8], doubling of the dose to 0.2 mg/kg weekly was tried, showing that in some patients the slope of decline in renal function improved [26]. An anecdotal report observed a similar response: decline of renal function was halted when the dose was increased to 0.4 mg/kg/biweekly (rate of GFR decline went from –6.2 ml/min to 2 ml/min) [27]. Clarke and co-workers studied five different dosing regimens of agalsidase-alfa up to 0.4 mg/kg weekly for 10 weeks [28]. They solely studied plasma GL-3 as outcome parameter and demonstrated that in all treatment regimens used a (similar) decline was noted. These results suggest that there might be a dose-dependent effect in some patients, but not always on surrogate endpoints. Phase I studies with both drugs support the hypothesis that GL-3 clearance is dose-dependent. In the phase I study of agalsidase-alfa, better clearance of urinary GL-3 was seen in the higher dosages studied (up to 0.1 mg/kg) [29]. Similarly, the phase I studies using agalsidase-beta showed improved clearance of renal, cardiac and skin tissue GL-3 at higher dosages (1.0 and 3.0 mg/kg vs. 0.3 mg/kg) [30]. No results are available in reports on larger groups of patients that were treated with higher dosages of agalsidase-beta than 1.0 mg/kg. Only a single patient with severe cardiac involvement is described, who was treated with 2.0 mg/kg of agalsidase-beta, and in whom it is impossible to address the influence of this higher dose [31]. Studies on dose reduction are very scarce as well. Apart from the comparative trial, in which 0.2 mg/kg of agalsidase-beta was administered, a dose reduction of agalsidase-beta has been tried in one other trial [32]. In this study, patients were treated for 6 months with the recommended dose of 1.0 mg/kg after which they were switched to the lower 0.3 mg/kg dose. Although GL-3 clearance in the kidney was maintained in the majority of patients, a subset demonstrated renal (and skin) GL-3 re-accumulation. No data can be found in the literature on clinical effects of lower dosage s of agalsidase-alfa. Publications addressing the comparison of outcomes of different dosages are extremely limited as well. Vedder and co-workers reported slightly better results on reduction in cardiac mass in patients treated with a higher dose, but clearly these results should be confirmed in larger cohorts of patients [33]. In conclusion, it is currently impossible to draw firm conclusions based on these small, usually underpowered, studies on the outcome of different dosages as well as differences in products. As a consequence, no clear insight can be obtained how choice of dose (or enzyme preparation) can positively influence treatment outcome. Collaborative initiatives will be needed to address these issues and it is surprising that these questions remain unanswered after almost a decade of ERT for Fabry disease.

30.3.2 Antibody Formation

Antibody formation towards α-Gal A has been shown to occur in a high percentage of male patients. In females, this phenomenon is very rare, which is hardly surprising since females have residual enzyme activity and thus exogenously administered protein is recognized as non-foreign. Studies have shown that the percentage of antibodies in male patients may vary between the two products: in the early clinical studies using agalsidase-alfa, 56% developed antibodies [1] vs. 88% [2] in the trial with agalsidase-beta. Obviously it is difficult to compare these data, because the employed assays were not identical. The only small study so far that compared the prevalence of antibody formation for both agalsidases using the same assay showed that indeed a higher percentage of patients using agalsidase-beta produced an immune response: of 28 male patients, 18 developed α-Gal A antibodies after 6 months of therapy (4/10 agalsidase-alfa 0.2 mg/kg, 6/8 agalsidase-beta 0.2 mg/kg and 8/10 agalsidase-beta 1.0 mg/kg) [34]. Antibodies were seen more frequently in patients treated with agalsidase-beta 1.0 mg/kg than in patients treated with agalsidase-alfa 0.2 mg/kg ($p=0.005$). The period of 6 months is relevant as most patients develop these IgG antibodies between 3 and 6 months after initiation of treatment and almost always within the first year. The direct clinical effects of antibodies are represented by allergic reactions, such as hives, fever, chills and aggravation of acroparesthesias, during or shortly after the infusion. Whether these antibodies also exhibit long-term negative effects has been debated. Most long-term follow-up studies have reported that antibodies do not seem to interfere with clinical outcome. However, the small groups of patients and the variation in the clinical outcome hamper the ability to draw a firm conclusion. In fact, it is very unlikely that the presence of antibodies does not interfere with efficacy of the exogenously administered enzymes. Several years ago, it has already been shown that the IgG antibodies directed towards the enzymes diminishes the activity of the enzyme in vitro and alters the targeting [34–36]. In the presence of antibodies towards the infused enzyme, the formed immune-enzyme complexes will be taken up by Fc-receptors present on phagocytes, e.g. granulocytes in the bloodstream and macrophages in the tissues rather than by the targeted cells through their mannose-6-phosphate receptor. Both the in vivo neutralization and the altered targeting result in less pronounced reduction of urinary GL-3 in the presence of antibodies, as compared to patients who do not exhibit an antibody response [34–36]. One may regard urinary GL-3 as an invalid marker of disease [37] and as such might claim that presence of antibodies does not influence outcome of disease. Yet in the Fabry mouse model, Ohashi and co-workers demonstrated that less enzyme was targeted to key organs in the presence of antibodies [38]. In a retrospective study of earlier clinical trials, Benichou et al. studied the (long-term) clinical outcome of Fabry patients on agalsidase-beta and the presence and titer of anti-agalsidase-beta antibodies [39]. They could not establish a correlation between anti-α-Gal A IgG titers and the onset of clinical events or the rate of change in estimated GFR during treatment. However, there was a clear trend towards an association between elevation of GL-3 and the presence of (high) titers of antibodies. More importantly, a relation between antibody titer and the recurrence of GL-3 accumulation in skin biopsies was established. This latter observation confirms the findings of Ohashi et al.: it is very likely that the antibody formation also has a negative effect on tissue level. Again it should be noted that the clinical consequences may only become apparent after a long period of time, given the slow progressive nature of the disease. One way to overcome the effect of the antibodies may be an increment in the dose, as shown in mice [38]. Also in humans, an increase in dose (agalsidase-alfa or beta at a dose of 0.2 mg/kg to agalsidase-beta 1.0 mg/kg) led to a subsequent reduction in GL-3 in the urine [33]. The observation that higher doses may be needed to overcome neutralization or mistargeting of infused proteins is not new: in hemophilia, antibody formation may lead to loss of function of infused factor VIII. A dose increase of the recombinant protein can help to overcome this problem, or the administration of specific drugs that eliminates the immune response [40].

The impact of antibodies on clinical outcome has also been demonstrated for other recombinant enzymes, used for treatment of lysosomal storage disorders, such as Pompe disease or mycopolysacharidosis (MPS)-I. In these diseases it has been shown to negatively influence treatment outcome. The development of anti agalsidase antibodies, their effect on long-term efficacy of ERT and explorations for immunosuppressive regimens deserve further study in Fabry disease.

30.4 Conclusions

The availability of enzyme replacement therapies for the treatment of Fabry disease has brought high expectations to the Fabry community. Although many patients benefit from therapy, it has become clear that there are individual limitations to the success of treatment. These limitations are largely unknown but some of these have been described here and encompass factors that are patient or treatment specific. In summary, it is clear that those patients with more severe disease at baseline, as evidenced by proteinuria, reduced GFR (below 55–70 ml/min) or with fibrosis at cardiac evaluation, probably fare worse than those without. It is at present unclear if such 'point of no return' also exists for cerebral complications. It is of interest to note that it is also unclear whether females have a better outcome of treatment than males.

Possible treatment related factors could be either enzyme preparation or dose. Although there is some (sometimes anecdotal) information that suggests that some patients may have an improved outcome with a higher dose, sound clinical studies supporting this view are lacking.

Antibodies towards the infused enzyme occur often in male patients and result in reduced efficacy on surrogate endpoints. There are no data demonstrating that antibody formation has an impact on clinical efficacy as well, but the repeatedly shown influence of antibodies on recurrence of GL-3 in urine as well as in skin biopsies suggests otherwise. This is supported by findings in other lysosomal storage disorders, in which antibodies may play an important role. The slow protracted course of Fabry disease and the limited efficacy of ERT in more affected patients makes it difficult to investigate this effect. Long term studies in large cohorts of patients are urgently needed to adequately address these questions.

References

1. Schiffmann R, Kopp JB, Austin HA III et al (2001) Enzyme replacement therapy in fabry disease: a randomized controlled trial. J Am Med Assoc 285(21):2743–2749
2. Eng CM, Guffon N, Wilcox WR et al (2001) Safety and efficacy of recombinant human ‡-galactosidase A replacement therapy in Fabry's disease. N Engl J Med 345(1): 9–16
3. Wilcox WR, Banikazemi M, Guffon N et al (2004) Long-term safety and efficacy of enzyme replacement therapy for Fabry disease. Am J Hum Genet 75(1):65–74
4. Germain DP, Waldek S, Banikazemi M et al (2007) Sustained, long-term renal stabilization after 54 months of agalsidase beta therapy in patients with Fabry disease. J Am Soc Nephrol 18(5):1547–1557
5. Schiffmann R, Ries M, Timmons M, Flaherty JT, Brady RO (2006) Long-term therapy with agalsidase-alfa for Fabry disease: safety and effects on renal function in a home infusion setting. Nephrol Dial Transplant 21(2):345–354
6. West M, Nicholls K, Mehta A et al (2009) Agalsidase-alfa and kidney dysfunction in Fabry disease. J Am Soc Nephrol 20(5):1132–1139
7. Altarescu G, Moore DF, Schiffmann R (2005) Effect of genetic modifiers on cerebral lesions in Fabry disease. Neurology 64:2148–2150
8. Ledvinova J, Poupetova H, Hanackova A, Pisacka M, Elleder M (1997) Blood group B glycosphingolipids in alpha-galactosidase deficiency (Fabry disease): influence of secretor status. Biochim Biophys Acta 1345(2):180–187
9. Linthorst GE, Folman CC, Aerts JM, Hollak CE (2003) Blood group does not correlate with disease severity in patients with Fabry disease (alpha-galactosidase A deficiency). Blood Cells Mol Dis 31(3):324–326
10. Deegan P, Marchesan D, Cox TM (2009) Studies on the serum phosphatase that abrogates uptake of mannose-6-phosphate-containing therapeutic lysosomal enzymes. Meeting of the European Study Group of lysosomal disease, Bad Honnef, 13 Sept 2009
11. Schiffmann R, Warnock DG, Banikazemi M et al (2009 Feb) Fabry disease: progression of nephropathy, and prevalence of cardiac and cerebrovascular events before enzyme replacement therapy. Nephrol Dial Transplant 24(7):2102–2111
12. Banikazemi M, Bultas J, Waldek S et al (2007) Agalsidase-beta therapy for advanced Fabry disease: a randomized trial. Ann Intern Med 146(2):77–86
13. Breunig F, Weidemann F, Strotmann J, Knoll A, Wanner C (2006) Clinical benefit of enzyme replacement therapy in Fabry disease. Kidney Intern 69:1216–1221

14. West M, Nicholls K, Mehta A et al (2009) Agalsidase-alfa and kidney dysfunction in Fabry disease. Am Soc Nephrol 20(5):1132–1139
15. Kunz R, Friedrich C, Wolbers M, Mann JF (2008) Meta-analysis: effect of monotherapy and combination therapy with inhibitors of the renin angiotensin system on proteinuria in renal disease. Ann Int Med 148(1):30–48
16. Beck M, Ricci R, Widmer U et al (2004) Fabry disease: overall effects of agalsidase-alfa treatment. Europ J Clin Invest 34(12):838–844
17. Koskenvuo JW, Hartiala JJ, Nuutila P et al (2008) Twenty-four-month alpha-galactosidase A replacement therapy in Fabry disease has only minimal effects on symptoms and cardiovascular parameters. J Inherit Metab Dis 31(3):432–441
18. Moon JC, Sachdev B, Elkington AG et al (2003) Gadolinium enhanced cardiovascular magnetic resonance in Anderson-Fabry disease. Evidence for a disease specific abnormality of the myocardial interstitium. Eur Heart J 24(23):2151–2155
19. Weidemann F, Niemann M, Breunig F et al (2009) Long-term effects of enzyme replacement therapy on fabry cardiomyopathy: evidence for a better outcome with early treatment. Circulation 119(4):524–529
20. Weidemann F, Niemann M, Herrmann S et al (2007) A new echocardiographic approach for the detection of non-ischaemic fibrosis in hypertrophic myocardium. EurHeart J 28(24): 3020–3026
21. Crutchfield KE, Patronas NJ, Dambrosia JM et al (1998) Quantitative analysis of cerebral vasculopathy in patients with Fabry disease. Neurology 50(6):1746–1749
22. Fellgiebel A, Muller MJ, Mazanek M, Baron K, Beck M, Stoeter P (2005) White matter lesion severity in male and female patients with Fabry disease. Neurology 65(4):600–602
23. Jardim LB, Aesse F, Vedolin LM et al (2006) White matter lesions in Fabry disease before and after enzyme replacement therapy: a 2-year follow-up. Arq Neuropsiquiatr 64(3B): 711–717
24. Vedder AC, Linthorst GE, Houge G et al (2007) Treatment of Fabry disease: outcome of a comparative trial with agalsidase alfa or beta at a dose of 0.2 mg/kg. PLoSONE 2(7):e598
25. Albrecht J, Dellani PR, Muller MJ et al (2007) Voxel based analyses of diffusion tensor imaging in Fabry disease. J Neurol Neurosurg Psych 78(9):964–969
26. Schiffmann R, Askari H, Timmons M et al (2007) Weekly enzyme replacement therapy may slow decline of renal function in patients with Fabry disease who are on long-term biweekly dosing. J Am Soc Nephrol 18(5):1576–1583
27. Torra R, Algaba F, Ars E, Santin S, Fernandez-Llama P, Ballarin J (2008) Preservation of renal function in a patient with Fabry nephropathy on enzyme replacement therapy. Clin Nephrol 69(6):445–449
28. Clarke JT, West ML, Bultas J, Schiffmann R (2007) The pharmacology of multiple regimens of agalsidase alfa enzyme replacement therapy for Fabry disease. GenetMed 9(8): 504–509
29. Schiffmann R, Murray GJ, Treco D et al (2000) Infusion of alpha-galactosidase A reduces tissue globotriaosylceramide storage in patients with Fabry disease. Proc Nat Acad Sci (USA) 97(1):365–370
30. Eng CM, Banikazemi M, Gordon RE et al (2001) A Phase 1/2 Clinical Trial of Enzyme Replacement in Fabry Disease: pharmacokinetic, Substrate Clearance, and Safety Studies. Amer J Hum Genet 68(3):711–722
31. Sheppard MN, Cane P, Florio R et al (2009) A detailed pathologic examination of heart tissue from three older patients with Anderson-Fabry disease on enzyme replacement therapy. Cardiovasc Pathol (epub 23/jul/09)
32. Lubanda JC, Anijalg E, Bzduch V, Thurberg BL, Benichou B, Tylki-Szymanska A (2009) Evaluation of a low dose, after a standard therapeutic dose, of agalsidase beta during enzyme replacement therapy in patients with Fabry disease. Genet Med 11(4):256–264
33. Vedder AC, Breunig F, Donker-Koopman WE et al (2008) Treatment of Fabry disease with different dosing regimens of agalsidase: effects on antibody formation and GL-3. Mol Genet Metab 94(3):319–325

34. Linthorst GE, Hollak CEM, Donker-Koopman WE, Strijland A, Aerts JMFG (2004) Enzyme therapy for Fabry disease: neutralizing antibodies toward agalsidase alpha and beta. Kidney Int 66(4):1589–1595
35. Whitfield PD, Calvin J, Hogg S et al (2005) Monitoring enzyme replacement therapy in Fabry disease–role of urine globotriaosylceramide. J Inherit Metab Dis 28(1):21–33
36. Ohashi T, Sakuma M, Kitagawa T, Suzuki K, Ishige N, Eto Y (2007) Influence of antibody formation on reduction of globotriaosylceramide (GL-3) in urine from Fabry patients during agalsidase beta therapy. Mol Genet Metab 92(3):271–273
37. Vedder AC, Linthorst GE, van Breemen MJ et al (2007) The Dutch Fabry cohort: diversity of clinical manifestations and Gb3 levels. J Inherit Metab Dis 30(1):68–78
38. Ohashi T, Iizuka S, Ida H, Eto Y (2008) Reduced alpha-Gal A enzyme activity in Fabry fibroblast cells and Fabry mice tissues induced by serum from antibody positive patients with Fabry disease. Mol Genet Metab 94(3):313–318
39. Benichou B, Goyal S, Sung C, Norfleet AM, O'Brien F (2009) A retrospective analysis of the potential impact of IgG antibodies to agalsidase beta on efficacy during enzyme replacement therapy for Fabry disease. Mol Genet Metab 96(1):4–12
40. Mendelsohn NJ, Messinger YH, Rosenberg AS, Kishnani PS (2009) Elimination of antibodies to recombinant enzyme in Pompe's disease. N Engl J Med 360(2):194–195

Chapter 31
Symptomatic and Ancillary Therapy

Catharina Whybra-Trümpler

Abstract Although enzyme replacement therapy has had a considerable impact on the management of patients with Fabry disease, it is essential that attention is also given to supportive therapy. In this chapter a general overview about ancillary therapy is given. The great variability of clinical symptoms faced by patients with Fabry disease need the involvement from many different specialists, as well as a wide range of concomitant treatments. Coordinating a good multidisciplinary approach for each patient and ensuring that treatment is made as convenient as possible may offer a more positive impact on the quality of life of those patients affected by Fabry disease.

Keywords Supportive therapy · Multidisciplinary approach · Concomitant medication

31.1 Supportive and Ancillary Therapy in Fabry Disease

As Fabry disease is a multisystemic disease, it is essential that attention is also paid to supportive therapy. Since the disease was first described in 1898 and up till the present there is no cure for the disease, the great variability of clinical symptoms need relief as a matter of course. To allow a multidisciplinary approach, it is of great importance to critically refer the patient to a respective specialist, for example, a cardiologist, a geneticist, a nephrologist, a pediatrician, a psychologist. As a result, a great variability of concomitant medications may be prescribed as shown summarized in Table 31.1.

C. Whybra-Trümpler (✉)
Universitätskinderklinik der Johannes Gutenberg Universität Mainz, Langenbeckstr. 1, Mainz, Germany
e-mail: c.whybra@web.de

D. Elstein et al. (eds.), *Fabry Disease*, DOI 10.1007/978-90-481-9033-1_31,

Table 31.1 Concomitant medications and recommendations

Acroparesthesias
Painful crisis: avoiding quick temperature changes,
Non-steroidal antiinflammatory drugs
Chronic pain: anticonvulsants (carbamazepine, gabapentin, phenytoin)

Hypohidrosis
Appropiate temperature and environment

Angiokeratomas
Cosmetic removal with argon laser therapy

Proteinuria
ACEI (Angiotensin Converting Enzyme Inhibitor) and/or
ARB (Angiotensin Receptor Blocker)

Renal failure
Dialysis, transplantation

Gastrointestinal symptoms
Pain relief, H2-blockers by gastric pain and reflux
Motility agents
Pancreatic enzyme supplementation

Hypertension
Regular monitoring and rigorous surveillance following general guidelines
(avoid ß-blockers: sinus bradycardia!)

Hyperlipidemia
Regular routine surveillance
Statin therapy

Lymphadenopathy
Compression stockings
Lymph drainage in some cases

Stroke prevention
Reducing general risk factors according to the AHA, e.g.

- Hypertension
- Diabetes mellitus
- Smoking
- Dyslipidemia

Aspirin, Clopidogrel

Depression
Anti-depressant drugs:

- SSRIs (selective serotonin reuptake inhibitors)
- SNRIs (serotonin norepinephrine reuptake inhibitors)

31.2 Pain Relief

The treatment of chronic neuropathic pain in patients with Fabry disease remains empiric [1]. Preventive pain therapy with *gabapentin, carbamazepine* and *amitriptyline* appears to be beneficial. One potential advantage of anticonvulsants is that compliance may be monitored and the risk of toxicity reduced by following serum levels. However, these levels do not have a direct correlation with neuropathic pain response.

Of the anticonvulsants, *gabapentin* is most often used [2, 3]. Advantages of gabapentin include low toxicity, a low incidence of drug interactions, and lack of liver metabolism. The nearly complete renal clearance is potentially a matter of concern in patients with Fabry disease, who are at risk regarding kidney disease. Therefore, renal function should be assessed before beginning gabapentin treatment and the dose should be adjusted accordingly, as renal function affects serum levels and half life.

In children less than 12 years old, the starting dose of *gabapentin* is 10–15 mg/kg/day divided into three doses. The dose may be slowly increased up to 50 mg/kg daily. For older children and adults the initial dose is typically 300 mg three times a day (900 mg total a day). The total maximum dose may be in the range of 1,800–2,400 mg/day.

A number of other anticonvulsants have been used for the treatment of neuropathic pain. Of the older drugs, carbamazepine and phenytoin have been used most often [4, 5].

However, phenytoin is not commonly used for chronic treatment in children because of concerns about adverse cosmetic effects that include hirsutism, gingival hyperplasia, and coarse facial features. In addition, chronic phenytoin treatment has been associated with the potential for cerebellar atrophy and peripheral neuropathy. Carbamazepine appears to be effective but causes induction of the P450 system in the liver, which can be a concern in patients on multiple drugs that are metabolized by the liver.

Amitriptyline at doses well below those used in the treatment of depression has been shown to be effective in the treatment of chronic neuropathic pain [6]. At the level of the lower doses used for neuropathic pain, serious side effects are uncommon. Nonetheless, an electrocardiogram should be obtained before and after beginning treatment since amitriptyline can cause adverse changes in cardiac conduction.

31.3 Kidney Function

Patients with Fabry disease are at high risk for progressive kidney failure. Only one study has directly examined the effectiveness of an angiotensin converting enzyme inhibitor (ACEI) and/or angiotensin receptor blocker (ARB) therapy [7]. In this non-randomized open-label study of 11 patients with Fabry disease and nephropathy (four and seven patients with Chronic Kidney Disease (CKD) stages 1 or 2 and CKD stages 3 or 4, respectively), all patients received ACE inhibitor and/or ARB therapy before starting enzyme replacement therapy, with careful dose titration determined empirically by baseline proteinuria, response to therapy, and induction of adverse effects (principally hypotension). Median initial blood pressure levels were 98/63 mmHg for patients with stage 1 or 2 disease, and 135/82 mmHg for those with stage 3 or 4 disease. At follow-up at 30 months, therapy resulted in stabilization of renal function and reductions in proteinuria. As an example, the urine protein to creatinine ratio decreased from 1.24 to 0.46 and the rate of decline of GFR was only –0.23 ml/min per 1.73 m^2/year among those with CKD stages 3 or 4 disease. This rate is superior to that described in patients who received enzyme replacement therapy, but not antihypertensive agents. In addition, blood pressure remained stable or minimally decreased with therapy (105/67 and 122/72 mmHg for those with stage 1 or 2 disease and stage 3 or 4 disease, respectively). Adverse effects include occasional episodes of hypotension that responded to dose adjustment and minor episodes of hyperkalemia.

Although further study in a larger number of patients is required, careful titration of ACE inhibitor/ARB therapy appears to help stabilize kidney function and decrease proteinuria in patients with Fabry disease, even in those with normal or low initial blood pressures [8].

General recommendations for the care of patients with chronic kidney disease should therefore be followed:

An angiotensin converting enzyme inhibitor (ACEI) or angiotensin receptor blocker (ARB) should be prescribed for the reduction of proteinuria and for blood pressure control.

Blood pressure control to a goal of <130/80 mmHg, as recommended for all patients with kidney disease.

31.4 Angiokeratomas

Cosmetic removal of the benign vascular skin lesions can be done by laser therapy. Argon laser therapy was one of the first techniques to be used clinically, although it is a continuous wave laser and leads to significant non-selective heating of surrounding tissues, which increases the risk of scarring. The variable pulse with neodymium: yttrium-aluminium garnet (Nd:YAG) laser appears to be an alternative option in the treatment of angiokeratomas [9]. The used of combined treatment with erbium: YAG and532 nm potassium titanyl phosphate lasers also leads to excellent cosmetic results without clinically visible scarring or recurrence. These procedures usually do not require anesthesia. Other treatments include fine-needle electrocautery or surgical removal, both of which require local anesthesia [10].

31.5 Lymphadenopathy

Lymphedema in Fabry disease can be complicated by erysipelas, with a risk of systemic infection. Thus, lymphedema may necessitate the use of compression stockings.

31.6 Pulmonary

There are no evidence-based recommendations for therapy for lung complications in patients with Fabry disease. Airway obstruction commonly occurs in patients with Fabry disease regardless of smoking history, and it increases with age [11]. Nevertheless, cigarette smoking is, of course, an aggravating factor. Those patients with moderate to severe obstruction should receive inhaled brochodilatators, such as long acting ß2-agnonists and atropine derivates. There is no evidence that steroids, either systemic or inhaled, are of any benefit for these patients, unless they have clinically apparent asthma. General measures, as in other chronic pulmonary diseases, immunization against influenza and pneumococcal infection are recommended.

31.7 Heart

All the usual measures for reducing cardiovascular risk are used in patients in Fabry disease, including statin therapy to lower lipid levels and antihypertensive treatment. Patients should be treated according to the recommendations of their cardiologist following the clinical signs and symptoms. Antianginal treatment should be given with care, as ß-blockers may aggravate the tendency for symptomatic bradycardia and AV conduction impairment. Dihidropyridine calcium channel blockers are relatively effective and safe. Anti-aggregation therapy should be offered to all symptomatic patients, regarding also the prothrombotic state associated with the endothelial dysfunction caused by the disease itself [12].

In patients with supraventricular rhythm disturbances, anticoagulant therapy should immediately be started. Pacemaker implantation is frequently required in patients with symptomatic bradycardia and/or AV conduction abnormalities.

Angiotensin-converting enzyme inhibitors or angiotensin receptor blockers should also be considered in asymptomatic individuals with left ventricular hypertrophy. The potential nephroprotective effects should also be considered. Patients with advanced congestive heart failure may be candidates for heart transplantation, as the intrinsic enzyme production within the graft should prevent its rapid deterioration [13].

Septal alcohol ablation may be effective in patients with LV outflow tract obstruction. Other treatment modalities (surgical myectomy, mitral valve replacement) should be considered in individuals with unsuitable septal branch anatomy [14].

31.8 Cerebrovascular

Standard ischemic stroke prevention measures are considered effective in secondary (and possibly primary) prevention for patients with Fabry disease, although this conclusion is based solely upon clinical experience [15].

The management of treatable risk factors that contribute to the development and progression of atherosclerotic cerebrovascular disease is important for reducing the risk of ischemic stroke. The major treatable risk factors for cerebrovascular atherosclerotic disease are similar to those for coronary atherosclerosis.

- Diabetes mellitus
- Smoking
- Dyslipidemia
- Hypertension

In adults, these measures include the use of anti-platelet agents (i.e. *aspirin* monotherapy, *clopidogrel* monotherapy, or the combination of aspirin with extended-release *dipyridamole*), antihypertensive agents and statins.

Accumulating evidence suggests that *aspirin* and *clopidogrel* in combination does not offer greater benefit for stroke prevention than either agent alone, but does substantially increase the risk of bleeding complications. This conclusion is supported by results from the MATCH trial [16]. In children, only *aspirin* therapy is suggested.

Additional American Heart Association (AHA) risk factor recommendations are as follows:

- Discontinue oral contraceptives and switch to another form of birth control
- Lower the homocysteine level when it is higher than normal with diet or supplementation of folate, vitamin B6, or vitamin B12
- Avoid triptans in children with hemiplegic migraine, basilar migraine, known vascular risk factors, or prior cardiac or cerebral ischemia
- Seek and treat iron deficiency, which may increase the risk of arterial ischemic stroke in conjunction with other risk factors
- Counsel children and their families regarding dietary improvement, the benefits of exercise, and avoidance of tobacco products.

31.9 Psychiatric Signs and Symptoms

Clinical observations and a few published reports have shown that a high proportion of patients with Fabry disease are also at risk of developing neuropsychiatric symptoms, such as depression, primary or secondary to the disease, suicidal tendencies and neuropsychological deficits. Depressive disorders are apparently most prevalent, whereas psychotic syndromes have been reported exceptionally. In most cases, depression is associated with feelings of hopelessness, passivity and pessimism, possibly leading to low treatment adherence and a high risk of substance abuse. As a matter of fact, there is very often a delay between the onset of symptoms and the diagnosis. This might contribute to severe psychosocial impairment as well. Psychotherapeutic and psychopharmacological treatment, especially SSRIs (selective serotonin reuptake inhibitors) and SNRIs (serotonin norepinephrine reuptake inhibitors) – the latter have also shown efficacy in the treatment of neuropathic pain – are promising to improve quality of life in patients with Fabry disease.

References

1. MacDermot J, MacDermot KD (2001) Neuropathic pain in Anderson-Fabry disease: pathology and therapeutic options. Eur J Pharmacol 429:121–125
2. Germain DP (2002) Fabry's disease (alpha-galactosidase-A deficiency): recent therapeutic innovations. J Soc Biol 196:183–190
3. Ries M, Mengel E, Kutschke G et al (2003) Use of gabapentin to reduce chronic neuropathic pain in Fabry disease. J Inherit Metab Dis 26:413–414
4. Lockman LA, Hunninghake DB, Krivit W, Desnick RJ (1973) Relief of pain of Fabry's disease by diphenylhydantoin. Neurology 23:871–875
5. Lenoir G, Rivron M, Gubler MC et al (1977) Fabry's disease. Carbamazepine therapy in acrodyniform syndrome. Arch Fr Pediatr 34:704–716
6. Saarto T, Wiffen PJ (2005) Antidepressants for neuropathic pain. Cochrane Database Syst Rev 3:CD005454
7. Tahir H, Jackson LL, Warnock DG (2007) Antiproteinuric therapy and Fabry nephropathy: sustained reduction of proteinuria in patients receiving enzyme replacement therapy with Agalsidase-beta. J Am Soc Nephrol 18:2609–2617
8. Wanner C, Breunig F (2007) Fabry nephropathy and the case for adjunctive renal therapy. J Am Soc Nephrol 18:2426–2428
9. Bechara FG, Huesmann M, Altmeyer P, Hoffmann K, Jansen T (2002) Angiokeratoma of the glans penis: successful treatment with Nd: YAG laser. Acta Paediatr Suppl 439:143
10. Mohrenschlager M, Brau-Falco M, Ring J, Abeck D (2003) Fabry disease: recognition and management of cutaneous manifestations. Am J Clin Dermatol 4:189–196
11. Brown LK, Miller A, Bhuptani A et al (1997) Pulmonary involvement in Fabry disease. Am J Respir Crit Care Med 155:1004–1010
12. DeGraba TT, Azhar S, Dignat George F et al (2000) Profile of endothelial and leukocyte activation in Fabry patients. Ann Neurol 47:229–233
13. Cantor WJ, Daly P, Iwannochko M, Clarke JT, Cusimano RJ, Butany J (1998) Cardiac transplantation for Fabry's disease. Can J Cardiol 14:81–84
14. Magage S, Linhart A, Bultas J et al (2005) Fabry disease: percutaneous transluminal septal myocardial ablation markedly improved symptomatic left ventricular hypertrophy and outflow tract obstruction in a classically affected male. Echocardiography 22:333–339
15. Moore DF, Kaneski CR, Askari H, Schiffmann R (2007) The cerebral vasculopathy of Fabry disease. J Neurol Sci 257:258–263
16. Diener HC, Bogousslavsky J, Brass LM et al (2004) Aspirin and clopidogrel compared with clopidogrel alone after recent ischaemic stroke or transient ischaemic attack in high-risk patients (MATCH): randomised, double-blind, placebo-controlled trial. Lancet 364:331–337

Chapter 32
The Price of Care Versus the Cost of Caring

Joe T.R. Clarke

Abstract The high drug costs of enzyme replacement therapy (ERT) of lysosomal storage diseases (LSD), including Fabry disease, make the overall per-patient costs of treatment extremely high. According to conventional cost-utility analyses, ERT does not meet generally accepted criteria for public reimbursement. However, research has shown that public involvement in healthcare resource allocation invariably includes consideration of other societal concerns, including severity of the disease, the potential for a positive response to treatment, and the life-threatening nature of the disease. The formal incorporation of societal values in decisions relating to financial support for expensive treatments for rare diseases is illustrated by the establishment of the Citizen's Council of the National Institute for Health and Clinical Excellence (NICE) in the UK. The need for ERT for LSD is generally deemed to be life-long, and other, non-medical, costs ultimately play a role in decisions by patients to continue treatment indefinitely.

Keywords Orphan drugs · Cost-utility · Cost-effectiveness · Social values · Lysosomal storage diseases · Fabry disease

32.1 Introduction

Enzyme replacement therapy (ERT) for lysosomal storage diseases (LSD), including Fabry disease, is extremely expensive for the individual patient. Drug costs exceeding $250,000 (US dollars) per year for the treatment of an adult patient are not unusual. The reason for the high costs is a matter of some debate. However, the implementation in 1984 of the terms of the Orphan Drug Act [1] in the United States

J.T.R. Clarke (✉)
Department of Pediatrics, Division of Clinical and Metabolic Genetics, Hospital for Sick Children and University of Toronto, Toronto, ON, Canada; Service de génétique médicale, Centre hospitalier universitaire, Sherbrooke, Canada
e-mail: jtrc@sickkids.ca

D. Elstein et al. (eds.), *Fabry Disease*, DOI 10.1007/978-90-481-9033-1_32,
© Springer Science+Business Media B.V. 2010

undoubtedly has been a major factor. According to the Act, which was introduced in an effort to encourage drug manufacturers to develop new and effective treatments for rare diseases, companies were accorded market exclusivity for a period of 7 years in the US, essentially eliminating any control on pricing that might have developed as a result as competition in the market place. Although the terms of the Act only apply to the US, the price set in that country became the international price.

Because costs to the individual are so high, third-party payers, including government-sponsored public drug reimbursement programs, inevitably became involved in covering the costs of treatment. Rare diseases, including all the LSD, are, by definition, rare. Thus, although the drug costs for treatment of the individual patient are generally exorbitant, the overall impact on public drug expenditures is, with some important exceptions, generally trivial. For example, the total drug costs of the treatment of all patients with Fabry disease with Fabrazyme or Replagal in Canada is still miniscule compared with total spending on prescription drugs, which was approximately $25 billion in 2008 (www.cihi.ca) when the total expenditure on the two drugs together was estimated to be less than $25 million (Clarke, unpublished data), i.e. not more than 0.1% of the total.

In order to ensure that the public is getting value for its tax support of public drug reimbursement programs, most governments have developed methods for assessing the cost-effectiveness of any investment in new drug therapies. Recognition of the need for some economically sound and equitable approach to the allocation of health care resources has generated rapidly growing interest in health technology assessment (HTA) throughout the western world. The total number of HTA reports increased more than 10-fold during the 15-year period ending in 2002 [2].

32.2 Evidence of the Effectiveness of ERT of Fabry Disease

The efficacy of ERT of Fabry disease was demonstrated in randomized, placebo-controlled clinical trials with agalsidase alfa [3, 4] or with agalsidase beta [5–7]. In addition, a wealth of information on the response to ERT has been reported. from observational studies of variable numbers of patients followed for different periods of time. A number of publications have emerged from the Fabry Outcome Survey (FOS), a large-scale observational database reporting on patients on treatment with agalsidase alfa [8–18]. The results of a 5-year follow-up of patients on agalsidase alfa showed a statistically significant reduction in left ventricular mass (LVM) in patients with baseline cardiac hypertrophy. The results of the study also showed an overall decrease of estimated glomerular filtration rate, as well as a significant improvement in pain and quality of life of patients receiving long-term ERT [19].

The results of similar open-label or long-term observational studies of the effectiveness of ERT with agalsidase beta have also been reported [20–27]. Only one head-to-head comparison of the relative efficacy of agalsidase alfa and agalsidase beta has been reported [28, 29]. The investigators were unable to demonstrate a significant difference in the efficacy of the two enzyme preparations administered at the same dose of 0.2 mg/kg every 2 weeks, but reported later that agalsidase beta administered at a higher dose of 1 mg/kg every 2 weeks had a more robust effect on decreasing urinary glycolipid excretion and produced a greater effect on the cardiomyopathy of the disease. This study has been criticized on methodological grounds [30], and the issue remains unresolved. An open-label study of the relative efficacy of different dosage regimens of agalsidase alfa showed that 0.1, 0.2, and 0.4 mg/kg administered weekly or biweekly produced similar reductions of plasma globotriaosylceramide levels in plasma [31]. What appears to be clear is that both enzyme preparations are apparently effective in preventing or retarding the progression of cardiac and renal complications of Fabry disease, though the relative effectiveness of the two treatment regimens remains unclear.

32.3 Cost-Effectiveness Analysis

A conventional approach to the evaluation of new therapies is to examine the cost-utility of the treatment which estimates the cost of the treatment in dollars per quality-adjusted life-year (QALY) [32, 33]. The drug cost of ERT is very high, running between $75,000 and $350,000 per patient-year, depending on the body weight of the patient [34]. According to a generally accepted threshold for assuming public payment for a new drug of $50,000–$150,000 per QALY [33], none of the newly developed treatments for LSD, including ERT or substrate reduction therapy (SRT), comes close to meeting this criterion for public reimbursement. In a detailed and rigorous assessment of the cost-effectiveness of ERT of Fabry disease, Moore and his colleagues showed clearly in quantitative terms the failure of the treatment to meet conventional criteria for cost-effectiveness [34]. This approach to decision-making regarding healthcare resource allocation is conceptually straight-forward and, given complete and accurate data, it is easy to compute. It also has the merit of permitting comparisons between completely different types of healthcare interventions.

Decisions based solely on cost-utility analysis are ultimately utilitarian: choices are made on the basis of the concept of distributive justice, or what produces the greatest good for the largest number of people. The experience of the State of Oregon is instructive in this regard. In the late 1980s, the state underwent a comprehensive analysis of cost-utility to guide decision-making regarding what healthcare interventions would be supported by the state-sponsored Medicaid program [35, 36]. The initial results of the analysis were recognized immediately to be seriously flawed, and the State went on to undertake a more elaborate process of ranking interventions involving extensive consultation with the public.

32.4 Importance of Social Values

The experience of the US state of Oregon showed that formal cost-effectiveness analysis, according to generally accepted techniques, often produces results that are clearly as odds with our intuitive feelings about resource allocation. The State of Oregon recognized this and embarked on an approach for which the theoretical foundation at the time was weak, but which ended up being more socially acceptable, despite some continuing debate about the ethical merits of the initiative. The Oregon experience underscored the fundamental importance of the role of societal values in resource allocation in general and with specific reference to health care spending in particular.

Concurrent with the emergence of the Oregon approach to health care resource allocation, the Norwegian economist, Eric Nord, published the results of a number of studies focused on describing and quantifying public attitudes towards the problem [37]. Many of his findings will not come as a surprise to the people of Oregon. What Nord and others have contributed is the theoretical foundation, based on formal research, for the way Oregon approached the crisis in Medicaid funding in the late 1980s. Nord's contribution is important because he provides the data to help us to reconcile the internal tension we experience between the desire to employ economically sound, utilitarian methods for making health care allocation decisions and the value we place on the life of the individual. One of Nord's most important observations was the somewhat surprising finding that some possibility, however small, of access by an individual to a particular medical treatment was, in the minds of the general public, more important than the extent to which that individual might be expected to benefit. The majority of people studied favored allocating most of a planned increase in access to treatment to patients with a lower initial health state than other patients for whom the potential improvement in Health-Related Quality of Life (HRQOL) from treatment is the same or even greater. The results of his research showed that in coming to decisions relating to health resource allocation, the public places more emphasis on disease severity than on potential for HRQOL gained. The results of the research, corroborated by subsequent studies by American, Peter Ubel [38, 39], were interpreted to underscore the importance the public assigned to fairness in health resource allocation decisions.

Resolution of the tension between escalating health care costs and the ethical imperative to ensure that access to health care resources is equitable is a major and growing challenge for health policy decision-makers in general and for those advising on reimbursement for ERT and SRT of LSD in particular. Assuming a fundamental commitment to the concept of health care as a 'public good', one of the most pressing challenges is to find an effective, efficient and credible way to involve the public in decisions concerning resource allocation [33]. Reliance on focus groups or public forums is an expensive and unwieldy process, and it begs the question – how many focus groups need to be convened to sample popular sentiments reliably. The usual standard of continuing to sample to saturation – i.e., until no ideas emerge that have not already been expressed – would simply be impractical, except perhaps when addressing some over-arching policy. It would certainly be impractical for addressing decisions concerning specific therapies.

In 2002, in response to the high priority it set on balancing the tension between efficiency and equity, The National Institute for Health and Clinical Excellence (NICE) in the UK (www.nice.org.uk) established a Citizen's Council comprised of 30 individuals, all 'ordinary members of the public', drawn from the population of England and Wales, to 'provide advice about the broad social values that NICE should adopt in preparing its guidance' to the National Health Service (NHS) on decisions relating to healthcare resource allocation. At the same time, NICE formally acknowledged the importance of social values in a document originally published in 2005 and in revised form in 2008 [40].

32.5 The Case of Rare Diseases

Policy decision-makers have been strongly influenced by the peculiar nature of rare diseases in general and the emergence of ERT for LSD in particular [41]. The LSD are generally recognized to be relentlessly progressive disorders causing serious morbidity and early mortality for which treatment prior to the introduction of ERT was limited to supportive measures often amounting to little more than palliative care. ERT represented the first primary treatment targeting the underlying metabolic defect and offering the possibility of significantly improving the quality of life and life expectancy of affected patients. Moreover, because they are rare, confident assessment of the impact of any new therapy is particularly difficult. Gathering enough patients to achieve sufficient statistical power to demonstrate significant clinical benefits is next to impossible to achieve in the course of short-term clinical trials. The most common causes of morbidity, such as the pain or gastrointestinal complaints of patients with Fabry disease, are often inherently difficult to quantify.

In response, in part, to mounting pressure from patient advocacy groups and treating physicians, and recognizing the special case of ERT for LSD, policy-makers have struggled to develop ways to provide patients with access to the treatment in a way that would not compromise a strongly held view that the allocation of public funds for the treatment of disease in general must meet commonly accepted criteria of equity. They are concerned about the precedent set by spending up to half a million dollars per year for the life-time of the patient with a LSD when a much larger number of patients with a more common condition might have to be denied access to another expensive treatment because the impact on total healthcare expenditures would be disastrous.

Although the marketplace may be an uncertain and imperfect way to control drug prices, all of the other approaches may be worse. Moreover, the cost of controlling the price of drugs with such small markets would almost certainly be prohibitive, considering the small contribution of spending on these products to total drug expenditures. The high per-patient costs are off-set by the small total numbers of patients. Hesitancy over paying for the treatments is as much a question of concerns about equity, as concerns about the effect on global drug spending.

32.6 Non-medical Costs

Most debate about the cost of ERT of LSD has focused on the material cost of the drug and to a lesser extent on the cost of support services, including the supplies necessary for intravenous infusions, home nursing, etc. However, what might be called the non-medical costs of treatment are not insignificant and have, in some cases, become so burdensome that patients elect to discontinue treatment or opt for another 'less costly' therapy, such as orally administered SRT, despite a potentially suboptimal response to the treatment. The need to undergo weekly or biweekly intravenous infusions is an unavoidable aspect of ERT. It often involves the need to travel to a hospital or infusion center, infusions sometimes taking hours, the need in some cases to employ subcutaneous venous access devices, and the side-effects of the enzyme infusion or the medications taken to prevent them. For children in school or adults with demanding careers, the cost may be considerable. The wide-spread adoption of home infusion programs is a reflection in part of the importance of this non-medical cost – the savings to hospitals or community infusion centers are trivial compared with the 'savings' to the patient who no longer needs to take the time and trouble to travel for ERT infusions [42–45]. Paradoxically, those patients who respond best to ERT may be those who find the personal, non-medical cost most irksome. At the other extreme, the parents of children with LSD involving progressive primary CNS involvement, who appear not to be benefiting significantly from ERT, may opt to discontinue the treatment because the perceived benefit is not considered to be commensurate with the personal, non-medical cost of the therapy. Efforts to decrease the non-medical costs need to be weighed against potential losses of efficacy, such as by shortening the duration of intravenous infusions, or the risk of serious infusion-related adverse reactions at home. What is needed is more research on predictors of adverse reactions, the effect of increasing infusion rates – i.e., decreasing the duration of infusions, the possibility of employing 'maintenance therapy' involving longer intervals between infusions [46], and the development of combined or adjuvant therapies designed to enhance mutant enzyme activity – so-called 'chaperone therapy', or to target potentially destructive secondary metabolic or cellular abnormalities.

32.7 Concluding Remarks

The emergence of ERT for LSD represents the first primary treatment for a class of rare, hereditary diseases previously associated with relentlessly progressive morbidity and early mortality. The very high drug costs of treatment have forced those administering public reimbursement programs to re-examine the basis of decisions relating to healthcare resource allocation. Discrepancies between the importance the public places on disease severity and the potential for treatment-related improvement of patients with rare, life-threatening diseases and decision-making on strictly utilitarian grounds employing conventional cost-utility criteria have resulted in innovative approaches to the evaluation of health care interventions. Further experience with such initiatives, including the Citizen's Council of the National Institute for Health and Clinical Excellence (NICE) of the UK, are expected to yield additional improvements in balancing the tension between equity and efficiency in this process.

References

1. Orphan Drug Act, Public Law 97-414. Sect. J(b) 1983 or Title 21, US Code, Sect. 360aa, note, Pub. L. No. 97–414 (1984, 1983)
2. Draborg E, Gyrd-Hansen D (2005) Time-trends in health technology assessments: an analysis of developments in composition of international health technology assessments from 1989 to 2002. Int J Technol Assess Health Care 21(4):492–498
3. Schiffmann R, Kopp JB, Austin HA III, Sabnis S, Moore DF, Weibel T et al (2001) Enzyme replacement therapy in Fabry disease: a randomized controlled trial. JAMA 285(21): 2743–2749
4. Hughes DA, Elliott PM, Shah J, Zuckerman J, Coghlan G, Brookes J et al (2008) Effects of enzyme replacement therapy on the cardiomyopathy of Anderson-Fabry disease: a randomised, double-blind, placebo-controlled clinical trial of agalsidase alfa. Heart 94(2):153–158
5. Feeny D, Furlong W, Boyle M, Torrance GW (1995) Multi-attribute health status classification systems. Health Utilities Index. Pharmacoeconomics 7(6):490–502
6. Eng CM, Guffon N, Wilcox WR, Germain DP, Lee P, Waldek S et al (2001) Safety and efficacy of recombinant human alpha-galactosidase A–replacement therapy in Fabry's disease. N Engl J Med 345(1):9–16
7. Banikazemi M, Bultas J, Waldek S, Wilcox WR, Whitley CB, McDonald M et al (2007) Agalsidase-beta therapy for advanced Fabry disease: a randomized trial. Ann Intern Med 146(2):77–86
8. Dehout F, Schwarting A, Beck M, Mehta A, Ricci R, Widmer U (2003) Effects of enzyme replacement therapy with agalsidase alfa on glomerular filtration rate in patients with Fabry disease: preliminary data. Acta Paediatr Suppl 92(443):14–15, discussion 5
9. Beck M, Ricci R, Widmer U, Dehout F, de Lorenzo AG, Kampmann C et al (2004) Fabry disease: overall effects of agalsidase alfa treatment. Eur J Clin Invest 34(12): 838–844
10. Dehout F, Roland D, Treille de Granseigne S, Guillaume B, Van Maldergem L (2004) Relief of gastrointestinal symptoms under enzyme replacement therapy [corrected] in patients with Fabry disease. J Inherit Metab Dis 27(4):499–505
11. Hoffmann B, Reinhardt D, Koletzko B (2004) Effect of enzyme-replacement therapy on gastrointestinal symptoms in Fabry disease. Eur J Gastroenterol Hepatol 16(10): 1067–1069
12. Hoffmann B, Garcia de Lorenzo A, Mehta A, Beck M, Widmer U, Ricci R (2005) Effects of enzyme replacement therapy on pain and health related quality of life in patients with Fabry disease: data from FOS (Fabry Outcome Survey). J Med Genet 42(3):247–252
13. Schwarting A, Dehout F, Feriozzi S, Beck M, Mehta A, Sunder-Plassmann G (2006) Enzyme replacement therapy and renal function in 201 patients with Fabry disease. Clin Nephrol 66(2):77–84
14. Hoffmann B, Beck M, Sunder-Plassmann G, Borsini W, Ricci R, Mehta A (2007) Nature and prevalence of pain in Fabry disease and its response to enzyme replacement therapy–a retrospective analysis from the Fabry Outcome Survey. Clin J Pain 23(6):535–542
15. Hoffmann B, Schwarz M, Mehta A, Keshav S (2007) Gastrointestinal symptoms in 342 patients with Fabry disease: prevalence and response to enzyme replacement therapy. Clin Gastroenterol Hepatol 5(12):1447–1453
16. Ramaswami U, Wendt S, Pintos-Morell G, Parini R, Whybra C, Leon Leal JA et al (2007) Enzyme replacement therapy with agalsidase alfa in children with Fabry disease. Acta Paediatr 96(1):122–127
17. Morel CF, Clarke JT (2009) The use of agalsidase alfa enzyme replacement therapy in the treatment of Fabry disease. Expert Opin Biol Ther 9(5):631–639
18. Pintos-Morell G, Beck M (2009) Fabry disease in children and the effects of enzyme replacement treatment. Eur J Pediatr 168(11):1355–1363

19. Mehta A, Beck M, Elliott P, Giugliani R, Linhart A, Sunder-Plassmann G, Schiffmann R, Barbey F, Ries M, Clarke JT; Fabry Outcome Survey investigators (2009) Enzyme replacement therapy with agalsidase alfa in patients with Fabry's disease: an analysis of registry data. Lancet 374(9706):1986–1996

20. Weidemann F, Breunig F, Beer M, Sandstede J, Turschner O, Voelker W et al (2003 Sep 16) Improvement of cardiac function during enzyme replacement therapy in patients with Fabry disease: a prospective strain rate imaging study. Circulation 108(11):1299–1301

21. Spinelli L, Pisani A, Sabbatini M, Petretta M, Andreucci MV, Procaccini D et al (2004) Enzyme replacement therapy with agalsidase beta improves cardiac involvement in Fabry's disease. Clin Genet 66(2):158–165

22. Wilcox WR, Banikazemi M, Guffon N, Waldek S, Lee P, Linthorst GE et al (2004) Long-term safety and efficacy of enzyme replacement therapy for Fabry disease. Am J Hum Genet 75(1):65–74

23. Bierer G, Balfe D, Wilcox WR, Mosenifar Z (2006) Improvement in serial cardiopulmonary exercise testing following enzyme replacement therapy in Fabry disease. J Inherit Metab Dis 29(4):572–579

24. Germain DP, Waldek S, Banikazemi M, Bushinsky DA, Charrow J, Desnick RJ et al (2007) Sustained, long-term renal stabilization after 54 months of agalsidase beta therapy in patients with Fabry disease. J Am Soc Nephrol 18(5):1547–1557

25. Wang RY, Abe JT, Cohen AH, Wilcox WR (2008 Oct 21) Enzyme replacement therapy stabilizes obstructive pulmonary Fabry disease associated with respiratory globotriaosylceramide storage. J Inherit Metab Dis (Epub ahead of print)

26. Wraith JE, Tylki-Szymanska A, Guffon N, Lien YH, Tsimaratos M, Vellodi A et al (2008) Safety and efficacy of enzyme replacement therapy with agalsidase beta: an international, open-label study in pediatric patients with Fabry disease. J Pediatr 152(4). 563–570, 570.e1

27. Imbriaco M, Pisani A, Spinelli L, Cuocolo A, Messalli G, Capuano E et al (2009) Effects of enzyme-replacement therapy in patients with Anderson-Fabry disease: a prospective long-term cardiac magnetic resonance imaging study. Heart 95(13):1103–1107

28. Vedder AC, Linthorst GE, Houge G, Groener JE, Ormel EE, Bouma BJ et al (2007) Treatment of Fabry disease: outcome of a comparative trial with agalsidase alfa or beta at a dose of 0.2 mg/kg. PLoS ONE 2(7):e598

29. Vedder AC, Breunig F, Donker-Koopman WE, Mills K, Young E, Winchester B et al (2008) Treatment of Fabry disease with different dosing regimens of agalsidase: effects on antibody formation and GL-3. Mol Genet Metab 94(3):319–325

30. Mehta A, Beck M, Kampmann C, Frustaci A, Germain DP, Pastores GM et al (2008) Enzyme replacement therapy in Fabry disease: comparison of agalsidase alfa and agalsidase beta. Mol Genet Metab 95(1–2):114–115

31. Clarke JT, West ML, Bultas J, Schiffmann R (2007) The pharmacology of multiple regimens of agalsidase alfa enzyme replacement therapy for Fabry disease. Genet Med 9(8):504–509

32. Drummond M, Brandt A, Luce B, Rovira J (1993) Standardizing methodologies for economic evaluation in health care. Practice, problems, and potential. Int J Technol Assess Health Care 9(1):26–36

33. Rawlins MD, Culyer AJ (2004 Jul 24) National Institute for Clinical Excellence and its value judgments. BMJ 329(7459):224–227

34. Moore DF, Ries M, Forget EL, Schiffmann R (2007) Enzyme replacement therapy in orphan and ultra-orphan diseases: the limitations of standard economic metrics as exemplified by Fabry-Anderson disease. Pharmacoeconomics 25(3):201–208

35. Hadorn DC (1991) The Oregon priority-setting exercise: quality of life and public policy. Hastings Cent Rep 21(3):S11–S16

36. Hadorn DC (1991 May 1) Setting health care priorities in Oregon. Cost-effectiveness meets the rule of rescue. JAMA 265(17):2218–2225

37. Nord E (1999) Cost-value analysis in health care. Cambridge University Press, Cambridge

38. Nord E, Pinto JL, Richardson J, Menzel P, Ubel P (1999) Incorporating societal concerns for fairness in numerical valuations of health programmes. Health Econ 8(1):25–39
39. Ubel PA (1999) The challenge of measuring community values in ways appropriate for setting health care priorities. Kennedy Inst Ethics J 9(3):263–284
40. National Institute for Health and Clinical Excellence (2008) Social value judgements: principles for the development of NICE guidance, London
41. Clarke JT, Amato D, Deber RB (2001 Sep 4) Managing public payment for high-cost, high-benefit treatment: enzyme replacement therapy for Gaucher's disease in Ontario. CMAJ 165(5):595–596
42. Milligan A, Hughes D, Goodwin S, Richfield L, Mehta A (2006) Intravenous enzyme replacement therapy: better in home or hospital? Br J Nurs 15(6):330–333
43. Linthorst GE, Vedder AC, Ormel EE, Aerts JM, Hollak CE (2006) Home treatment for Fabry disease: practice guidelines based on 3 years experience in The Netherlands. Nephrol Dial Transplant 21(2):355–360
44. Hughes DA, Mlilligan A, Mehta A (2007) Home therapy for lysosomal storage disorders. Br J Nurs 16(22). 6–9, 1384
45. Cousins A, Lee P, Rorman D, Raas-Rothschild A, Banikazemi M, Waldek S et al (2008) Home-based infusion therapy for patients with Fabry disease. Br J Nurs 17(10):653–657
46. Lubanda JC, Anijalg E, Bzduch V, Thurberg BL, Benichou B, Tylki-Szymanska A (2009) Evaluation of a low dose, after a standard therapeutic dose, of agalsidase beta during enzyme replacement therapy in patients with Fabry disease. Genet Med 11(4):256–264

Summary: Fabry Disease, a Uniquely Different Lysosomal Storage Disorder

Deborah Elstein

Abstract Lysosomal storage disorders (LSDs) can be viewed as unified by their pathology; however, clinical presentation in each of the LSDs is uniquely variable, often even among those with the same genotype Nonetheless, there are areas of commonality within the sub-types of LSDs (infantile, juvenile and late-onset forms) as well as among the various LSDs. Having said that, Fabry disease may, nonetheless, be the one LSD that is least like the others, possibly because it is X-linked. This chapter will review what is currently known about Fabry disease and put this in the context of the other LSDs.

Keywords Lysosomal storage diseases · Fabry disease · Diagnosis · Clinical symptoms · Enzyme replacement therapy

Introduction

Lysosomal storage disorders (LSDs) can be viewed as unified by their pathology which involves abnormal accumulation of partially degraded glycosphingolipids derived from the plasma membranes of eukaryotic cells and intracellular lysosomal and Golgi apparatus, in various organs. In each of these diseases a specific lysosomal hydrolase which should have been destined for post-translational modification and catabolism is putatively way-laid (by virtue of mis-folding) because of mutation(s) in its sequence. Virtually all of the LSDs can be considered within the context of the sequential breakdown of ganglioside A1 (GA1), myelin gangliosides (GM1, GM2, and GM3) and globoside, all of which devolve on the lactosylceramide pathway that would normally produce ceramide and eventually sphingosine.

D. Elstein (✉)
Gaucher Clinic, Shaare Zedek Medical Cente, Jerusalem, Israel
e-mail: elstein@szmc.org.il

D. Elstein et al. (eds.), *Fabry Disease*, DOI 10.1007/978-90-481-9033-1,

LSDs can also be viewed clinically as so rare as to often escape the immediate attention and care of medical practitioners ('the diagnostic odyssey') which inadvertently leads to widening of the therapeutic gap as symptoms and signs progress and in many cases become irreversible.

Finally, LSDs had been difficult to manage historically because of the multiple organs involved and the fact that symptomatic treatment and palliation did not in fact impact the trajectory of the disease. However, within the past 2 decades, there has been a radical change in the natural course of several of these LSDs by virtue of the commitment of some pharmaceutical companies to take on the challenge of producing specific enzyme replacement therapy (ERT), substrate reduction therapy (SRT), and most recently, pharmacological chaperones (PC). Moreover, with better understanding of the underlying mechanisms and concerted efforts to identify patients prior to onset of irreversible organ damage, particularly neurological and cognitive deterioration, the future for patients with LSDs can be viewed with greater, albeit guarded, optimism.

Fabry disease is well-positioned within the above overview of LSDs: importantly, it has been targeted for ERT, SRT, and PC. Nonetheless, it is distinctly different than most LSDs by virtue of the myriad of organs involved that are not comparable to other LSDs vs. other organs that are critically involved in other LSDs but are spared in Fabry disease. This chapter will compare Fabry disease to the bulk of other LSDs in order to highlight its unique pathology.

Diagnosis

Deficient enzyme production in many LSDs is generally interpreted as <15% of enzymatic activity relative to that in unaffected individuals. It has been presumed that in cases with even abysmal levels of activity, should exogenous enzyme be provided continually, some normalization of pathology can be achieved; males with classic Fabry disease, however, lack (or have undetectable levels of) α-galactosidase A activity. This may imply something about the early evolution of Fabry organ pathology in utero.

Accumulated storage material in LSDs is seen to be the nexus for system pathology, yet there is no apparent correlation between the degree of accumulation and organ involvement. This is a conundrum that appears to be common to Fabry disease as well.

There are apparently only rare instances of tight genotype-phenotype correlation among the LSDs. Fabry disease is marked by more than 300 mutations and almost as many private and rare genotypes, making prediction of disease severity highly problematic even between patients with the same genotype. As in other LSDs, epigenetic and environmental factors including life cycle events also impact the phenotype.

Early identification of pre-symptomatic patients is a goal of the medical community, and for most LSDs, screening of at-risk populations, as well as large-scale screening of newborns and even amniotic fluid, is available. In the case of Fabry disease, screening of the extended pedigree of an index case (male or female) as well newborn screening is encouraged. The rationale for extensive newborn screening for Fabry disease is the probability that disease prevalence may be greater than suspected based on current numbers of identified patients, and since, unlike some LSDs where there is also some ethnic predilection such as among Ashkenazi Jews for Tay-Sachs disease and Gaucher disease, GM1 gangliosidosis in natives of Malta, or Metachromatic Leukodystrophy among Navajo Indians and Muslim Arabs, Fabry disease is panethnic. Moreover, with the availability of the Chamoles filter paper method of screening many LSDs simultaneously, and efficient multiplexing, accurate and timely evaluations are realistic expectations.

It should be noted that whereas most LSDs are recessive disorders, Fabry disease (and Hunter syndrome) is an X-linked disorder.

For many LSDs, there are no adjunct lab measures to support enzyme and mutation analysis and assess disease severity changes over time relative; for Fabry disease as well as four Mucopolysaccharidoses (MPS) disorders and Gaucher disease, there are enzyme or macrophage biomarkers, and for Fabry disease and six other LSDs, there are substrate markers.

Clinical Features

Clinical presentation in each of the LSDs is uniquely variable, often even among those with the same genotype Among all LSDs, there is probably only one well-described example of tight genotype-phenotype correlation: D409H homozygosity and the Gaucher cardiac variant. Nonetheless, there are areas of commonality within the sub-types of each LSD (infantile, juvenile and late-onset forms) as well as among the various LSDs. Having said that, Fabry disease may nonetheless be the one LSD that is least like the others, possibly because it is X-linked, although MPS II (Hunter syndrome) is also X-linked and shares many features with other MPSs, especially MPS I (the Hurler-Scheie syndromes).

Among some LSDs it is axiomatic that the earlier the onset of symptomatic disease, which usually means emergence of neurological signs, the more probable a severe and fulminant course. In Fabry disease, many of the symptoms and signs that are seen in the youngest boys (and sometimes girls), particularly those of a gastrointestinal etiology, albeit very debilitating, are not actually indices or predictors of ultimate disease severity. In addition, cardiac involvement in Fabry disease although progressive (in most affected boys) from before puberty and is a marker of overall disease severity, the aggressive effects of renal involvement which usually only manifest in young adulthood, intervene and dominate the clinical picture so that the sequelae of proteinuria and hypertension are more often the cause of severe morbidity and eventual mortality.

Clinical disease severity in LSDs is invariably correlated with progressive and devastating neurological involvement, marked by intellectual decline (with only a few exceptions), neurogenic spasticity, problems with speech and hearing, disrupted gait, and eventually clonus and seizures. This clinical trajectory is true in all the infantile forms of LSDs that are fatal within the first decade of life. There is no acute infantile form that is lethal in Fabry disease and this is unique among the LSDs. With regard to central nervous system involvement, Fabry disease has predominantly small vessel involvement that occurs after the first decade of life and is expressed as abnormal vasodilatative and vasoconstrictive forces and result in thrombosis or thromboembolism. Unlike in other LSDs, ischemic and hemorrhagic strokes in Fabry disease, often with consequent white matter lesions, as well as the predictable clinical consequences of strokes, can be seen in many adult patients (males more than females).

Delayed acquisition of developmental milestones and/or regression and/or impaired intellectual ability is usually evident within the 1st year of life among the infantile and juvenile forms of the LSDs. For the chronic forms of some LSDs including Fabry disease and Gaucher disease (but not in the late-onset forms of Tay-Sachs disease or Metachromatic Leukodystrophy where cognitive regression often leads to confusion and dementia in early adulthood), cognitive function is unaffected. It therefore is to be recommended that for children with Fabry disease who are incapacitated by their disease to the extent that they are unable to attend school regularly, home instruction should be instituted to prevent cognitive decline.

Neuropathic pain, while rare in other LSDs, is very common in Fabry disease and often is an early manifestation (even in young children); acroparesthesia, another finding that is common in Fabry disease but much less so in other LSDs, is both an early and concerning complaint of patients but is not correlated with involvement of other organs such as the heart, kidney, or lungs.

The eyes are noted to be affected in virtually all LSDs, particularly corneal opacities are commonly seen because of storage material as in Fabry disease, but also gaze palzies (horizontal or vertical) and nystagmus are present in many infantile forms but not so in Fabry disease.

There is progressive hearing loss in several LSDs including in Fabry disease where it is because of sensori-neurological involvement.

Peripheral neuropathy including autonomic involvement (hypohidrosis, orthostatic hypotension, and the gastrointestinal disturbances) is basic to the issues that reduce quality of life for patients with Fabry disease, but it is relative rare among LSDs other than in Niemann-Pick disease, Krabbe disease, and Metachromatic Leukodystrophy.

Involvement of the skin such as angiokeratoma (albeit in areas that are mostly clothed) is an overt sign of Fabry disease that has no parallel among other LSDs. There are, however, examples of discoloration of the skin such as the ochre color of patients with Niemann-Pick type A who also may have xanthomas.

The facial dysmorphism (coarsening) that is pathognomonic of some of the LSDs, and is actually an interesting feature of commonality that may help in diagnosis of MPSs, is less dramatic in Fabry disease males and has been described as 'gargoyloid' facies.

Cardiomyopathy with fatal congestive heart disease is noted in infantile forms of some LSDs like GM1 gangliosidosis, but cardiac involvement which is progressive and marked by left ventricular hypertrophy is nearly universal in Fabry disease and this is unique. There are some examples of cardiac valve involvement in LSDs such as in a cardiac variant of Gaucher disease with progressive calcification of heart valves, and some cardiac valvular disease in the MPSs, especially MPS I and II.

Storage in the glomerular and tubular apparatus of the kidney is not a universal finding in LSDs: the kidneys may actually be small albeit fatty in Niemann-Pick disease and there may be hyper-filtration in MPS II and in a benign form in Gaucher disease. In Fabry disease renal end-stage failure is a major component of the pathology, it is both age-related and a marker of severity once proteinuria is detectable.

Hepatosplenomegaly which is characteristic of Gaucher disease and less massively in patients with the sub-types of Niemann-Pick disease as well as some of the MPS disorders, is distinctly uncommon in Fabry disease. Abnormal liver function is rarely noted in LSDs other than the neonatal jaundice of Niemann Pick disease, whereas hypersplenism is characteristic of Gaucher disease but no other LSD.

There seems to be a degree of pulmonary infiltrative disease in many LSDs especially infants with Niemann-Pick (type A) but also in the adults with Niemann-Pick (type B); pulmonary involvement in Gaucher disease and some of the MPSs is a very poor prognostic sign. The etiology of lung involvement may be accumulation of storage material in the alveolar and/or macrophages of the lungs, and/or in the epithelial and smooth muscle cells. Progression of lung pathology is unabated by symptomatic treatment but also disease-specific therapy seems not to greatly alter the course especially in the younger patients who are severely affected with Gaucher disease; this is equally true in pediatric and adult patients with Fabry disease.

Skeletal involvement takes a myriad of pathological forms among the LSDs. Avascular necrosis seen in some of the chronic forms such as Gaucher disease and also in younger patients with MPS I (Hurler and Scheie sub-groups), II (Hunter syndrome), and IV (Morquio syndrome), but is virtually missing among the remaining LSDs. The joint and muscle pain of Fabry disease, on the other hand, may be vascular in origin and/or due to lack of exercise (walking, climbing stairs) and/or because of intolerance due to cardiac and pulmonary involvement. In contradistinction, the lack of joint (especially shoulder) mobility seen in MPS I, II, and especially VII (Maroteaux-Lamy syndrome) is dissimilar because it may be due to storage in these sites and is not correlated with severity of other organs or with age. Neuromotor decline and gait/ataxia abnormalities may mark the disease course of many older patients with LSDs but this is not seen in Fabry disease.

Finally, adult patients with Fabry disease describe long-standing feelings of depression. This is quite distinct from behavioral changes and emotional lability which precedes the dementia of late-onset Metachromatic Leukodystrophy. It is also dissimilar to the psychiatric disturbances that mark the early stages of late-onset forms of Tay-Sachs disease as well as Metachromatic Leukodystrophy. In the LSDs with intellectual decline from childhood, the patient can not be described as feeling depressed; in LSDs such as type 1 Gaucher disease where intelligence is not affected, depression is rather infrequent. However, in Fabry disease (and in MPS IV and IX) where intelligence is intact, depression is no doubt a reflection of the reality of living with a multi-systemic disorder that is not sufficiently appreciated by those with whom the patient comes in contact.

Management

Beyond recommendations for symptomatic therapy and palliation, beyond physio-therapy, and beyond ancillary treatments which should include vitamin supplementation as needed, non-specific management of LSDs can probably be as exclusive or as inclusive as required by the condition of any individual patient. There may also be a place for non-traditional, alternative forms of medicine such as acupuncture, herbal medicine, and even ozone therapy. However, the great advantage that LSDs enjoy over other rare disorders is that enzyme replacement therapy (ERT) and substrate reduction therapy (SRT) are currently available. Infusible ERT, since its seminal trials in Gaucher disease type 1, has been the immediate therapeutic goal for other LSDs including Fabry disease and MPS I, II, and VI. In general, these molecules are safe, although there are some inimical issues such as those related to infusions per se, to antibody formation, and even to the high cost of ERT. Efficacy is also considered good, although here too there are problems of not all patients responding optimally, of some organ systems (beside the central nervous system) being more impervious to improvement, and of course, not actually curing the underlying disease.

SRT with miglustat has the one advantage of being capable of traversing the blood-brain barrier, and although its safety is not as high as for ERT, it provides hope for patients with neurological forms such as the late-onset form of Tay-Sachs disease, Niemann-Pick disease type C, and Gaucher disease type 3; there may be a rationale for the use of glucosylceramide synthase inhibitors in Fabry disease based on animal studies.

Finally, because of the possible chaperoning effects of SRT, new classes of pharmacological chaperones have been developed for use in both neurological and non-neurological forms of various LSDs including Fabry disease, although the disappointing results in Gaucher disease trials needs to be taken into consideration.

Summary

Fabry disease is a rather prevalent rare disease, but it has stymied researchers and clinicians since its recognition. The extent of the multi-system involvement is particularly confusing since specific ERT does not seem to halt progression of any of these. There are no acute forms with early demise, but rather an inexorable and irreversible worsening of all systems from early childhood to a pain-filled adulthood. This is still the sad reality for patients with Fabry disease. As in the Dedication page at the start of this textbook, I would like to conclude by quoting Orison Swett Marden: *'There is no medicine like hope, no incentive so great, and no tonic so powerful as expectation of something better tomorrow.'* We pray for a better tomorrow.

Fabry Patient Associations

AIPAF Onlus – Italian Association of Anderson-Fabry Patients
Via Tino Corzani
3 - 47026 San Pietro in Bagno - Forlì - Cesena
Italy
info@aipaf.org
www.aipaf.org
Tel: +39 (0)543 917434
Fax: +39 (0)543 901260

APL – Associação Portuguesa das Doenças Do Lisosoma
Av. Defensores de Chaves, 33-5°
1000-111 Lisboa
Portugal
geral@aplisosoma.org
www.aplisosoma.org
Tel: 213 194 710
Fax: 213 194 719

BOKS, Belgian organization for metabolic disease
Floralaan 35A
B 9120 Beveren
Belgium
www.boks.be
Tel: 03 775 48 39

Brazilian Association of Fabry Disease (ABRAFF)
Rua Irene Palma
212 - Ch.São José 13054-060
Brazil
Fabry@fabry.org.br
www.fabry.org.br
Tel: 19 3224-4210
Fax: 19 3224-4210

Canadian Fabry Association
9011 - 142 Street NW
Edmonton, Alberta T5R 0M6
Canada
amkoning@telus.net
www.fabrycanada.com
Tel: 780-489-0012
Fax: 780-443-4959

Canadian Organization for Rare Disorders (CORD)
151 Bloor Street West, Suite 600
Toronto, Ontario M5S 1S4
Canada
info@raredisorders.ca
www.raredisorders.ca
Tel: 416-969-7464 (877) 302-7273
Fax: (416) 969-7420

CLIMB National Information Centre for Metabolic Diseases
Climb Building,
176 Nantwich Road
Crewe, CW2 6BG
Great Britain
info.svcs@climb.org.uk
www.climb.org.uk
Tel: 0800 652 3181

Danish Organization of Fabry Patients
www.fabry.dk

Fabry Disease Patient Association – France
Mme Nathalie Triclin
9 rue de la Gare
08160 Vendresse
contact@apmf-fabry.org
www.apmf-fabry.org

Fabry – Hungary
www.fabry.mnsza.hu

Fabry International Network
Søre Titlestad 111
FANA, 5243
Norway
finpresident@myconnect.org
www.fabryintnetwork.com

Fabry Onlus – Italian Fabry Patient Group
Gruppo Italiano Pazienti Fabry
C/da Caravotti 3
66020 Paglieta (CH)
Italy
www.fabryonlus.org
Tel: +39 0872.809890
Fax: +39 0872.808605

Fabry Patient Association – Norway
www.fabry.no

Fabry Suisse
Willikon 58
CH-8618 Oetwil am See
Switzerland
info@fabrysuisse.ch
www.fabrysuisse.ch
Tel: +41 (0)44 929 05 74

Fabry Support Center of China
zhangasiaafrica@sina.com
www.fabry.org.cn

Fabry's Support Group
PO Box 269
Willoughby NSW 2068
Australia
info@fabry.net.au
www.fabry.net.au
Tel: 03 9497 8017

Fabry Support & Information Group (FSIG)
108 NE 2nd St. Ste C
P.O. Box 510
Concordia, MO 64020
info@fabry.org
www.fabry.org
Tel: 660-463-1355 866-30-FABRY (32279)
Fax: 660-463-1356

Fabry Support & Informatie Groep Nederland
Boelenkamp 10
8431 BL Oosterwolde
Netherlands
FSIGN@fabry.nl
www.fabry.nl
Tel: 06-25488090

Lysosomal Disease New Zealand
125 Cuba St
Petone
Lower Hutt City
New Zealand
john.forman@xtra.co.nz

www.ldnz.org.nz
Tel: 04 566 7707
Fax: 04 566 7717

MPS Society – UK
MPS House, Repton Place
White Lion Road
Amersham, Buckinghamshire, HP7 9LP
Great Britain
mps@mpssociety.co.uk
www.mpssociety.co.uk
0845 389 9901

MPS Society – Spain
info@mpsesp.org
www.mpsesp.org/
Tel: 617 080 198

Morbus Fabry Selbsthilfegruppe e.V.
Ditmar Basalla
Guilleaumestr. 13
51065 Köln
Gemany
info@fabry-selbsthilfegruppe.de
www.fabry-selbsthilfegruppe.de
Tel.: +49 (0) 221 - 222 73 93

National Fabry Disease Foundation
4301 Connecticut Ave. N.W.
Suite 404
Washington, DC 20008-2369
Tel: 800-651-9131
Fax: 800-651-9135
info@TheNFDF.org
www.thenfdf.org
Tel: 800-651-9131

National Organization for Rare Disorders (NORD)
P.O. Box 1968
(55 Kenosia Avenue)
Danbury, CT 06813-1968
orphan@rarediseases.org
http:////www.rarediseases.org
Tel: 203-744-0100 Voice Mail 800-999-NORD (6673)
Fax: 203-798-2291

National Tay-Sachs and Allied Diseases Association
2001 Beacon Street
Suite 204
Brighton, MA 02135
info@ntsad.org
http:////www.ntsad.org
Tel: 617-277-4463 800-90-NTSAD (906-8723)
Fax: 617-277-0134

New England Fabry Support Group
www.nefsg.org

Nordic Fabry
Christina Graef Christensen,
Ravnstrupvej 9
4684 Holmegaard
Denmark
formand@fabry.dk
www.fabry.dk
Tel: 5556 2212

VML – Vaincre les Maladies Lysosomales
2 Ter Avenue De France
91300 MASSY
France
www.vml-asso.org
Tel: 01 69 75 40 30

Index